DEPARTMENT OF ANESTHESIOLOGY

Second Edition

COMMON PROBLEMS IN

PEDIATRIC ANESTHESIA

Second Edition

COMMON PROBLEMS IN
PEDIATRIC ANESTHESIA

LINDA STEHLING, M.D.
Former Professor of Anesthesiology and Pediatrics
State University of New York
Health Sciences Center at Syracuse
Syracuse, New York
Medical Consultant
Blood Systems, Inc.
Scottsdale, Arizona

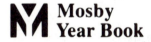
Mosby
Year Book

St. Louis   Baltimore   Boston   Chicago   London   Philadelphia   Sydney   Toronto

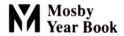
Mosby
Year Book

Dedicated to Publishing Excellence

Sponsoring Editor: Susan M. Gay
Assistant Editor: Sandra E. Clark
Associate Managing Editor, Manuscript Services: Deborah Thorp
Senior Production Assistant: Maria Nevinger
Proofroom Manager: Barbara Kelly

Mosby–Year Book, Inc.
11830 Westline Industrial Drive
St. Louis, MO 63146

1 2 3 4 5 6 7 8 9 0   CL MV   96 95 94 93 92

Library of Congress Cataloging-in-Publication Data
Common problems in pediatric anesthesia / [edited by] Linda Stehling.
 —2nd ed.
   p.   cm.
   Includes bibliographical references and index.
   ISBN 0-8016-6495-0
   1. Pediatric anesthesia—Complications—Case studies.
 I. Stehling, Linda C., 1942-
   [DNLM: 1. Anesthesia—in infancy & childhood.   WO 440 C734]
 RD139.C65   1992
 617.9′6798—dc20
 DNLM/DLC   92-18735
 for Library of Congress   CIP

CONTRIBUTORS

J. CHRISTIAN ABAJIAN, M.D.
Associate Professor
University of Vermont
College of Medicine
Burlington, Vermont

MICHAEL D. ABRAMOWITZ, M.D.
Associate Clinical Professor
George Washington University
Attending Anesthesiologist
Fairfax Hospital
Falls Church, Virginia

J. MICHAEL BADGWELL, M.D.
Associate Professor of Anesthesiology and
*   Pediatrics*
Texas Tech University Health Sciences
*   Center*
Lubbock, Texas

LAWRENCE S. BERMAN, M.D.
Associate Professor of Anesthesiology and
*   Pediatrics*
University of Florida School of Medicine
Gainesville, Florida

FREDERIC A. BERRY, M.D.
Professor of Anesthesiology and Pediatrics
University of Virginia Health Sciences
*   Center*
Charlottesville, Virginia

DEREK BLACKSTOCK, M.B.,
 F.F.A.R.C.S.I., F.R.C.P.C.
Clinical Assistant Professor
Univeristy of British Columbia
Vancouver, British Columbia, Canada

JAMES W. BLAND JR., M.D.
Professor of Anesthesiology
Associate Professor of Pediatrics
Emory University School of Medicine
Egleston Children's Hospital
Atlanta, Georgia

DESMOND J. BOHN, M.D., B.CH.,
 F.R.C.P.C.
Assistant Director
Pediatric Intensive Care Unit
Hospital for Sick Children
Associate Professor of Anaesthesia
University of Toronto
Toronto, Ontario, Canada

BARBARA W. BRANDOM, M.D.
Associate Professor
Department of Anesthesiology
University of Pittsburgh School of Medicine
Pittsburgh, Pennsylvania

JOHN T. BRITTON, M.D.
Assistant Professor of Anesthesiology and
*   Pediatrics*
Children's National Medical Center
The George Washington University School of
*   Medicine*
Washington, D.C.

T.C.K. BROWN, M.D., F.A.N.Z.C.A.,
 F.C.A.(U.K.)
Director of Anaesthesia
Royal Children's Hospital
Melbourne, Australia

ROBERT M. BRUSTOWICZ, M.D.
Assistant Professor of Anaesthesia
Harvard Medical School
Senior Associate in Anesthesia
Children's Hospital
Boston, Massachusetts

FREDERICK A. BURROWS, M.D.,
 F.R.C.P.C.
Associate Professor of Anaesthesia
The Hospital for Sick Children
University of Toronto
Toronto, Ontario, Canada

RICHARD S. CARTABUKE, M.D.
*Assistant Clinical Professor of
Anesthesiology
Ohio State University
Attending Anesthesiologist
Children's Hospital
Columbus, Ohio*

ROBERT P. CASTLEBERRY, M.D.
*Attending Pediatrician
The Children's Hospital
Professor of Pediatrics
University of Alabama at Birmingham
Birmingham, Alabama*

JON-BRUCE CHOPYK, M.D.
*Staff Anesthesiologist
Memorial Hospital
Hollywood, Florida*

D. RYAN COOK, M.D.
*Professor of Anesthesiology and
Pharmacology
University of Pittsburgh
Children's Hospital of Pittsburgh
Pittsburgh, Pennsylvania*

CHARLES J. COTÉ, M.D.
*Associate Professor of Anaesthesia
Harvard Medical School
Associate Anesthetist
Massachusetts General Hospital
Boston, Massachusetts*

PETER N. COX, M.B., CH.B.,
F.F.A.R.C.S. (LOND), F.R.C.P.(C)
*Assistant Director
Pediatric Intensive Care Unit
Hospital for Sick Children
Toronto, Ontario, Canada*

ROBERT E. CREIGHTON, M.D.,
F.R.C.P.C.
*Senior Anaesthetist
The Hospital for Sick Children
Associate Professor of Anaesthesia
University of Toronto
Toronto, Ontario, Canada*

PETER J. DAVIS, M.D.
*Associate Professor of Anesthesiology,
Critical Care Medicine and Pediatrics
University of Pittsburgh School of Medicine
Attending Anesthesiologist
Children's Hospital of Pittsburgh
Pittsburgh, Pennsylvania*

JAMES H. DIAZ, M.D., M.H.A.
*Section Head
Pediatric Anesthesia
Medical Director
Respiratory Therapy
Department of Anesthesiology
Ochsner Clinic and Alton Ochsner Medical
Foundation
Clinical Associate Professor of
Anesthesiology
Tulane University School of Medicine
New Orleans, Louisiana*

BURTON S. EPSTEIN, M.D.
*Professor of Anesthesiology
George Washington University School of
Medicine and Health Sciences
Washington, D.C.*

LYNNE R. FERRARI, M.D.
*Director, Pediatric Anesthesia
Massachusetts Eye and Ear Infirmary
Harvard Medical School
Boston, Massachusetts*

ROBERT B. FORBES, M.D., F.R.C.P.C.
*Associate Professor
Department of Anesthesia
University of Iowa College of Medicine
Iowa City, Iowa*

M. LIZANNE FOX, M.D.
*Instructor of Anesthesiology
The Children's Hospital
Harvard Medical School
Boston, Massachusetts*

GERALD V. GORESKY, M.D., C.M.,
F.R.C.P.C.
*Associate Professor
Department of Anaesthesia
University of Calgary
Calgary, Alberta, Canada*

NISHAN G. GOUDSOUZIAN, M.D., M.S.
*Associate Professor of Anesthesia
Harvard Medical School
Boston, Massachusetts*

CHARLES M. HABERKERN, M.D.
*Assistant Professor
Anesthesiology and Pediatrics
University of Washington
Children's Hospital Medical Center
Seattle, Washington*

STEVEN C. HALL, M.D.
Associate Professor of Clinical Anesthesia
Children's Memorial Hospital
Northwestern University Medical Center
Washington, D.C.

RAAFAT S. HANNALLAH, M.D.
Professor of Anesthesia and Pediatrics
George Washington University Medical
Center
Vice Chairman
Director of Research
Department of Anesthesia
Children's National Medical Center
Washington, D.C.

JEAN F. HARRINGTON, M.D.
Associate Professor of Clinical Anesthesia
and Pediatrics
University of Cincinnati College of Medicine
Cincinnati, Ohio

DAVID J. HATCH, M.B.B.S., F.C.ANAES
Portex Professor of Pediatric Anaesthesia
Institute of Child Health
University of London
London, England

PAUL R. HICKEY, M.D.
Director, Cardiac Anesthesia Service
Harvard Medical School
The Children's Hospital
Boston, Massachusetts

GEORGE M. HOFFMAN, M.D.
Assistant Professor of Anesthesiology and
Pediatrics
Medical College of Wisconsin
Assistant Chief
Department of Anesthesiology
Associate Director
Pediatric Intensive Care Unit
Children's Hospital of Wisconsin
Milwaukee, Wisconsin

INGRID HOLLINGER, M.D.
Professor of Anesthesiology
Albert Einstein College of Medicine
Montefiore Medical Center
Bronx, New York

ROBERT S. HOLZMAN, M.D.
Assistant Professor of Anaesthesia
Harvard Medical School
Boston, Massachusetts

MADELYN KAHANA, M.D.
Assistant Professor of Anesthesia and
Pediatrics
University of Cincinnati College of Medicine
Cincinnati, Ohio

HELEN W. KARL, M.D.
Assistant Professor of Anesthesiology
University of Washington School of Medicine
Seattle, Washington

THOMAS P. KEON, M.D.
Associate Professor of Anesthesiology
University of Pennsylvania School of
Medicine
Philadelphia, Pennsylvania

BABU V. KOKA, M.D.
Assistant Professor of Anesthesia
Harvard Medical School
Senior Associate in Anesthesia
Children's Hospital
Boston, Massachusetts

GOPAL KRISHNA, M.D.
Director, Section of Pediatric Anesthesia
and Critical Care
Indiana University School of Medicine
Indianapolis, Indiana

GEOFFREY A. LANE, M.B., F.F.A.R.C.S.
Associate Clinical Professor of
Anesthesiology and Pediatrics
The University of Colorado Health Sciences
Center
Medical Director
Ambulatory Surgery
The Children's Hospital
Denver, Colorado

JERROLD LERMAN, M.D., F.R.C.P.C.
Anaesthetist-in-Chief
The Hospital for Sick Children
Associate Professor of Anaesthesia
Univeristy of Toronto
Toronto, Ontario, Canada

LETTY M.P. LIU, M.D.
Associate Professor of Anaesthesia
Chief of Pediatric Anesthesia
Harvard Medical School
Massachusetts General Hospital
Boston, Massachusetts

CHARLES H. LOCKHART, M.D.
Clinical Professor of Anesthesiology and
Pediatrics
University of Colorado School of Medicine
Chairman, Department of Anesthesiology
The Children's Hospital
Denver, Colorado

JAMES C. LOOMIS, M.D.
Valley Anesthesia Consultants
Phoenix, Arizona

ANNE M. LYNN, M.D.
Associate Professor
Anesthesiology and Pediatrics
University of Washington
Children's Hospital and Medical Center
Seattle, Washington

ANGELA MACKERSIE, M.SC., M.B.B.S.,
F.C. ANAES
Consultant Anaesthetist
Hospital for Sick Children
London, England

THOMAS J. MANCUSO, M.D.
Assistant Professor of Anesthesiology and
Pediatrics
Emory University School of Medicine
Egleston Children's Hospital
Atlanta, Georgia

WILLIS ALEXANDER McGILL, M.D.
Professor of Anesthesia and Pediatrics
George Washington University Medical
Center
Chairman, Department of Anesthesiology
Children's Hospital
Washington, D.C.

ROBERT B. MESROBIAN, M.D.
Staff Anesthesiologist
Fairfax Hospital
Falls Church, Virginia

JEFFREY P. MORRAY, M.D.
Associate Professor of Anesthesiology and
Pediatrics
University of Washington School of Medicine
Associate Director
Pediatric Intensive Care Unit
Children's Hospital and Medical Center
Seattle, Washington

LUCILLE A. MOSTELLO, M.D.
Assistant Director of Anesthesiology and
Pediatrics
George Washington University
Washington, D.C.

ETSURO K. MOTOYAMA, M.D.
Professor and Vice Chairman
Department of Anesthesiology/Critical Care
Medicine
Professor of Pediatrics
University of Pittsburgh School of Medicine
Children's Hospital of Pittsburgh
Pittsburgh, Pennsylvania

DAVID J. MURRAY, M.D.
Associate Professor of Anesthesia and
Pediatrics
University of Iowa College of Medicine
Iowa City, Iowa

TAE HEE OH, M.D.
Professor of Anesthesiology
Yale University School of Medicine
New Haven, Connecticut

ROBERT C. PASCUCCI, M.D.
Instructor in Anaesthesia (Pediatrics)
Harvard Medical School
Associate Director-MICU
Associate in Anaesthesia
Children's Hospital
Boston, Massachusetts

RAMESH I. PATEL, M.D.
Associate Professor of Anesthesiology
George Washington University
Staff Anesthesiologist
Children's Medical Center
Washington, D.C.

PATRICIA HARPER PETROZZA, M.D.
Director of Neuroanesthesia
Wake Forest University Medical Center
Winston-Salem, North Carolina

MARY ANN PUDIMAT, M.D.
Assistant Professor
Georgetown University Medical Center
Washington, D.C.

LINDA JO RICE, M.D.
Associate Professor of Anesthesiology
Assistant Professor of Pediatrics
George Washington University
Children's National Medical Center
Washington, D.C.

JESSE D. ROBERTS, JR., M.D., M.S.
Assistant in Anesthesia and Pediatrics
Harvard University
Massachusetts General Hospital
Boston, Massachusetts

MARK A. ROCKOFF, M.D.
  Associate Professor of Anaesthesia
    (Pediatrics)
  Harvard Medical School
  Acting Anesthesiologist-in-Chief
  Clinical Director
  Children's Hospital
  Boston, Massachusetts

DAVID A. ROSEN, M.D.
  Associate Professor
  Department of Anesthesia
  Instructor of Pediatrics and Communicable
    Disease
  University of Michigan
  CS Mott Children's Hospital
  Ann Arbor, Michigan

KATHLEEN R. ROSEN, M.D.
  Assistant Professor
  Department of Anesthesia
  Instructor of Pediatrics and Communicable
    Disease
  University of Michigan
  CS Mott Children's Hospital
  Ann Arbor, Michigan

MARK A. ROSEN, M.D.
  Associate Professor of Clinical Anesthesia
    and Obstetrics, Gynecology and
    Reproductive Sciences
  University of California at San Francisco
  San Francisco, California

HENRY ROSENBERG, M.D.
  Professor and Chairman
  Department of Anesthesiology
  Hahnemann University
  Philadelphia, Pennsylvania

RICHARD B. SIEGEL, M.D.
  Pediatric Anesthesiologist
  The Children's Hospital
  Birmingham, Alabama

MICHAEL SMITH, M.D., F.R.C.P.(C.)
  Clinical Assistant Professor
  University of British Columbia
  Department of Anesthesia
  British Columbia's Children's Hospital
  Vancouver, British Columbia, Canada

SULPICIO G. SORIANO, M.D., M.S. Ed.
  Instructor in Anaesthesia
  Harvard Medical School
  Assistant in Anesthesia
  Children's Hospital
  Boston, Massachusetts

LINDA STEHLING, M.D.
  Former Professor of Anesthesiology and
    Pediatrics
  State University of New York
  Health Sciences Center at Syracuse
  Syracuse, New York
  Medical Consultant
  Blood Systems, Inc.
  Scottsdale, Arizona

DAVID J. STEWARD, M.B., F.R.C.P.(C)
  Professor of Anesthesiology
  University of Southern California
  Director, Department of Anesthesiology
  Children's Hospital of Los Angeles
  Los Angeles, California

SUSAN G. STRAUSS, M.D.
  Assistant Professor
  University of Washington
  Children's Hospital and Medical Center
  Seattle, Washington

BRAD W. WARNER, M.D.
  Assistant Professor of Surgery
  University of Cincinnati College of Medicine
  Division of Pediatric Surgery
  Children's Hospital Medical Center
  Cincinnati, Ohio

SUSAN PRINCE WATSON, M.D.
  Pediatric Anesthesiologists, PA
  Le Bonheur Children's Medical Center
  Clinical Associate Professor of
    Anesthesiology and Pediatrics
  University of Tennessee
  Memphis, Tennessee

NORBERT J. WEIDNER, M.D.
  Assistant Professor of Anesthesiolgoy
  Children's Hospital Medical Center
  Cincinnati, Ohio

KIM R. WEIGERS, M.D.
  Senior Instructor
  University of Colorado Health Sciences
    Center
  The Children's Hospital
  Denver, Colorado

LEILA G. WELBORN, M.D.
  Associate Professor of Anesthesia and
    Pediatrics
  George Washington University
  Children's National Medical Center
  Washington, D.C.

HELEN R. WESTMAN, M.D.
Clinical Associate Professor
Department of Anesthesia
University of Pittsburgh
Children's Hospital
Pittsburgh, Pennsylvania

CATHERINE E. WOOD, M.B., Cн.B.,
F.C.Aɴᴀᴇs.
Lecturer, Department of Anaesthesia
University of Calgary
Alberta, Canada

MASAO YAMASHITA, M.D.
Anesthetist-in-Chief
Ibaraki Children's Hospital
Mito, Ibaraki, Japan

MYRON YASTER, M.D.
Associate Professor of Anesthesiology,
Critical Care Medicine and Pediatrics
The Johns Hopkins Hospital
Baltimore, Maryland

ALFONSO E. YONFA, M.D.
Pediatric Anesthesiologist
The Children's Hospital
Birmingham, Alabama

FOREWORD TO THE SECOND EDITION

Dr. Stehling's first edition of *Common Problems in Pediatric Anesthesia* fitted easily into the literature of the rapidly growing field. Neither voluminous text nor stripped-down guidebook, the series of succinct, definitive descriptions of individual problem situations was certainly a sparkling contribution.

During the decade that has intervened, the appearance of new agents, new methods of patient management, new diseases, and new surgical procedures, as well as recent information on familiar pathologic conditions, all provide ample justification for this second edition. While many of the articles are of necessity partly repetitious, nearly all have been reworked and bibliographies updated. New articles on AIDS, patients undergoing MRI examinations, masseter spasm, and other topics have been introduced. Although several articles concern closely related problems, such as those on infant gastrointestinal lesions and several on cardiac anomalies, repetition has been artfully avoided. It is interesting to find, however, how nicely the new techniques and agents have been introduced, such as trends toward regional anesthesia, the extended use of opioids, and successive forms of relaxants.

In this edition, as in the last, it is impressive to find that there are so many pediatric anesthesiologists now present who have the experience and capability to write with authority on the many common (and uncommon) conditions described.

I have really enjoyed reading this book, and turned each page with interest and expectation.

ROBERT M. SMITH, M.D.
Chief of Anesthesia, 1946–1980
The Children's Hospital
Boston, Massachusetts

FOREWORD TO THE FIRST EDITION

This book presents in a refreshingly direct way a wide variety of pediatric problems with which the anesthesiologist might be faced. It describes the anaesthetic management of these problems, each chapter being an account of the way in which one expert responds to the challenge of a specific situation. The topics chosen by the editor are wide ranging. Some relate to surgical conditions, the correction of which may give rise to an anesthetic problem that may tax the anesthesiologist's ingenuity; some relate to diseases that may influence the management of anesthesia for unrelated surgical procedures. The choice both of subjects and of experts to deal with them has been wise.

The problem-oriented approach in a book on pediatric anesthesia is particularly apt. It is the experience of many teachers in this field that trainees (and, indeed, established practitioners who are occasional pediatric anaesthetists) do not have the same basic familiarity with pediatric medicine that they have with adult medicine, and therefore are less confident in their approach to children presenting with specifically pediatric disease. This book should be of great value to these practitioners and enable them to face such patients much more competently. The editor is to be congratulated on recognizing a need for a book of this nature; many anesthesiologists will have cause to be grateful for the clear and specific accounts of the management of those conditions that are dealt with in this work.

G. Jackson Rees, M.B.
Consultant Anaesthetist
Royal Liverpool Children's Hospital Liverpool, England

PREFACE TO THE SECOND EDITION

Enormous changes have taken place in the practice of medicine in the last decade. The words oximetry and capnography did not appear in the first edition of *Common Problems in Pediatric Anesthesia*. Pulse oximetry and capnography are now a standard of care. New anesthetic agents and muscle relaxants were introduced. Not only have preoperative medications changed, the routes of administration are different. Few authors recommend intramuscular premedication; oral, intranasal, transdermal, rectal, or intravenous administration is usually preferred. Regional anesthesia is being employed more often in children and techniques of postoperative pain management have been extended to include this group. A quiet revolution, perhaps appreciated even more by children than the avoidance of injections, has occurred in the practice of withholding oral intake prior to elective surgery. Less frequently are children forced to starve for 8 to 12 hours, as was formerly the custom.

The number and variety of procedures performed in outpatient centers has increased dramatically. A disadvantage of this practice is the minimal contact anesthesiologists have with patients prior to surgery. Often little time is available for establishing rapport or reviewing the child's medical history. While *Common Problems in Pediatric Anesthesia* is not meant to substitute for more extensive textbooks of anesthesiology and pediatrics, it does provide concise descriptions of many congenital and acquired disorders and operative procedures with important anesthetic implications. Children presenting for the same surgical procedure may require totally different anesthetic management and monitoring. One child can be an outpatient and another will require hospitalization. The anesthesiologist must be able to make these determinations rapidly.

New surgical procedures have been devised and old ones modified. Liver transplantation and autologous bone marrow harvesting are now relatively commonplace. For the first edition, I elected to omit discussion of procedures that could only be performed in specialized centers by uniquely trained personnel. Many hospitals now have surgeons who perform procedures formerly undertaken in only a few institutions. Not all of these hospitals have anesthesiologists with fellowship training in pediatric anesthesia. In addition, children who previously had cardiac surgery, organ transplantation, or extensive reconstructive procedures frequently go to community hospitals for "common" operations, such as hernia repair and myringotomy. A thorough knowledge of the physiologic alterations associated with the child's underlying disease and the changes induced by prior surgery is critical.

When *Common Problems in Pediatric Anesthesia* was published in 1982, the medical community was unaware that blood transfusion could transmit the human immunodeficiency virus and cause AIDS. More conservative transfusion practices, evident in many chapters in this edition, undoubtedly reflect concerns about transfusion-transmitted disease.

With all of these changes in mind, I once again called upon a group of friends and a few strangers to give of their time and talent. Many of the original contributors totally revised their chapters. New topics and new authors were added. Each contributor was asked to provide a brief discussion of the unique aspects of each case and to outline an approach to anesthetic management. In a few cases I asked too much; the topic could not be adequately covered in a brief discussion. Some chapters are, therefore, longer than others. However, they were so thoughtfully and thoroughly prepared that excision of sections for the sake of brevity was unthinkable. In all cases, the authors were asked to emphasize safe approaches to patient management and to discuss the techniques they would personally use. Readers are frequently cautioned to employ techniques and agents with which they are most familiar and comfortable. That is sound advice and should be followed.

I am most grateful to each of the contributors. I hope that I did not lose many friends while wielding my editorial pen. The kind words of Bob Smith mean a great deal to me. Dr. Smith's contributions to pediatric anesthesia are legion and will continue to be evident for many decades. The staff at Mosby-Year Book, Inc. were extremely helpful and made possible the short gestation period of the book. Last, and never least, I wish to thank my husband and friend, Howard Zauder, for serving as surrogate editor and devoting almost as much effort to the project as I did. We spent our time profitably if even one child benefits from the recommendations contained herein.

LINDA STEHLING, M.D.

PREFACE TO THE FIRST EDITION

The perioperative course of each patient is unique. However, certain problems and complications are often associated wtih specific disease processes and surgical procedures and should be anticipated. It is the intent of this volume to present many of the common situations with which the anesthesiologist who deals with children may be confronted. Although the book was prepared for clinicians, residents in training and nurse anesthetists may find it useful.

This is not a textbook of pediatrics or anesthesiology. It is a selection of case studies and suggested techniques of management. Each author was asked to present a safe approach to the anesthetic care of the child presented. Neither the editor nor the contributors offer these recommendations as *the* way to manage an individual patient. Often there are several equally acceptable anesthetic techniques. The one chosen is influenced to a great extent by the preferences and experience of the anesthesiologist as well as the individual characteristics of the patient, the surgeon, and the hospital. Procedures which should only be performed in specialized centers by personnel uniquely trained are not included (e.g., corrective surgery for complex congenital cardiac defects and craniofacial dysostoses). Many medical and surgical disease processes are omitted.

Neonatal physiology, invasive monitoring, and anesthetic systems are topics that are covered extensively elsewhere and are not discussed in depth here. In most cases the number of references is minimal. Textbooks, review articles, and monographs devoted to the anesthetic management of children should be familiar to the reader.

The text is divided into three sections: procedures in neonates, in infants, and in children. Although most of the procedures in the first two groups are age-related, many of the disorders can occur in children of any age.

The majority of the case presentations are based on the editor's own clinical experience. The illustrations provided by numerous surgical colleagues have been of great value. In many instances no descriptions of the surgical lesions can compare with photographs.

The help of the contributors is sincerely appreciated; each devoted considerable time to providing the reader with a concise description of the problems (existing and potential) and a safe method of managing them. Each author approached the case in his own way, armed with his clinical experience, a case discussion prepared by the editor, and a brief description of the intentions and expectations for the book. There is minimal repetition and overlap despite the fact that the contributors were not aware of the content of other chapters. However, each chapter is meant to stand alone, and some things common to many clinical situations are repeated.

LINDA STEHLING, M.D.

CONTENTS

1

Neonatal Resuscitation

An infant girl is born by cesarean delivery performed for fetal distress. She is cyanotic and has irregular respirations. Heart rate, 80. The obstetrician asks you to resuscitate the infant.

Recommendations by Mark A. Rosen, M.D.

The transition from fetal to extrauterine life involves major physiologic changes in the respiratory and circulatory systems. Although these changes most often occur spontaneously, some infants require assistance to safely and successfully make the complex transition from a dependent fetus to an independent neonate. Resuscitation is required more often in the first few minutes after birth than at any other time in life. Prompt and appropriate resuscitative efforts are mandatory to treat this patient, who has suffered intrauterine asphyxia, diagnosed by a history of fetal distress and hypoventilation, bradycardia, and cyanosis at birth.

FETAL PHYSIOLOGY

In utero, blood is oxygenated in the placenta and returns to the fetal heart via the umbilical and hepatic veins, ductus venosus, and inferior vena cava. A majority of the blood is shunted at the atrial level to the left heart or diverted from pulmonary perfusion by shunting across the ductus arteriosus. With arrest of umbilical blood flow at cord clamping and/or vasoconstriction of the umbilical vessels, the neonate's systemic vascular resistance increases, left atrial pressure rises as pulmonary venous blood flow increases, and atrial shunting of blood ceases. With lung expansion and increases in pH and Pao_2, the neonatal pulmonary vascular resistance falls. Pulmonary perfusion increases, and shunting across the ductus arteriosus decreases. Eventually, ductal shunting ceases.

In utero, the fetal lung is filled with an ultrafiltrate of plasma, a substantial portion of which is removed before, during, and immediately after birth. Neonatal ventilatory efforts usually occur

1

within seconds after delivery. The first several breaths establish the functional residual capacity, and within 90 seconds after delivery, most neonates establish regular, rhythmic ventilation.

NEWBORN RESUSCITATION

Preparation for newborn resuscitation requires the availability of qualified personnel with adequate supplies, drugs, equipment, and monitoring devices. It is important to anticipate neonatal depression, which can be associated with a wide variety of antepartum and intrapartum factors (Table 1–1).

The initial steps in routine management of all neonates just after delivery include suctioning the airway, preventing heat loss, placing the neonate in a head-down position to allow gravity drainage of pulmonary fluid, providing tactile stimulation to initiate ventilation, and evaluating the neonate's condition. The neonate should be placed under a radiant warmer, the skin wiped dry, and the wet towel removed. Towel drying decreases evaporative heat loss. The room should be warm and without draft to decrease convective heat loss. As a consequence of a large surface area-to-volume ratio, infants cool quickly. Premature and small-for-gestational-age infants have less adipose tissue to act as insulation and are at increased risk for cold stress, which is associated with increased morbidity and decreased survival. Thermal maintenance under radiant heat is critical since it minimizes oxygen requirements and improves response to resuscitation.

Gentle suctioning of the mouth, nose, and hypopharynx clears the airway and may be a useful stimulus for ventilation. However, excessive suctioning should be avoided since it can induce vagal responses from posterior pharyngeal stimulation, breath holding, or laryngospasm. If suctioning the oropharynx and drying the skin do not induce ventilation, tactile stimulation such as firmly rubbing the back, slapping the soles of the feet, or flicking the heels is indicated. If a neonate remains apneic after one or two brief attempts, such efforts should not persist since appropriate resuscitative efforts would be delayed. Gentle stimulation is appropriate to support early ventilatory efforts, but not to initiate ventilation in an apneic neonate.

Simultaneous with administration of the routine care, the condition of the newborn should be evaluated. Ventilation, heart rate, and color are assessed as a guide to resuscitative efforts. Constant reappraisal throughout the resuscitation is essential.[1]

If ventilation is inadequate and unresponsive to tactile stimulation or the heart rate is below 100 beats/min, positive-pressure ventilation with 100% oxygen should be initiated with a bag and face mask. Excessive inspiratory pressures should be avoided. The head is best placed in a neutral position, with the neck slightly extended. A rolled blanket or towel under the shoulders with no more than a 1- to 2-cm elevation may be useful for infants with large occiputs due to molding or edema. Adequacy of positive-pressure ventilation can be assessed by chest movement, auscultation in the axillae, prompt improvement in heart rate and color, and pulse oximetry. The trachea should be intubated if it is anticipated that prolonged positive-pressure ventilation will be required or if bag and mask ventilation is ineffective.

After 15 to 30 seconds of positive-pressure ventilation, if the heart rate is below 60 beats/min or remains between 60 and 80 beats/min and is not increasing, external cardiac massage should be initiated and continued until the heart rate is above 80 beats/min. The newborn's sternum is compressed with the tips of the middle and ring fingers and the index finger is used to identify the

TABLE 1–1.

Factors Predisposing to Neonatal Depression

Antepartum factors
  Pre-eclampsia or eclampsia
  Hypertension
  Diabetes mellitus
  Chronic renal disease
  Maternal malnutrition or severe obesity
  Sickle cell disease
  Anemia
  Rh or ABO incompatibility
  Heart disease
  Pulmonary disease
  Second- or third-trimester bleeding
  Drug or ethanol abuse
  Drug therapy
  Maternal infection
  Uterine or pelvic anatomic abnormalities
  Previous fetal or neonatal deaths
  Oligohydramnios or polyhydramnios
  Multiple gestation
  Postmaturity
  Prematurity
  Intrauterine growth retardation
Intrapartum factors
  Meconium-stained amniotic fluid
  Breech or other abnormal presentation
  Forceps delivery
  Cesarean section
  Prolapsed umbilical cord
  Nuchal cord
  Prolonged general anesthesia
  Excessive administration of sedatives or opioids to the
    mother
  Anesthetic complications
  Prolonged or precipitous labor
  Uterine hypertonia
  Abnormal heart rate or rhythm
  Prolonged rupture of membranes
  Abruptio placentae
  Placenta previa

proper position, one finger breadth below an imaginary line drawn between the nipples. Firm support for the back is necessary and can be provided by the other hand if the surface on which the baby lies is not rigid. The sternum is depressed 0.5 to 0.75 in. at a rate of 120 times per minute. This should be accompanied by positive-pressure ventilation at a rate of 40 to 60 breaths per minute, preferably through an endotracheal tube. Monitoring by assessing peripheral pulses, stopping to assess spontaneous cardiac rhythm, and ideally monitoring the electrocardiograph (ECG) and blood pressure with an indwelling catheter are advocated. Improper technique risks pneumothorax and liver laceration.

If cyanosis or bradycardia persists, the possibility of metabolic acidosis, pneumothorax, diaphragmatic hernia, or congenital heart disease must be considered.[2] Tension pneumothorax can occur spontaneously, in association with meconium aspiration, or with excessive airway pressures administered during resuscitation. When it is suspected, a 22-gauge needle connected to a three-way stopcock and syringe is inserted in the second intercostal space in the midclavicular line. If air is aspirated, an appropriately sized chest tube is inserted.

Epinephrine, sodium bicarbonate, tromethamine, volume expanders, dopamine, naloxone, dextrose, as well as other drugs should be readily available for neonatal resuscitation. The preferred route for drug therapy is by catheter in an umbilical artery or vein. However, it is important to remember that epinephrine can be administered through an endotracheal tube.

Epinephrine, 0.1 to 0.3 mL/kg of a 1:10,000 solution, is administered for asystole or heart rates that remain below 80 beats/min after 30 seconds of adequate ventilation and chest compression. Epinephrine can be administered intravenously, intratracheally, or through an umbilical artery catheter and may be repeated every 3 to 5 minutes if necessary. However, if the heart rate remains below 100, the diagnosis of metabolic acidosis and/or hypovolemia should be considered. Treatment with bicarbonate and/or volume expanders may be indicated. If repeated doses of epinephrine are required to maintain a heart rate greater than 100 to 120 beats/min, an isoproterenol infusion should be initiated.

Sodium bicarbonate is administered to correct neonatal acidosis, thereby reversing both cardiac failure and pulmonary vasoconstriction associated with asphyxia. In addition, sodium bicarbonate administration may partially expand the circulatory volume. A 4.2% solution of sodium bicarbonate is administered slowly at a dose of 2 mEq/kg and a rate of 1 mEq/kg/min for documented severe metabolic acidosis, that is, a base deficit greater than 15 mEq. If blood gas analysis is not immediately available, sodium bicarbonate may be administered to neonates who remain severely depressed despite adequate ventilation. Effective ventilation must precede and accompany bicarbonate administration to minimize the risk of intracranial hemorrhage, which has been associated with bicarbonate administration to preterm neonates. An alternative to sodium bicarbonate is tris hydroxymethyl aminomethane (THAM), which has the advantage of reducing Pa_{CO_2}. It is particularly useful in critical circumstances of combined severe respiratory and metabolic acidosis.

Volume expanders are administered for evidence of acute bleeding or signs of hypovolemia such as hypotension, pallor, poor capillary refill, tachycardia with faint pulses, and tachypnea. Hypovolemia should be suspected in asphyxiated newborns or neonates born following cord compression, abruptio placentae, or placenta previa. Appropriate volume expanders are 5% albumin solutions or other plasma substitutes and isotonic crystalloid, 10 mL/kg, administered over a period of 5 to 10 minutes and repeated if signs of hypovolemia persist. In the unlikely event that blood is required, it should be cytomegalovirus (CMV)-seronegative and irradiated. It can be type O, Rh-negative, and may be crossmatched against the mother's blood. If there is little or no improvement, consideration should be given to additional treatment of acidosis and inotropic support of the circulation.

Dopamine, 5 μg/kg/min increased to 20 μg/kg/min, is indicated when a neonate remains hypotensive with poor perfusion after epinephrine, volume expanders, and bicarbonate have been appropriately administered. Higher doses have been used but are controversial. Isoproterenol infusions, 0.5 to 1 μg/kg/min, are reserved for infants unresponsive to dopamine.

Naloxone, 0.01 mg/kg, is used to treat neonatal respiratory depression associated with maternal opiate administration. It is contraindicated in newborns of narcotic-addicted mothers. The route of administration may be intravenous, intramuscular, subcutaneous, or intratracheal. The sign of narcotic depression in a neonate is hypoventilation. Commonly, a neonate will be vigorous at birth, with a high Apgar score at 1 minute, and subsequently become lethargic, even apneic, within a few minutes.

Dextrose is indicated for hypoglycemia, which should be suspected in neonates with intrauterine growth retardation, those born with severe asphyxia, and those born to diabetic mothers. Glucose can be measured by heel stick during resuscitation. Blood glucose levels less than 30 mg/dL should be treated. Ten percent dextrose in water ($D_{10}W$) can be administered intravenously or into an umbilical artery catheter at a dose of 2 to 3 mL/kg over a 5-minute period. An infusion of $D_{10}W$ is then started and blood glucose determinations made.

A common outcome of intrauterine asphyxia, meconium aspiration requires expert and prompt management to avoid the risks associated with meconium aspiration pneumonitis.[3, 4] In managing this baby, it would be important to know whether the amniotic fluid was clear or meconium stained. Immediate endotracheal intubation and tracheal and bronchial suctioning should be performed when babies are born with meconium-stained amniotic fluid. The tracheal tube is used as a suction catheter to remove particulate meconium that cannot be dislodged with smaller catheters. This procedure should be repeated until meconium is no longer recovered. An assistant should continuously monitor the neonate's condition. Suctioning should be temporarily interrupted to ventilate with 100% oxygen when the heart rate decreases below 80. Tracheal aspiration is resumed when the rate is above 100. The gastric contents should also be aspirated. Further therapy consists of chest physiotherapy, ultrasonic mist, and possibly steroids and antibiotics.

SUMMARY

Skillful resuscitation of the depressed newborn is essential to maximize the potential for a normal outcome. Optimal resuscitation should begin without delay and with an appropriate level of intensity to evaluate the newborn; establish a patent airway; ensure adequate ventilation; restore normal blood volume, cardiac output, and acid-base and electrolyte status; and provide thermal maintenance.

REFERENCES

1. Bloom RS, Cropley CC: *Textbook of Neonatal Resuscitation*. Dallas, American Heart Association, 1987.
2. Gregory GA: Unusual cases of neonatal respiratory failure in the delivery room, in Shnider SM, Levinson G (eds): *Anesthesia for Obstetrics*. Baltimore, Williams & Wilkins, 1987.
3. Gregory GA, Gooding CA, Phibbs RH, et al: Meconium aspiration in infants: Prospective study. *J Pediatr* 1974; 85:848.
4. Ting P, Brady JP: Tracheal suction in meconium aspiration. *Am J Obstet Gynecol* 1975; 122:767.

2

Diaphragmatic Hernia

A 4-hour-old, 3.5-kg male infant is transferred from an outlying hospital with a diagnosis of diaphragmatic hernia. Hemoglobin, 16 g/dL; hematocrit, 48%.

Recommendations by David J. Steward, M.B.

The infant with congenital diaphragmatic hernia who has severe respiratory distress in the first hours of life is one of the most demanding patients for the pediatric surgeon, anesthesiologist, and intensivist. The mortality rate for babies with this condition, even when all the recent therapeutic advances are applied, is still extremely high. For these reasons, treatment of congenital diaphragmatic hernia should only be attempted in hospitals with staff and facilities to provide all aspects of critical neonatal care.

THE ANATOMIC DEFECT

The basic problem is the associated hypoplasia of the lungs, which determines whether survival is possible. Severe pulmonary hypoplasia is present in many infants. Indeed, there may be insufficient lung tissue to provide for essential gas exchange. The defect in the diaphragm that allows herniation of the abdominal contents into the thorax requires repair at some stage, but it is now established that the infant's respiratory status will not be improved by the operation.

The most common site of the defect is the left posterolateral aspect of the diaphragm. The stomach, large and small intestine, and sometimes the liver or spleen herniate into the thorax through the foramen of Bochdalek. The x-ray findings (Fig 2–1) are usually diagnostic but can be confused with lung cysts or congenital lobar emphysema. Correct diagnosis is essential because the management of babies with other conditions differs from that outlined here.

If a gastric tube has been employed, it may be seen to double back into the stomach within the thorax. Alternatively, a small amount of radiopaque contrast medium may be instilled via the gastric

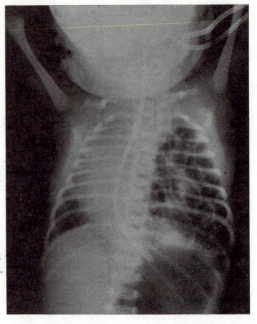

FIG 2–1.
Chest x-ray of a newborn with a congenital diaphragmatic hernia. Note the appearance of gas-filled abdominal viscera in the left thorax that are displacing the heart to the right. A gastric tube has been passed into the stomach, which also appears to be air-filled and should be evacuated immediately.

tube to outline the position of the abdominal viscera. Antenatal diagnosis is also possible. While diagnosis by ultrasound examination of the fetus has permitted very early postnatal intervention, it has not improved the overall results of treatment.[1] Antenatal diagnosis does, however, introduce the possibility of fetal surgery to correct the lesion in utero.

Infants with congenital diaphragmatic hernia also commonly have other defects. These most frequently involve the central nervous system, alimentary tract, and cardiovascular system and include spina bifida, hydrocephalus, malrotation of the gut, esophageal atresia, and patent ductus arteriosus (PDA).

In recent years, basic questions have been asked concerning the etiology of the syndrome of congenital diaphragmatic defcct and the associated pulmonary hypoplasia. Under question is the previously held dogma that compression of the developing lungs with resultant pulmonary hypoplasia is the sole mechanism for the disease. An alternative view is that the primary disease process involves both the lungs and the diaphragm.[2]

While it had been difficult to determine reliable prognostic indicators in any particular baby, some progress has been made in the objective assessment of patients with this disease. Attempts had been made to assess the severity of the pulmonary hypoplasia by following the level of arterial oxygenation and/or the acid-base status of the infant; however, these indices are unreliable. The use of a plot of the arterial carbon dioxide tension against a respiratory index (mean airway pressure multiplied by the respiratory rate) has enabled investigators to classify the severity of the disease and to follow its progress with treatment.[3] Patients with lower arterial carbon dioxide tensions and respiratory indicies, that is, those with more compliant respiratory systems, have a better prognosis.

There has also emerged the surprising fact that reduction of the hernia and repair of the diaphragm does not improve but, indeed, compromises the infant's ventilatory function. It has been demonstrated that total thoracic compliance is markedly reduced following surgical correction,[4] thus confirming the clinical observation that the patient's condition very frequently deteriorates following surgery. It is therefore the current recommendation that the initial approach to the patient with congenital diaphragmatic hernia be nonsurgical.[5]

EARLY MANAGEMENT

The immediate treatment for the infant in distress with congenital diaphragmatic hernia is intubation of the trachea and gentle intermittent positive-pressure ventilation (IPPV) with oxygen. A gastric tube is passed for decompression of the stomach and bowel. The patient should not be allowed to struggle and gasp, and IPPV should never be applied via a face mask since increased distension of the intrathoracic abdominal viscera may result and further compromise ventilation. After intubation, the infant should be sedated with a large dose of fentanyl, and a fentanyl infusion, 20 µg/kg/hr, should be initiated. This drug has been demonstrated to have a favorable effect on pulmonary vascular resistance. Muscle relaxation can be accomplished with vecuronium, 0.1 mg/kg. This management permits optimal ventilation and prevents struggling, thus minimizing the metabolic demands and also decreasing the risk of pneumothorax. Tension pneumothorax, a common complication in infants with congenital diaphragmatic hernia, must be anticipated. If any doubt exists as to its presence, bilateral chest drains should be inserted.

It is most important that the infant be constantly maintained in a warm environment in an incubator set at 35 to 36° C to prevent cold stress and a fall in core temperature. The gases to the ventilator circuit should be warmed and humidified.

Ventilation should be continued with the rate and volume adjusted to keep the arterial PCO_2 below 40 mm Hg and the preductal PO_2 above 60 mm Hg, if possible. High ventilatory pressures should be avoided to prevent further pulmonary damage. In some infants it may be impossible to achieve these objectives with conventional mechanical ventilation. In such instances it may be necessary to resort to high-frequency ventilation or, if this fails, to extracorporeal membrane oxygenation (ECMO). Emergency surgery is not recommended.

Monitoring with a pulse oximeter, arterial and central venous pressure catheters, and a urinary catheter should be employed. Frequent blood gas and acid-base determinations are essential. Cardiac ultrasound examination has been recommended to detect other congenital anomalies and to assess ventricular function.

Patients with congenital diaphragmatic hernia are prone to hypoxic cardiomyopathy, and in such cases afterload reduction with sodium nitroprusside or nitroglycerine may be beneficial.[6] Some patients require inotropic support and pulmonary vasodilators to increase cardiac output and improve pulmonary blood flow. Heparinization is required in patients receiving ECMO to maintain the activated clotting time at 150 to 200 seconds. An increased dose of fentanyl is also required since the drug is adsorbed onto the plastic components of the ECMO circuit.

During the preoperative stabilization period air should be continuously aspirated from the stomach and intrathoracic portion of the bowel to decompress the lungs. In many cases the mediastinal shift will progressively decrease.

When cardiopulmonary function is improved and stable, consideration can be given to closure of the diaphragmatic defect. The criteria for surgery include the ability to ventilate the patient with a low mean airway pressure and to achieve very acceptable blood gas parameters. This may be possible after 24 hours or more of intensive respiratory care, and the operation may be performed either in the operating room or in a special area of the neonatal intensive care unit.

ANESTHETIC MANAGEMENT

Anesthetic management for surgical repair should consist of continued ventilatory support and supplemental doses of fentanyl and muscle relaxant. No attempt should be made to further expand the lungs when the hernia is reduced because this may cause increased and unnecessary pulmonary damage. Blood loss is usually minimal, but additional fluid infusions may be required to replace losses into the bowel. The systemic blood pressure should be carefully monitored and used as a guide to fluid replacement.

Repair of the diaphragmatic defect has been performed with the patient still receiving ECMO. In these infants great care must be taken not to disturb or kink the indwelling cannulas. Pulse oximetry may be unreliable due to the weak pulsatile signal, and frequent blood gas determinations should be made. Despite heparinization, bleeding is not usually a significant problem. The patient should be kept in the intensive care unit where ventilatory support is continued until there are clear indications for weaning and subsequent extubation.

THE FUTURE

At the present time, there are unresolved questions regarding the optimal management of patients with congenital diaphragmatic hernia. The role of ECMO remains to be precisely defined. This therapy is extremely expensive and cannot offer any lasting hope to the infant with a degree of pulmonary hypoplasia incompatible with life. The best possible criteria to determine who might benefit from such technology must be developed. It is still not clear whether ECMO will significantly increase the numbers of patients with borderline pulmonary function who can be salvaged.

The possible role of fetal surgery for congenital diaphragmatic hernia is also undetermined. Initial clinical experience with this approach was reported in 1990[7] and established that fetal congenital diaphragmatic hernia repair is feasible in selected cases. The fetal lungs grew quickly following decompression, and postnatal pulmonary function was good. This would support the theory that compression of the developing lungs is indeed a major cause of the pulmonary hypoplasia. However, fetal surgery introduces a host of additional problems and potential complications for both the infant and the mother. Further conclusions must await more extensive clinical experience.

REFERENCES

1. Adzick NS, Harrison MR, Glick PL, et al: Diaphragmatic hernia in the fetus: Prenatal diagnosis and outcome in 94 cases. *J Pediatr Surg* 1985; 20:357–361.
2. Iritani I: Experimental study on embryogenesis of congenital diaphragmatic hernia. *Anat Embryol* 1984; 169:133–139.

3. Bohn D, James I, Filler R, et al: The relationship between Pa_{CO_2} and ventilation parameters in congenital diaphragmatic hernia. *J Pediatr Surg* 1984; 19:666–671.
4. Sakai H, Tamura M, Hosokawa Y, et al: Effect of surgical repair on respiratory mechanics in congenital diaphragmatic hernia. *J Pediatr* 1987; 111:432–438.
5. Bohn D, Tamura M, Perrin D, et al: Ventilatory predictors of pulmonary hypoplasia in congenital diaphragmatic hernia, confirmed by morphologic assessment. *J Pediatr* 1987; 111:423–431.
6. Hazebroek FHJ, Tibboel D, Bos AP: Congenital diaphragmatic hernia: Impact of preoperative stabilization. A prospective pilot study in 13 patients. *J Pediatr Surg* 1988; 23:1139–1146.
7. Harrison MR, Langer JC, Adzick NS, et al: Correction of congenital diaphragmatic hernia in utero, V. Initial clinical experience. *J Pediatr Surg* 1990; 25:47–57.

3

Omphalocele

A 3-kg newborn is transferred from an outlying hospital for repair of an omphalocele. The defect is large, with small- and large-bowel herniation (Fig 3–1). The infant has a very large tongue. A glucose sample drawn when he was 3 hours old was reported to be 18 mg/dL. He received an unknown amount of 50% glucose intravenously. Hemoglobin, 16 g/dL; hematocrit, 48%. Surgical closure of the defect is indicated as soon as possible.

Recommendations by Nishan G. Goudsouzian, M.D.

The association of exomphalos, macroglossia, and somatic gigantism (EMG syndrome), more frequently known as Beckwith-Wiedemann syndrome, is an unusually complex congenital finding commonly associated with severe hypoglycemia.[1] It is genetically transmitted as an autosomal dominant trait with variable expressivity and incomplete penetration.[2] Infants so diagnosed are usually oversized for gestational age. They have a very large, muscular tongue, occasionally a cleft palate, and usually visceromegaly involving the liver, kidneys, and pancreas.[3, 4] The umbilical abnormalities vary from a simple umbilical hernia to a large omphalocele.

As growth occurs, gigantism becomes apparent with advanced bone age. Occasionally hemihypertrophy ensues. Affected children tend to develop malignant neoplasms such as Wilms' tumor, adrenal carcinoma, and nephroblastoma.[5] Some are also polycythemic. Other malformations such as microcephalus, facial flame nevi, and/or earlobe grooves may be present.

The characteristic hypoglycemia that occurs in some patients is believed to be secondary to hyperinsulinism from hyperplasia of the islet cells in the pancreas or else due to nesidioblastosis, or diffuse proliferation of the islet cells. Growth hormone levels are within the normal range, but increased somatomedin levels have been described. Repeated and often undetected episodes of hypoglycemia are probably a cause of retardation in some of these patients.

Once the critical early months have passed, the symptoms often improve, allowing healthy further development and a normal mental status. The hypoglycemia will usually resolve spontaneously

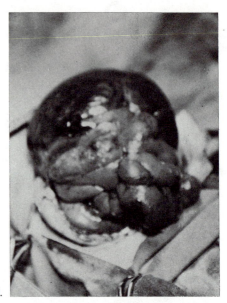

FIG 3–1.
Ruptured omphalocele in a newborn.
The liver and intestines are herniated.

within these first months of life.[6] With growth, the protuberance of the tongue diminishes due to enlargement of the oral cavity and repositioning of the hyoid bone. With time the hyoid moves posteriorly and inferiorly to permit gradual accommodation of the tongue in the oral cavity.

There is no specific treatment for Beckwith-Wiedemann syndrome. The management of these infants is supportive and is geared toward treating the hypoglycemia and the ruptured omphalocele.

PREANESTHETIC EVALUATION AND MANAGEMENT
Hypoglycemia

Hypoglycemia is usually defined as a blood glucose level less than 30 mg/dL in full-term infants during the first 72 hours and less than 40 mg/dL thereafter. In a premature infant, a blood glucose level of less than 20 mg/dL in the first 72 hours is considered hypoglycemic. These levels represent general guidelines for clinical management. No specific value can be considered hypoglycemic in any case, rather, the clinician must recognize that falling blood glucose levels can induce neurologic dysfunction of varying degrees in affected infants.[7] The clinical features of hypoglycemia are nonspecific in infancy but include irritability, twitching, and convulsions. Pallor, lethargy, hypothermia, sweating, and apneic or cyanotic spells are also indicative of hypoglycemia. In the presence of any of these symptoms, frequent determinations of the blood glucose concentration should be made. Of greatest importance is the realization that even one episode of hypoglycemia with seizures can result in permanent brain damage.

Infants at risk for hypoglycemia must be monitored frequently. Blood glucose levels should be estimated every half hour until the infant is stabilized and every 2 hours thereafter. In general, it is wise to start treatment if a blood glucose level of less than 40 mg/dL is detected and imperative that the infant not be left unattended after a hypoglycemic episode. The immediate symptoms may be temporarily relieved by intravenous glucose, but a rebound hypoglycemic episode may follow the release of additional insulin.

Treatment is usually initiated with the administration of one or two "miniboluses" of 200 mg/kg of 10% glucoses (2 mL/kg) injected over a period of 1 minute followed by a glucose infusion at a rate of 8 to 10 mg/kg/min. Occasionally, larger amounts of glucose will be required.[7, 8] If intravenous glucose infusion is inadequate to eliminate symptoms and maintain constant normal blood glucose concentrations, hydrocortisone, 5 mg/kg/12 hr, or prednisone, 2 mg/kg/day, should be administered. In an emergency when there is no intravenous access, intramuscular glucagon will produce a temporary release of glucose from the liver. After therapy has been started, blood glucose should be measured every 2 hours until a level of over 40 mg/dL is maintained. Subsequently, blood levels should be measured every 6 hours and treatment gradually reduced. Treatment may be discontinued after the blood glucose has reached normal values and the infant remains asymptomatic for 1 to 2 days.

Ruptured Omphalocele

The infant with a ruptured omphalocele is a candidate for semi-emergent surgery. The longer the bowel is exposed to the atmosphere, the greater the chances for infection and infarction of the bowel. The hours spent stabilizing the patient can be invaluable in preparing for both surgery and the postoperative state. As in the case of any child with a congenital anomaly, a thorough examination must be performed to detect any other anomalies.

Preoperative management of the omphalocele consists of minimizing evaporative fluid loss from the exposed intestine. This is especially important if the peritoneal membranes have already ruptured. A temporary solution is to cover the intestine with a large saline-soaked gauze pad and a polyurethane sheet. It is imperative to replace the exudative and evaporative fluid loss with appropriate intravenous fluids.

OTHER PREOPERATIVE CONSIDERATIONS

A secure intravenous catheter should be inserted and an intravenous solution of 10% to 20% glucose administered at a rate of 10 mg/kg/min. Because of the need for repeated blood sampling, an arterial cannula should be inserted percutaneously or by cutdown. If the arterial cannula cannot be inserted, a central venous catheter may be used for obtaining the blood samples.

With the catheter secured, blood gases, electrolytes, and glucose determinations should be performed. If the blood glucose content is less than 30 mg/dL, the rate of glucose administration should be increased. If the child is hypotensive, systolic blood pressure less than 50 mm Hg, a normal saline solution with 5% albumin can be administered. Once the infant's general condition is stabilized and the hypoglycemia corrected, he can be transported to the operating room.

Macroglossia, in most situations, does not present a specific problem. If marked, however, it can cause respiratory obstruction. The obstruction can be relieved by holding the infant in the prone position. In the presence of a concomitant omphalocele, however, the prone position is inadvisable. Preoperative endotracheal intubation then becomes necessary.

ANESTHETIC MANAGEMENT

The operating room should be warmed or an overhead warmer used. All monitoring devices should be at hand: precordial stethoscope, blood pressure cuff, temperature probe, pulse oximeter, and an arterial pressure transducer. A humidified gas flow system should be used.

If the child does not have a nasogastric tube in place, one should be inserted to empty the stomach. Urine output should be observed; it is one of the most important signs of adequate hydration.

Because of macroglossia, an awake intubation is usually indicated. Oxygenation should be monitored throughout by pulse oximetry. A no. 0 Miller blade and a 3-mm endotracheal tube is appropriate. If necessary, a stylette should be used to give the correct curvature to the endotracheal tube. A trained assistant should be present to hold the infant's shoulders and stabilize the head during intubation. Occasionally, cricoid pressure is required to bring the larynx into view. The tube should be placed orotracheally. At the end of the surgical procedure, if the child requires postoperative ventilation, the tube can be replaced with a nasotracheal tube.

Once the trachea is intubated, thiopental, 4 mg/kg, should be administered, followed by pancuronium or vecuronium, 0.05 mg/kg. Nitrous oxide should be avoided to prevent further distension of the bowel from diffusion of the gas into its lumen. The infant will probably tolerate an air-oxygen mixture with the addition of 0.5% halothane or isoflurane. If he becomes hypotensive on this regimen, the rate of fluid infusion should be increased and use of the halogenated agent discontinued until his condition is stabilized. The anesthetic can be supplemented and modified with fentanyl, 2 to 10 µg/kg, according to the requirements of the patient and the planned postoperative care.[9]

A special problem with these infants is respiratory embarrassment when the bowel is tucked snugly inside the abdominal cavity. If ventilation is difficult, primary fascial closure of the abdomen should probably not be attempted. Rather, staged silicone elastomer repair is performed, whereby a Silastic mesh is sutured into the abdominal wall and then closed over as a sac containing all the viscera. The clinical decision between primary closure or the use of Silastic mesh hinges on a number of considerations. Generally speaking, if tucking the viscera into the abdominal cavity raises the intragastric pressure to more than 20 mm Hg or the central venous pressure increases by more than 4 mm Hg, then a staged closure may be in order.[10] An alternative approach, less popular nowadays, is to close only the skin over the viscera and repair the hernia at 6 months to 1 year of age.[11]

During the anesthetic procedure, vital signs and laboratory values should be followed closely and treatment altered accordingly. It is not unusual for infants with ruptured omphaloceles to require large volumes of intravenous crystalloid or albumin because of the large exudative loss.

At the end of the surgical procedure the respiratory parameters should be re-evaluated by blood gas determinations. If they are satisfactory, extubation can be planned following reversal of pancuronium or vecuronium with atropine and neostigmine. Postoperative respiratory support is generally required, however, to offset the effects caused by compression of the lung when the abdominal viscera are pushed upward against the diaphragm.

POSTOPERATIVE TREATMENT

In the postoperative period, the infusion of glucose should be continued and the rate of administration adjusted according to the blood glucose concentration, which may fluctuate widely at this time.

The ventilator setting should be adjusted to provide a Pao_2 in the range of 65 to 90 mm Hg, a $Paco_2$ of about 30 to 40 mm Hg, and a pH of 7.3 to 7.4. Some infants will need additional doses of pancuronium to remain in phase with the ventilator and to maintain optimum gas exchange.

If a Silastic mesh is used for abdominal closure, the fluid volume requirements will be high because of oozing from the pouch that covers the intestine. The pouch is usually tightened every second day by the surgeon. This does not require general anesthesia but should be performed in a sterile fashion, preferably in the operating room. It is imperative that the stomach contents be emptied before each of these procedures to decrease the possibility of regurgitation. Three to four separate tightening procedures are usually required. The last step, skin closure and removal of the Silastic pouch, will require general anesthesia. On average, complete closure can be accomplished in about 10 days. It is important that the Silastic mesh not be tightened too rapidly if respiratory embarrassment and ischemia of the bowel are to be prevented. It is not unusual to notice venous congestion of the legs after each tightening, a condition that generally clears in several hours. It is interesting to note that as the viscera are forced into the abdomen, the abdominal muscles gradually stretch to accommodate the additional visceral mass.

Of additional concern in infants with large omphaloceles is delayed initiation of intestinal function. If this condition persists, hyperalimentation is generally in order.

Hypoglycemia corrects itself spontaneously in some infants. When prolonged therapy is required, however, a secure intravenous catheter, preferably central, is invaluable for ensuring uninterrupted glucose administration. It can also be used as a site for rapid treatment of the condition. Maintaining peripheral intravenous access in infants requiring concentrated glucose solutions is a difficult task. In infants with persistent hypoglycemia, steroid therapy, diazoxide, or even partial pancreatectomy are sometimes indicated.

The growth and development of the infant should be followed carefully, especially if he has other associated anomalies such as microcephaly. He should be monitored carefully for the development of neoplasms and appropriate diagnostic and radiologic procedures performed at regular intervals.

REFERENCES

1. Engström W, Lindham S, Schofield P: Wiedemann-Beckwith syndrome. *Eur J Pediatr* 1988; 147:450–457.
2. Niikawa N, Ishikiriyama S, Takahashi S, et al: The Wiedemann-Beckwith syndrome: Pedigree studies on five families with evidence for autosomal dominant inheritance with variable expressivity. *Am J Med Genet* 1986; 24:41–55.
3. Sotelo-Avila C, Gonzalez-Crussi F, Fowler JW: Complete and incomplete forms of Beckwith-Wiedemann syndrome: Their oncogenic potential. *J Pediatr* 1980; 96:47–50.
4. Takato T, Kamei M, Kato K, et al: Cleft palate in the Beckwith-Wiedemann syndrome. *Ann Plast Surg* 1989; 22:347–349.
5. Lodeiro JG, Byers JW, Chuipek S, et al: Prenatal diagnosis and perinatal management of the Beckwith-Wiedemann syndrome: A case and review. *Am J Perinatol* 1989; 6:446–449.
6. Meizner I, Carmi R, Katz M, et al: In utero prenatal diagnosis of Beckwith-Wiedemann syndrome; a case report. *Eur J Obstet Gynecol Reprod Biol* 1989; 32:259–264.
7. Cornblath M, Schwartz R, Aynsley-Green A, et al: Hypoglycemia in infancy: The need for a rational definition. *Pediatrics* 1990; 85:834–837.
8. Fanaroff AA, Martin RJ: *Behrman's Neonatal-Perinatal Medicine*. St Louis, Mosby–Year Book, 1983, pp 864–866.

9. Gurkowski MA, Rasch DK: Anesthetic considerations for Beckwith-Wiedemann syndrome. *Anesthesiology* 1989; 70:711–712.
10. Yaster M, Scherer TLR, Stone MM, et al: Prediction of successful primary closure of congenital abdominal wall defects using intraoperative measurements. *J Pediatr Surg* 1989; 24:1217–1220.
11. Martin LW, Torres AM: Omphalocele and gastroschisis. *Surg Clin North Am* 1985; 65:1235–1244.

4

Gastroschisis

A 6-hour-old, 2.6-kg baby is transferred from a rural hospital for repair of a gastroschisis.

Recommendations by Myron Yaster, M.D.

The perioperative anesthetic management of a child born with a gastroschisis or omphalocele has more to do with the child's gestational age, lung maturity, and the presence or absence of associated anomalies than with the defect itself. Indeed, despite the anatomic differences between omphalocele and gastroschisis, the anesthetic management is virtually the same.

GASTROSCHISIS

The embryogenic event that results in gastroschisis remains unclear. The most widely held view is that it is the consequence of an intrauterine vascular accident resulting in interruption of the abdominal wall musculature. Because it is a vascular accident, other major congenital anomalies are rarely associated with the defect. The herniated, or eviscerated, bowel consists of small intestine and rarely involves the liver. Furthermore, since the bowel is not covered by any membrane or sac in utero, it is "burned" by the amniotic fluid. This results in an atretic bowel with thickened and adherent loops covered by a gelatinous layer. It is subject to tremendous postnatal evaporative fluid losses as well as infection. In gastroschisis, the umbilical cord is almost always found to the left side of the herniated bowel.

These defects are being diagnosed with increased frequency in utero via abdominal ultrasound, thus permitting transfer of the infants to tertiary-care facilities *prior to birth* in the safest and most effective transport vehicle available, namely, the child's mother. Obviously, this significantly reduces transport-related complications and hastens definitive repair.

THE SURGICAL REPAIR

The optimal method of operative management of congenital abdominal wall defects remains controversial. Two options exist: primary fascial closure and staged repair using either a silicone elastomer pouch or primary skin closure. Primary fascial closure of gastroschisis carries the risk of placing the abdominal contents under pressure and leading to a reduction in cardiac output, hypotension, bowel ischemia, venous stasis, and postoperative respiratory and renal failure.[1] When primary fascial closure cannot be achieved, either because of the large size of the defect or because it critically compromises respiratory or cardiovascular function, the alternative approach is a staged repair. Staged silicone elastomer repair carries an increased risk of infection as well as the need for multiple anesthetic and surgical procedures. Skin closure with secondary ventral herniorrhaphy incurs the same risks.

Traditional criteria for determining the type of repair are based on the size of the defect, the presence of associated congenital anomalies, and clinical observations of the infant's respiratory rate, pulmonary compliance, blood pressure, skin color, and peripheral perfusion during fascial approximation. Unfortunately, these clinical observations may not be reliable, particularly in paralyzed, anesthetized infants.

ANESTHETIC MANAGEMENT

The newborn with an abdominal wall defect is transported to the operating room with the exposed bowel covered with sterile moist gauze and plastic sheeting to reduce heat and fluid loss from the exposed bowel. A nasogastric tube should be inserted prior to transport to decompress the stomach and to limit further abdominal distension.

Once in the operating room, the infant is intubated and anesthetized with fentanyl, 10 to 12.5 µg/kg. Pancuronium and oxygen are also administered.[2] Fentanyl clearance as well as analgesic requirements may be significantly decreased in infants with gastroschisis if the intra-abdominal pressure increases. Increases in intra-abdominal pressure, over 15 to 20 mm Hg, markedly reduce liver and splanchnic blood flow. This magnitude of increase in intra-abdominal pressure has been documented to occur following closure of abdominal wall defects such as gastroschisis. The decreased liver blood flow reduces fentanyl biotransformation and thereby anesthetic requirements. The fentanyl dose may therefore be dependent on the type of surgery being performed as well as the neonate's postnatal age and physical condition.

Aside from routine monitoring, catheters are placed in the right radial artery and the internal jugular vein. Intragastric pressure is measured by a fluid-filled, 12 F oral gastric tube. Successful management of infants with omphalocele or gastroschisis can often be determined by intraoperative measurement of intragastric and central venous pressures (Fig 4–1).[1, 3, 4] In this treatment algorithm, primary repair is always attempted. However, if the intragastric pressure rises above 20 mm Hg and/or the central venous pressure increases by 4 mm Hg or more following closure of the abdominal fascia, the primary repair is abandoned and a staged repair with a silicone elastomer chimney performed. This algorithm avoids the consequences of acutely elevating intra-abdominal pressure, specifically bowel ischemia and infarction, renal failure, acidosis, and hypotension.

Following surgery, the patient is taken to the neonatal intensive care unit, intubated, and placed

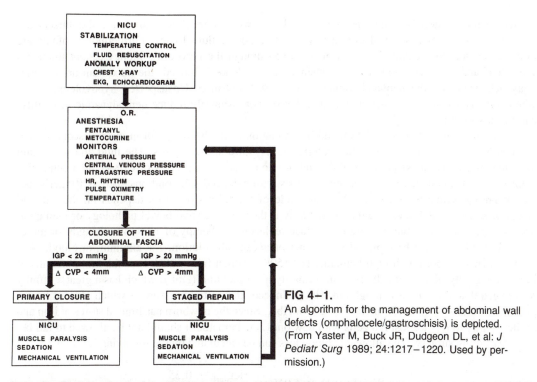

FIG 4–1.
An algorithm for the management of abdominal wall defects (omphalocele/gastroschisis) is depicted. (From Yaster M, Buck JR, Dudgeon DL, et al: *J Pediatr Surg* 1989; 24:1217–1220. Used by permission.)

on controlled mechanical ventilation. Infants treated with a staged repair have their silos gradually reduced over 2 to 10 days. Central venous and intragastric pressure determinations may be used to guide this therapy as well.[3]

FLUID THERAPY

Newborn infants with abdominal wall defects have significantly increased fluid requirements because of increased insensible losses that occur when eviscerated bowel is exposed to the environment.[5] Additionally, they have enormous "third-space" losses due to the traumatized, inflamed bowel and adynamic ileus that develops perioperatively. Obviously, fluid requirements are greater in gastroschisis than omphalocele because the herniated viscera lack a protective covering and suffer chemical burns.

Intraoperative intravenous fluid therapy provides the infant with maintenance requirements of water, electrolytes, and glucose to replace preoperative deficits and ongoing intraoperative "third-space" and blood loss. Maintenance fluid requirements are calculated from the assumption that 100 mL of water is required for every 100 calories consumed. The newborn's energy and fluid requirements are 100 calories (mL)/24 hr in the unanesthetized state or approximately 4 mL/kg/hr. Under anesthesia, however, these basal caloric requirements are significantly reduced.[6]

Since the majority of newborns presenting with gastroschisis are stabilized in the neonatal intensive care unit prior to surgery, the logical presumption is that preoperative fluid deficits are nonexistent. Unfortunately, this may not be true. Most newborns are fluid restricted in the nursery despite the presence of a surgical emergency and third-space fluid losses. Furthermore, infants are rarely given solutions containing electrolytes, even though the newborn's kidney cannot tolerate a water load and will waste sodium even when water overloaded. Indeed, the maximum urine osmolality achievable by the neonatal kidney is only 800 mOsm/L. Unsuspected hypovolemia, even when combined with drugs such as fentanyl that do not ordinarily reduce hemodynamic instability, can be catastrophic.

Surgical trauma and manipulation and inflammation of the bowel result in internal sequestration of functional extracellular fluids, often referred to as "third-space" losses. The fluid and salt within the "third space" act as sequestered fluid and are nonfunctional in terms of extracellular fluid. Replenishment of this interstitial water and salt loss with balanced salt solutions such as Ringer's lactate or normal saline is essential. The magnitude of the third-space loss depends on the site and extent of injury. Abdominal surgery, particularly if there is extensive bowel pathology or manipulation as in gastroschisis, may require third-space replacement therapy of 10 to 40 mL/kg/hr or more.

All blood loss must be replaced with either balanced salt solution, 5% albumin, or blood. Normally, infants are born with high hematocrits (>50%), which fall to 30% over the first 3 months of life. Additionally, these red cells contain primarily hemoglobin F (HbF), which has a greater affinity for oxygen than does adult hemoglobin (HbA). Indeed, the partial pressure at which 50% of hemoglobin is saturated (P_{50}) is 19 for HbF vs. 27 for HbA. Since the newborn has limited stores of iron and limited ability to replace lost red cells with new ones, the hematocrit should not be allowed to fall below 35% during surgery. The allowable blood loss can be calculated by the following formula[7]:

$$\text{Weight (kg)} \times \text{EBV} \times \frac{\text{Hct}_{\text{start}} - 0.35}{\text{Hct}_{\text{average}}}$$

where EBV = estimated blood volume and $\text{Hct}_{\text{average}} = (\text{Hct}_{\text{start}} + 0.35)/2$.

Ideally, blood should be replaced with fresh whole blood since it contains platelets and clotting factors as well as red cells. Unfortunately, this is rarely if ever available. Red blood cells are usually used instead. This component typically has a hematocrit of 60% to 70% and little if any factors V and VIII.

MONITORING

Critically ill neonates undergoing emergency surgery require as much if not more monitoring during anesthesia and surgery than do critically ill adults because the margin of error is so small and because disaster can strike so quickly. Unfortunately, compromises are often made because of the technical difficulty in monitoring small children and because once positioned and draped on the operating room table, observation, palpation, and even auscultation are often difficult if not impossible. Meticulous attention to detail is absolutely necessary. Despite this, it must be emphasized that no machine can replace a vigilant anesthesiologist who will evaluate, interpret, and analyze the patient's condition.

Unquestionably, the single most important monitor in pediatric anesthesia remains the precordial or esophageal stethoscope. It provides beat-to-beat, breath-by-breath information on the patient's condition. For example, the first indication of cardiovascular deterioration may be a change in heart sounds, from brisk and close to muffled and distant. Loss of breath sounds may indicate a mechanical disconnection or an endobronchial intubation well before a mechanical alarm sounds. Despite its importance, this low-technology, inexpensive monitor is rapidly being discarded by anesthesiologists in favor of more "glitzy" and expensive monitors.

Just a hair's breadth less important than the precordial stethoscope is the pulse oximeter.[8] This noninvasive, beat-to-beat monitor of oxygen saturation has revolutionized anesthesia monitoring and should be utilized not only in the operating room but in transport to and from the operating room as well. In neonates, the probe is preferentially placed on the right hand, earlobe, or tongue.[9] Newborns can easily shunt venous, desaturated blood across the ductus arteriosus, which causes blood distal to the left subclavian artery to become desaturated. The right hand or buccal mucosa will be perfused with preductal arterial blood, and pulse oximetry will reflect preductal and most importantly coronary and cerebral oxygen saturation.[9] This is critical because newborns, particularly premature neonates, are at risk for developing retinopathy of prematurity, "retrolental fibroplasia," if exposed to high oxygen concentrations. If the sensor is postductal, that is, on the left hand or the feet, low arterial oxygen saturations may be measured and too much oxygen administered. On the other hand, one must *never compromise oxygen delivery to the neonate's brain in order to protect the eyes.*

The next most important monitor is blood pressure. Newborns, particularly premature newborns less than 1.5 kg, may have normal systolic blood pressures of only 40 mm Hg. Blood pressure measurement and control become Herculean tasks. Indeed, this is the reason that many pediatric anesthesiologists prefer fentanyl-based anesthetics to inhalation agents when providing anesthesia for newborns. An adequately sized blood pressure cuff, a Doppler ultrasonic transducer, or an automatic blood pressure device is necessary for noninvasive blood pressure determinations. However, for most major surgery, continuous invasive intra-arterial monitoring is indicated. Catheterization of the radial artery is accomplished either percutaneously or by cutdown. The temporal arteries must be avoided as an intra-arterial site because of the catastrophic brain embolization associated with their use. Alternative catheterization sites include the dorsalis pedis, the posterior tibial, and the umbilical arteries. The arterial catheter provides beat-to-beat monitoring and a means to frequently sample for blood gases, hematocrit, and glucose. It is also a sensitive guide of the patient's intravascular volume status.

It is extremely difficult to judge intravascular volume clinically in the neonate. During the surgical repair of gastroschisis, third-space fluid losses may approach 100 to 200 mL/kg. The arterial waveform is one of the best signs of early intravascular volume depletion (Fig 4–2). The anesthesiologist looks for either a change in the shape of the arterial waveform, that is, decreased area under the curve, or the development of respiratory variation in the waveform. During positive-pressure ventilation, decreased venous return will cause a dramatic fall or drift in the arterial waveform with each breath. Typically, this fall occurs when the intravascular volume has been depleted.

In adults, the more commonly used monitors of intravascular volume are a central venous or a pulmonary artery catheter. Historically, central venous pressure measurements have been considered not only technically difficult to obtain but also useless in infants. Experiments done in the 1960s during exchange transfusions demonstrated little correlation with blood loss of as much as 20% of the estimated blood volume and central venous pressure as measured by umbilical central venous catheters. Unfortunately, these experiments have never been repeated with central venous catheters

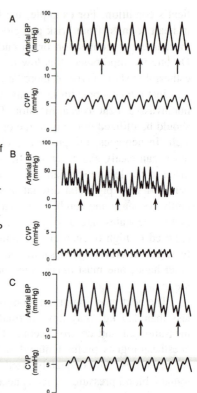

FIG 4–2.
Representation of a calibrated paper recording of transduced and amplified arterial and central venous pressure *(CVP)* waveforms of a neonate undergoing an exploratory laparotomy for necrotizing enterocolitis. *Arrows* represent controlled positive-pressure breaths. **A,** with the abdomen closed, systolic arterial pressure averages 70 mm Hg and CVP, 5 mm Hg. There is minimal effect on blood pressure with each positive-pressure breath. **B,** with the abdomen open, systolic arterial pressure falls to 55 mm Hg and CVP to 0 to 2 mm Hg. The arterial pressure waveform changes; the dicrotic notch separates, and there is "loss of volume under the curve." Each positive-pressure breath produces an exaggerated fall (10 to 20 mm Hg) ("pulsus paradoxus") in arterial blood pressure. This is consistent with intravascular hypovolemia. **C,** following an intravenous fluid bolus of 20 mL/kg of Ringer's lactate the arterial waveform no longer changes with ventilation, and blood pressure returns to normal. (From Yaster M: The anesthetic management of newborn surgical emergencies, in Rogers MC, Tinker JH, Covino BG, et al (eds): *The Principles and Practice of Anesthesiology,* St Louis, Mosby–Year Book, 1992. Used by permission.)

placed in the internal or external jugular vein and pressure transduced with modern equipment. In our experience, central venous pressure measurement is not only useful but essential in managing children with abdominal wall defects. It serves as a guide to intravascular volume and reflects intragastric pressure. Typically, we aim for central venous pressures of 4 to 9 mm Hg throughout surgery.

As described above, primary closure of an abdominal wall defect may result in dangerously elevated intra-abdominal pressure. This increase in intra-abdominal pressure can be measured by increases in intragastric and central venous pressure. Why central venous pressure rises in patients with increased intra-abdominal pressure is unclear. Presumably, the increase in right atrial pressure is due to increased pleural pressure transmitted from the abdomen by the cephalad movement of the diaphragm. Alternatively, the elevated central venous pressure may be secondary to decreased right ventricular compliance or possibly to decreased myocardial contractility. Finally, one of the other advantages of a central venous catheter is its utility in treating hypovolemia. These are large-bore catheters that are securely inserted within the vascular tree, usually via the internal jugular vein, and are a reliable means of administering fluids and vasoactive drugs.

One of the mainstays in the assessment of volume status is the measurement of urine output, or lack thereof. Bladder catheterization is easily accomplished with a 5 F feeding tube, not a balloon-tipped Foley catheter. The catheter is secured to the skin with tape and connected to a calibrated urinometer by low-volume tubing. Minimum acceptable urine output ranges between 0.5 and 1.0

mL/kg/hr. Unfortunately, in very small children, this small volume of urine may take hours to travel the length of the operating room table to reach the urinometer. Because of this, measurement of urine output during surgery is of marginal value.

Respiratory monitoring is essential. Despite the many technical problems involved in measuring end-tidal carbon dioxide concentrations (P_{ETCO_2}) through small uncuffed endotracheal tubes, particularly when utilizing Mapleson circuits, P_{ETCO_2} determination together with pulse oximetry remains mandatory for the provision of safe anesthesia.

Last, but not least, is temperature monitoring. All newborns are at extraordinarily high risk of becoming cold during transport and in the operating room. To minimize this risk, we routinely wrap children in plastic bags, use overhead warmers and heated water mattresses, turn the temperature of the operating room up, warm intravenous fluids, and use heated, humidified gases. Temperature is monitored with either a rectal or a nasopharyngeal probe.

SUMMARY

Invasive monitoring has contributed much to the survival of newborns with gastroschisis. In contrast to neonates with omphaloceles who frequently have significant associated anomalies, these babies usually have no other malformations and do well.

REFERENCES

1. Yaster M, Buck JR, Dudgeon DL, et al: Hemodynamic effects of primary closure of omphalocele/gastroschisis in human newborns. *Anesthesiology* 1988; 69:84–88.
2. Yaster M: The dose response of fentanyl in neonatal anesthesia. *Anesthesiology* 1987; 66:433–435.
3. Yaster M, Scherer TL, Stone MM, et al: Prediction of successful primary closure of congenital abdominal wall defects using intraoperative measurements. *J Pediatr Surg* 1989; 24:1217–1220.
4. Yaster M: The anesthetic management of newborn surgical emergencies, in Rogers MC, Tinker JH, Covino BG, et al (eds): *The Principles and Practice of Anesthesiology.* St Louis, Mosby–Year Book, 1992.
5. Mollitt DL, Ballantine TV, Grosfeld JL, et al: A critical assessment of fluid requirements in gastroschisis. *J Pediatr Surg* 1978; 13:217–219.
6. Lindahl SG: Energy expenditure and fluid and electrolyte requirements in anesthetized infants and children. *Anesthesiology* 1988; 69:377–382.
7. Furman EB, Roman DG, Lemmer LA, et al: Specific therapy in water, electrolyte and blood-volume replacement during pediatric surgery. *Anesthesiology* 1975; 42:187–193.
8. Cote CJ, Goldstein EA, Cote MA, et al: A single-blind study of pulse oximetry in children. *Anesthesiology* 1988; 68:184–188.
9. Jobes DR, Nicolson SC: Monitoring of arterial hemoglobin oxygen saturation using a tongue sensor. *Anesth Analg* 1988; 67:186–188.

5

Encephalocele

An 8-hour-old, 3-kg girl is scheduled for repair of a large occipital encephalocele. Hemoglobin, 15 g/dL; hematocrit, 45%.

Recommendations by
Angela Mackersie, B.S., M.B.B.S., F.C. Anaes.

Ideally, the encephalocele would be diagnosed antenatally and the infant delivered in a hospital where pediatric surgeons and anesthesiologists are readily available. If not, it may be necessary to transfer the infant to another institution shortly after birth.

ENCEPHALOCELES

Encephaloceles are herniations of the cranial contents through bony defects in the skull. Occipital lesions occur between the lambda and foramen magnum, but encephaloceles also occur in the parietal, frontal, and basal areas. Typically the contents are a combination of cerebrospinal fluid (CSF) and protruding neural tissue. In occipital lesions this is usually derived from the occipital lobes but is often associated with dysraphic disturbances of the cerebellum and superior mesencephalon. The neural structures are usually connected to the underlying brain by a narrow neck of tissue. The covering tissues vary from a flimsy meningeal sac with predominantly CSF contents to a well-formed skin complete with hair, although the latter is usually sparse and coarse (Fig 5–1).

The lesion occurs at the time of anterior neural tube closure about the 26th day of gestation. Lesions involving only meningeal structures can occur at a later developmental stage. Some infants with encephaloceles will also have associated malformations of neural origin, such as hydrocephalus, spina bifida, or microcephaly. Associated anomalies of non-neural origin are cleft lip and palate as well as cardiac and renal defects. The Meckel-Gruber association consists of occipital encephalocele, polydactyly, polycystic kidneys, and occasionally microcephaly, micrognathia, cleft lip and

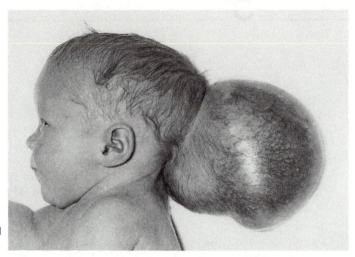

FIG 5–1.
A 3-kg girl with a large occipital encephalocele.

palate, cardiac anomalies and ambiguous genitalia. In a large rectrospective survey of births in U.S. Army hospitals, 40% of newborns with encephaloceles had associated anomalies.[1]

Occipital encephaloceles account for more than three quarters of all encephaloceles in Caucasians. In non-caucasians encephaloceles arising from other areas may predominate, for example, frontal lesions are far more common among Southeast Asians.[2] As with all neural tube defects, there is considerable geographic variation in the incidence not only between countries but also within individual countries. Europe has a higher incidence than the United States, and there is some evidence for a decreasing incidence from the east to west coast of the United States. The survey of infants born in the U.S. Army hospitals, a population representative of the U.S. population as a whole, showed a lower incidence of encephaloceles and a higher incidence of hydrocephalus in the Pacific region.[1] With the frequent movement of service personnel, many infants may have been conceived in one area and born in another, thus nullifying the geographic effects. Great Britain has one of the highest rates of neural tube defects in the world, especially in Wales, Northern Ireland, and Scotland, where the Celts predominate. In India, another country with a significant incidence of infants with these defects, the highest rate is in the Sikh community of the North.

While much is known about the incidence of neural tube defects, anencephaly, spina bifida, and encephaloceles, there are still many unanswered questions.[3] Several areas of the world have reported a spontaneous decrease in the incidence of these lesions that cannot be explained by antenatal diagnosis and therapeutic abortion. Approximately 10% of neural tube defects result from a genetic mutation or chromosomal abnormality, while the remainder have a multifactorial causation. It is this larger group that characteristically produces regional and geographic variations, while those that are genetically caused appear to have a similar incidence worldwide. However, genetic factors must have some importance even in the multifactorial group since there is an increased incidence in females as well as in siblings of affected infants. Recent work from the Medical Research Council Vitamin Research Group in the United Kingdom[4] showed a 72% reduction in the incidence of neural tube defects in pregnancies conceived after treatment with daily folic acid supplements. There was no such benefit from multivitamin preparations.

Maternal serum α-fetoprotein levels or ultrasound may be used for antenatal screening of neural tube defects. The former is only reliable for open defects, which are less likely to occur with encephaloceles than with other lesions. Ultrasound will not only diagnose the presence of an encephalocele but also give an indication of the contents of the lesion and the presence of other nervous system abnormalities such as microcephaly, hydrocephalus, spina bifida, or the polycystic kidneys of the Meckel-Gruber syndrome.[5] Ultrasound can therefore contribute to assessment of the likely viability of the infant. A positive ultrasound examination or raised α-fetoprotein level at 12 to 14 weeks enables discussion of therapeutic abortion. Ultrasound examination late in pregnancy permits planning of the optimal mode of delivery and its timing. Nonvaginal delivery may be recommended either because of the risk of rupture of a meningeal lesion or because of the risk of pelvic disproportion with a large solid lesion. To minimize the detrimental effect of raised ventricular pressure on cerebral function, some obstetricians and pediatricians recommend early delivery when hydrocephalus is present. However, the risks of prematurity may outweigh any advantage of early delivery.

Minimal postnatal investigation prior to surgery should consist of ultrasonography to diagnose the contents of the lesion and the size of the ventricles. Ideally, a computed tomographic (CT) scan or magnetic resonance imaging (MRI) should be performed to allow optimal assessment of any intracranial abnormality.

Neurosurgical management is recommended for nearly all cases of occipital encephalocele, except when there is gross microcephaly verging on anencephaly. The latter infants may be regarded as potential organ donors. Early surgery is recommended for all large lesions and when the covering is very delicate and there is a risk of rupture and meningitis. Lesions that ruptured during delivery or are likely to rupture even with meticulous nursing care should have urgent closure performed. Others can be delayed a few days.

PREOPERATIVE PREPARATION

Preoperative evaluation should include a full physical examination to determine the presence of any coexisting pathology. An assessment of the difficulty of intubation must be made, with the size of the encephalocele, its exact position and nature of the tissues, as well as any associated anomalies such as cleft lip and palate or micrognathia taken into consideration. Crossmatched blood must always be available. Atropine, 0.2 mg, is administered intramuscularly three quarters of an hour preoperatively. It is essential that secretions be minimized in infants turned prone to prevent dislodgement of the the endotracheal tube. Vitamin K, 1 mg, is given if not administered previously.

ANESTHETIC MANAGEMENT

The position for intubation should be planned. While many authors suggest the left lateral position, optimal conditions can be obtained with the infant supine. Several "donut" head rings of suitable internal diameter are stacked to encase the occipital lesion. A foam pad or folded blanket is placed under the body of the infant to provide support. The front of the head, neck, and body should be in a neutral position. This position is not only optimal for intubation but helps to ensure an unobstructed airway during preoxygenation and induction of anesthesia.

All neonates requiring surgery, unless able to feed, require intravenous fluids preoperatively to maintain blood glucose and electrolyte balance. Infants with encephaloceles may be slow to feed because of an obtunded neurologic state due to either hydrocephalus or a primary cerebral abnormality. Raised intracranial pressure is unlikely to be of clinical importance because of the ability to decompress the cranial contents into the encephalocele. A 3-kg infant is not at particularly high risk from spontaneous hypoglycemia. If the encephalocele is very large, the true weight of the baby may well be a few hundred grams less than measured and should be considered when blood volume and drug dosages are calculated.

Intravenous access should be secured prior to induction of anesthesia. Awake intubation is the safest option if there is any doubt about the ease of intubation or the abilities of an inexperienced anesthesiologist. Inhalation induction with oxygen and low concentrations of halothane or intravenous induction with thiopental 2 to 3 mg kg, can be utilized in appropriate cases. Once the ability to inflate the lungs with a mask has been demonstrated, succinylcholine, 1 to 2 mg/kg, can be administered for rapid intubation under optimal conditions. Alternatively, atracurium, 0.4 to 0.5 mg/kg, could be used, but the longer period of mask ventilation may result in a rise in intracranial pressure and splinting of the diaphragm due to distension of the stomach.

A Silastic reinforced tube is best for all neurosurgical procedures in children, especially in those operated upon in the prone position. A 3.0-mm tube is likely to be the correct size for a 3-kg infant, but because of the thicker wall of the reinforced tube, the larger external diameter may be too big, and a 2.5-mm tube should be instantly available. A small leak around the tube is advisable, but a large leak can lead to difficulty in ventilating the prone infant. A subsequent rise in carbon dioxide levels could result in poor surgical conditions. Fixation of the tube is critical, and ventilation of both lungs should be checked with the head flexed because this is the likely position in the prone patient. Three times the internal diameter of the tube in centimeters is a good guide to the usual length from tube tip to the lips in small children and infants. In a 3-kg baby the difference between an apparently well-positioned and a malpositioned tube is only a few millimeters. Silastic tubes are much easier to secure than are plastic tubes with a smooth surface, which makes fixation difficult.

Minimal monitoring requirements include electrocardiography (ECG), noninvasive blood pressure monitoring, and pulse oximetry, along with an esophageal stethoscope and nasopharyngeal temperature probe. End-tidal carbon dioxide concentrations should be used if appropriate equipment is available. The additional dead space of conventional apparatus may detract from an otherwise optimal anesthetic technique and prevent moderate hypocapnia. Direct arterial pressure monitoring is advisable for infants with large lesions, especially when a significant amount of neural tissue is present. It also enables blood gas analysis to be performed. The narrow neck of the lesion is often associated with abnormal blood vessels (Fig 5–2), which may make it difficult to control bleeding, especially if the vessels enter the skull through a small bony defect. Commonly there is a hemangiomatous malformation in the skin and underlying tissues that may increase blood loss. Venous access must therefore be adequate to keep up with large losses. Two large peripheral cannulas should be inserted, preferably into the long saphenous veins. Alternatively, a central venous catheter is placed via the femoral vein.

Careful positioning of the patient is essential to achieve optimum operating conditions. The infant should be supported with a soft roll under the chest and pelvis when turned prone to facilitate unrestricted ventilation and prevent inferior vena caval compression. The head should be positioned in a manner that will result in unobstructed venous drainage and a resultant rise in cerebral venous pressure. The position of the endotracheal tube should be checked at this time since its position may

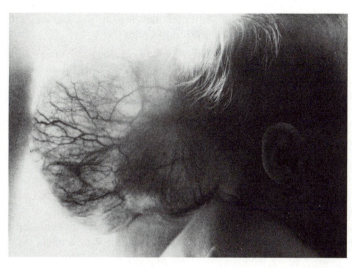

FIG 5–2.
A transilluminated view of the encephalocele demonstrates the abnormal leash of vessels in the neck of the lesion.

have been altered during the change in patient position. Use of an infant ventilator will allow intermittent positive-pressure ventilation without positive end expiratory pressure. If there is any doubt about compliance or adequacy of ventilation, manual ventilation should be instituted.

Temperature control in the prone position is difficult because the infant is raised off the hot air or water mattress by the chest and pelvic supports. Heat losses can be minimized by covering the body with foil or plastic bubble sheeting under Webril. A sterile adhesive plastic drape over the infant's head prevents evaporative loss with the inevitable CSF spillage. Heat loss occurring through the head and the encephalocele may account for almost half the surface area of a 3-kg baby. The normal surface area of the head of a baby is 18% of the total area, double that of an adult. All fluids administered intraoperatively should be warmed to prevent a further decrease in temperature.

Anesthesia is maintained with nitrous oxide or air and oxygen sufficient to provide adequate oxygenation as demonstrated by pulse oximetry. Hyperoxia is to be avoided since even a 3-kg infant may be susceptible to the adverse effects of high oxygen concentrations common in premature infants. The mixture should be supplemented as required with low-dose isoflurane. Apart from dissection of the surrounding skin, the lesion is unlikely to have significant innervation, and surgical stimulation is minimal. Opiate analgesia with fentanyl, 1 to 3 μg/kg, should be administered only if postoperative ventilation is planned. Adequate muscle relaxation is best achieved with atracurium, 0.3 to 0.4 mg/kg.[6] Neuromuscular blockade should be monitored with a peripheral nerve stimulator to avoid overdosage. Newborn infants may be more sensitive to nondepolarizing relaxants in the presence of hypothermia.

Maintenance fluids are continued during surgery with either 5% or 10% dextrose in 0.9% NaCl at 10 mL/hr, depending on the preoperative blood sugar content. Volume replacement with human albumin solution should be adequate for a blood loss of less than 50 mL, which represents 20% of this patient's estimated blood volume. For larger losses blood transfusion will be required to maintain the hemoglobin and hematocrit within the normal range for newborns. While the use of cutting diathermy throughout dissection markedly reduces blood loss in this type of surgery, difficulty in gaining control of the abnormal vessels around the neck of the lesion may occasionally lead to sudden massive blood loss. Excessive CSF drainage from the ventricles may lead to low intracranial pressure with a fall in blood pressure and require a rapid transfusion of colloid.

At the end of the procedure, unless the temperature of the infant has fallen markedly or postoperative ventilation had been planned, residual muscle relaxation should be reversed with atropine, 0.025 mg/kg, and neostigmine, 0.05 mg/kg. Once adequate ventilation is established and the infant has returned to her preoperative state she may be extubated in the left lateral position. The cerebral abnormality in these infants often leads to defective temperature regulation. Therefore, postoperative care should be provided either under a radiant heater or in an incubator until normal thermoregulation has been demonstrated. Apnea monitoring is mandatory, and oxygen should be administered as required to maintain normal oxygen saturation. No additional respiratory support should be required. However, if there is a major associated intracranial lesion with obtunded responses or primary respiratory pathology, ventilatory support may be required either as continuous positive airway pressure (CPAP) or by intubation and mechanical ventilation.

Postoperative fluid administration should be continued until adequate oral intake is achieved. Feeding, either orally or through a nasogastric tube, can usually be started within 4 to 6 hours.

Should analgesia be required, a single dose of codeine phosphate, 1 mg/kg, is usually adequate if there is no history of irregular or depressed respiration and the infant is vigorous. Where cerebral irritation is present from contamination of the CSF with blood, resulting in a "jittery" infant, a single dose of phenobarbital, 1.5 mg/kg, is indicated.

REFERENCES

1. Wiswell TE, Tuttle DJ, Northam RS, et al: Major congenital neurologic malformations. A 17 year survey. *Am J Dis Child* 1990; 144:61.
2. David DJ, Proudman TW: Cephalocoeles: Classification, pathology and management. *World J Surg* 1989; 13:349.
3. Sellar MJ: Unanswered questions on neural tube defects. *Br Med J* 1987; 294:1.
4. MRC Vitamin Research Group: Prevention of neural tube defects: Results of the Medical Research Council Vitamin Study. *Lancet* 1991; 338:131.
5. Graham D, et al: The role of ultrasound in the prenatal diagnosis and management of encephalocele. *J Ultrasound Med* 1982; 1:111.
6. Nightingale DA: Use of atracurium in neonatal anaesthesia. *Br J Anaesth* 1986; 58:32S.

6

Tracheoesophageal Fistula

A 16-hour-old, 3.2-kg infant boy with a presumptive diagnosis of tracheoesophageal fistula is transferred to the neonatal intensive care unit from an outlying hospital. He is in no respiratory distress. Pulse, 140; temperature, 36.4° C; hemoglobin, 16.2 g/dL; hematocrit, 50%. He was observed to choke and "turn blue" during his first (and only) feeding. Attempts at inserting a small nasogastric tube were unsuccessful. If radiographic examinations confirm the diagnosis, the surgeon would like to proceed with surgery as soon as possible.

Recommendations by Thomas P. Keon, M.D.

Esophageal atresia with tracheoesophageal fistula is a congenital malformation that occurs with an incidence of 1:3,000 to 1:4,000 live births. Although this anomaly was accurately described in 1698 by Thomas Gibson, an English physician, the first survivor was reported in 1939 by Drs. Logan and Ladd, who performed an initial gastrostomy shortly after birth with delayed ligation of the tracheoesophageal fistula.[1]

EMBRYOLOGY AND ANATOMY

The defect occurs between the 21st and 34th days of fetal development as a result of imperfect division or septation of the foregut into the trachea anteriorly and the esophagus posteriorly. Esophageal atresia results when the tracheal structure consumes most of the endoderm, and the fistula results when the esophageal and tracheal ridges fail to develop and leave a communication between the two structures. No common environmental or genetic cause has been found to account for the development of this anomaly.

Different anatomic variations of the anomaly have been described (Fig 6–1). The most common variation, occurring in 90% of cases, is proximal esophageal atresia with a tracheoesophageal

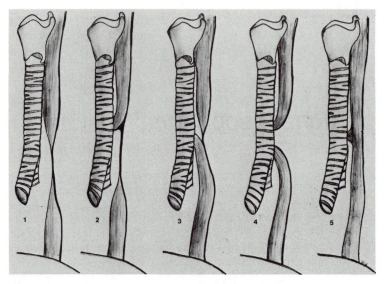

FIG 6−1.
Major types of esophageal atresia and tracheoesophageal fistula.

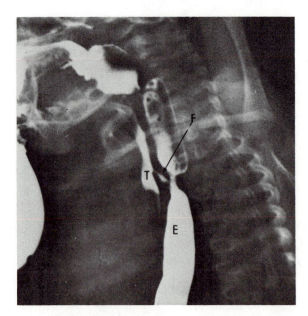

FIG 6−2.
Radiograph illustrating a tracheoesophageal fistula *(F)* between the trachea *(T)* and the distal esophageal *(E)* segment.

fistula between the posterior aspect of the trachea and the distal portion of the esophagus (Fig 6–2). The fistula usually originates near the carina, and the proximal esophageal pouch ends blindly in the mediastinum at the level of the second or third thoracic vertebra. Many anatomic variations occur, and Kluth, in 1976, described 97 different anatomic types and subtypes of congenital esophageal anomalies; therefore, an anatomic description of the lesion is appropriate rather than designating the lesion with numbers or letters.[2]

DIAGNOSIS AND PREOPERATIVE MANAGEMENT

The diagnosis should be suspected when maternal polyhydramnios and premature labor occur. Esophageal obstruction in the fetus that prevents swallowing of amniotic fluid may result in both conditions. The inability to pass a gastric tube in the delivery room may be the first sign. Early diagnosis of the lesion is important to prevent pulmonary damage that results from aspiration of gastric and oral secretions.

The newborn infant with excessive salivation, frequent coughing, choking and cyanosis with feeding, and respiratory distress should be investigated. Confirmation of the diagnosis can be demonstrated by radiologic evidence of the radiopaque catheter curled in the proximal part of the esophageal pouch. Air in the intestines confirms the presence of a fistula between the trachea and the distal portion of the esophagus, whereas a gasless intestine suggests esophageal atresia without a tracheoesophageal fistula.

Associated congenital anomalies are present in approximately 50% of infants. Congenital heart lesions occur in 20% to 25% and include ventricular septal defect, patent ductus arteriosus, atrial septal defect, coarctation of the aorta, truncus arteriosus, the tetralogy of Fallot, transposition of the great arteries, and tricuspid atresia.[3] The incidence of musculoskeletal anomalies is 20% to 30% and includes vertebral malformations, radial amelia, polydactyly, wrist anomalies, and knee malformations. Fifteen percent to 20% of the infants have gastrointestinal anomalies, including imperforate anus, malrotation of the gut, duodenal atresia, annular pancreas, and Meckel diverticulum. Among the genitourinary anomalies, which occur in 10% to 15%, are renal agenesis, lobulation, malposition, hydronephrosis, ureteral anomalies, and hypospadias.

The VATER association is a nonrandom occurrence of defects which include a combination of vertebral defects (V), anal atresia (A), tracheoesophageal fistula (TE), and radial and renal anomalies (R). This entity has not been recognized as a specific syndrome, and its components have been variable. The VACTERL association has also been proposed, with C referring to cardiovascular anomalies and L to limb defects.[4]

Preoperatively, the infant is cared for in a semisitting position with a suction catheter, or Replogle tube, in the proximal part of the esophageal pouch. Urgent surgical intervention is necessary to prevent pulmonary aspiration and pneumonitis. Occasionally, in the face of prematurity and severe respiratory failure secondary to pneumonitis and atelectasis, a gastrostomy is performed and the thoracotomy postponed until improvement in respiratory function occurs. The thoractomy is performed through a right chest incision using an extrapleural approach to ligate the fistula and undertake primary anastomosis of the esophagus.

Preanesthetic evaluation of the infant should include a thorough evaluation of pulmonary status and a search for associated congenital abnormalities. Cardiac evaluation includes auscultation for murmur, electrocardiography, a chest film, and echocardiography. Ultrasonagraphy is important in the diagnosis of any associated renal or genitourinary disorder.

ANESTHETIC MANAGEMENT

The operating room and appropriate equipment for the neonate should be prepared. The following measures are necessary to maintain body temperature: operating room temperature of 26 to 28° C; an overhead radiant warmer during induction and preparation; warming blanket; heated, humidified inspired gases; and wrapping of all exposed skin. The breathing system must have minimal dead space.

The precordial stethoscope is secured in the left axilla. Conventional, noninvasive monitoring devices and a right radial artery catheter are employed.

Venous access should be established prior to induction of anesthesia with a plastic cannula. Atropine, 0.02 mg/kg, should be administered intravenously. The pharnyx is suctioned prior to laryngoscopy, and the use of an oxyscope laryngoscope permits placement of a 3.0-mm endotracheal tube while the infant continues to breathe oxygen-enriched air. After intubation, low concentrations of isoflurane should be administered with oxygen while the endotracheal tube is positioned. The endotracheal tube is advanced gently into the right main bronchus and then withdrawn to a position just above the carina. This position is desired because the fistula is usually just proximal to the carina on the posterior aspect of the trachea. Rotation of the endotracheal tube such that the bevel faces posteriorly may help to prevent intubation of the fistula itself. The tube should be taped securely in this position after ausculation of the chest confirms bilateral air entry. Rarely, progressive gastric dilatation occurs and requires repositioning of the tube for satisfactory pulmonary ventilation.

After placement of the endotracheal tube and induction of anesthesia with an inhalation agent, a nondepolarizing muscle relaxant such as pancuronium, 0.1 mg/kg, is administered and ventilation controlled. In infants who do not tolerate potent inhalation agents, incremental doses of fentanyl, total of 10 to 15 μg/kg, can be administered. The inspired oxygen concentration should be titrated to maintain the infant's arterial saturation, as measured by pulse oximetry, between 92% and 99%. Increased inspired oxygen concentrations will be necessary when the right lung is compressed and retracted.

Air entry and heart sounds must be monitored continuously with the stethoscope secured in the left axilla. The anesthesiologist should observe the surgical field because airway obstruction can occur from surgical traction and compression of the trachea. The surgeon must be alerted to surgical maneuvers that result in impairment of ventilation. In some infants it will be necessary to remove surgical packs and permit intermittent ventilation of the right lung to correct hypoxemia and hypercarbia. Because airway obstruction may also occur due to accumulation of tracheal secretions and blood, intermittent suctioning of the endotracheal tube will be necessary during the procedure.

Initial maintenance fluid should consist of 4 mL/kg/hr of 10% dextrose in lactated Ringer's solution. An intraoperative serum glucose measurement permits adjustment of the glucose concentration administered. "Third-space" fluid requirements are usually no more than 5 mL/kg/hr, but signs of hypovolemia dictate the administration of additional crystalloid solution. Blood transfusion is rarely necessary, but crossmatched blood should be available and may be given to maintain a hematocrit value greater than 40%. The arterial cannula allows continuous blood pressure monitoring and sampling of blood for blood gases, glucose, hematocrit, electrolytes, and acid-base status.

Full-term infants free of pulmonary or cardiac complications can usually be extubated in the operating room at the end of the operation. The action of the nondepolarizing muscle relaxant is reversed with atropine, 0.02 mg/kg, and neostigmine, 0.07 mg/kg. Criteria for extubation include normal neuromuscular function as evidenced by sustained tonus of the extremities, a regular respiratory pattern, and eye opening. Premature infants and infants not satisfying the criteria for extubation should be returned to the neonatal intensive care unit for continued controlled ventilation and intensive monitoring.

HAZARDS IN NEONATES WITH LOW PULMONARY COMPLIANCE

Neonates with respiratory distress syndrome or pulmonary disease requiring high-pressure ventilation pose special problems in the operating room when a gastrostomy is created. The danger to patients with increased pulmonary resistance is not gastric distension, but sudden loss of intragastric pressure. In the presence of poor lung compliance, the esophageal fistula and stomach function in continuity with the tracheobronchial tree. The placement of a gastrostomy results in an acute loss of effective ventilating pressure.[5] The patient deteriorates immediately, and resuscitation can only be accomplished by maneuvers to immediately occlude the fistula and restore the required high inflation pressures. These maneuvers have included the placement of a Fogarty balloon catheter through a bronchoscope via the trachea and retrograde placement of a similar catheter through the stomach.[6, 7] The most prudent way to manage these patients is to perform thoracotomy and ligation of the fistula prior to placement of the gastrostomy.

POSTOPERATIVE MANAGEMENT

Tracheomalacia may be present because the developing fetal trachea is compressed by the dilated and hypertrophied proximal esophageal pouch. Airway obstruction or retained secretions may require reintubation of the infant. The head should be maintained in a neutral position and laryngoscopy and intubation undertaken after the administration of appropriate doses of atropine, thiopental, and succinylcholine. A marked catheter is utilized for suctioning the posterior portion of the pharynx to prevent disruption of the esophageal anastomosis.

The overall survival rate with this anomaly is now reported to be between 80% and 90%.[8] Mortality is directly related to the severity of associated congenital anomalies, and the survival rate for term infants without serious associated problems approaches 100%.

Postoperative surgical complications include leak at the anastomotic side, esophageal stricture, gastroesophageal reflux, and thoracic cage deformity in adolescence. Nevertheless, 90% of patients are asymptomatic after 15 to 25 years, and correction of this congenital anomaly can be a satisfying surgical and anesthetic accomplishment.

REFERENCES

1. Ashcraft KW, Holder TM: The story of esophageal atresia and tracheoesophageal fistula. *Surgery* 1969; 65:332.
2. Kluth D: Atlas of esophageal atresia. *J Pediatr Surg* 1976; 11:901.
3. Greenwood RD, Rosenthal A: Cardiovascular malformations associated with tracheoesophageal fistula and esophageal atresia. *Pediatrics* 1976; 57:87.
4. Khoury MJ, Cordero JF, Greenberg F, et al: A population study of the VACTERL association: Evidence of its etiologic heterogeneity. *Pediatrics* 1983; 71:815.
5. Templeton JM Jr, Templeton JJ, Schnaufer L, et al: Management of esophageal atresia and tracheoesophageal fistula in the neonate with severe respiratory distress syndrome *J Pediatr Surg* 1985; 20:394.
6. Karl HW: Control of life-threatening air leak after gastrostomy in an infant with respiratory distress syndrome and tracheoesophageal fistula. *Anesthesiology* 1985; 62:670.
7. Filston HC, Chetwood WR, Schkolne B, et al: The Fogarty balloon catheter is an aid to management of the infant with esophageal atresia and tracheoesophageal fistula complicated by severe RDS or pneumonia. *J Pediatr Surg* 1982; 17:149.
8. Spitz L, Kiely E, Brereton RJ: Esophageal atresia: Five year experience with 148 cases. *J Pediatr Surg* 1987; 22:103.

7

Duodenal Atresia and Trisomy 21

A 24-hour-old, 3.5-kg boy with trisomy 21 is scheduled for exploratory laparotomy. He has been vomiting bile-stained fluid. The abdomen is not distended. The presumptive diagnosis is duodenal atresia. Temperature, 37° C; pulse, 170; respirations, 45; hemoglobin, 18 g/dL; hematocrit, 55%.

Recommendations by Jesse D. Roberts, Jr., M.D., M.S.

Trisomy 21 (Down syndrome) is the most common chromosomal defect and has an incidence of 1 in 660 to 1,000 live deliveries. Approximately 5% to 7% of patients with trisomy 21 develop duodenal atresia.[1] The presenting sign of duodenal atresia is bilious vomiting in an infant without abdominal distension. A flat plate of the abdomen classically reveals a "double-bubble" sign (Fig 7–1) with air in the stomach and proximal portion of the duodenum, but not in the distal part of the bowel.

PREOPERATIVE ASSESSMENT

Preoperative considerations in the patient with intestinal obstruction include assessment of intravascular volume and metabolic status. Protracted vomiting can produce dehydration secondary to decreased fluid intake as well as ongoing fluid loss. The patient's heart rate is within the normal statistical limits and suggests adequate intravascular volume; however, determination of intravascular fluid status requires further investigation.

Even in the newborn, the physical examination may provide important information about the state of hydration. With progressive dehydration, one would expect to find dryness of the mucosal membranes, decreased urine production, sunken fontanelles, decreased skin turgor, poor capillary refill, tachycardia, and hypotension. The patient's weight should be compared with his birth weight. A normal newborn is expected to lose approximately 1% of body weight per day for the first week

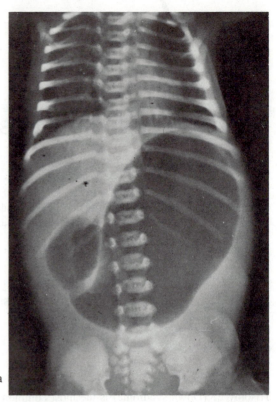

FIG 7–1.
Classic "double-bubble" sign seen on a radiograph of a neonate with duodenal atresia.

of life. If this patient's weight is significantly different from that obtained at birth, dehydration should be expected. If the infant's urine volume has been less than 0.5 to 1.0 mL/kg/hr, hypovolemia should be presumed. Treatment of hypovolemia is imperative prior to the induction of anesthesia.

Protracted vomiting can also lead to hypochloremic metabolic alkalosis. With progression of dehydration, metabolic acidosis may develop secondary to poor tissue perfusion. Because this patient has been vomiting, serum electrolyte levels should be determined. If the degree of dehydration is thought to be severe, an arterial blood sample should be obtained for assessment of pH and gas tensions. Correction of acidosis prior to surgery is advisable. Although an elevated blood urea nitrogen (BUN) level may suggest dehydration, interpretation in the newborn can be influenced by the ingestion of blood at the time of delivery.

Term newborn infants have limited glucose stores. Glucose requirements can usually be met by glycogenolysis within the first few hours of life. However, if caloric intake is subsequently inadequate, hypoglycemia will ensue. Hypoglycemia may initially produce no symptoms in the newborn.[2] This patient should have a blood glucose determination preoperatively. If present, hypoglycemia should be corrected by bolus administration of an intravenous solution containing 10% dextrose,[3] and the glucose level should be reassessed to determine the adequacy of treatment.

Aspiration pneumonitis is another potential complication in infants with doudenal atresia and is characterized by tachypnea, respiratory distress, and occasionally cyanosis. A newborn with aspiration pneumonitis may not become hyperthermic, but rather may demonstrate temperature instability or hypothermia. If the patient's respiratory rate is abnormal or rales and rhonchi are ausculated, a chest x-ray is indicated. An orogastric tube should be placed prior to surgery to decrease proximal intestinal distension and the risk of aspiration.

Cardiac lesions occur in 30% to 50% of patients with trisomy 21.[4] These include endocardial cushion defects (40%), ventricular septal defects (30%), patent ductus arteriosus (12%), and tetralogy of Fallot (8%). In the perinatal period, these lesions may produce cyanosis by increasing the right-to-left shunting of deoxygenated blood at an intracardiac or pulmonary level. With time, pulmonary vascular resistance may decrease and produce congestive heart failure by increasing left-to-right shunting of blood. Persistent cyanosis and polycythemia may also develop. The hyperviscosity of polycythemia can produce increased pulmonary vascular resistance, hypoglycemia, renal dysfunction, and occasionally seizures.[5] Although newborns with Down syndrome often have high hematocrits,[6] this patient's value is within normal limits.

The patient should be examined carefully for signs indicative of a cardiac lesion such as tachypnea, cyanosis, an active precordium, or a murmur. Electrocardiography may show left-axis deviation (0 to −90 degrees) and right or left ventricular hypertrophy in children with endocardial cushion defects.[7] Determination of preductal and postductal oxygen saturation by pulse oximetry or measurement of arterial blood gases in the upper and lower extremities may be useful. Evaluation by a pediatric cardiologist is recommended. Patients with cardiac lesions should receive antibiotics prior to surgery to prevent bacterial endocarditis.

Infants with trisomy 21 may develop primary pulmonary hypertension[8, 9] or pulmonary hypertension secondary to chronic aspiration, obstructive apnea, or increased pulmonary blood flow associated with cardiac anomalies. Manifestations include cyanosis and a murmur consistent with mitral regurgitation.

Some authors have stated that infants with trisomy 21 exhibit an exaggerated response to treatment with atropine; others disagree.[10, 11] The newborn's cardiac output is dependent upon heart rate, and concerns about this unproven adverse effect should not preclude the administration of atropine in a bradycardic infant with associated hypotension.

Although Down syndrome is associated with hypothyroidism,[12, 13] clinical assessment of thyroid function is difficult in the perinatal period. Early signs of hypothyroidism include lethargy, inactivity, hypotonia, and hypothermia. However, these symptoms are nonspecific and encountered in many sick newborns with normal thyroid function. In the newborn, a large anterior and posterior fontanelle and delayed bone age may be more specific for hypothyroidism.[7]

Airway management and endotracheal intubation are often complicated in patients with trisomy 21. Abnormalities of the upper airway include a relatively large tongue and a narrow short palate. The incidence of congenital subglottic stenosis[14] also appears to be higher in these children.

Several coagulation factors are present in lower concentrations in neonates,[15, 16] including those requiring vitamin K for their normal functional activity. In the confusion occasionally associated with the birth of a sick infant, prophylactic vitamin K administration may be forgotten. During the preoperative evaluation, the anesthesiologist should confirm that vitamin K was indeed administered.

ANESTHETIC MANAGEMENT

Prior to transporting the patient to the surgical suite, the operating room temperature should be raised to no less than 30° C. A warming blanket should be used beneath the patient and a radiant warmer used during induction and surgical preparation. Additionally, all lavage and intravenous fluids should be warmed prior to use. A coaxial or circle anesthetic circuit can be employed with measures to ensure adequate airway humidification. Increasing the water vapor content of the inspired gases provides a means of decreasing insensible water loss and also prevents cooling due to the heat of vaporization utilized to humidify inspired dry gases.

In addition to noninvasive monitors, an intra-arterial catheter should be placed for blood pressure and blood gas tension determinations. In the perinatal period, an umbilical arterial catheter or postductal peripheral arterial cannula can be utilized. A bladder catheter may be useful for assessing urinary output and therefore the adequacy of fluid replacement.

The airway should be secured in a manner that decreases the chance for aspiration of gastric contents. The stomach is first aspirated with a suction catheter. Following preoxygenation and application of cricoid pressure, a rapid-sequence induction utilizing sodium thiopental and succinylcholine is performed, and an uncuffed orotracheal tube is placed. Although patients with trisomy 21 occasionally have subglottic stenosis, the endotracheal tube size is usually that expected from the patient's physical size.[11] However, smaller tubes must be readily available. Awake intubation should be attempted if physical examination raises concerns over the ease of securing the airway. Once the airway is established, end-tidal CO_2 can be monitored and an esophageal stethoscope placed for auscultation of breath and heart sounds.

Controlled ventilation is required because surgical retraction within the upper abdominal quadrants may impede respiratory function and lead to atelectasis. Manual ventilation allows breath-to-breath assessment of the patency of the airway.

Anesthesia can be maintained with a balanced technique employing fentanyl and a muscle relaxant, or an inhalation agent can be administered. To reduce bowel distension, nitrous oxide should not be used. The inspired oxygen concentration should be adjusted by utilizing air to produce a Pao_2 of 68 to 80 mm Hg.

After approximately 34 weeks of gestation, neonatal renal tubular function is fairly well developed. As a result, in most normal newborns nonelectrolyte solutions are used for maintenance fluids within the first 24 hours of life. As discussed above, protracted vomiting may lead to electrolyte abnormalities necessitating the administration of fluids containing electrolytes. During this procedure, third-space fluid loss as well as increased insensible losses due to operative exposure will necessitate a replacement rate of approximately 10 mL/kg/hr. This is in excess of three times the normal maintenance requirement of 80 mL/kg/day for a newborn during the first 24 hours of life. Urine output should be maintained between 0.5 and 1.0 mL/kg/hr.

POSTOPERATIVE MANAGEMENT

The patient should be returned to the neonatal intensive care unit following the operation. Continued monitoring of intravascular volume status is important because additional third-space fluids may collect postoperatively. Muscle relaxation should be reversed and assisted ventilation decreased as the patient's ventilatory status returns toward normal.

REFERENCES

1. Jones KL: Down syndrome (trisomy 21), in *Smith's Recognizable Patterns of Human Malformation,* ed 4. Philadelphia, WB Saunders Co, 1988.
2. Fluge G: Clinical aspects of neonatal hypoglycemia. *Acta Paediatr Scand* 1974; 63:826–832.
3. Lilien LD, Pildes RS, Srinivasan G, et al: Treatment of neonatal hypoglycemia with minibolus and intravenous glucose infusion. *J Pediatr* 1980; 97:295.
4. Greenwood RD, Nadas AS: The clinical course of cardiac disease in Down's syndrome. *Pediatrics* 1976; 58:893–897.
5. Gross GP, Hathaway WE, McGaughey HR: Hyperviscosity in the neonate. *J Pediatr* 1973; 82:1004–1012.
6. Lappalainen J, Louvalainen K: High hematocrits in newborns with Down's syndrome. *Clin Pediatr* 1972; 11:472–474.
7. Rudolph AM (ed): *Rudolph's Pediatrics,* ed 19, Norwalk, Conn, Appleton & Lange, 1991.
8. Chi TL, Krovetz LJ: The pulmonary vascular bed in children with Down syndrome. *J Pediatr* 1975; 86:533–538.
9. Wilson SK, Hutchins GM, Neil CA: Hypertensive pulmonary vascular disease in Down syndrome. *J Pediatr* 1979; 95:722–726.
10. Mir GH, Cumming GR: Response to atropine in Down's syndrome. *Arch Dis Child* 1971; 46:61–65.
11. Kobel M, Creighton RE, Steward DJ: Anaesthetic consideration in Down's syndrome: Experience with 100 patients and a review of the literature. *Can Anaesth Soc J* 1982; 29:593–599.
12. King SL, Ladda RL, Kulin HE: Hypothyroidism in an infant with Down's syndrome. *Dis Child* 1978; 132:96–97.
13. Levin S, Schlesinger M, Handzel S, et al: Thymic deficiency in Down's syndrome. *Pediatrics* 1979; 63:80.
14. Steward DJ: Congenital abnormalities as a possible factor in the aetiology of post-intubation subglottic stenosis. *Can Anaesth Soc J* 1970; 17:388–392.
15. Shapiro AD, Jacobson LJ, Armon ME, et al: Vitamin K deficiency in the newborn infant: Prevalence and perinatal risk factors. *J Pediatr* 1986; 109:675–680.
16. Andrew M, Paes B, Milner R, et al: Development of the human coagulation system in the full-term infant. *Blood* 1987; 70:165–172.

8

Excision of a Sacrococcygeal Teratoma

A 4-kg, 1-day-old girl with a large sacrococcygeal teratoma (Fig 8–1) is admitted for excision of the tumor. Hemoglobin, 14.3 g/dL; hematocrit, 45.6%.

Recommendation by Leila G. Welborn, M.D.

Sacrococcygeal teratomas are most commonly seen in infancy and early childhood, a large portion being present at birth.[1-3] Most infants with sacrococcygeal teratomas are full term. Teratomas occur more frequently in twins or in families in which there is a history of twins. The tumor is seen predominantly in girls, with a ratio of four females to one male. Affected males are more likely to have malignant tumors. A tumor diagnosed before the age of 4 months is likely to be benign; after the age of 4 months it is more likely to be malignant. All sacrococcygeal masses should be excised before the child is 4 months of age, if possible. If the tumor proves to be a teratoma, the whole tumor mass and entire coccyx must be removed. The cure rate for benign sacrococcygeal teratoma is over 90%; however, it is near zero for malignant teratoma. In the malignant group, treatment has altered radically over the last two decades with the introduction of multiagent chemotherapy and delayed surgery. α-Fetoprotein assay became available in 1978 and is used as a tumor marker to monitor response and as an indicator of tumor relapse.[4, 5]

The incidence of associated congenital abnormalities in this group of patients is high. Malformations usually occur in the long axis of the child; for example, spina bifida, cleft palate, meningocele, and undescended testicles.

The differential diagnosis of sacrococcygeal teratoma can be difficult. Lipomas, lipomeningoceles, meningocele, hemangiomas, epidermal cysts, sarcomas, and rectal duplications may all present as skin-covered caudal masses in the neonate. The most common diagnostic confusion is between meningocele and sacrococcygeal teratoma.

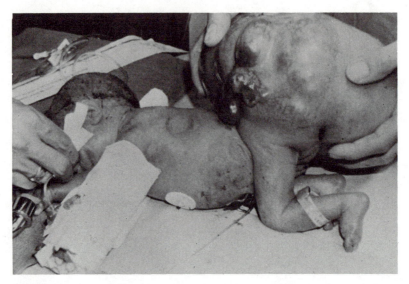

FIG 8–1.
Sacrococcygeal tumor in a neonate.

Altman et al.[1] have classified these tumors according to their location as follows:

- Type I.   Predominantly external (sacrococcygeal) with only minimal presacral components
- Type II. Presenting externally but with significant intrapelvic extension
- Type III. Apparent externally, but the predominant mass is pelvic and extends into the abdomen
- Type IV. Presacral with no external presentation

The type I lesion is the most common, but the incidence of malignancy is higher in types II, III, and IV. Benign tumors are generally noninvasive and cystic and contain calcifications.

The surface of the lesion may exhibit erosions that bleed profusely because of the extreme vascularity of the tumor. Death from spontaneous hemorrhage, even prior to surgical intervention, has been reported. Thus, hemorrhage is the major cause of operative mortality in the newborn period. Preoperative vascular mapping may be used to assist the surgeon in delineating areas of potential bleeding.

Any sacrococcygeal teratoma, regardless of type, can have an intraspinal component. Radiographs of the spine may demonstrate changes consistent with an intraspinal mass. A sacrococcygeal teratoma with an intraspinal component may cause lower motor neuron signs and can also be associated with congenital or acquired changes in the sacrum and coccyx.

PREOPERATIVE EVALUATION

The anesthesiologist should have an opportunity to evaluate the patient and to inform the parents of the anticipated anesthetic risks and complications prior to the day of surgery. The child should be fully evaluated for associated anomalies, particularly cardiac malformations. A chest x-ray is indicated to exclude the possibility of pulmonary metastases.

ANESTHETIC MANAGEMENT

The major problems are those of intraoperative positioning and excessive blood loss. General considerations common to management of any neonate are thermoregulation and fluid and electrolyte therapy.

Careful observation and monitoring of vital signs are essential. Standard monitors include an esophageal stethoscope, electrocardiogram (ECG), blood pressure cuff, nasopharyngeal thermistor probe, an infrared carbon dioxide analyzer, and pulse oximeter. Placement of the pulse oximeter probe on the lower extremity will facilitate assessment of the adequacy of circulation during surgical intervention. Because of the anticipated blood loss, an arterial cannula should be inserted to permit continuous monitoring of arterial blood pressure and obtain blood for determining blood gas, electrolyte, and glucose concentrations. A central venous pressure catheter is useful for assessing central blood volume. In addition, a urinary catheter should be inserted to monitor output and facilitate management. At least one large-bore intravenous cannula is essential for rapid transfusion.

In anticipation of a long procedure, the patient should be positioned on a carefully padded operating table. Pressure points such as the arms, feet, and head should be meticulously padded.

The areas of concern regarding thermoregulation are transport, environmental temperature in the operating room, humidification and heating of anesthetic gases, warming of intravenous fluids and blood, and postoperative transport. The newborn has a relatively large body surface area, high metabolic rate, and immature thermoregulatory mechanisms, therefore, heat is lost rapidly. A temperature reduction of 1° C induces a 12% increase in the oxygen requirement. Measures to minimize thermal stress include heating the operating room to a temperature of 27° C, placing a heating blanket on the operating table, using overhead infrared heating lamps, heating and humidifying inspired gases, using a blood warmer for the administration of fluid and blood components, and wrapping the extremities with Webril and plastic wrap.

Because of the malformation, positioning of the baby for intubation may pose a problem. Awake intubation performed in the lateral position following preoxygenation is the preferred technique. If the anesthesiologist is unable to intubate the patient in this position, an assistant can hold the baby in her stretched arms during the intubation. Alternatively, the baby can be placed with the defect protruding through the opening of a ring cushion made of foam rubber or other suitable material.

Because of the cardiovascular depressant effects of halothane and the likelihood of hypotension secondary to hemorrhage during the procedure, the technique of choice is nitrous oxide and oxygen, a nondepolarizing muscle relaxant such as pancuronium, and a narcotic such as fentanyl. Ventilation should be controlled during the procedure. The dose of long-acting muscle relaxant must be titrated carefully because of the extreme variability in response of infants. The initial dose is one third to one half the usual dose used in older patients.[6] A dose of fentanyl in the range of 1 to 4 μg/kg can be repeated every 30 minutes as needed. Newborn infants are highly sensitive to narcotics; therefore these agents should be used with great caution. Respiratory depression may well outlast analgesic activity in the postoperative period.[7]

The greatest potential intraoperative problem is sudden, massive, and uncontrollable hemorrhage, which can be a fatal complication. Blood replacement in excess of twice the patient's blood volume is not unusual. In a series of six consecutive sacrococcygeal teratoma excisions, the average amount of blood transfused was 300 mL, and the average rate of infusion was 7 mL/kg/min. One of the patients had a cardiac arrest during the procedure and four patients had multiple episodes of severe hypotension, presumably due to inadequately replaced blood volume and a reduction in venous drainage secondary to position. Other possible causes of hypotension are hypocalcemia and decreased myocardial contractility associated with rapid transfusion. The surgical team must be aware of the potential requirement for rapid and extensive resuscitation, and there should be a plan of management for turning the patient supine to facilitate resuscitation.

Blood loss should be estimated by direct measurement of blood in suction bottles and on sponges, as well as evaluation of nonmeasurable sites such as drapes, the floor, and surgeons' gowns. Serial hematocrit determinations can be most informative; however, the contribution of intraoperative hemodilution must be taken into account.

Massive blood replacement often alters the coagulation system and lowers the ionized calcium level, thus necessitating ready availability of laboratory support services. Coagulation studies are useful in defining the coagulopathy and determining hemotherapy. The blood bank must be able to provide appropriate component therapy, including platelets and fresh frozen plasma.

POSTOPERATIVE CARE

The patient should be transported to the intensive care area of the nursery with continuous monitoring of the ECG and intra-arterial pressure as well as pulse oximetry. The endotracheal tube should be left in place and the child ventilated manually with an Ambu bag in a warmed transport incubator. An extra endotracheal tube and laryngoscope should be available in case the child is accidentally extubated while being transported.

When the child's cardiovascular system is stable and the recognized criteria are met, she can be weaned from the respirator.

REFERENCES

1. Altman P, Randolh JG, Lilly JR: Sacrococcygeal teratoma: American Academy of Pediatrics Surgical Section Survey—1973, *J Pediatr Surg* 1974; 9:389–398.
2. Bale PM: Sacrococcygeal development. Abnormalities and tumors in children. *Perspect Pediatr Pathol* 1984; 1:1–56.
3. Ein SH, Mancer K, Adeyemi SD: Malignant sacrococcygeal teratoma—Endodermal sinus, yolk sac tumor in infants and children: A 32-year review. *J Pediatr Surg* 1985; 20:473–477.
4. Tsuchida Y, Hasegawa H: The diagnostic value of alpha-fetoprotein in infants and children with teratoma. *J Pediatr Surg* 1983; 18:152–155.
5. Raney RB, Chatten J, Littman P: Treatment strategies for infants with malignant sacroccocygeal teratoma. *J Pediatr Surg* 1981; 16:573–577.
6. Goudsouzian NG, Martyn JAJ, Liu LMP, et al: The dose response effect of long-acting nondepolarizing neuromuscular blocking agents in children. *Can Anaesth Soc J* 1984; 31:246–250.
7. Hertzka RE, Gauntlett IS, Fisher DM, et al: Fentanyl-induced ventilatory depression: Effects of age. *Anesthesiology* 1989; 70:213–218.

9

PDA Ligation

A 6-day-old infant, 1600 g, is scheduled for patent ductus arteriosus ligation. He was intubated in the delivery room, transferred to the premature intensive care unit (ICU), and continues to require mechanical ventilation. Attempts at pharmacologic closure of the defect have been unsuccessful, and the infant remains in a state of congestive heart failure. Hemoglobin, 13.5 g/dL; hematocrit, 40.5%.

Recommendations by James C. Loomis, M.D.

Persistent patency of the ductus arteriosus (PDA) is the most common cardiovascular anomaly encountered in premature infants.[1] The incidence varies with the gestational age at birth, ranging from approximately 1:2000 in term infants to 20% to 45% in those weighing less than 1500 g.[2, 3] Besides prematurity, other factors that may contribute to persistent PDA include the presence of respiratory distress syndrome (RDS), excessive intravenous (IV) fluid administration, neonatal asphyxia, and persistent or recurrent episodes of hypoxemia and acidosis.[4, 5, 6, 7]

CLINICAL MANIFESTATIONS OF PDA

A patent ductus allows shunting of blood between the systemic and pulmonary circulations in the direction of the pressure gradient. As the pulmonary vascular resistance decreases during the first few days of life, the magnitude of the pressure gradient from the systemic to the pulmonary circulation will generally increase, resulting in an increasing left-to-right shunt. In a small percentage of infants, for example, those with persistent fetal circulation or congenital diaphragmatic hernia with hypoplastic pulmonary vasculature, persistence of high pulmonary vascular resistance may cause continued right-to-left shunting.[8]

In the more common situation with a large left-to-right shunt, congestive heart failure, manifested by tachypnea, fluid retention, hepatomegaly, and cardiomegaly, may result. Increased pulmonary vascularity may be evident on chest radiographs. Overcirculation of the lungs can contribute to respiratory dysfunction because of pulmonary interstitial edema, decreased compliance, and increased airway resistance. A PDA is a frequent cause of persistent RDS and failure to wean from ventilatory support in the preterm infant.[3, 4]

The diagnosis of PDA in the premature infant should be suspected on the basis of the aforementioned physical signs and the presence of a typical continuous murmur. Because of the low-resistance shunt through the pulmonary vasculature, the systemic arterial pulse pressure is often wide, giving the impression of "bounding" peripheral pulses. Analysis of the pressure wave form from a systemic arterial catheter will show a rapid downslope and a low diastolic pressure.[9] Confirmation of the diagnosis is now generally made by echocardiography, which demonstrates left heart volume overload by a ratio of left-atrial-to-aortic-root diameter that is greater than normal.[10] In most cases, real-time two-dimensional (2D) echocardiography allows direct visualization of the patent ductus and estimation of its size.[11] Cardiac catheterization and aortography are now rarely required for diagnosis of a PDA in the premature infant.

PHARMACOLOGIC THERAPY

Pharmacologic closure of a PDA in the neonate may be attempted by use of an inhibitor of prostaglandin synthesis, such as indomethacin.[12, 13] Prostaglandin activity is one of the major factors controlling patency of the ductus arteriosus. Administration of indomethacin orally or intravenously in a dose of 0.1–0.2 mg/kg every 12–24 hours for up to three doses will produce functional closure of the ductus in 50% to 70% of infants.[14, 15] It is less likely to be effective in the very immature infant (less than 1000 g) or in the infant older than 4 to 6 weeks at the time of treatment. In low doses, indomethacin seems to be fairly safe, but in the higher dose range it may cause renal damage or bone marrow suppression.[12, 13] Indomethacin is contraindicated in the infant with renal insufficiency, bleeding disorders, thrombocytopenia, or significant jaundice. When indomethacin therapy is contraindicated or unsuccessful in the infant with a PDA and congestive heart failure, surgical closure of the ductus is indicated.[16, 17]

PREOPERATIVE EVALUATION

In addition to PDA, the premature infant is subject to a number of other medical problems, which include respiratory distress syndrome, sepsis, temperature instability, hyperbilirubinemia, hypoglycemia, hypocalcemia, intracranial hemorrhage, and retinopathy of prematurity (retrolental fibroplasia). During preoperative assessment, it is necessary to evaluate the infant for these and other problems that may influence anesthetic management or may require treatment during the perioperative period.

Because of the difficulties and risks of transporting a critically ill newborn infant who requires ventilatory support to the operating room for surgery, PDA ligation is commonly carried out in the neonatal ICU. Performing such a procedure outside the usual operating room environment requires careful preparation and cooperation among the surgical, intensive care, and anesthesia personnel.

Surgical instruments, equipment, and supplies must be assembled. A surgical area must be designated that provides adequate light, temperature control, and limited traffic, to assure aseptic technique. Several large series of successful ductus ligations in neonatal ICUs have been reported.[18, 19]

ANESTHETIC MANAGEMENT

Respiratory support should be optimized before beginning surgery. The endotracheal tube should be checked for proper position and secure fixation and it should be thoroughly suctioned. Recent arterial blood gas measurements, hematocrit reading, and blood chemical analyses should be examined to assure that the infant is adequately prepared for surgery. Blood for immediate transfusion, though not usually necessary during an uncomplicated ductus ligation, should be available in the event of a surgical complication. A secure intravenous cannula is required for administration of drugs, intravenous fluids, and blood.

The critically ill premature infant in a neonatal ICU will generally have in use most of the monitoring devices required for safe anesthetic management. Pulse oximetry, intra-arterial blood pressure monitoring, electrocardiography, and body temperature measurement are routinely performed. The use of an esophageal stethoscope and, if available, capnography will be useful in assuring the adequacy of ventilation during thoracotomy and lung retraction. Ventilation during surgery can usually be maintained with the infant ventilator, most commonly a pressure-limited flow generator type, already supporting the infant's respiration. Some anesthesiologists prefer to change to manual ventilation during the critical parts of the procedure. Oximetric measurements should be constantly monitored to assure adequate oxygenation without the use of excessive inspired oxygen concentration for prolonged periods, which is potentially toxic to the lung or the immature retina.

In the neonatal ICU environment, anesthesia is normally provided by using intravenous agents alone, unless special provision has been made to deliver inhalation anesthetics through the ventilator. The usual approach is to administer a large dose of an opiate, most commonly fentanyl, along with a nondepolarizing neuromuscular blocking agent, while ventilation is maintained with a mixture of air and oxygen. This combination is generally well tolerated, even by the critically ill infant with congestive heart failure. Ten years ago, Robinson and Gregory[20] reported the use of high dose fentanyl, 30–50 µg/kg, in a series of premature infants undergoing PDA ligation. They observed only modest decreases in heart rate and blood pressure, even with these large doses of fentanyl. Because of aggressive fluid restriction and diuresis commonly used to treat congestive heart failure in these infants, the authors recommended intravascular volume expansion with 10 mL/kg of Ringer's lactate, before or concurrent with the administration of fentanyl. A modest decrease in heart rate may sometimes occur with high-dose fentanyl, but can be prevented by the administration of glycopyrrolate or atropine or by the selection of pancuronium, with its vagolytic effect, as the neuromuscular blocking agent. The dose of fentanyl required to block the response to surgical incision in the premature infant may be lower than 30–50 µg/kg. A dose of 10–20 µg/kg may be adequate to prevent any increase in heart rate or blood pressure, particularly in the more immature and critically ill infant.[21]

Some respiratory depression may persist postoperatively even with short-acting opiates such as fentanyl. This should not be a problem since the infant with congestive heart failure and respiratory insufficiency will certainly require an extended period of postoperative ventilatory support. Surprisingly, the infants in the Robinson and Gregory[20] series were reported to be awake and making ventilatory efforts within an hour after surgery, even with the large doses of fentanyl employed.

Significant physiologic changes can be anticipated during the surgical procedure. As the chest is opened and the lung retracted, the magnitude of intrapulmonary shunting will increase and the compliance will decrease, usually requiring an increased F_{IO_2} and inflating pressure to maintain adequate oxygenation and ventilation. When the ductus is isolated and occluded, there is often a moderate increase in blood pressure, especially the diastolic pressure, as the large low-resistance shunt through the lung is eliminated. This change in blood pressure is rarely of sufficient magnitude to require treatment.

COMPLICATIONS

Surgical complications during PDA ligation are unusual. Those occasionally seen include damage to surrounding structures, such as the recurrent laryngeal nerve or the thoracic duct. Of more immediate concern to the anesthesiologist is the possibility of sudden massive hemorrhage that may occur if the ductus, aorta, or pulmonary artery is torn during dissection, or if the ligating suture cuts through the ductal wall when it is tightened. Even such a major complication need not be fatal if the hemorrhage is rapidly controlled and the anesthesiologist has adequate venous access and blood ready for immediate transfusion.

POSTOPERATIVE CARE

After PDA ligation, the infant with significant preoperative respiratory disease or congestive heart failure will require a period of ventilatory support before the improved hemodynamics will result in improved respiratory function. Because of the effects of surgical incision and retraction trauma to the lung, an increased level of support is sometimes required for 12 to 24 hours. In most cases, the benefit of decreasing pulmonary blood flow to a normal level will lead to rapid improvement. Failure of the respiratory status to improve in 24 to 48 hours after an uncomplicated PDA ligation should suggest another etiology for the infant's pulmonary problems, such as infection or bronchopulmonary dysplasia. When congestive heart failure does not improve, especially if a murmur persists, echocardiography should be repeated to identify another cardiac lesion, such as a ventricular septal defect.

REFERENCES

1. Baylen B, Emmanouilides GC: Patent ductus arteriosus in the newborn, in Thibeault DW, Gregory GA (eds): *Neonatal Pulmonary Care*. Menlo Park, Addison-Wesley Publishing Co, 1979, pp 318–333.
2. Siassi BG, Blanco C, Cabal L, et al: Incidence and clinical features of patent ductus arteriosus in low-birth-weight infants: A prospective analysis of 150 consecutively born infants. *Pediatrics* 1976; 57:347.
3. Zachman RD, Steinmetz GP, Botham RJ, et al: Incidence and treatment of the patent ductus arteriosus in the ill premature neonate. *Am Heart J* 1974; 87:697.

4. Thibeault DW, Emmanouilides GC, Nelson RJ, et al: Patent ductus arteriosus complicating the respiratory distress syndrome in premature infants. *J Pediatr* 1975; 86:120.

5. Neal WA, Bessinger FB, Hunt CE, et al: Patent ductus arteriosus complicating respiratory distress syndrome. *J Pediatr* 1975; 86:127.

6. Steveson JG: Fluid administration in the association of patent ductus arteriosus complicating respiratory distress syndrome. *J Pediatr* 1977; 90:256.

7. Bell EF, Warburton D, Stonestreet BJ, et al: Effect of fluid administration on the development of symptomatic patent ductus arteriosus and congestive heart failure in premature infants. *N Engl J Med* 1980; 302:598–604.

8. Sapire DW: *Understanding and Diagnosing Pediatric Heart Disease.* Norwalk, Conn, Appleton & Lange, 1991, p 117.

9. Milstein JM, Riemenschneider TA, Goetzmann BW, et al: Assessment of patent ductus arteriosus shunting using diastolic pressure analysis. *J Pediatr* 1979; 94:122.

10. Baylen BG, Meyer RA, Kaplan S, et al: The critically ill premature infant with patent ductus arteriosus and pulmonary disease—an echocardiographic assessment. *J Pediatr* 1975; 86:423.

11. Heymann MA: Patent ductus arteriosus, in Adams FH, Emmanouilides GC, Riemenschneider TA (eds): *Heart Disease in Infants, Children and Adolescents.* Baltimore, Williams & Wilkins, 1989, pp 209–224.

12. Friedman W, Hirschlan M, Provitz M, et al: Pharmacologic closure of patent ductus arteriosus in the premature infant. *N Engl J Med* 1976; 295:526–529.

13. Heymann M, Rudolph A, Silverman N: Closure of the ductus arteriosus in premature infants by inhibition of prostaglandin synthesis. *N Engl J Med* 1976; 295:530–533.

14. Holiday HL, Hirata T, Brady JP: Indomethacin therapy for large patent ductus arteriosus in the very low birth weight infant: Results and complications. *Pediatrics* 1979; 64:154.

15. Brash AR, Hickey DE, Graham TP, et al: Pharmacokinetics of indomethacin in the neonate: Relation of plasma indomethacin levels to response of the ductus arteriosus. *N Engl J Med* 1981; 305:67–72.

16. Edmunds LH, Gregory GA, Heymann MA, et al: Surgical closure of the ductus arteriosus in premature infants. *Circulation* 1973; 48:856–863.

17. Hall GS, Helmsworth JA, Schreiber JT, et al: Premature infants with patent ductus arteriosus and respiratory distress syndrome: Selection for ductal ligation. *Ann Thorac Surg* 1976; 22:146–150.

18. Oxnard SC, McGough EC, Jung AL, et al: Ligation of the patent ductus arteriosus in the newborn intensive care unit. *Ann Thorac Surg* 1977; 23:564–567.

19. Coster DD, Gorton ME, Grooters RK, et al: Surgical closure of the patent ductus arteriosus in the neonatal intensive care unit. *Ann Thorac Surg* 1989; 48:386–389.

20. Robinson S, Gregory GA: Fentanyl-air-oxygen anesthesia for ligation of patent ductus arteriosus in preterm infants. *Anesth Analg* 1981; 60:331–334.

21. Yaster M: The dose response of fentanyl in neonatal anesthesia. *Anesthesiology* 1987; 66:433–435.

10

Necrotizing Enterocolitis

A 1-week-old, premature, 1.2-kg boy is brought to the operating room for exploratory laparotomy. The presumed diagnosis is necrotizing enterocolitis. He is intubated and mechanically ventilated. Hemoglobin, 14 g/dL; hematocrit, 45%; blood pressure, 40/20 mm Hg; pulse, 180; temperature, 36.7°C.

Recommendations by Madelyn Kahana, M.D., and Brad W. Warner, M.D.

Necrotizing enterocolitis (NEC) is one of the most common life-threatening disorders of the neonatal period. In the United States alone, it is estimated that 2,000 to 4,000 newborn infants each year develop NEC, an incidence of 1% to 8% of neonates admitted to intensive care units. NEC is second only to respiratory distress syndrome[1] as a leading cause of death in the neonate. It is also the cause of significant long-term morbidity in the form of short-gut syndrome.

The etiology of NEC remains elusive and probably multifactorial. Although multiple risk factors have been proposed, the only two that are consistently found in carefully controlled prospective studies are low birth weight and prematurity. Since NEC can occur in epidemics as well as in sporadic cases, an infectious causative agent has been sought but never identified.

The time of onset of NEC is quite variable, 1 day to 3 months, but is usually noted between the third and tenth days of life. The clinical presentation varies from subtle feeding intolerance to frankly bloody stools, abdominal distension, and shock. In the majority of cases abdominal distension, vomiting, and blood per rectum are noted. The infant may show signs of peritonitis consisting of edema and erythema of the abdominal wall and tenderness to palpation. Laboratory findings are nonspecific and are associated with other conditions that are present in the sick neonate. Leukopenia, thrombocytopenia, elevated prothrombin and partial thromboplastin times, hypofibrinogenemia, and metabolic acidosis are frequently identified in patients requiring surgical intervention.

TABLE 10–1.

Heart Rates in Normal Children

Age	Range (Beats/min)	Mean (Beats/min)
Premature	120–180	150
Newborn–3 mo	100–180	140
3 mo–2 yr	100–160	130
2 yr–10 yr	60–140	80
>10 yr	50–100	75

On plain radiography of the abdomen, pneumatosis intestinalis, gas within the bowel wall, remains the diagnostic hallmark of NEC and is present in up to 98% of cases. Patients who require laparotomy and bowel resection frequently also have pneumoperitoneum, signaling a perforated viscus.

NEC is successfully managed without surgery in over 50% of cases. The bowel should be decompressed with a nasogastric tube and the feedings withheld. Vigorous volume resuscitation is indicated to compensate for the large amount of "third-space" loss into the bowel lumen, bowel wall, peritoneal cavity, and extracellular fluid compartment. This resuscitation should be accomplished with a balanced salt solution to meet the physiologic end points of stable vital signs, adequate peripheral perfusion, and a urine output of 1 to 2 mL/kg/hr (Table 10–1 and Fig 10–1). The nonoperatively managed infant with NEC should be carefully monitored for the development of a gangrenous bowel and/or perforation. For the first several days, platelet count, white blood cell (WBC) count, acid-base status, and plain radiographs should be followed at least every 6 hours. Monitoring every 12 to 14 hours is indicated as the infant improves. A minimum of 7 to 10 days of bowel rest and broad-spectrum antibiotic therapy are recommended.

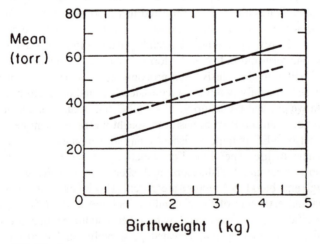

FIG 10–1.
Range of normal mean arterial pressure.

TABLE 10–2.

Preoperative Evaluation of the Infant With Necrotizing
Enterocolitis

Assess intravascular volume status
Evaluate concurrent pulmonary dysfunction
Laboratory studies
    Electrolytes, blood urea nitrogen, creatinine, glucose,
      calcium
    Arterial blood gases
    Coagulation profile
    Complete blood count, differential, platelet count
Radiographs
    Chest
    Abdomen

PREOPERATIVE PREPARATION

For the infant who requires urgent laparotomy for perforation or an ischemic bowel, aggressive preoperative volume resuscitation is imperative. Preoperative assessment should focus on evaluation of the patient's intravascular volume status, laboratory assessment of coagulation, the examination of coexisting pulmonary dysfunction, and acid-base status (Table 10–2). Because most infants with NEC are 28 to 32 weeks postconceptual age, infant respiratory distress syndrome (IRDS) frequently complicates their care. These infants are generally intubated and require mechanical ventilatory support. Significant deterioration in the patient's respiratory status may occur in the perioperative period with restriction of chest wall movement by abdominal distension and/or the development of pulmonary edema. Massive pulmonary hemorrhage is also seen in the very sick neonate with IRDS and NEC and is often a fatal event.

INTRAOPERATIVE PREPARATION

In preparation for exploratory laparotomy (Table 10–3), it is imperative to have an adequate supply of blood components including red blood cells, platelets, cryoprecipitate, and fresh frozen plasma, as dictated by preoperative coagulation parameters. Even in the rare patient with normal preoperative coagulation results, blood components should be easily accessible because intraoperative blood loss can be excessive. The operating suite should be warmed to 30 to 32°C. A warming blanket should be on the operating table. A system for warm humidification of anesthetic gases should be set up if at all possible. Plastic wrap or reflective blanket material should be available to wrap the patient's extremities and head to reduce temperature loss during laparotomy. Overhead warmers are ineffective in this setting. In addition to the usual intraoperative monitors, central venous and arterial catheter placement may be indicated. A urinary catheter should be inserted preoperatively to allow adequate assessment of intraoperative urine output. Either a circle system or mod-

TABLE 10–3.

Priorities for Intraoperative Management for the Neonate
With Necrotizing Enterocolitis

Adequate venous access
Attention to temperature control
Warm room (30–32°C)
Warming blanket
Warm anesthetic gases
Warm intravenous fluids
Wrapping the baby's extremities and head
Warm irrigation fluid
Adequate monitoring
Electrocardiogram (ECG)
Noninvasive blood pressure (NIBP)
Precordial or esophageal stethoscope
Pulse oximeter
Urinary catheter
Optional
Arterial catheter
Central venous catheter
Blood component availability
Volume resuscitation

ified Mapleson circuit can be used. The currently available anesthesia ventilators may be inadequate in the very ill child, and in this circumstance, ventilation by hand is preferred.

ANESTHETIC MANAGEMENT

Only after preparation of the operating room is complete and the blood components are available is the neonate brought to the surgical suite. This minimizes exposure time to a rather cold environment and preoperative heat losses. Monitors are placed, the infant's extremities and head are wrapped, and invasive monitors are inserted. Arterial catheter placement and monitoring facilitates the intraoperative assessment of intravascular volume repletion and allows for blood gas measurements. In the hypovolemic neonate, the arterial pressure trace has a characteristic pattern. Following a positive-pressure breath, the height of the waveform diminishes (Fig 10–2). The respiratory variation seen in the arterial pressure trace is an early signal that additional intravascular volume is required. As the volume status of the neonate is further compromised, the arterial waveform may be lost entirely. Despite its value, placement of an arterial cannula in the sick neonate can be difficult, is not mandated, and should not inordinately delay surgery.

Similarly, a central venous catheter provides reliable venous access for vasoactive drugs as well as for volume administration but can be supplanted by adequate peripheral venous access. In infants with significant coagulopathy, peripheral access is preferred. Because aggressive volume administration is required during laparotomy for NEC, *it is imperative to have adequate venous access.*

The tenuous nature of the sick neonate's hemodynamic status usually dictates a narcotic-relax-

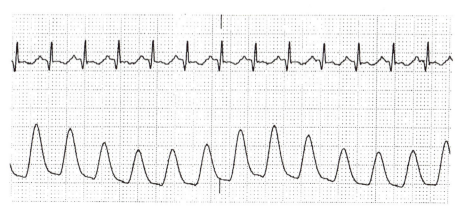

FIG 10–2.
Respiratory variation of arterial waveforms.

ant anesthetic technique.[2] Nitrous oxide is best avoided to minimize bowel distension. Volatile anesthetic agents may be tolerated by some patients.

Volume Resuscitation

The critical issue in the perioperative management of these children is not the anesthetic technique but rather meticulous attention to volume resuscitation upon which their very survival depends. The history of fluid and electrolyte management in the perioperative period for all patients is much like the course of a pendulum—swinging between salt restriction[3] and the recommended use of balanced salt solutions.

In the 1940s, because investigators found low urine chloride values, surgical patients were believed not to tolerate a salt load.[3] Glucose and water solutions were recommended. In the 1950s there were a multitude of reports of hyponatremia complicating postoperative care with dire consequences.[4] In the 1960s Shires et al.[5] first recommended balanced salt solution as the preferred perioperative fluid based upon estimated losses of extracellular fluid in patients during operation and trauma. These recommendations have remained the standard of care for the adult patient, while the neonate has long been viewed as a different animal with peculiar needs. Although the physiology of the neonate is in phases of transition from intrauterine to extrauterine life and maturation from fetus to neonate, the fundamental perioperative requirement for balanced salt solution resuscitation is much the same as in the adult.

The early work with urinary electrolytes has evolved into an expanding knowledge of the perioperative stress response that should guide modern perioperative fluid management. During surgery or other significant stress, there is an elaboration of hormones teleologically designed to promote survival and defend the intravascular space and cardiac output. Catecholamines, aldosterone, and arginine vasopressin (antidiuretic hormone [ADH]) are liberated for this purpose and are present for up to 5 days following a stressful event.[6] The most persistent of these hormones is ADH, which peaks 6 to 12 hours postoperatively and returns to prestress levels at 5 days.[7] The administration of large quantities of free water during the peak secretion of ADH invariably results in a drop in serum sodium, sometimes to levels causing neurologic symptoms and seizures.[8] This phenomenon has well been described in the neonate[9] and in the adult.

The limited function of the neonatal kidney has also been used to advocate salt restriction in this patient population. Although renal blood flow (RBF) and the glomerular filtration rate (GFR) are low in the preterm infant, particularly before 34 weeks of postconceptual age, free water clearance is well above adult levels.[8] The maximum concentrating ability of the newborn kidney is limited to 500 to 600 mOsm/L, so excessive fluid restriction in these infants is not well tolerated. Minimum acceptable urine output is 1 to 2 mL/kg/hr. The premature infant also has an obligate sodium loss, perhaps because the renal tubules are less responsive to aldosterone. Fractional excretion of sodium is greater than 5 in the healthy preterm newborn. Sodium deprivation is therefore also not well tolerated in the premature infant. This intolerance is exaggerated when there are excessive sodium losses, such as in "third-space" loss. These data further support the aggressive use of balanced salt solution in the perioperative period.

Volume resuscitation with a balanced salt solution such as Ringer's lactate or normal saline or with colloid solutions is the current gold standard for perioperative fluid management in the preterm infant with NEC. Sufficient balanced salt solution should be administered to maintain circulating blood volume and adequate urine flow even if the fluid volume required exceeds predictions. It is not uncommon to administer in excess of 100 mL/kg of balanced salt solution during laparotomy for NEC in the sick neonate.

It is important to emphasize the consequences of error in volume resuscitation. Excessive volume replacement can and does result in peripheral and pulmonary edema. Hypoxemia and reduced lung compliance occur, and peak airway pressure increases. In the absence of renal failure, this condition generally responds promptly to diuresis. Inadequate volume resuscitation results in insufficient perfusion of the kidney, brain, heart, and liver. Devastating consequences result. Renal failure, liver dysfunction or failure, and impaired cardiac performance respond to appropriate support and therapy with much less predictability. Multisystem organ failure can result, and death is likely. Err, therefore, if unsure, with *more,* not less.

In addition to balanced salt solution, the premature infant may require continuation of a basal glucose infusion of 4 to 7 mg/kg/min to maintain an adequate serum glucose concentration. The need for intraoperative glucose administration requires monitoring of the serum glucose level during surgery, and again, the needs of each individual patient will vary.

Hypocalcemia is the other important electrolyte abnormality that may require intraoperative treatment. The neonate is commonly modestly hypocalcemic, which can be significantly aggravated by rapid transfusion of blood components. If untreated, hypocalcemia results in reduced cardiac output and hypotension.

The administration of blood components must be guided by individual patient needs. The hematocrit should be sufficient to ensure oxygen delivery; coagulation factors and platelets must be adequate for hemostasis. It is important to recall that the ill premature infant requires hematocrit values of 40% or greater to ensure acceptable oxygen delivery because of his underlying pulmonary pathology and limited cardiac reserve. Intraoperative transfusion practice and fluid management should be continued into the immediate postoperative period because "third-space" losses continue for 24 to 48 hours, as does the stress response.

POSTOPERATIVE CARE

Optimal postoperative care of the infant with NEC demands repeated examination of the patient for signs of inadequate intravascular volume and frequent monitoring of serum electrolytes. If his course is uncomplicated, the neonate will begin to excrete excess extracellular fluid at 24 to 48 hours postoperatively, as does the adult. Because of limited RBF and GFR, this may require additional time or augmentation with judicious use of loop diuretics.

On the third to fifth postoperative day, if the infant has shown clinical signs of improvement, he is returned to the operating room for placement of a central catheter for aggressive parenteral nutrition. Antibiotics and bowel rest are continued for 14 to 21 days. Refeeding is begun slowly with dilute elemental formula at that time.

Survival of the premature infant with NEC depends as much upon the skill of the anesthesiologist as it does upon that of the surgeon. Without appropriate and aggressive management of perioperative fluid losses, the infant with NEC will not survive.

REFERENCES

1. Brans YW, et al: Perinatal mortality in a large perinatal center: Five year review of 31,000 births. *Am J Obstet Gynecol* 1982; 148:284.
2. Anand KJS, Sippell WG, Aynsley-Green A: Randomized trial of fentanyl anesthesia in preterm babies undergoing surgery: Effects of the stress response. *Lancet* 1987; 1:243.
3. Coller FA, et al: Post operative salt intolerance. *Ann Surg* 1944; 119:533.
4. Zimmerman B, Wangensteen OH: Observations on water intoxication in surgical patients. *Surgery* 1952; 31:654.
5. Shires T, Williams J, Brown F: Acute change in extracellular fluids associated with major surgical procedures. *Ann Surg* 1961; 154:803.
6. Weissman C: The metabolic response to stress: An overview and update. *Anesthesiology* 1990; 73:308.
7. Deutsch S, Goldberg M, Dripps R: Post operative hyponatremia with the inappropriate release of antidiuretic hormone. *Anesthesiology* 1966; 27:250.
8. Ekblad H, Kero P, Takala J: Water, sodium, and acid-base balance in premature infants: Therapeutic aspects. *Acta Paediatr Scand* 1987; 76:47.
9. Anand KJS, Aynsley-Green A: Measuring the severity of surgical stress in newborn infants. *J Pediatr Surg* 1988; 23:297.

11

Pierre Robin Syndrome

A 10-day-old, 3-kg girl with Pierre Robin syndrome is scheduled for creation of lip-tongue adhesion. She is severely micrognathic and has a cleft palate. She has had several apneic episodes and is unable to feed without becoming cyanotic. Hemoglobin, 14 g/dL; hematocrit, 42%.

Recommendations by Ingrid Hollinger, M.D.

Congenital micrognathia with glossoptosis is a relatively rare condition that occurs once in 50,000 births[1] and is referred to as Pierre Robin syndrome (Fig 11–1). An associated cleft palate is found in more than 50% of patients,[2-4] and congenital cardiac and skeletal defects are present in 25% to 30%.[5] Patients should be screened for Stickler syndrome, which includes myopia in infancy, retinal detachment, and preventable blindness.[2-4] Associated choanal atresia should be excluded by passing a catheter through each nostril.[4]

PATHOLOGY

Depending on the degree of microretrognathia, severe respiratory difficulties may be present soon after birth. The tongue is displaced posteriorly and may be hyperplastic. In the supine position, this causes obstruction of the oral and nasal pharynx, thus preventing normal breathing (Fig 11–2). Increasing inspiratory efforts create negative pressure in the pharynx, which further enhances the already severe obstruction.[1] Unrelieved upper airway obstruction may result in the development of cor pulmonale and congestive heart failure.[6] These respiratory problems are frequently compounded by aspiration when the infant attempts to feed.[2, 4] Placing the infant in a prone position allows the tongue to fall forward and partially relieves the airway obstruction. Insertion of an oropharyngeal or nasopharyngeal airway will, in most instances, clear the airway.

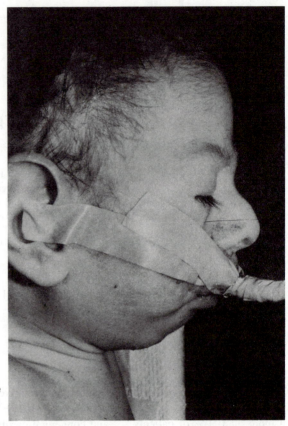

FIG 11–1.
Two-month-old infant with typical features of Pierre Robin syndrome: retropositioned mandible, birdlike face.

Nevertheless, swallowing is impaired, and aspiration pneumonitis is frequent. Weight gain is usually poor, and "glossoptotic cachexia" may develop.[2, 4, 7, 8] Pierre Robin, in his original report, considered this lesion incompatible with survival after the second year of life.[4] As recently as 20 years ago, mortality in infants with this syndrome was as high as 50% despite treatment.[3, 4, 9]

With intensive nursing care in a constantly maintained prone position and gavage feeding, the majority of these infants can be managed conservatively.[2, 7] Surgical intervention becomes necessary when retrognathia is more than 1 cm in relation to the maxilla and/or when recurrent obstruction or aspiration episodes occur despite proper positioning.[4] Most infants are operated on between 2 weeks and 2 months of age, the younger usually because of recurrent life-threatening obstructive episodes, the older ones because of chronic aspiration with pneumonitis and failure to thrive due to feeding problems.[4] Glossopexy by creation of a lip-tongue adhesion has become the preferred method of surgical treatment[4, 10, 11] (Fig 11–3). Tracheostomy, with its inherent problems in the neonate, is rarely performed.[4] Because most micrognathic mandibles have normal growth potential, to a large extent the deformity tends to correct itself within the first few months of life if nutrition can be maintained and if hypoxic episodes can be avoided.[2, 4, 7, 8, 12]

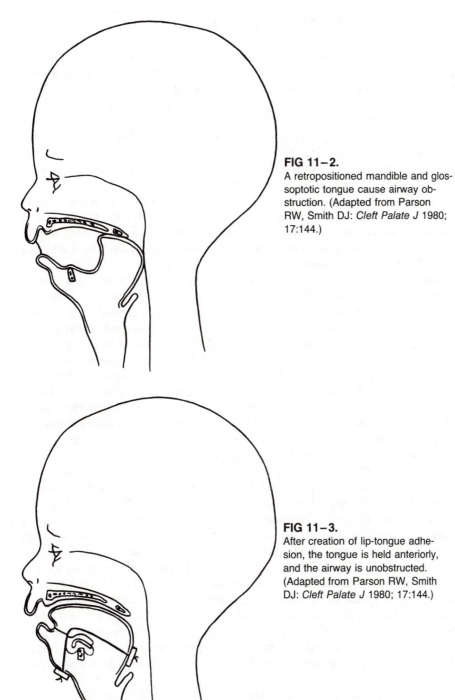

FIG 11–2.
A retropositioned mandible and glossoptotic tongue cause airway obstruction. (Adapted from Parson RW, Smith DJ: *Cleft Palate J* 1980; 17:144.)

FIG 11–3.
After creation of lip-tongue adhesion, the tongue is held anteriorly, and the airway is unobstructed. (Adapted from Parson RW, Smith DJ: *Cleft Palate J* 1980; 17:144.)

ANESTHETIC MANAGEMENT

Anesthetic management presents several challenges.[10, 13, 14] Foremost is the maintenance of an adequate airway prior to endotracheal intubation since these patients usually become obstructed immediately when they are turned supine. In addition, all the problems of anesthesia in the neonate have to be considered, including transitional circulation, sensitivity to inhalation agents and muscle relaxants, the danger of hyperoxia, and thermal instability.

Sedation should not be administered preoperatively because relaxation during sleep tends to aggravate the existing airway obstruction.[13] Atropine, 0.1 to 0.02 mg/kg or a minimum of 0.1 mg, should be administered intramuscularly 30 minutes prior to induction to block parasympathetic reflexes and reduce oral secretions, which are frequently copious.

The infant should be brought to the operating room in a prone position. The operating room temperature should be 26 to 28°C and a warming blanket and an overhead heating lamp used to allow free access to the infant without a fall in body temperature. Noninvasive monitoring devices are positioned while the patient is maintained prone. If no intravenous access has been established prior to arrival in the operating room, it should be established at this time.

Infants with micrognathia often present a formidable obstacle to endotracheal intubation.[4, 8, 13, 14] Prior to any attempt at laryngoscopy, a surgeon capable of performing tracheostomy in an infant must be present in the operating room. A tracheostomy tray must be open and appropriately sized tracheostomy tubes ready. Several sizes and styles of oropharyngeal airways and an assortment of laryngoscope blades should be readily available. We have found a Robertshaw or Wis-Hipple blade, slightly larger than predicted by age, to be useful.[13] Introduction of the laryngoscope blade on the extreme right side (retromolar) with concurrent adjustment of the larynx by cricoid pressure often results in improved visualization.[15] In small infants an awake intubation should be performed.[10, 13, 14] The infant is preoxygenated in the prone position and then turned supine and restrained, with the head extended by an assistant. A small towel roll is placed under the shoulders. Complete airway obstruction frequently occurs the moment the infant is turned supine. Insertion of an oropharyngeal airway or introduction of the laryngoscope blade displaces the tongue anteriorly and allows the infant to breathe. Oxygen can be insufflated via a catheter held next to the laryngoscope blade or with an Oxyblade. The larynx is often at a lower position than anticipated, and with gentle pressure on the cricoid by an assistant the arytenoids and the posterior aspect of the cords may become visible.[13, 14] Because of the anterior position of the larynx, the endotracheal tube may have to be curved slightly, with the help of a stylet, in order to place it through the cords. If the larynx cannot be visualized, the endotracheal tube can be placed blindly by following breath sounds. Application of topical lidocaine jelly to anesthetize the tongue and pharynx greatly facilitates awake laryngoscopy. Special care is needed during blind intubation to avoid trauma to the laryngeal structures. With experience, an ultrathin fiber-optic bronchoscope can be used after topical anesthesia of the nose and pharynx to perform an awake nasal intubation with surprising ease.[14] As soon as proper endotracheal tube position has been ascertained by auscultation of the chest, anesthesia is induced with halothane and nitrous oxide via a nonrebreathing system. We prefer the Jackson Rees modification of the Ayres T-piece with a heated in-line cascade humidifier. The infant then is allowed to breathe spontaneously and the endotracheal tube securely taped.

In older infants, inhalation induction with halothane and oxygen should be carried out with an oropharyngeal or nasopharyngeal airway in place. Adequate time for the laryngoscopy can be achieved by deepening the level of anesthesia. Because the breath sounds and the movement of air bubbles in the pharynx are useful guides for intubation, the child should be allowed to breath spontaneously. Muscle relaxants should not be used since airway obstruction is more likely to occur when soft tissues are relaxed.[13, 14] After intubation, nitrous oxide can be added to the anesthetic mixture.

In the neonate, halothane may cause severe hypotension, particularly in the presence of dehydration. This can occur despite an inadequate depth of anesthesia. Should it occur, halothane use should be discontinued. Nitrous oxide and oxygen and ketamine, 0.5 to 1.0 mg/kg intravenously, with controlled ventilation but without the use of relaxants provide adequate anesthesia.

The surgical site is usually infiltrated with 0.5% lidocaine, with the addition of epinephrine, 1:200,000 to 1:400,000. No more than 0.3 mL/kg of the 1:200,000 solution may be used in any 10-minute period, and the surgeon should be informed of the maximum permissible volume before the start of infiltration.[16]

Surgery is ordinarily completed in less than an hour with minimal blood loss. At the conclusion of the procedure, a traction suture should be placed through the base of the tongue. Nasopharyngeal airways should be inserted bilaterally and position confirmed by direct visualization. Upon awakening, the infant is extubated in the operating room and observed for airway obstruction. Only after patency of the airway has been ascertained is the patient transferred to the recovery room and placed in a high-humidity hood for several hours. During this interval the child is cared for in either a prone or lateral position. From the recovery room, the patient should be transferred to an intensive care unit. The nasopharyngeal airways are left in place for 3 to 4 days until all edema has resolved. Oral feedings are withheld and the infant fed by gavage.[10] These babies are kept in the hospital 2 to 4 weeks until they feed well orally, show satisfactory weight gain, and have no recurrent episodes of respiratory obstruction. The management described has successfully been used in 26 patients referred from our craniofacial center over the last 12 years with no mortality and only minor morbidity. No patient required tracheostomy, and there were no anesthetic complications.

REFERENCES

1. Fletcher MM, Blum SL, Blanchard CL: Pierre Robin syndrome: Pathophysiology of obstructive episodes. *Laryngoscope* 1969; 79:547.
2. Dennison WM: The Pierre Robin syndrome. *Pediatrics* 1965; 36:336.
3. McEvitt WG: Micrognathia and its management. *Plast Reconstr Surg* 1963; 41:450.
4. Randall P: The Robin anomalad: Micrognathia and glossoptosis with airway obstruction, in Converse JM (ed): *Reconstructive Plastic Surgery*, ed 2, vol 4. Philadelphia, WB Saunders Co, 1977.
5. Pearl W: Congenital heart disease in the Pierre Robin syndrome. *Pediatr Cardiol* 1982; 2:307–309.
6. Dykes EH, Raine PH, Arthur DS, et al: Pierre Robin syndrome and pulmonary hypertension. *J Pediatr Surg* 1985; 20:49–52.
7. Lewis MB, Pashayan HM: Management of infants with Robin anomaly. *Clin Pediatr* 1980; 19:519.
8. Mallory SB, Paradise JL: Glossoptosis revisited on the development and resolution of airway obstruction in the Pierre Robin syndrome. *Pediatrics* 1979; 64:946.
9. Williams AJ, Williams MA, Walker CA, et al: The Robin anomalad (Pierre Robin syndrome), a follow-up study. *Arch Dis Child* 1981; 56:663–668.
10. Routledge RT: The Pierre Robin syndrome: A surgical emergency in the neonatal period. *Br J Plast Surg* 1960; 13:704.

11. Parsons RW, Smith DJ: A modified tongue-lip adhesion for Pierre Robin anomalad. *Cleft Palate J* 1980; 17:144.
12. Randall P, Krogman WM, Jahina S: Pierre Robin and the syndrome that bears his name. Presented at the Convention of the American Cleft Palate Association, 1964.
13. Wilton TN: Anesthesia and the neonate. *Br J Anaesth* 1960; 32:116.
14. Rasch DK, Browder F, Barr M, et al: Anaesthesia for Treacher Collins and Pierre Robin syndromes: A report of 3 cases. *Can Anaesth Soc J* 1986; 33:364–370.
15. Bonfils P: Schwierige Intubation bei Pierre Robin Kindern. *Anaesthesist* 1983; 32:363–367.
16. Johnston RR, Eger EI, Wilson C: A comparative interaction of epinephrine with enflurane, isoflurane and halothane in man. *Anesth Analg* 1976; 55:709.

12

Inguinal Hernia

A 2-week-old boy weighing 2.3 kg is scheduled for bilateral inguinal herniorrhaphy prior to discharge from the hospital where he has been since birth. His Apgar scores were 4 at 1 minute and 7 at 5 minutes. His trachea was intubated in the delivery room and extubated shortly afterward. At no time was he mechanically ventilated. Hemoglobin, 11.2 g/dL; hematocrit, 35%.

Recommendations by Tae Hee Oh, M.D.

Inguinal herniorrhaphy is the most frequently performed operation in infancy and childhood. The overall incidence of inguinal hernia and hydrocele in infants is reported to be from 4.8% to as high as 30% in prematurely born infants.[1, 2] In infancy, inguinal hernia may result in incarceration, intestinal obstruction, or cryptorchism. Thus it should be repaired as soon as possible to avoid complications, especially incarceration, which is reported to occur in 31%.[2]

Many investigators have reported serious postoperative complications, mainly apnea and bradycardia, following inguinal herniorrhaphy in these "nursery graduates."[3, 4] In general, it is recommended that elective repair be postponed until the infant reaches 44 to 60 weeks' gestational age.[3, 5-9] The optimal time for repair is still controversial, but I would administer general anesthesia whenever the repair is performed.

PREOPERATIVE EVALUATION AND PREPARATION

A review of the gestational and neonatal history of the infant is important to the identification of additional abnormalities such as patent ductus arteriosus (PDA), respiratory distress syndrome (RDS), and bronchopulmonary dysplasia (BPD). Pathophysiology related to neonatal respiration, circulation, oxygenation, the hepatorenal system, and heat regulation is of major concern. The common denominators contributing to anesthetic risks in premature infants include prematurity of multiple organ systems, the presence of pulmonary disease, and deterioration of oxygen delivery capacity.

Immaturity of the central nervous system, particularly the vasomotor and respiratory centers, frequently results in apnea and bradycardia. Apneic episodes are common in premature infants, the incidence correlating inversely with gestational age and weight. All infants weighing less than 1,000 g will have at least one apneic spell, although only 2% of infants weighing less than 2,500 g are affected. Several anesthesiologists have reported that premature infants, regardless of a previous history of apnea/bradycardia, are prone to develop postoperative cardiorespiratory complications or even cardiac arrest following otherwise uneventful anesthesia for inguinal herniorrhaphy.[8, 9] Since this patient never required mechanical ventilation, RDS and abnormal pulmonary function are not problems.

Premature infants have a higher fraction of fetal hemoglobin and a lower concentration of red cell 2,3-diphosphoglycerate (2,3-DPG) than do full-term infants. The oxyhemoglobin dissociation curve therefore shifts to the left, and the amount of available oxygen in the tissue decreases. Blood-oxygen affinity remains high and the P_{50} value low, in the range of 19 to 24 mm Hg, until about 10 weeks of age. At that time, the P_{50} abruptly rises to 29 to 33 mm Hg, and the oxygen affinity of blood decreases. Therefore, the tissue oxygenation of anemic infants less than 3 months of age is handicapped by the reduced blood oxygen with anemia per se and decreased oxygen unloading ability at the tissue level. Hypoxia and metabolic acidosis may result. Recently, infants with hemoglobin levels less than 10 g/dL were reported to more frequently develop postoperative apnea and bradycardia than were nonanemic infants.[10]

ANESTHETIC MANAGEMENT

Infants of this age require no premedication. The patient should be adequately hydrated before surgery but should not be fed milk for at least 4 hours. Clear liquid or dextrose water may be offered 2 hours before induction of anesthesia.

The infant should be placed in a warm incubator during transportation from the neonatal intensive care unit (ICU) to the operating room by a nurse or a member of the anesthesia team. His heart rate and respiration should be monitored using an electrocardiogram (ECG) and apnea monitor during transportation. A face mask and bag with oxygen should be available at all times.

In the operating room an intravenous catheter should be placed if it was not already done in the ICU. Dextrose, 2.5% in water, with one-half normal saline is used for intravenous infusion. Regional techniques such as caudal, spinal, and epidural anesthesia have been introduced for these premature infants undergoing inguinal herniorrhaphy.[11, 12] However, I would choose general anesthesia with controlled ventilation. I consider regional anesthesia to be in an experimental stage, with further investigation needed to document its benefits in premature infants. In my opinion, well-controlled general endotracheal anesthesia outweighs the value of any other type of anesthesia. Securing the airway by endotracheal intubation is safer than administering anesthesia by mask. Awake endotracheal intubation may be indicated. In my experience, the endotracheal tube size should not be smaller than 3.0 mm internal diameter. Even in a neonate less than 1,000 g, a 3.0-mm tube can be used. It is extremely difficult to pass a suction catheter into a 2.5-mm tube to aspirate secretions or condensed humidified water accumulated in the airway. To prevent severe bradycardia during laryngoscopy, atropine, 0.15 mg, must be administered intravenously. In our institution, for infants and children we use primarily the Mapleson D system modified with an attached apparatus for a humidifier and scavenging device. Noninvasive monitoring is employed, including a precordial stethoscope, blood pressure cuff, ECG, oximeter, thermometer, nerve stimulator, and oxygen concentration analyzer.

Initially anesthesia is maintained with nitrous oxide and oxygen, but extreme care should be taken with certain anesthetic agents such as ketamine and halothane. Ketamine is a potent respiratory depressant in infants. Because respiratory depression caused by ketamine may persist for a prolonged period, this agent is not usually recommended unless postoperative ventilatory assistance is planned. Despite its myocardial depressant action, halothane is most frequently used. A relatively low concentration of halothane is required to maintain an adequate level of anesthesia in premature infants. A muscle relaxant, either pancuronium or vecuronium, 0.05 mg/kg, should be administered to ensure adequate muscle relaxation while halothane-nitrous oxide-oxygen anesthesia is maintained. To avoid bowel distension, nitrous oxide may be replaced with air or nitrogen. If the infant does not tolerate halothane, as evidenced by hypotension and a decreased heart rate, halothane may be replaced by either a lower concentration of isoflurane or a small dose of fentanyl, up to 5 μg/kg. After surgery, the trachea should be extubated when the infant is fully awake and normothermic and the neuromuscular blockade has been completely reversed. If any residual effect of anesthetics or muscle relaxant is suspected, the infant should be transported to the ICU intubated for postoperative ventilatory assistance.

Recently in our institution 47 premature infants who underwent herniorrhaphy were studied for postoperative complications. We found that 43% had untoward events. The most common complication was apnea/bradycardia. None of the babies required treatment for the complications longer than 24 hours, and none had a cardiac arrest. We concluded, however, that prematurely born infants who undergo herniorrhaphy must be placed in a monitored bed in the neonatal ICU in the postoperative period.

REFERENCES

1. Harper RG, Garcia A, Sin C: Inguinal hernia: A common problem of premature infants 1000 grams or less at birth. *Pediatrics* 1975; 56:112–115.
2. Rescorla FG, Grosfeld JL: Inguinal hernia in the perinatal period and early infancy: Clinical considerations. *J Pediatr Surg* 1984; 19:332–337.
3. Gregory GA, Steward DJ: Life-threatening perioperative apnea in the ex-"premie" (editorial). *Anesthesiology* 1983; 59:495–497.
4. Kattwinkel J: Apnea in the neonatal period. *Pediatr Rev* 1980; 2:115.
5. Kurth CD, Spitzer AR, Broennle AM, et al: Postoperative apnea in preterm infants. *Anesthesiology* 1987; 66:483–488.
6. Liu LM, Coté CJ, Goudsouzian NG, et al: Life-threatening apnea in infants recovering from anesthesia. *Anesthesiology* 1983; 59:506–510.
7. Mayhew J, Bourke D, Guinee W: Evaluation of the premature infant at risk for postoperative complications. *Can J Anaesth* 1987; 34:627–631.
8. Steward DJ: Preterm infants are more prone to complications following minor surgery than are term infants. *Anesthesiology* 1982; 56:304–306.

9. Welborn LG, Ramirez N, Oh TH, et al: Postanesthetic apnea and periodic breathing in infants. *Anesthesiology* 1986; 65:658–661.
10. Welborn LG, Hannallah RS, Luban NLC, et al: Anemia and postoperative apnea in former preterm infants. *Anesthesiology* 1991; 74:1003–1006.
11. Gallagher TM, Crean PM: Spinal anesthesia in infants born prematurely. *Anaesthesia* 1989; 44:434–436.
12. Harnik EV, Hoy GR, Potolicchio S, et al: Spinal anesthesia in premature infants recovering from respiratory distress syndrome. *Anesthesiology* 1986; 64:95–99.

13

Pyloric Stenosis

A 5-week-old, 4-kg boy is admitted with a 2-week history of persistent vomiting. His skin turgor is poor and he is not very active. Blood pressure, 65/38 mm Hg; pulse, 140; respirations, 42; temperature, 37°C; hemoglobin, 12 g/dL; hematocrit, 36%; Na, 130 mEq/L; K, 3.1 mEq/L; Cl, 87 mEq/L; CO_2, 34, mmol/L. The surgeon would like to proceed with pyloromyotomy if you concur.

Recommendations by Ramesh I. Patel, M.D.

First described in 1788, pyloric stenosis occurs in approximately 0.3% of live births.[1] It is a benign hypertrophy of the pyloric smooth muscle that, if not diagnosed and treated, results in serious metabolic sequelae.[2] The onset of symptoms commonly occurs between 2 and 8 weeks of age, but has been reported to occur at birth and as late as the fifth month of life. The incidence is four times greater in boys than in girls.[3] It occurs more frequently in whites than in blacks, in firstborn children, and in infants whose parents, particularly the mother, had pyloric stenosis.[1, 4] The etiology of pyloric stenosis is controversial. Primary muscle disease, allergy-induced hypertrophy, elevated prostaglandin E_2, and abnormalities of peptide-containing nerve fibers have all been implicated. Two percent of children with pyloric stenosis develop jaundice as a result of a glucuronyl-transferase deficiency. The jaundice resolves rapidly following pyloromyotomy.[5]

PATHOPHYSIOLOGY

The pathologic findings of pyloric stenosis consist of hypertrophy of the circular and longitudinal fibers of the pylorus and an associated edema of the pyloric mucosa. The size of the tumor does not correlate well with the duration or severity of symptoms.[6] Although the stenosis may be present at birth, symptoms generally do not appear until later. As milk or curd pass through the narrow pylorus, they irritate the mucosa, leading to mucosal swelling. The combination of stenosis and mucosal swelling causes the pyloric passage to narrow, resulting in delayed gastric emptying, gastric dilatation, regurgitation, and nonbilious projectile vomiting. Persistent vomiting leads to dehydration, weight loss, anemia, electrolyte imbalance, and alkalosis. The typical derangement is a hypochloremic, hypokalemic metabolic alkalosis.

PREANESTHETIC EVALUATION

When evaluating the infant with pyloric stenosis, the parents should be asked about the frequency and usual quantity of vomitus, fluid intake and urine output over this period, and a change in mental status. Urine output may be gauged by inquiring about the frequency of diaper changes. After obtaining this information, a review of systems should be performed in the usual manner.

On physical examination, this child has a pulse of 140; blood pressure, 65/38 mm Hg; respirations, 42; and a temperature of 37°C. The normal pulse rate for a 5-week-old child is about 120, with a range of 80–160.[7] Therefore, a pulse of 140 is in the normal range, particularly if the child is crying. Normal blood pressure in infants of this age is 80 [±16]/46 [±16].[7] The patient's blood pressure is at the lower limit of the normal range. The child is not very active and has poor skin turgor. All these symptoms and signs suggest dehydration. Other signs of dehydration are depressed fontanelles, sunken eyeballs, dry mucous membranes, decreased salivation, vasoconstriction, rapid "thin" pulse, mottled skin color, scanty urine output, and high specific gravity of the urine. It should be recalled that neonates and infants can concentrate urine only up to 500–700 mOsm/L.

The hemoglobin and hematocrit values of 12 g/dL and 36% in this child are related to three factors: age, dehydration, and anemia. There is normally a reduction in hemoglobin levels between the second and fourth months of life. Anemia can also occur as result of poor oral intake in pyloric stenosis. Dehydration can cause hemoconcentration and an apparent increase in the hematocrit. Therefore, the hematocrit and hemoglobin values must be reassessed after the child is adequately hydrated.

Vomiting results in a loss of water, H^+, Na^+, Cl^-, and K^+, which gives rise to dehydration, metabolic alkalosis, hyponatremia, hypochloremia, and hypokalemia. The effects of hydrogen ion loss elevating the serum HCO_3^- precede the alteration in other serum electrolytes.[8] Arterial blood gas analysis will confirm metabolic alkalosis and may show compensatory respiratory acidosis. Patients with severe dehydration have a normal pH or even metabolic acidosis.

The diagnosis of pyloric stenosis is made by obtaining the suggestive history and palpation of a firm, olive-shaped mass in the upper abdomen. Abdominal ultrasonography is commonly used to confirm the diagnosis. A barium swallow roentgenogram is reserved for those patients who present confusing diagnostic features.

PREOPERATIVE PREPARATION

A thorough knowledge of the pathophysiology is necessary to correct the fluid and electrolyte deficits that characterize pyloric stenosis. The interrelationships between dehydration, hypokalemia, hypochloremia, and metabolic alkalosis should be considered. The level of serum bicarbonate rises because of loss of H^+ due to vomiting. The body tries to compensate for the resulting metabolic alkalosis through the respiratory and renal systems. Hypoventilation and limited retention of carbon dioxide cause compensatory respiratory acidosis. The renal adjustment consists of excreting HCO_3^- in place of Cl^-. The kidneys seem to preferentially conserve volume over Na^+, over H^+, over K^+, and HCO_3^- over Cl^-.[9] Sodium is excreted along with HCO_3^- as the preferential cation. However, as hyponatremia develops, the body tries to conserve sodium; K^+ and H^+ are then used to excrete bicarbonate, thus worsening the existing hypokalemia and metabolic alkalosis. Due to excretion of H^+, there is a paradoxical acidic urine, in spite of the systemic alkalosis. Hence, in pyloric stenosis, urine is alkaline initially and becomes acidic when hyponatremia develops. The paradoxical aciduria may worsen the existing alkalemia. The hypokalemia is due to loss of K^+ secondary to vomiting, systemic alkalosis in which intracellular H^+ is exchanged for extracellular K^+, and urinary excretion of K^+. Serum chloride and bicarbonate levels provide an index for assessing the severity of metabolic alkalosis.

Volume and electrolyte deficits of Na^+, Cl^-, and K^+ must be fully corrected to restore acid-base balance. In children who are severely dehydrated, this may require two to three days. However, most patients are ready for surgery within 24 hours.

This infant is not very active, has poor skin turgor, and borderline low blood pressure; therefore, a bolus of 10-20 mL/kg of normal saline or lactated Ringer's solution should be administered. Response to the fluid bolus is monitored, and the subsequent rate of fluid therapy adjusted accordingly. Potassium is added to the fluids only when the child has begun to urinate. Maintenance requirements of fluids and electrolytes in an infant are: water, 100 mL/kg/day; sodium, 3 mEq/kg/day; chloride, 3 mEq/kg/day; and potassium, 2–3 mEq/kg/day. Surgery may be safely performed when vital signs are stable, pH is between 7.3 and 7.5, serum chloride is more than 88 mEq/L, bicarbonate is less than 30 mmol/L, potassium is more than 3.0 mEq/L, urine output is 1 to 2 mL/kg/hour, and the specific gravity of the urine is less than 1.020. Generally, all of the above parameters correct simultaneously.

Pyloric stenosis can be a medical emergency, but it is never a surgical emergency. Patients should not be taken to the operating room until the fluid, electrolyte, and acid–base imbalances have been corrected. The morbidity and mortality in children with pyloric stenosis occur because of preoperative dehydration and electrolyte imbalance, and from aspiration of gastric contents during intraoperative vomiting and regurgitation.

ANESTHETIC MANAGEMENT

In addition to the potential problems associated with anesthetizing any newborn such as hypothermia and a labile cardiovascular system, the anesthesiologist must also be prepared to deal with the consequences of upper gastrointestinal tract obstruction. The child is brought to the operating room after the anesthesiologist has ascertained that the following equipment is readily available: suction, endotracheal tubes of different sizes, laryngoscope, warming blanket, and radiant heat lights. Monitors should include a precordial stethoscope, blood pressure cuff, electrocardiograph, pulse oximeter, capnograph, and an axillary temperature probe.

The infant is placed in the supine position. The nasogastric tube, if present, should be suctioned. Otherwise, oxygen is administered by mask and intravenous atropine 0.02 mg/kg (minimum dose, 0.1 mg) is given through an indwelling intravenous catheter. The infant is then placed in the left lateral position. A lubricated large-bore oral gastric tube is inserted to decompress the stomach. The infant is then turned supine and preoxygenation continued.

The choices for intubation are awake intubation or rapid-sequence induction with cricoid pressure. An awake intubation requires the help of an assistant, who stabilizes the body and head of the child. If the child is too vigorous, or if awake intubation is unsuccessful, one should proceed with a rapid sequence induction. The key is to know when to cease attempts at awake intubation. Blood in the pharynx makes rapid-sequence intubation difficult; thus, attempts at awake intubation should be abandoned in favor of the rapid-sequence induction before pharyngeal bleeding occurs. Propofol, 2 mg/kg, or thiopental, 3 to 4 mg/kg followed by succinylcholine, 2 mg/kg, is used for induction of anesthesia. Normally, a 3.0 to 3.5 mm endotracheal tube is used for a 5-week-old child. Anesthesia is maintained with nitrous oxide, oxygen and low-dose halothane or isoflurane. Atracurium or vecuronium is used for muscle relaxation. Opioids should be avoided.

The surgical procedure, named after Fredt-Ramstedt, consists of an incision of about 5 cm in the right upper quadrant of the abdomen. The pylorus is split up to the mucosa and the abdomen is then closed. The muscle relaxant should be reversed with atropine, 0.02 to 0.03 mg/kg, and neostigmine, 0.07 mg/kg. The stomach is again carefully decompressed. The endotracheal tube is removed when the infant is breathing well, coughing, opening his eyes, grimacing and when the reversal of muscle relaxation is adequate. The postoperative analgesic effect of local infiltration of 0.25% bupivacaine before surgical closure is controversial.[10, 11]

POSTANESTHETIC CARE

Supplemental oxygen should be administered during transport from the operating room and in the recovery room.[12, 13] The two main risks to the child in the recovery room are respiratory depression and reactive hypoglycemia. Respiratory acidosis occurs as a compensation for metabolic alkalosis. If left undisturbed and unstimulated during recovery, the patient may hypoventilate while the Pco_2 returns to its high preoperative level. Following general anesthesia the child has a depressed respiratory center and can breathe only at a Pco_2 higher than the preoperative value. Higher levels of Pco_2 act as a respiratory depressant and may lead to respiratory arrest.

Reactive hypoglycemia occurs in glycogen-depleted infants. Continuous infusion of a glucose-containing solution leads to the increased secretion of insulin. Hypoglycemia may occur in infants whose hepatic glycogen stores have been depleted if the glucose infusion is stopped before oral intake is adequate. Hypoglycemia may cause unexplained respiratory arrest and seizures. To prevent hypoglycemia, glucose-containing solutions should be administered intravenously until adequate oral intake is tolerated by the infant. Feeding should be started with plain water and, if well tolerated, advanced to dilute formula.

REFERENCES

1. Daly AM, Conn AW: Anaesthesia for pyloromyotomy: A review. *Can Anaesth Soc J* 1969; 16(4):316–320.
2. Eikenbary KF: Pyloric stenosis. Its anesthetic management and a case study. *J Am Assoc Nurse Anesth* 1978; 46(5):517–521.

3. Conn AW: Anaesthesia for pyloromyotomy in infancy. *Can Anaesth Soc J* 1963; 10(1):18–29.
4. Gibbs MK, Van Herrclen JA, Lynn MB: Congenital hypertrophic pyloric stenosis: Surgical experiences. *Mayo Clin Proc* 1975; 50:312–316.
5. Wooley MM, Felsher BF, Asch MJ, et al: Jaundice, hypertrophic pyloric stenosis and hepatic glucuronyl transferase. *J Ped Surg* 1974; 9:359–363.
6. Garcia VF, Randolph JG: Pyloric stenosis: Diagnosis and management. *Ped Rev* 1990; 11:1292–1296.
7. Smith RM: *Anesthesia for Infants and Children,* ed 4. St Louis, CV Mosby Co, 1980, p 18.
8. Touloukiam RJ, Higgins E: The spectrum of serum electrolytes in hypertrophic pyloric stenosis. *J Pediatr Surg* 1983; 18:394–397.
9. Bennett EJ: *Fluids for Anesthesia and Surgery in the Newborn and the Infant.* Springfield, Ill, Charles C Thomas, 1975, p 121.
10. McNicole LR, Martin CS, Smart NG, et al: Perioperative bupivacaine for pyloromyotomy pain (letter). *Lancet* 1990; 335:54–55.
11. Sury MRJ, Mcluckie A, Booker PD: Local analgesia for infant pyloromyotomy. Does wound infiltration with bupivacaine affect postoperative behavior? *Ann Royal Coll Surg* (Engl) 1990; 72:324–328.
12. Patel R, Norden J, Hannallah RS: Oxygen administration prevents hypoxemia during post-anesthetic transport in children. *Anesthesiology* 1988; 69:616–618.
13. Motoyama EK, Glazner CH: Hypoxemia after general anesthesia in children. *Anesth Analg* 1986; 65:267–272.

14

Inguinal Hernia and Prematurity

A 3-month-old boy is scheduled for bilateral inguinal hernia repair. The left inguinal hernia has become increasingly more difficult to reduce. The patient was born at an estimated gestational age of 30 weeks and was hospitalized for 6 weeks for treatment of prematurity, respiratory distress syndrome, and periodic apnea. Mechanical ventilation was required for one week. Weight, 4 kg; hemoglobin, 9 g/dL; hematocrit, 27%. The parents ask if the surgery can be performed on an outpatient basis.

Recommendations by J. Christian Abajian, M.D.

The growing knowledge and expertise of neonatal intensive care unit (NICU) personnel has led to continued improvement in the survival rate of infants born prematurely. This in turn has led to problems previously not experienced by the anesthesiologist and surgeon. Infants in the NICU are often ill with such diseases as respiratory distress syndrome, bronchopulmonary dysplasia, recurrent apneic episodes, bradycardia, sepsis, necrotizing enterocolitis, retinopathy of prematurity, anemia, and congestive heart failure. Other abnormalities such as congenital heart disease or anatomic congenital anomalies such as laryngomalacia are also associated with premature birth. Many of these conditions necessitate ventilatory support, leading to possible complications of mechanical ventilation, including pneumothorax and tracheal stenosis. If a surgical emergency such as incarcerated inguinal hernia is superimposed, all the ingredients for potential disaster are present. Hence the frequently used term *high-risk infant* is applied. Meeting the criteria for discharge from the NICU does not eliminate the risk presented by these infants, for many of the previously mentioned diseases have residual effects lasting for months.

INGUINAL HERNIA

The incidence of inguinal hernia in the premature infant varies from 13% of infants born at less than 32 weeks gestational age,[1] to as high as 30% of infants with birth weight less than 1000 g.[2] Bilateral presentation is reported to range from 44% to 55% in this group, compared to 8% to 10% in older infants and children.[2] Incarcerated inguinal hernia in an infant is considered a surgical emergency. While nonoperative reduction is often successful, this only converts an emergent case into a semielective one. Many pediatric anesthesiologists have recommended delaying surgery in the high-risk infant until after 60 weeks postconceptual age, that is, gestational age plus age since birth, to minimize the risk of postoperative apnea, a complication frequently seen following the administration of general anesthesia to these patients.[3, 4] This conservative approach may not always be an option, as delay can lead to an increased risk of testicular infarction or intestinal complications.

PREOPERATIVE EVALUATION

Preoperative evaluation of the patient should include calculation of the postconceptual age, 42 weeks in this case, and an assessment as to the presence and severity of any residual problems that may have been present in the NICU. More often than not these will be respiratory in nature. Some infants require oxygen therapy and apnea monitoring even after discharge from the hospital. Infants younger than 45 weeks gestational age are prone to retinopathy of prematurity. While this is a multifactorial disease, care should be taken to avoid excessive arterial oxygen concentrations if oxygen therapy is necessary.

A history of prolonged intubation and mechanical ventilation in the NICU should alert the anesthesiologist to the possibility of subglottic stenosis and the need to have an appropriate selection of endotracheal tubes available. Eliciting a history of stridor may be a clue to the presence of this occult problem. Circulatory problems would likely be related to the presence of congenital heart disease, persistence of a patent ductus arteriosis, or anemia. Recent data suggest that preterm infants with hematocrits of less than 30% receiving general anesthesia have an increased incidence of postoperative apnea, and recommendations were to postpone elective surgery until the hematocrit is greater than 30%.[5]

THE CASE FOR SPINAL ANESTHESIA

The use of spinal anesthesia for surgery in post-premature infants was first described as a safe and reliable alternative to general anesthesia in 1984.[6] Thirty six of 78 infants reported were classified as high-risk infants because they had been delivered prematurely and/or because they had been treated for neonatal respiratory distress syndrome. Since that report, numerous others have been published supporting the safety efficacy of regional anesthetic techniques for this group of infants.[7-14] While no anesthetic technique is free from complications, published data and our own experience suggest that the incidence and severity of complications are less with regional anesthetic techniques.[12, 15]

Life-threatening apnea has been reported to have occurred after spinal anesthesia in two post-premature infants.[16] A careful review of this report shows the title to be misleading as both infants developed the apnea after multiple doses of oral codeine phosphate, 9 and 32 hours following spinal anesthesia. In addition, both infants were being treated with theophylline for apnea at the time of surgery. A review of published cases and personal experience with 166 cases of spinal anesthesia in post-premature infants with a mean postconceptual age of 44.5 weeks has revealed no evidence of postoperative apnea when there was no concurrent history of apnea and only the spinal anesthetic was administered. Recent work attempting to elucidate the pathogenesis of postoperative apnea in former premature infants has demonstrated that airway obstruction is frequently a major component.[17] It is unlikely that the metabolized spinal anesthetic will have any chronic effects on the airway musculature, perhaps explaining the marked reduction in the incidence of apnea following spinal anesthesia without sedation.

ANESTHETIC MANAGEMENT

The patient should fast for a minimum of two hours before coming to surgery. The operating room should be heated to 26° to 28°C, and an overhead radiant heat source should be available to prevent heat loss during administration of the spinal anesthetic. A suitable infant breathing circuit should be immediately available to support respiration in the event of respiratory embarrassment from an excessively high spinal anesthetic. While it is unnecessary to administer atropine preoperatively, a dose in the range of 0.02 mg/kg should be readily available to treat bradycardia that is unrelated to hypoxemia, should this occur during surgery.

Pulse oximetery and ECG monitoring should be established before positioning the infant for lumbar puncture (LP). Placing the baby in a sitting posture with the chin extended offers the least likelihood for oxygen desaturation.[18] The increased hydrostatic pressure may also facilitate the flow of cerebral spinal fluid (CSF). If difficulty with the LP is encountered, moving the child to the lateral decubitus position with the knees flexed and the chin extended may be helpful. Following a sterile "prep" and the use of a small amount of local anesthetic for cutaneous anesthesia, a 22-gauge 4 cm or a 25-gauge 2.5 cm styletted[19] spinal needle is used for the LP. While a great deal has been written about which interspace to use for LP, and where the spinal cord ends in adults (L2) and infants (L3), the actual interspace at which the LP is made is of little consequence. Without X-ray confirmation, no one really knows *for sure* which interspace is being used. A study currently in progress has thus far demonstrated a 20% error rate in needle placement for lumbar disc surgery where the surgeon has asked for X-ray confirmation of the surgical site.

Lumbar puncture is a frequently performed procedure in the NICU and is often delegated to the most junior members of the medical staff. It is a procedure that has stood the test of time and has an extremely low complication rate. While an attempt should be made to be below the L3 level, it is more important to make a cautious approach, to remove the stylet frequently to check for CSF, and to keep the needle in the midline to minimize the incidence of a "bloody tap." The latter occurs in approximately 5% of lumbar punctures in this age group. Should this occur, it may make it more difficult to obtain and clearly identify CSF, even at a different spinal level. If CSF cannot be obtained, an attempt at caudal anesthesia may prove successful. When both techniques fail and surgical conditions permit, delaying the procedure for 24 hours and attempting the LP again is preferable to using general anesthesia in this patient.

TABLE 14–1.

Mean Dose of 1% Tetracaine in Former Preterm and Term Infants Undergoing Inguinal Hernia Surgery

Weight Range, g	Preterm Infants (Mean Postconceptual Age, 44.4 wk)		Term Infants (Mean Postconceptual Age, 50.1 wk)	
	Dose, mg/kg	No. of Cases	Dose, mg/kg	No. of Cases
<3000	0.56	65	0.58	3
3000–3999	0.47	38	0.47	29
4000–4999	0.42	13	0.42	44
>5000	0.37	13	0.36	65

Table 14–1 lists and compares dosage recommendations for hernia surgery in term and preterm infants. A 1% tetracaine solution made hyperbaric with an equal volume of 10% dextrose was used in all cases. Since the doses in each weight range are essentially identical for both groups, it would appear that weight, and not the degree of prematurity, is a determining factor. The calculated dose is rounded to the nearest quarter milligram and drawn up in a 1 mL tuberculin syringe; a short, fine-gauge needle is used to minimize the dilutional effects that a larger needle may have on the small doses being administered. When the procedure is expected to last longer than 30 minutes, the addition of 0.02 mL of 1:1000 epinephrine should produce approximately 90 minutes of surgical anesthesia. While increasing the dose has been reported to prolong anesthesia, the incidence of high spinal anesthesia requiring airway management also increases.[20] Recent experience with continuous spinal and caudal anesthesia in this age group indicates that these techniques may permit longer surgical times without posing the risk of respiratory compromise from high levels of spinal anesthesia.[21, 22]

Once a free flow of CSF is obtained, the medication is injected over 3 to 5 seconds and the needle and syringe removed as a single unit. Checking for backflow before and after the injection is unnecessary and may dislodge the needle in a squirming infant. After the needle is removed, the infant should be placed supine and his legs observed for signs of motor weakness. This is usually apparent in 1 to 3 minutes. Attempts should be made to soothe the infant if necessary. If IV access was not previously established, using an anesthetized lower extremity will be less painful for the infant. The blood pressure cuff and pulse oximeter sensor are best located on a lower extremity to prevent motion artifact. Unlike what occurs in the adult, clinically significant falls in blood pressure are rarely seen following spinal or caudal anesthesia in infants and young children.[23, 24] If there is a fall in blood pressure, it is easily treated with fluid administration. Lactated Ringer's solution at normal maintainence infusion rates is usually all that is necessary. Elevation of the infant's legs for placement of a cautery pad on the back has been cited as a cause for high spinal anesthesia.[25] While this is difficult to prove, care should be taken not to elevate the extremities too soon after injection of the spinal anesthetic agent or for too long a period.

Accurate assessment of the spinal dermatome level is not crucial. A level that is above T_{10} and yet not so high as to cause respiratory distress is all that is important. Pinching or pricking with a needle only upsets an infant who is just settling down. A level below T_{10} is likely to be inadequate for surgery. If the level is inadequate and at least ten minutes has elapsed since injection of the tetracaine, the spinal may be repeated using the same dose, or the level can be supplemented with a caudal block. Local infiltration by the surgeon may be effective in some situations, but is more likely to be accompanied by excessive movement of the patient.

The vast majority of infants this size will fall asleep as the spinal level is established. Sudden apnea and a falling arterial oxygen saturation are indicative of too high a level of anesthesia. This problem may be managed by assisting ventilation by mask or by endotracheal intubation. There may be a noticeable decrease in the volume of the infant's cry, and in some situations the torso and extremities become pallid. These signs may occur despite normal values for pulse, blood pressure, and arterial oxygen saturation. On occasion, "blow by" oxygen therapy may be indicated to maintain the oxygen saturation values above 90%. During the surgical prep, the infant's hands should be restrained to prevent him from contaminating the surgical site. The large surgical drape should be brought over the "ether screen" and tucked under the infant's arms to allow freedom of movement without risk of contamination. A cloth cap should be placed on the infant's head to minimize heat loss. A nipple stuffed with gauze or the patient's own pacifier, moistened with sugar water, may be used to comfort the fussy infant. If the abdomen appears distended, an 8 F feeding tube can be passed through the nose to decompress the stomach.

Traction on the hernia sac during surgery may cause discomfort and awaken a sleeping infant. Having a syringe of 0.25% bupivicaine readily available on the surgical field will enable the surgeon to inject or drip this solution onto the base of the sac to minimize this stimulus. The solution may also be used during wound closure to provide postoperative pain relief. Seldom do these measures fail to comfort the infant. In one series, 122 of 166 high-risk infants received only unsupplemented spinal anesthesia. When those methods fail to comfort the infant, intravenous midazolam, 0.05 to 0.1 mg/kg, may be administered. Some authors have recommended small doses of intravenous ketamine, 0.25 mg/kg, for sedation.[10, 12] Whatever the choice, once parenteral medication has been given the likelihood for intraoperative and postoperative apnea is increased. *Narcotics are even more likely to produce this complication and should be avoided.* Should it become necessary to induce general anesthesia, surgery must be temporarily halted. If significant quantities of sugar water have been given, an attempt should be made to empty the stomach with nasogastric suction prior to the induction of anesthesia.

POSTOPERATIVE CARE

In the recovery room, the infant should be monitored with pulse oximetery and, if necessary, oxygen administered to maintain saturation values above 90%. If the infant received no supplementary anesthetic agents or sedative drugs during surgery, and had previously been at home, no overnight stay is necessary. He may be discharged once the spinal anesthetic has worn off, as evidenced by withdrawal of the foot in response to a toe pinch, and oral feeding is tolerated. Voiding before discharge is not a requirement. These criteria are usually met within two hours of arrival in the recovery room.

If any supplementary agents or sedatives were used during surgery, the monitoring recommendations for patients receiving general anesthesia apply. That is, apnea monitoring should be provided for 12 to 24 hours postoperatively for any infant less than 60 weeks postconceptual age. The use of narcotics for postoperative pain control is strongly discouraged. Wound infiltration with

TABLE 14–2.

Advantages of Spinal Anesthesia for High-Risk Infants

Preserves protective airway reflexes
Eliminates the need for endotracheal intubation
Rapid return to the pre-anesthestic state
Frequently eliminates the need for depressant
  medications
Decreased incidence of postoperative apnea
A safe, reliable, and simple technique

0.25% bupivicaine at the time of closure, plus acetaminophen, administered orally or rectally should control pain in the vast majority of infants.

SUMMARY

H. Tyrrell-Gray must have had a vision of the NICU and its graduates when he wrote in *The Lancet* in 1909, "The *advantages* to be gained by the use of spinal anesthesia have so far impressed me that I am convinced it will occupy an important place in the surgery of children in the future."[26] The ability of anesthesiologists to use both spinal and caudal anesthetic techniques with minimal imbalance of the fragile physiologic states of such infants has been a major advance. (Table 14–2).

The disadvantages of regional anesthesia often revolve around the ability to deal with an awake infant in the operating room setting. Some infants cry during the lumbar puncture. While crying is a normal occurrence in the nursery or procedure room on a pediatric ward, it runs counter to the operating room environment. The temptation to administer potentially depressant medications should be resisted. Adequate explanation of the advantages this technique offers to the high risk infant should easily satisfy the concerns of the surgical team as well as those of anxious parents.

Once skills for performing lumbar puncture in infants are perfected, use of this technique should not delay the start of surgery, a commonly held misconception. Resistance by surgeons who are accustomed to general anesthesia is slowly being overcome.[12, 13, 27] Absolute contraindications to spinal anesthesia are infection at the LP site and parental refusal. The surgeon can often reassure anxious parents that the anesthesiologist's choice is the correct one. Relative contraindications to spinal anesthesia in adults include coagulopathy, neurologic disorders, allergy to local anesthetics, hypovolemia, and anatomical abnormalities of the spine. However, it should be noted that spinal anesthesia has been used successfuly in infants with spina bifida, congenital heart disease, and neurological disease. When selecting any anesthetic technique, the risks and benefits must be carefully weighed in light of the patient's physical condition.

REFERENCES

1. Peevy KJ, Speed FA, Hoff CJ: Epidemiology of inguinal hernia in preterm infants. *Pediatrics* 1986; 77:246–247.
2. Harper RG, Garcia A, Sia C: Inguinal hernia: A common problem of premature infants weighing 1000 grams or less at birth. *Pediatrics* 1975; 56:112–115.

3. Steward DJ: Preterm infants are more prone to complications than are term infants. *Anesthesiology* 1982; 56:304–306.

4. Gregory GA, Steward DJ: Life threatening perioperative apnea in the ex-"premie". *Anesthesiology* 1983; 59:495–498.

5. Welborn LG, Hannallah RS, Luban NLC, et al: Anemia and postoperative apnea in former preterm infants. *Anesthesiology* 1991; 74:1003–1006.

6. Abajian JC, Mellish RWP, Browne AF, et al: Spinal anesthesia for surgery in the high risk infant. *Anesth Analg* 1984; 63:359–362.

7. Blaise GA, Roy WL: Spinal anesthesia in children. *Anesth Analg* 1984; 63:1140–1141.

8. Harnik EV, Hoy GR, Potolicchio S, et al: Spinal anesthesia in premature infants recovering from respiratory distress syndrome. *Anesthesiology* 1986; 64:95–99.

9. Webster AC, McKishnie JD, Kenyon CF, et al: Spinal anaesthesia for inguinal hernia repair in high risk neonates. *Can J Anaesth* 1991; 38:281–286.

10. Schwartz N, Eisenkraft JB, Dolgin S: Spinal anesthesia for the high risk infant. *Mt Sinai J Med* 1988; 55(5):399–403.

11. Gallagher TM, Crean PM: Spinal anaesthesia in infants born prematurely. *Anaesthesia* 1989; 44:434–436.

12. Veverka TJ, Henry DN, Milroy MJ, et al: Spinal anesthesia reduces the hazard of apnea in high-risk infants. *Am Surg* 1991; 57(8):531–535.

13. Gunter JB, Watcha MF, Forestner JE, et al: Caudal epidural anesthesia in conscious premature and high risk infants. *J Pediatr Surg* 1991; 26:9–14.

14. Spear RM, Deshpande JM, Maxwell LG: Caudal anesthesia in the awake, high risk infant. *Anesthesiology* 1988; 69:407–409.

15. Welbourn LG, Rice LJ, Hannallah RS, et al: Postoperative apnea in former preterm infants: Prospective comparison of spinal and general anesthesia. *Anesthesiology* 1990; 72:838–842.

16. Cox RG, Goresky GV: Life-threatening apnea following spinal anesthesia in former premature infants. *Anesthesiology* 1990; 73:345–347.

17. Kurth CD, LeBard SE: Association of postoperative apnea, airway obstruction and hypoxemia in former preterm infants. *Anesthesiology* 1991; 75:22–26.

18. Gleason CA, Martin RJ, Anderson JV, et al: Optimal position for a spinal tap in preterm infants. *Pediatrics* 1983; 71:31–35.

19. Shaywitz BA: Epidermoid spinal cord tumors and previous lumbar punctures. *J Pediatr* 1972; 80:638–640.

20. Ramamoorthy C, Sukhani R, Black PR: Pediatric spinals without supplement: In search of the optimal drug and dose. *Anesthesiology* 1991; 75:A915.

21. McDonald T, Berkowitz R, Santini J, et al: Single dose and continous microcatheter spinal anesthesia in former preterm infants. *Anesthesiology* 1991; 75:A911.

22. Henderson KH, Sethna NF, Berde CB: Continious caudal anesthesia with 2- chloroprocaine for premature infants undergoing inguinal hernia repair. *Anesthesiology* 1991; 75:A916.

23. Dohi S, Naito H, Takahashi T: Age related changes in blood pressure and duration of motor block in spinal anesthesia. *Anesthesiology* 1979; 50:319–322.

24. Broadman LM, Hannallah RS, Norden JM, et al: "Kiddie caudals": Experience with 1154 consecutive cases without complications. *Anesth Analg* 1987; 66:S18.

25. Wright TE, Orr RJ, Haberkern CM, et al: Complications during spinal anesthesia in infants. High spinal blockade. *Anesthesiology* 1990; 73:1290–1291.

26. Tyrrel-Gray H: A study of spinal anesthesia in infants and children. *Lancet* 1909; 3:913–919.

27. Sartorelli KH, Abajian JC, Kreutz JM, et al: Improved outcome utilizing spinal anesthesia in high risk infants. *J Pediatr Surg* 1991; In Press.

15

Cleft Lip

A 3-month-old, 5-kg girl with bilateral cleft lip is scheduled for repair. She also has bilateral club feet and a cleft palate. Hemoglobin, 9 g/dL; hematocrit, 27%.

Recommendations by David J. Hatch, M.B.

Fusion of the medial and lateral nasal swellings in the fetus is normally complete by 35 days of intrauterine life. Failure of lip fusion, which may be unilateral or bilateral, may impair subsequent closure of the palatal shelves, which do not normally fuse until the eighth or ninth intrauterine week. Therefore, cleft lip is frequently associated with cleft palate (CL/P).

CLEFT LIP AND CLEFT PALATE

The incidence of CL/P is approximately 1 in 1,000 live births in Caucasian babies, in whom it is approximately twice as common as in black infants. Genetic influences are stronger in the case of CL/P than for the anomaly of isolated cleft palate, and its occurrence is more frequent in boys than in girls. Twenty-five percent of cases are bilateral, and 85% of these are associated with a cleft palate. The presence of other congenital abnormalities is more frequent with isolated cleft palate than with CL/P, although this possibility should always be borne in mind since up to 10% of children with CL/P have other congenital anomalies. Over 100 syndromes have been described in association with CL/P, but fortunately they are all rare. Some, however, have important anesthetic implications (Table 15–1).

Although there have been suggestions that environmental factors are involved in the etiology of CL/P, the only clear associations are related to maternal phenytoin or alcohol ingestion. Some progress has been made in identifying "candidate genes" for CL/P, although the etiology is almost certain to be heterogeneous, with other modifying genes playing some part.[1, 2]

The cleft lip deformity varies in severity from a small notch in the vermillion border to a com-

TABLE 15–1.

Cleft Lip/Palate Syndromes With Anesthetic Implications

Syndrome	Problem
Ectrodactyly-ectodermal dysplasia, clefting syndrome (EEC syndrome)	Maxillary hypoplasia
Fetal trimethadione effects	Congenital heart disease (CHD)
Kniest	Kyphoscoliosis
Miller	CHD
Mohr	Maxillary and mandibular hypoplasia
Orofaciodigital	Renal anomalies
Shprintzen	Micrognathia plus CHD
4-p	Micrognathia plus CHD

plete separation of the lateral and medial elements that extends into the floor of the nose. Other secondary anomalies that may be present include defects of tooth development in the area of the cleft, i.e., deformed, supernumerary, or absent teeth, and deformity of the nasal ala cartilage. Bilateral clefts are frequently associated with a deficiency of the central columella and elongation of the vomer, which causes protrusion of the anterior aspect of the premaxillary process (Fig 15–1). In other cases the premaxilla is completely absent (Fig 15–2).

The common time for surgical repair of a cleft lip is about 3 months after birth. In recent years, however, interest has been expressed in neonatal repair, and it seems likely that this will become increasingly popular in the future.[3] Although there is no evidence that surgical results are better after neonatal repair, the advantages in terms of bonding between mother and child are obvious. Neonatal repair must clearly be performed in centers equipped to deal with the problems of the new-

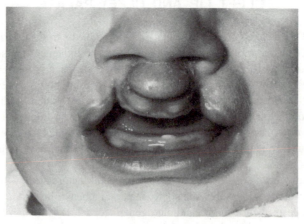

FIG 15–1.
Bilateral cleft lip with a prominent premaxilla.

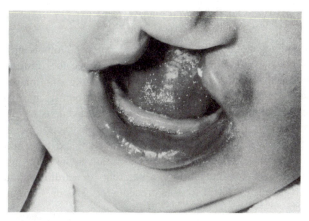

FIG 15–2.
Bilateral cleft lip with an absent premaxilla.

born. The operation is straightforward, and blood transfusion is virtually never required. It could be argued that centers that are not equipped to deal with the problems of young infants probably should not embark on repair of cleft lip even at 3 months of age. Cardiac murmurs are sometimes not apparent in the immediate newborn period. Therefore, one theoretical disadvantage of neonatal repair is the failure to immediately detect congenital heart disease in the unlikely event that it is present.

PREOPERATIVE ASSESSMENT

Careful preoperative assessment is essential at any age. When the operation is performed after the infant is 3 months of age, it is important for the anesthesiologist to obtain information about any preoperative feeding difficulties or history of aspiration. With modern nursing techniques, the use of thickened formula, and the upright position for feeding, aspiration is seldom a serious problem.

One disadvantage of surgery at 3 months is the physiologic anemia of infancy, which is most marked at this age. The normal hematocrit ranges from 30% to 42%. Although a hematocrit down to 25% is acceptable, the threshold for blood transfusion is reduced by the pre-existing anemia. It would be unwise to embark on this surgery if the infant has a hemoglobin content of 9 g/dL without a full hematologic profile to exclude rarer causes of anemia. Blood should be available, although it is unlikely that it will be required.

Preoperative assessment should also be directed to the possibility of coexisting congenital anomalies. The presence of bilateral club feet increases the likelihood of there being other anomalies, particularly cardiac or renal. Routine urinalysis should therefore be performed, and a preoperative electrocardiograph (ECG) and chest x-ray would be advisable. Since there is an increased risk of postoperative apnea in ex–premature infants, it is also important for the anesthesiologist to know the postconceptual age of the infant. In ex–premature babies younger than 60 weeks postconceptual age, apnea monitoring should be carried out for at least 12 to 18 hours after surgery, and nonurgent surgery such as this should probably be delayed until 44 weeks postconceptual age.[4, 5] Time should be taken at the preoperative visit to reassure the parents and discuss any underlying fears.

ANESTHETIC MANAGEMENT

The period of preoperative starvation is regularly debated. Withholding solid food for 6 hours and clear fluids for 4 hours is common and safe practice. Since the cardiac output of an infant is more rate-dependent than that of an adult, atropine, 0.02 mg/kg, minimum of 0.1 mg, should be given either intramuscularly a half to three quarters of an hour before anesthesia or intravenously at induction. Anesthesia can be induced by an inhalation or intravenous technique. Halothane is the agent of choice for inhalation induction in infants. Airway obstruction occurring during induction can be overcome with raised airway pressure via a tightly applied face mask. Intubation using a straight-blade laryngoscope can be performed with the infant under deep inhalation anesthesia, although the MAC of halothane for intubation exceeds that for cardiorespiratory depression at this age. A preformed RAE tube is excellent for this procedure, a 3.5- or 3.0-mm internal diameter size probably being required.

In the absence of micrognathia or other upper airway problems there is no objection to the use of muscle relaxants for intubation, the author's preference still being succinylcholine. Those not confident of judging when muscle relaxants can be used with safety in this situation should not proceed unsupervised. Relaxants should be avoided if there is any doubt about the ability to inflate the child's lungs. Although a protruding or absent premaxilla is disconcerting to the inexperienced, there is seldom difficulty if the correct intubating technique is used. With proper head positioning and adequate mouth opening, the laryngoscope blade should never come in contact with the upper alveolar margin. Some prefer, however, to protect the gums with a gauze pack. Because of the relative ease of bronchial intubation, particularly when an RAE tube is used, the chest should be carefully auscultated immediately after intubation.

In an otherwise healthy infant, intravenous access need not be established until after induction. This is kinder to the infant and easier for the anesthesiolgist. A 22-gauge cannula is usually inserted into a vein in the hand or foot, although the presence of bilateral clubfeet probably makes this site unsuitable. Veins may be readily visible on the dorsum of the hand or even on the ventral surface of the wrist. Gentle squeezing of the wrist for 1 to 2 minutes may enable the deeper veins on the hand to be palpated even though they are not visible. Transillumination may help in difficult cases, but it is no substitute for experience. The composition of the crystalloid maintenance fluid used varies from center to center, the author's preference being for 4% glucose in 0.18% NaCl. The rate should be calculated at 4 mL/kg/hr, adjusted to include the period of preoperative starvation.

Monitoring should include ECG, noninvasive blood pressure, and pulse oximetry. Measurement of end-tidal carbon dioxide is highly desirable. Despite these sophisticated monitors, the precordial stethoscope still provides one of the most reliable continuous monitors of heartbeat and respiration and can be applied before induction of anesthesia without disturbing the infant. For continuous use, a molded earpiece is essential. Although temperature control is less critical at 3 months than in the newborn, temperature should be monitored and steps taken to minimize heat loss. A warm air mattress is the most efficient and safest way of providing additional heat and allows the operating room to be maintained at a temperature tolerable to staff. Covering all areas outside the surgical field is very important, as is the warming of inspired gases.

Insertion of a gauze throat pack minimizes the risk of aspiration of blood, stabilizes the tracheal tube in the midline, and thus provides minimal distortion of the surgical field. The eyes should be protected. Jackson Rees' modification of Ayre's T-piece, a Bain coaxial T-piece system, or a pediatric circle can all be used satisfactorily for this case.

Although in the past this procedure has been carried out successfully with the child breathing spontaneously, most pediatric anesthesiologists would use controlled ventilation. The newer generation of ventilators for use with the T-piece or Bain system do not rely on the fresh gas flow (FGF) to inflate the chest, and FGF can therefore be reduced to the minimum level required for gas exchange. Using a flow of 1,000 plus 200 mL/kg allows conservation of anesthetic gases and provides optimum retention of heat and water vapor in the upper airways.

Since the surgeon is likely to use epinephrine for hemostasis, enflurane or isoflurane are safer maintenance agents than halothane.[6] Muscle relaxation with one of the newer nondepolarizing relaxants, atracurium or vecuronium, is satisfactory, and both these drugs are suitable for administration by continuous infusion. Atracurium is infused at 8 μg/kg/min after an initial bolus of 0.5 mg/kg and vecuronium at 1.5 to 2 μg/kg/min following a bolus 0.1 mg/kg. Adequacy of neuromuscular blockade can be monitored by peripheral nerve stimulation using the post-tetanic twitch count (PTC).[7] The PTC should be maintained between 5 and 10 for easy reversal.

Blood loss is seldom a problem with an experienced surgeon. The child's blood volume is estimated at 75 mL/kg or just under 400 mL. Even allowing for the pre-existing mild anemia, a loss of 10% of the blood volume, 40 mL, can be allowed without transfusion of red cells. Since only 5% to 10% of fetal hemoglobin remains at this age, oxygen transport should be adequate. The increasing hazards of blood transfusion have led to a more conservative approach to red blood cell replacement. The hematocrit can probably be allowed to fall to around 23% quite safely.

At the end of the procedure, the anesthetic should be discontinued and the muscle relaxant reversed with intravenous atropine, 0.02 mg/kg, and neostigmine, 0.05 mg/kg. The throat pack should be removed and any remaining blood in the mouth or pharynx gently aspirated. To avoid laryngospasm, the tracheal tube should not be removed until the infant is fully awake and objecting to its presence. Oxygen enrichment is advisable for the first 15 minutes or so in the recovery area, and careful assessment of airway patency is essential. In the straightforward case there should be no difficulty with the airway postoperatively, but problems can arise in the presence of micrognathia or other airway anomaly. In rare cases, a tongue stitch may be required for the first few hours after surgery.

Analgesic requirements are minimal and can be met by the use of a mild oral analgesic. The infant should be returned to her mother as soon as possible. Oral feeding can usually be recommenced within 2 hours. The first feeding should be clear liquid. If this is tolerated, normal feeding can be gradually reintroduced.

REFERENCES

1. Carter CO, Evans K, Coffey R, et al: A three generation family study of cleft lip with or without cleft palate. *J Med Genet* 1982; 19:246–261.
2. Holder SE: Cleft lip—is there light at the end of the tunnel? *Arch Dis Child* 1991; 66:829–832.
3. Desai SN: Cleft lip repair in newborn babies. *Ann R Coll Surg Engl* 1990; 72:101–103.
4. Kurth CD, Spitzer AR, Broennle AM, et al: Post operative apnea in preterm infants. *Anesthesiology* 1987; 66:483–488.

5. Welborn LG, de Soto H, Hannallah RS, et al: The use of caffeine in the control of post-anesthetic apnea in former premature infants. *Anesthesiology* 1988; 68:796–798.
6. Johnston RR, Eger EI II, Wilson C: A comparative interaction of epinephrine with enflurane, isoflurane and halothane in man. *Anesth Analg* 1976; 55:709–712.
7. Ridley SA, Hatch DJ: Post-tetanic count and profound neuromuscular blockade with atracurium infusion in paediatric patients. *Br J Anaesth* 1988; 60:31–35.

16

Laryngoscopy and Bronchoscopy

A 3-month-old, 4.8-kg girl with a history of stridor since birth is scheduled for laryngoscopy and bronchoscopy. The child is slightly micrognathic, but otherwise normal on physical examination. Hemoglobin, 9.5 g/dL; hematocrit, 29%. The otolaryngologist prefers to perform the procedure in the outpatient surgery center.

Recommendations by
Derek Blackstock, M.B., F.F.A.R.C.S.I., F.R.C.P.C.

Several features in this patient's history deserve further comment. It is essential that the etiology of the stridor be determined so that any required therapy can be initiated or the parents can be reassured that no treatment is indicated.

ANEMIA

The normal hemoglobin concentration of a newborn is 16 to 18 g/dL and decreases to 9 to 11 g/dL in the first three months of life. This gradual reduction allows the infant to adapt to the so-called physiologic anemia and is usually well tolerated. There is an increase in 2,3-diphosphoglycerate and a decrease in the concentration of hemoglobin F, both of which improve oxygen delivery to the tissues. The decrease in oxygen carrying capacity due to anemia is partly compensated by the increased flow associated with decreased viscosity. The principal mechanism supporting oxygen delivery to the tissues in anemic patients is increased cardiac output. It is important, therefore, to maintain normal cardiac function. As the newborn or young infant has a fixed stroke volume, it is essential that a normal or slightly elevated heart rate be maintained to preserve cardiac output and ensure normal tissue oxygenation. As the heart rate is already high in the first months of life, a further increase in cardiac output by increasing tachycardia is limited.

The lowest acceptable level of hemoglobin concentration in a patient requiring a general anesthetic is not known. With increasing anemia, any decrease in cardiac output or reduction in alveolar ventilation will result in very rapid tissue hypoxia. When the hemoglobin level is below 8 g/dL, oxygen transport is very dependent on an elevated cardiac output. Oxygen delivery to the myocardium becomes inadequate below 5 g/dL and ischemia and decreased myocardial contractility occur. Drugs that reduce myocardial function should be used cautiously, especially in the first three months of life, when the myocardium contracts poorly.

STRIDOR

Stridor is the sound produced when airflow becomes turbulent in a narrowed segment of the airway.[1, 2] It is the most common symptom in children with airway obstruction. The respiratory tract changes with the respiratory cycle in the infant. During inspiration the extrathoracic airway constricts, whereas the intrathoracic airway expands. The reverse is true during expiration. Theoretically, constriction of the extrathoracic airway will produce inspiratory stridor, as the airway is smallest during the inspiratory part of the respiratory cycle. Constriction of the intrathoracic airway during exhalation usually produces expiratory stridor. Stridor throughout the respiratory cycle can occur when there is obstruction at the laryngeal level. When both extrathoracic and intrathoracic lesions are present, localization of the obstruction can be difficult based only on clinical assessment, and an accurate diagnosis may only be made following bronchoscopy.

In an otherwise healthy 3-month-old, the most likely structural abnormalities are congenital anomalies, stenosis, endobronchial masses, or extrinsic compression by other structures. Abnormal airway dynamics are associated with laryngomalacia, tracheomalacia, or vocal cord paralysis.

In the newborn and young infant, the airway is poorly supported as the cartilaginous structures are not well developed, and changes in transmural pressure can distort the larynx, trachea, or bronchi to a greater degree than in older children and adults. It is important to differentiate between structural abnormalities and abnormal airway dynamics. Dynamic changes in the airway associated with respiration can only be assessed adequately while the patient is breathing spontaneously; this presents an interesting challenge for the anesthesiologist.

ENDOSCOPIC EXAMINATION

Complete endoscopic examination should be performed in children with laryngeal stridor to ensure that there are no additional abnormalities in the lower airway, since many children have multiple abnormalities.[3] Whether bronchoscopy is performed on an outpatient basis depends on many factors, including the experience of the endoscopist, the condition of the patient, the difficulty of the examination, and the type and size of instrumentation used.

In our hospital, a rigid bronchoscope with a ventilating sidearm is preferred by the surgical staff because of the superior optics. The bronchoscopy is performed in the operating room, usually with the patient under general anesthesia. Fiberoptic bronchoscopy is commonly performed in the intensive care unit and medical clinics and both local anesthesia and ketamine are used.

In low-risk patients only, fiberoptic laryngoscopy and bronchoscopy may be performed on an outpatient basis. Following a straightforward rigid bronchoscopy, patients who have no increase in symptoms in the postoperative period and are otherwise stable may be discharged the same day. It is important to have suitable facilities to observe, treat, or admit patients in whom increasing airway obstruction develops following a more difficult procedure. All other patients are admitted for careful observation in the postanesthesia area and, if required, are transferred to the intensive care unit (ICU).

When a supraglottic abnormality or vocal cord paralysis is suspected based on the history and physical examination, a preliminary examination using a flexible fiberoptic bronchoscope with an external diameter of 3.5 to 4 mm may be undertaken using local anesthesia. [4] Observation of the vibrating structures in the airway provides valuable information if the patient has stridor at the time of examination. A decline in oxygen saturation frequently occurs with a flexible bronchoscopy, especially in infants younger than 12 months, when the instrument is located in the midtrachea.[5] With the recent introduction of a 2.7-mm instrument, premature infants can be examined. However, this bronchoscope lacks a suction port and the tip of the instrument cannot be directed.

A rigid bronchoscope is required to visualize the posterior wall of the larynx and upper trachea, for operative procedures such as removal of foreign bodies, biopsy, or diagnosis of the origin of hemoptysis, and when surgical procedures for vascular rings or innominate artery compression are planned. The rigid bronchoscope has the added advantage that it can be used to secure the airway under direct vision. This is particularly important when there is distortion of the normal anatomy by tumor or by edema associated with bacterial or viral infection, or when there is the possibility a foreign body may change position and occlude the airway during induction of anesthesia. It is important not to pass the bronchoscope through an area of narrowing in the trachea or main-stem bronchi, as this may cause edema and subsequent life-threatening airway obstruction.

The use of the Storz bronchoscope with a jet injector for ventilation can be extremely hazardous, as high inflation pressures can occur when the 3- and 4-mm bronchoscopes are used. An infant is less likely to have an adequate leak around the bronchoscope and minor alterations in technique may produce large changes in airway pressure and ventilation. As there is a real risk of serious barotrauma with the jet ventilator, we do not advocate its routine use in the pediatric population.

ANESTHETIC TECHNIQUE

Reliable identification of normal adult and pediatric patients at risk of airway compromise is not always possible before induction of general anesthesia.[6, 7] This is also true in patients with abnormal airways. When airway obstruction is life-threatening, whatever the cause, awake layrngoscopy following oxygenation and application of topical anesthesia is the safest technique. Equipment to perform tracheostomy, cricothyroidotomy or rigid bronchoscopy should be readily available for all cases in which there is risk of airway compromise.

When the degree of respiratory distress is not severe, or there is an anatomical abnormality of the airway, mask induction with halothane in oxygen provides some safety should the airway suddenly become obstructed. Intravenous atropine, 20 μg/kg, is administered to all infants before induction of anesthesia. As the level of anesthesia is gradually deepened, respiration may be gently assisted to assess the ease of ventilation of the lungs. The application of positive airway pressure with a face mask will usually minimize the inspiratory stridor during spontaneous ventilation by decreasing the pressure gradient in the upper airway. This is particularly helpful in the young patient with laryngotracheomalacia.[8] If it is not possible to maintain the airway in this way, the anesthetic should be aborted and the patient awakened. Further investigation is required before anesthesia is attempted.

Failure to ventilate with positive airway pressure and a face mask is an unusual occurrence in normal infants and children with moderate degrees of micrognathia. The Pierre Robin syndrome includes severe micrognathia, and intubation or ventilation is often impossible. In these cases, awake assessment of the airway is advisable. The Treacher Collins syndrome also includes micrognathia. Although intubation is frequently difficult, the problems are often less severe than in infants with the Pierre Robin syndrome.

Deep anesthesia with halothane coupled with topical anesthesia of the larynx and bronchi, is a safe method of anesthesia for bronchoscopy in older infants and children. Spontaneous respiration can also be preserved. This technique is particularly useful if there is distortion of the airway by tumor or infection or if a foreign body is present. In such cases, the use of muscle relaxants is contraindicated. Paradoxical breathing is common at end-tidal concentrations of 1% halothane. This becomes more marked with increasing depths of anesthesia, and hypercarbia commonly occurs.[9] In addition, myocardial depression can occur with deep halothane anesthesia in infants less than 6 months of age and may be accompanied by severe hypotension. To avoid hypotension associated with high concentrations of halothane, succinylcholine, 2 mg/kg, can be administered intravenously for muscle relaxation. This allows passage of the bronchoscope under light general anesthesia.[10]

Pretreatment with atropine prevents the occurrence of bradyarrhythmias and is strongly recommended in all cases. Before passage of the bronchoscope the lungs are ventilated with 100% oxygen, and the larynx is sprayed with lidocaine to establish topical anesthesia. The total dose should not exceed 5 mg/kg, and a maximum dose of 1.5 mg/kg should be used to spray directly into the trachea. After an intubating dose of succinylcholine infants do not develop a phase II block, and incremental doses or an infusion to a maximum dose of 5 mg/kg may be given as required. The incidence and significance of masseter spasm following succinylcholine in young infants is controversial. For short procedures where rapid return to normal muscle function is required, succinylcholine remains a useful drug.

The use of the Storz pediatric rigid open bronchoscope and rod lens telescope permits good visualization of the airway while the telescope is in place. However, if the 2.5-, 3-, and 3.5-mm internal diameter bronchoscopes are used, there is increased resistance to breathing, as the lumen of the bronchoscope is partly occluded by the telescope. Inspiration is assisted by hand ventilation using a Jackson-Rees T-piece system attached directly to the bronchoscope system. This avoids the additional dead space introduced when a flexible extension is inserted between the anesthetic circuit and bronchoscope, but requires close cooperation between the endoscopist and anesthesiologist. Exhalation may be inadequate as the elastic recoil of the lungs may not fully expel gas during expiration. This will lead to serious overinflation of the lungs and possible barotrauma. Both inspiration and expiration are impaired with the 2.5 mm bronchoscope, and the telescope must be removed at regular intervals to permit adequate ventilation. The use of continuous pulse-oximetery, and end-tidal CO_2 sampling allows rapid confirmation of hypoxia and hypercarbia.

As the succinylcholine wears off, spontaneous ventilation is reestablished, and the dynamics of the larynx, trachea, and bronchi can be assessed. The endoscopist can also visualize vocal cord function by withdrawing the bronchoscope above the vocal cords as the patient is allowed to awaken. Oxygen is administered during this period via the bronchoscope. Laryngospasm may occur as the depth of anesthesia is reduced, and the anesthesiologist should be prepared to administer an additional small dose of muscle relaxant if a decrease in oxygen saturation occurs. With adequate topical anesthesia of the larynx, it is usually possible to ventilate the lungs with positive airway pressure alone, and additional muscle relaxant is seldom required. Reintubation of the trachea with either the rigid bronchoscope or an endotracheal tube is occasionally required.

COMPLICATIONS

The most common complications of pediatric bronchoscopy are bradycardia associated with airway manipulation and hypotension caused by halothane. Postoperative stridor and dyspnea following instrumentation are frequent, and infants should receive moist oxygen during recovery. Persistent symptoms can be treated with racemic epinephrine solution, 11.25 mg, (0.5 mL) added to 2.5 mL normal saline, via a nebulizer driven with oxygen. The nebulized dose is delivered for 10 to 15 minutes and may be repeated as necessary. Patients should be admitted following racemic epinephrine treatment and closely observed. After discontinuation of oxygen therapy, oxygenation should be confirmed by pulse oximetry before discharge from the recovery area.

With the development of pediatric fiberoptic bronchoscopes, a decreasing number of patients require general anesthesia for endoscopy. Those high-risk patients who require rigid instrumentation for diagnosis and treatment deserve careful preoperative assessment.

SUMMARY

With careful selection of appropriately sized equipment, close cooperation between the endoscopist and anesthesiologist, and modern monitoring of oxygenation, ventilation, blood pressure, temperature, and ECG, serious complications such as pneumothorax, pneumomediastinum, cardiac arrest, or death are very rare.[9]

The final decision to discharge the child on the day of surgery depends on the confirmed diagnosis, the difficulty of the procedure, and the presence or absence of increased airway compromise after bronchoscopy. The competence of the parents and the distance the family lives from the hospital also influence the decision.

REFERENCES

1. Holinger LD: Etiology of stridor in the neonate, infant and child. *Ann Otol Rhinol Laryngol* 1980; 89:397–400.
2. Maze A, Bloch E: Stridor in pediatric patients. *Anesthesiology* 1979; 50:132–145.
3. Gonzales C, Reilly JS, Bluestone CD: Synchronous airway lesions in infancy. *Ann Otol Rhinol Laryngol* 1987; 96:77–80.
4. Hawkins DB, Clark RW: Flexible laryngoscopy in neonates, infants, and young children. *Ann Otol Rhinol Laryngol* 1987; 96:81–85.
5. Schnapf BM: Oxygen desaturation during fiberoptic bronchoscopy in pediatric patients. *Chest* 1991; 99; 3:591–594.

6. Oates JD, Macleod AD, Oates PD, et al: Comparison of two methods for predicting difficult intubation. *Br J Anaesth* 1991; 66:305–309.

7. Kanter RK, Pollack MM, Wright WW, et al: Treatment of severe tracheobronchomalacia with continuous positive airway pressure (CPAP). *Anesthesiology* 1982; 57:54–56.

8. Lindahl SGE, Yates AP, Hatch DJ: Respiratory depression in children at different end-tidal halothane concentrations. *Anaesthesia* 1987; 42:1267–1275.

9. Puhakka H, Kero P, Valli P, et al: Pediatric bronchoscopy: A report of methodology and results. *Clinical Pediatr* 1989; 28(6):253–257.

17

Cleft Palate and Goldenhar Syndrome

A 4-month-old boy with Goldenhar syndrome is scheduled for cleft palate repair. Hemoglobin, 10 g/dL; hematocrit, 30%.

Recommendations by Robert S. Holzman, M.D.

Surgical correction of congenital anomalies early in life tends to minimize psychological problems for the child and family. Moreover, early repair may prevent secondary anatomical distortions that can result from uncorrected defects.[1-3] Much family support is required for what are often staged or recurrent procedures drawn out over years. Initial repairs may be followed by additional procedures to correct physiologic or cosmetic deformities during subsequent growth and development, including nasal tip correction, revision of the vermilion border, and pharyngeal flap for velopharyngeal insufficiency. A multidisciplinary approach is most useful, with the close cooperation of plastic surgeons, anesthesiologists, oral surgeons, dentists, otolaryngologists, speech pathologists, psychologists, psychiatrists, dysmorphologists, social workers, nurses, and medical illustrators or photographers.

The face develops from a combination of upper midline structures that arise from the frontal prominence as well as lateral and middle facial structures from the branchial arches. Midline or paramedian fusion defects may result in cleft palate (Fig 17–1).

The branchial arches are bars of mesenchymal tissue that are separated from each other by clefts. The first branchial arch gives rise to the maxilla, mandible, zygoma, and a portion of the temporal bone, along with the incus and the malleus. The muscles of mastication—mylohyoid, tensor tympani, tensor palatini, and anterior belly of the digastric—also derive from the first arch, and are innervated by the trigeminal nerve (V). The 2nd branchial arch gives rise to the stapes, styloid process of the temporal bone, stylohyoid ligament, and a portion of the body of the hyoid. The muscles that develop from the 2nd arch are the stapedius, stylohyoid, posterior belly of the digas-

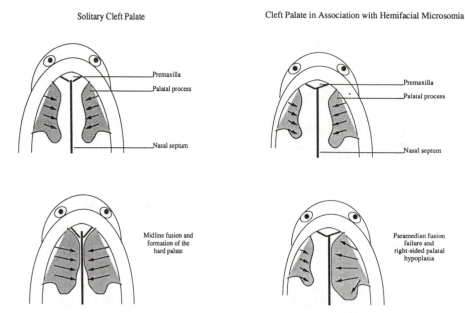

Solitary Cleft Palate

Cleft Palate in Association with Hemifacial Microsomia

Premaxilla

Palatal process

Nasal septum

Midline fusion and formation of the hard palate

Paramedian fusion failure and right-sided palatal hypoplasia

FIG 17–1.
Solitary cleft palate and soft palate in association with hemifacial microsomia.

tric, auricular, and all the muscles of facial expression that receive their innervation from the facial nerve. (VII). The 1st branchial pouch gives rise to the eustachian tube and middle ear, and the 1st branchial cleft, between the 1st and 2nd arches, forms the external ear, which is the only normal structure to arise from a branchial cleft. The various arch components, especially the 1st and 2nd, may give rise to obvious as well as quite subtle anatomic abnormalities that are important because of their airway implications.

GOLDENHAR SYNDROME

The Goldenhar syndrome, oculoauriculovertebral dysplasia, is characterized by preauricular appendages and fistulas, associated with mandibulofacial dysostosis (Fig 17–2). It was originally thought to be distinct from—but now is thought to be a continuum of—the first and second branchial arch syndrome.[4,5] The defect may originate as early as the seventh to eighth week of development; hence, it is frequently associated with other anomalies of early development.[6] Micrognathia, unilateral mandibular hypoplasia, and cleft palate can be found in association with vertebral abnormalities such as the Klippel-Feil anomalad and a 35% incidence of congenital heart disease.[7]

In hemifacial microsomia (HFM) the structures involved are also from the first and second branchial arches, including the intervening first cleft; this involvement may cause bilateral, as well as the more common unilateral, deformity. Hemifacial microsomia is characterized by ear abnormalities and hypoplasia of the mandibular condyle and ramus. Various gradations exist depending

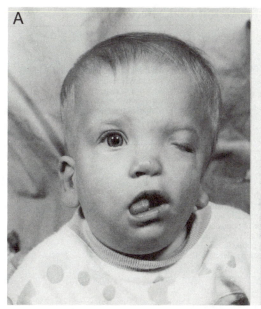
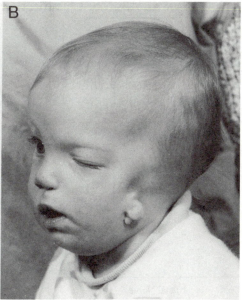

FIG 17–2.
Child with hemifacial microsomia, showing typical features of ear deformity and facial asymmetry **(A)**. **B,** micrognathia becomes more evident when patient is viewed in profile.

on the severity of the hypoplasia.[8] The chin is usually deviated toward the affected side, and mandibular mobility may be impaired not only due to the bony abnormalities but also because of abnormal development of the muscles of mastication and developmental effects on innervation.

At Children's Hospital, the clinical features of Goldenhar syndrome are incorporated into the OMENS (**o**rbital distortion, **m**andibular hypoplasia, **e**ar anomaly, **n**erve involvement, **s**oft tissue deficiency) classification[9] (Fig 17–3) and are viewed as a variant of HFM. In a series of 154 patients, the degree of mandibular hypoplasia correlated with the severity of orbital, auricular, neural, and soft tissue involvement (Fig 17–4). This has also been predictive of treatment effectiveness: types M_1 and M_{2A} have been treated with an activator appliance and surgical elongation, while types M_{2B} and M_3 have been treated with mandibular and temporomandibular joint reconstruction.

The classically described features of Goldenhar syndrome, vertebral anomalies, rib deformities, and epibulbar dermoids in association with mandibular hypoplasia, were found in only 3 of the 154 patients with HFM. Sixteen had two of the three features, and 32 demonstrated only one of the three "classical" features. Palatal deviation occured in one-third of patients[9] and overt palatal defects were found in 12%.[2] These defects are not etiologically the same as the isolated midline cleft palate. Hypoplasia of the palatal muscles, usually appreciated during the operative repair, argues for the embryologic relationship of hypoplasia of a proximal branch of the facial nerve innervating the levator veli palatini (see Fig 17–1).

The anesthetic plan must account for requirements of the cleft palate repair and the potential difficulties associated with Goldenhar syndrome or HFM.

O.M.E.N.S. Classification for Hemifacial Microsomia

Orbit

Oo: Normal orbital size and position
O1: Abnormal orbital size
O2: Abnormal orbital position. Arrow denotes
     relative position of affected side (i.e. O2↑
     denotes superior position)
O3: Abnormal orbital size and position

Ear

Eo: Normal ear
E1: Mild hypoplasia and cupping with all
     structures present
E2: Absence of external auditory canal with
     variable hypoplasia of the concha.
E3: Malpositioned lobule with absence auricle.
     Lobular remnant usually inferiorly and
     anteriorly displaced.

Mandible

Mo: Normal Mandible
M1: Mandible and glenoid fossa small; short ramus
M2: Mandibular ramus short/abnormally shaped
  2A Glenoid fossa in anatomically acceptable
      position with reference to opposite TMJ
  2B TMJ is inferiorly, medially, and anteriorly
      displaced; severely hypoplastic condyle
M3: Complete absence of ramus, glenoid fossa,
     and TMJ.

Facial Nerve

N7o: No facial nerve involvement
N71: Upper facial nerve involvement
      (temporal and zygomatic branches)
N72: Lower facial nerve involvement
      (buccal, mandibular and cervical branches)
N73: All branches of the facial nerve affected.
      Other nerve involvement may be
      designated (i.e. trigeminal N5, hypoglossal
      N12)

Soft Tissue

So: No obvious soft tissue or muscle deficiency
S1: Minimal subcutaneous/muscle deficiency
S2: Moderate-between the two extremes, S1
     and S3
S3: Severe soft tissue deficiency due to
     subcutaenous and muscular hypoplasia

FIG 17–3.
OMENS (*orbit*, *m*andible, *e*ar, facial *n*erve, *s*oft tissue) classification for hemifacial microsomia.

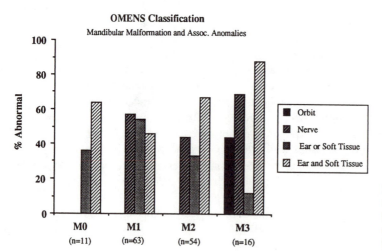

FIG 17–4.
OMENS (*orbit*, *m*andible, *e*ar, facial *n*erve, *s*oft tissue) classification of mandibular malformation and associated anomalies.

ANESTHETIC MANAGEMENT

Anesthesia consultation should be obtained by the plastic surgeon, ideally with individuals who are experienced with management of congenital abnormalities of the head and neck in children. Well-prepared parents will have already seen the pediatrician, and in all likelihood, a dysmorphologist, perhaps in a multidisciplinary craniofacial clinic. They will probably have a good understanding of the issues that a pediatric anesthesia consultant will discuss with them, such as the need for special airway equipment, possible awake laryngoscopy and intubation, and considerations for postoperative ventilatory support and monitoring in an intensive care setting. In this regard, a complete workup may have already been done by pediatric specialists, including evaluation for associated congenital anomalies such as the Klippel-Feil anomalad and congenital heart disease. The anesthesiologist, as part of this team, must be aware of the potential for these and other associated anomalies.[10]

Children with branchial arch anomalies present challenges for airway management. The defect in hemifacial microsomia is usually unilateral; therefore, the unaffected side may provide a reasonable approach for laryngoscopy and intubation. The mask fit can be difficult due to unilateral or bilateral mandibular and maxillary hypoplasia. Cervical spine abnormalities and macrostomia can make the mask fit and intubation difficult. In addition, there is the risk of spinal cord trauma.

Options for endotracheal intubation in children with midface and branchial arch anomalies are no different than those for the adult patient with the recognized difficult airway: awake intubation with either direct vision or "blind" methods, administration of a general anesthetic with or without spontaneous respiration, and tracheotomy, either awake or with a general anesthetic.

I prefer an anesthetic induction designed to preserve spontaneous ventilation. In one large series, 23 of 28 patients with Goldenhar syndrome underwent induction with spontaneous respirations, regardless of whether or not they had had tracheal intubation for surgery.[11] A sufficient depth of anesthesia needs to be achieved to permit direct laryngoscopy or fiberoptic bronchoscopy for visualization of the airway. While high doses of volatile agents are associated with apnea and bradycardia in young babies, routine use of an anticholinergic and slow, progressive administration of the agent tend to minimize these side effects. Halothane remains a safe volatile agent for anesthetic induction, even in children with cyanotic congenital heart disease.[12] Supplemental local anesthesia by mucosal application can be extremely helpful in preserving respiratory function while attenuating protective airway reflexes. This can be accomplished by allowing the baby to suck on a gloved finger lubricated with 2% lidocaine jelly. The lidocaine will dissolve in the oral secretions, and topically anesthetize the oral mucosa. Laryngoscopy is helpful in determining the potential for visualization prior to attempted intubation. If visualization proves not to be difficult, a muscle relaxant may be utilized. Doxapram, in divided doses up to 2 mg/kg as a respiratory stimulant during a volatile agent induction, may be useful to preserve ventilatory drive while the anesthetic state is deepened.[13-15] The intravenous catheter is placed following induction, and atropine or glycopyrrolate are given for their antisialagogic and/or anticholinergic cardiac effects. If an awake intubation is to be performed, atropine is administered intramuscularly prior to endoscopy.

It is important to differentiate the difficult airway from the difficult intubation: one does not necessarily follow from the other. In fact, difficulty with ventilation by mask is much more hazardous than the difficult intubation. The mask fit will be related to facial anatomy. Many of these patients do not have normal jaw or midfacial architecture, and maneuvers such as building up the cheeks with gauze, application of "upside-down" masks, insertion of a dental roll in the cleft palate, and other innovative techniques may become necessary to establish an effective mask seal and patent upper airway. A shortened endotracheal tube passed transnasally, with connection to the anesthesia circuit via a 15-mm connector, may also be useful for pharyngeal insufflation should the mask fit prove difficult. A variety of laryngoscope blades should be available, as should the Jackson infant anterior commissure laryngoscope. With current instrumentation, fiberoptic bronchoscopy is possible for intubation with a size 2.5-mm endotracheal tube. The endotracheal tube should be placed transorally because passage transnasally will interfere with the surgical repair. A tracheal guidewire may be passed via the suction port of a flexible pediatric bronchoscope, and an endotracheal tube threaded over the wire.[16] The laryngeal mask airway has also been used successfully for cleft palate repair in a baby with Pierre Robin syndrome when endotracheal intubation proved impossible.[17] Finally, tactile intubation with palpation of the epiglottis by two fingers, followed by insertion of the curved endotracheal tube around the base of the tongue, tracing the curvature of the palpating fingers, was described in the days before pediatric laryngoscopes were available; this technique may still be successfully applied today.

If intubation through the supraglottic larynx proves impossible, then an infraglottic retrograde approach using an epidural needle and catheter placed through the cricothyroid membrane with a modified Seldinger technique can be successfully carried out with a 20 gauge needle and a 0.021-in. guidewire. Insertion into the Murphy eye of the endotracheal tube rather than the larger end-hole allows an additional 1 cm of tube to pass into the larynx before wire withdrawal. This technique has been successfully applied in a 5-month-old infant with Goldenhar syndrome.[18]

Occlusion of the lumen by secretions or blood is more common with smaller endotracheal tubes. Kinking of warm, small-diameter endotracheal tubes may also occur with the weight of surgical drapes. We tend to avoid the RAE endotracheal tube in infant sizes as passage of a suction catheter around the preformed curve can prove difficult. For fixation, we frequently wire transoral tubes to the lower teeth or place a circummandibular wire in edentulous infants. Tubes may also be sutured to the base of the tongue. The midtracheal placement of the tube should be checked by placing the child's head into extension and flexion and listening to breath sounds. Changes in position of the head and neck during these procedures can result in caudad or cephalad motion of the tube, and right mainstem intubations or extubations of the trachea can occur.

Usual noninvasive monitors are applied. The breathing circuit used makes relatively little difference, regardless of patient size, so long as controlled ventilation is used. The circuit should be long enough to enable the operating table to be turned 90 degrees following induction without tension on the tubing.

Temperature may be measured in the rectum or axilla. It may be advantageous to monitor both and follow the temperature gradient between the core and the periphery. Heat loss is rarely a problem, and frequently for these procedures, heat retention tends to be the problem. The patient is fully covered except for the face and temperatures in patients of 38° to 38.5° C are common at the completion of surgery. While hypothermia is a rare finding, patient temperature may decrease rapidly during the last 10 minutes in the operating room when drapes are being removed and radiant heat loss takes place.

Many anesthetic maintenance strategies are acceptable for these procedures, and all have their advocates and detractors. In the absence of a history of abnormal ventilatory control in babies in this age group, once the airway is secured, I prefer to use a narcotic-based technique with fentanyl, a low-maintenance concentration of volatile agent, and pancuronium as the muscle relaxant.

Following anesthetic induction and endotracheal intubation, the surgeon will place the infant at the edge of the head of the table. Positioning and symmetry are key elements of the surgical repair. The eyes are allowed to remain closed in a natural position following lubrication; occasionally they will be sutured by the surgeon. They should not be taped. After placing the mouth gag and a throat pack with an extraoral tag, lidocaine, 0.5% with epinephrine 1:200,000 is injected for local control of bleeding. This will decrease anesthetic requirements, and impose some considerations for anesthetic technique. While it is rare to encounter ventricular irritability with halothane and exogenous epinephrine in this concentration and age group,[19-21] we generally change to isoflurane following induction with halothane.

When surgery is finished, the surgeon removes the throat pack, passes a suction catheter into the stomach under direct vision, and removes the mouth gag. A long tongue stitch may be placed to facilitate mechanical clearing of the airway. The anesthesiologist should take advantage of the opportunity to examine the airway at the end of surgery while the mouth gag is still in place, and check for uvular edema or swelling of the supraglottic structures, which may influence the timing of extubation. Massive macroglossia and airway obstruction have been reported after cleft palate repair,[22] as has delayed postintubation croup.[23]

We administer humidified oxygen in the postanesthesia care unit (PACU). Airway edema following use of a mouth gag is a common occurrence, and an oxygen-enriched atmosphere is helpful should the airway worsen during the initial postoperative period. For postextubation croup, racemic epinephrine may be used in dilute mixtures, with some respect for the fact that it works by mucosal vasoconstriction, and rebound may occur.

Depending on the difficulty of the intubation, the immediate perioperative anatomical changes, amount of edema, and concurrent medical problems, planning for the intensive care unit (ICU) may be appropriate, where full-time physician and specialized nursing care are invaluable. Extubation may need to be accomplished in the ICU several days following the procedure after edema clears. Near-prone positioning may help to sustain a natural airway. Respiratory inductance plethysmography in conjunction with pulse oximetry has been found useful for perioperative monitoring of patients with Goldenhar syndrome.[24]

REFERENCES

1. Pigott RW: Objectives for cleft palate repair. *Ann Plast Surg* 1987; 19:247–259.
2. Mulliken JB, Kaban LB: Analysis and treatment of hemifacial microsomia in childhood. *Clin Plast Surg* 1987; 14:91–100.
3. Kaban LB, Moses MH, Mulliken JB: Surgical correction of hemifacial microsomia in the growing child. *Plast Reconstruct Surg* 1988; 82:9–19.
4. Aleksic S, Budzilovich G, Reuben R, et al: Congenital trigeminal neuropathy in oculoauriculovertebral dysplasia-hemifacial microsomia (Goldenhar-Gorlin syndrome). *J Neurol Neurosurg Psychol* 1975; 38:1033–1035.
5. Scholtes JL, Veyckemans F, van Obbergh L, et al: Neonatal anaesthetic management of a patient with Goldenhar's syndrome with hydrocephalus. *Anaesth Intensive Care* 1987; 15:338–340.

6. Fiore C, Santoni G, Lungarotti S, et al: A propos d'un cas atypique de syndrome de Goldenhar. *Opthalmologica* 1983; 186:162–168.
7. Ward CF: Pediatric head and neck syndromes, in Katz J, Steward DJ (eds): *Anesthesia and Uncommon Pediatric Diseases.* Philadelphia, WB Saunders, 1987, pp 255–256.
8. Murray JE, Kaban LB, Mulliken JB, et al: Analysis and treatment of hemifacial microsomia, in Caronni EP (ed): *Craniofacial Surgery.* Boston, Little Brown, 1985, pp 378–379.
9. Vento AR, LaBrie RA, Mulliken JB: The O.M.E.N.S. classification of hemifacial microsomia. *Cleft Palate-Craniofacial J* 1991; 28:68–76.
10. Stehling L: Goldenhar syndrome and airway management (letter.) *AJDC* 1978; 132:818.
11. Madan R, Trikha A, Venkataraman RK, et al: Goldenhar's syndrome: An analysis of anaesthetic management. *Anaesthesia* 1990; 45:49–52.
12. Hensley FA, Larch DR, Stauffer RA, et al: The effect of halothane/nitrous oxide/oxygen mask induction on arterial hemoglobin saturation in cyanotic heart disease. *Anesthesiology* 1985; 63:A3.
13. Gupta PK, Moore J: The use of doxapram in the newborn. *Br J Obstet Gynaecol* 1973; 80:1002–1006.
14. Zuccaro GM, Zocche GP, Musto P: Considerazioni sull'impiego del doxapram in anestesia infantile e neonatale. *Minerva Anestes* 1970; 36:325–332.
15. Fisher B, Rodarte A: Use of doxapram to increase respirations without a concomitant increase in intracranial pressure. *Crit Care Med* 1987; 15:1072–1073.
16. Scheller JG, Schulman SR: Fiber-optic bronchoscopic guidance for intubating a neonate with Pierre-Robin syndrome. *J Clin Anesth* 1991; 3:45–47.
17. Beveridge ME: Laryngeal mask anaesthesia for repair of cleft palate. *Anaesthesia* 1989; 44:656–657.
18. Cooper CMS, Murray-Wilson A: Retrograde intubation: Management of a 4.8-kg, 5-month infant. *Anaesthesia* 1987; 42:1197–1200.
19. Ueda W, Hirakawa M, Mae O: Appraisal of epinephrine administration to patients under halothane anesthesia for closure of cleft palate. *Anesthesiology* 1983; 58:574–576.
20. Funakoshi Y, Iwai S, Kaneda H, et al: Hemodynamic effects of locally applied epinephrine used with various general anesthetic techniques. *J Oral Surg* 1977; 35:713–718.
21. Wallbank WA: Cardiac effects of halothane and adrenaline in hare-lip and cleft palate surgery. *Br J Anaesth* 1970; 42:548–552.
22. Bell C, Oh TH, Loeffler JR: Massive macroglossia and airway obstruction after cleft palate repair. *Anesth Analg* 1988; 67:71–74.
23. Pechter EA, Lesavoy MA: Postintubation croup in two consecutive patients undergoing cleft lip and/or palate repair. *Ann Plast Surg* 1985; 14:81–84.
24. Aoe T, Kohchi T, Mizuguchi T: Respiratory inductance plethysmography and pulse oximetry in the assessment of upper airway patency in a child with Goldenhar's syndrome. *Can J Anaesth* 1990; 37:369–371.

18

Phocomelia

A 5-month-old boy, 5 kg, with upper extremity phocomelia and deformed lower extremities is scheduled for surgery on both feet (Fig 18–1). He is known to have a systolic murmur. Hemoglobin, 11.5 g/dL; hematocrit, 34.5%.

Recommendations by Helen R. Westman, M.D.

Phocomelia is a developmental anomaly characterized by absence of the proximal part of a limb or limbs. The hands or feet are attached to the trunk by a single, small, irregularly shaped bone. Phocomelia may be partial or complete. There are usually no associated congenital anomalies. The systolic murmur in this child most likely represents a second congenital anomaly unrelated to the phocomelia.

PREOPERATIVE EVALUATION

Preoperative evaluation should center on the general physical status of the patient, an awareness of the technical problems associated with this deformity, and an adequate cardiac evaluation. The hematocrit and hemoglobin values are acceptable. Urinalysis is required by law in some states, but a clean catch urine at this age is difficult to obtain. In view of his heart murmur, a chest x-ray could possibly provide useful information. He should be seen by a pediatric cardiologist and evidence of cardiac failure should be sought. On physical examination, the most frequent finding indicative of cardiac failure is an enlarged liver. If a structural defect is discovered, subacute bacterial endocarditis (SBE) prophylaxis may be indicated. The most frequent cardiac lesions are atrial and ventricular septal defects. If either is present, intravenous catheters must be carefully checked for air bubbles to prevent air entry into the cerebral circulation.

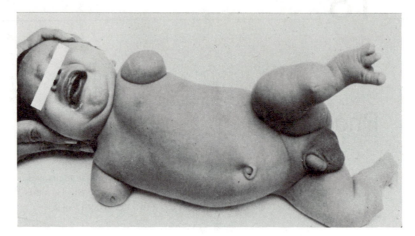

FIG 18–1.
Infant with quadrimelic phocomelia.

ANESTHETIC MANAGEMENT

Preoperative sedation should not be required. The infant is not yet old enough to have separation anxiety. Other medications, such as the SBE prophylaxis, can be given after induction, but prior to endotracheal intubation.

Certain problems are common to all infants in the operating room. Heat loss, choice of breathing circuits, laryngeal anatomy, monitoring, fluid replacement, and the type of anesthesia all need to be considered. This child's care may be further complicated by his heart lesion and the technical problems secondary to phocomelia and the surgical sites.

Heat loss is a constant problem. Infants are prone to hypothermia because of their relatively greater surface area, lack of subcutaneous fat, and inadequate shivering mechanism. With moderate hypothermia, oxygen consumption can be increased to twice normal, reversal of muscle relaxants is inadequate, and postoperative respiratory embarassment is common. The room should be warmed to 28°C or higher. Heating lamps and a warming mattress should be used. Warmed humidified gases can be supplied by use of a heated humidifier. Intravenous fluids should also be warmed.

A Jackson-Rees or Bain anesthesia breathing circuit should be used. An adult circle absorber is cumbersome to use, and the excessive work of spontaneous breathing for an infant may lead to acidosis and cardiovascular collapse.[1] Provision of a secure airway by endotracheal intubation is recommended. A 3.5 to 4.0 mm oral tube and a no. 1 Flagg, Phillips, or Miller laryngoscope blade are appropriate on the basis of the patient's age and weight.

Adequate monitoring will be difficult in this case, but every effort should be made. Heart tones and breath sounds are readily accessible with a precordial stethoscope. Placement of ECG leads should present no problem, and either rectal or esophageal temperature can be monitored. Monitoring blood pressure will be somewhat more difficult. With bilateral upper arm phocomelia, the only sites for the cuff are the upper thighs. It may not be possible to use a cuff at all if the surgeons wish to use bilateral tourniquets. The problem can be solved, however, by limiting surgery to one limb at a time so that one thigh is available for blood pressure monitoring and the other for tourniquet placement. This necessitates removal and replacement of tourniquets, reprepping and draping of the extremities, and some increase in operating time, but is a small price to pay for adequate monitoring of blood pressure. Probe placement for pulse oximetry also presents a problem. The solution, as with blood pressure monitoring, is to alternate limbs. There will be signal interferences during blood pressure measurements. Alternative sites for probe placement include the nose, ear lobe, and the penis.[2] Signal interference is common when infrared heating lamps are in use and with high intensity OR lighting. The probe can be shielded by covering it with a used alcohol aluminum foil packet.[3] Placement of an arterial catheter would not only be impractical and require use of a temporal or femoral artery, but is unwarranted in view of the limited extent of the surgery. Bladder catheterization should be considered if the procedure is anticipated to last longer than four hours or if major blood loss is expected.

Fluid replacement should consist of 5% dextrose in quarter normal saline (D5.2NS) for the maintenance and deficit replacement. Ringer's lactate solution is administered for third space loss, 0 in this case, and for blood loss, 2–3 mL/mL blood loss. Placement of an intravenous cannula can be one of the most difficult aspects of anesthetic management in any infant, but venous access is mandatory. Resuscitation may be necessary if the child's heart cannot compensate for the demands placed upon it. Transfusion may also be required if tourniquets are not used or are ineffective during the procedure. Unfortunately, because of the planned surgery, the saphenous and other lower extremity veins are not available for use. The most readily available site for catheter placement in this 5-month-old infant is the head. The parents should be informed preoperatively that the scalp will be shaved. Using a rubber band as the tourniquet, a 20- or 22-gauge plastic catheter can usually be inserted without undue difficulty. Straight steel needles are not recommended. Care should be taken that an artery is not cannulated. Arteries are superficial in the scalp and can easily be mistaken for veins. Alopecia may result. The external jugular vein can also be cannulated. This may be easier to accomplish with the patient awake and crying and creating greater venous pressure. However, movement will increase the difficulty. Internal jugular cannulation in a child this age should only be attempted by an anesthesiologist experienced in the procedure. A femoral vein can be used as an alternative to internal jugular cannulation. Occasionally, there will be a vein available on the appendages or the chest wall. If all else fails, a cutdown on the external jugular or femoral vein should be performed by a pediatric surgeon. Placement of the intravenous catheter is generally easier and more successful if attempted after induction of anesthesia.

Inhalation induction with halothane and nitrous oxide–oxygen is appropriate. Intramuscular atropine is occasionally indicated during induction to treat bradycardia prior to intravenous placement. Intubation may be accomplished following vascular cannulation using a nondepolarizing muscle relaxant such as atracurium. Intubation with deep halothane is not recommended because of the significant myocardial depressant effects of halothane in this age group. Intramuscular ketamine can be used for induction if the heart lesion is such that cardiac output may be compromised by inhalation anesthesia. Following intubation and vascular cannulation, halothane, 0.3% to 0.5%, and nitrous oxide–oxygen, and a nondepolarizing muscle relaxant such as atracurium, 0.3–0.5 mg/kg[4] are used for maintenance of anesthesia. Anesthesia could also be maintained with a balanced technique employing a narcotic, muscle relaxant, and nitrous oxide. Alfentanil may be the narcotic of choice in this age group.

The halothane should be discontinued 5 to 10 minutes prior to the end of surgery. After the dressings are in place, the atracurium should be reversed with neostigmine, 0.07 mg/kg, and atropine, 0.03 mg/kg and the patient extubated when fully reactive.

REFERENCES

1. Graff TD, Holzman RS, Benson DW: Acid–base balance in infants during halothane anesthesia with the use of an adult circle-absorption system. *Anesth Analg* 1964; 43(5):583–589.
2. Robertson RE, Kaplan RF: Another site for the pulse oximeter probe. *Anesthesiology* 1991; 74:198.
3. Zablocki AD, Rasch DK: A simple method to prevent interference with pulse oximetry by infrared heating lamps. *Anesth Analg* 1987; 66:915.
4. Cook DR, Marcy JH: Pediatric anesthetic pharmacology, in Cook DR, Marcy JH, eds: *Neonatal anesthesia,* California, 1988, Appleton Davies, Inc.
5. Killian A, Davis PJ, Stiller RL, et al: Influence of gestational age on pharmacokinetics of alfentanil in neonates. *Dev Pharmacol Ther* 1990; 15:82–85.

19

Muscle Biopsy

A 5-month-old, 5-kg boy is scheduled for a quadriceps muscle biopsy. The child is hypotonic, and the presumed diagnosis is Werdnig-Hoffmann disease. Hemoglobin, 11 g/dL; hematocrit, 33%.

Recommendations by Helen W. Karl, M.D.

Severe type I spinal muscular atrophy (SMA) of childhood, often known as Werdnig-Hoffmann disease, is a degenerative lower motor neuron disorder that results in rapidly progressive skeletal muscle weakness. It is inherited as an autosomal recessive abnormality of chromosome 5q,[1] which changes neurofilament metabolism, thereby causing degeneration of anterior horn cells in spinal cord and brain stem motor nuclei.[2]

SPINAL MUSCULAR ATROPHY

SMA is currently the most common cause of infant mortality due to an inherited disease. Recent advances in genetic mapping now allow prenatal diagnosis; thus, the number of infants born with this disorder is likely to decrease.[1] SMA type I is distinguished from the related disorders SMA types II and III on the basis of severity and age of onset; all three forms are probably due to different mutations at the same gene locus.[1]

SMA must be differentiated from other conditions that cause generalized hypotonia in infants: primary central nervous system (CNS) diseases and motor unit disorders. The latter category includes other less common anterior horn cell disorders, defects in presynaptic or postsynaptic neuromuscular transmission, and myopathies.[3] No study of anesthetic management of infants with Werdnig-Hoffmann disease has been reported; thus, the recommendations outlined below are based on medical descriptions of the disease[4-6] and on extrapolation from what is known about the anesthetic management of patients with related diseases.[7]

Infants with severe SMA are often noted to have generalized weakness at birth; in fact, careful questioning of the mother may reveal that she noticed a decrease in the strength of fetal movements as gestation progressed. Some infants with the disorder appear completely normal at birth. In these patients, the illness presents in the first few months of life with an acute loss of strength or a more gradual progression of delayed development of motor skills, feeding problems, or respiratory insufficiency.[4-6] There may be a family history of muscle weakness, failure to thrive, or sudden infant death syndrome (SIDS).

Infants with severe SMA have decreased respiratory reserve due to muscle weakness, decreased fetal lung development,[4] and/or parenchymal compromise from chronic aspiration. Throughout their lives, they have frequent respiratory infections and usually die of respiratory failure during the first or second year.[5]

There is no medical treatment specific for SMA. However, increased understanding of secondary metabolic defects in SMA type II has led to the development of palliative treatments that may be extended to infants with SMA type 1.[8] Cloning the gene whose mutation is the basis for all SMAs and investigation of its product may soon allow even more specific approaches to therapy as well as an understanding of the neurobiological requirements for maintenance of neuronal integrity.

PREOPERATIVE EVALUATION

On physical examination, these infants appear alert due to preservation of facial and extraocular muscle activity, but they exhibit severe generalized weakness. This weakness affects axial muscles more than extremities and the proximal portions of lower extremities more than the distal arms. Deep tendon reflexes are absent.[5] Preoperatively, particular attention should be given to examination of the chest. In most infants with SMA, intercostal muscles are severely affected and the diaphragm is relatively spared. This results in a narrow upper thorax with plastic bowing of the ribs often described as a "bell-shaped" chest.[5, 9] On inspiration there may be intercostal retractions as well as paradoxical flattening of the chest and distension of the abdomen. The infants usually have a weak cry and an ineffective cough and may have associated bulbar weakness with difficulty in swallowing secretions.

Because of the decreased respiratory reserve, measurement of oxygen saturation while the infant is breathing room air is the most important form of preoperative evaluation beyond the history and physical examination. Oxygen saturation less than 95%, tachypnea greater than 40 breaths per minute, or a history of frequent respiratory infections should prompt a preoperative chest radiograph. In addition to evidence of pulmonary parenchymal problems, the chest x-ray may show thinning or bowing of the ribs.[9, 10] Electrocardiography (ECG) is not required preoperatively; cardiac muscle is unaffected by SMA, and the ECG is normal except for a fasiculation-induced tremor of the isoelectric line.[5] Laboratory examinations obtained during initial medical evaluation of these infants may include a plasma creatine kinase concentration that is usually normal.

Sensory and motor nerve conduction studies are usually normal in infantile SMA and serve to differentiate this disorder from peripheral neuropathies. Electromyographic (EMG) changes distinguish SMA from myopathies, muscular dystrophies, and abnormalities of neuromuscular transmission.[3] EMG is noninvasive and is the most sensitive indicator of SMA. Muscle biopsy is used to provide additional confirmation of the diagnosis.[3] Because of the anesthetic implications of this and other neuromuscular diseases and of the high specificity of EMG in diagnosing this particular disorder,[3] EMG results and interpretation should be available for review by the anesthesiologist prior to induction of anesthesia for muscle biopsy.

NEUROMUSCULAR BLOCKADE

There have been no reports describing experience with neuromuscular blocking agents in infantile SMA; however, the possibility of the more common complications of their administration, particularly hyperkalemia, prolonged paralysis, and malignant hyperthermia, must be considered. Severe succinylcholine-induced hyperkalemia leading to cardiac arrest has been reported in other degenerative diseases of motor neurons such as acute idiopathic anterior horn cell disease as well as in muscular denervation, paraplegia, and hemiplegia.[7] Administration of succinylcholine is therefore contraindicated in patients with Werdnig-Hoffmann disease, and the benefits of its administration should be considered carefully in any infant or child,[11] particularly those with a family history of neuromuscular disease or SIDS.

Patients with amyotrophic lateral sclerosis, a disease also characterized by progressive anterior horn cell degeneration, have been reported to have increased sensitivity to nondepolarizing neuromuscular blocking agents.[7] If relaxants of this type are used, reduced doses and careful monitoring should be employed. Of particular note is the importance of complete return of neuromuscular function prior to tracheal extubation because of the limited respiratory reserve and increased risk of aspiration of gastric contents in these patients.

Malignant hyperthermia is rare, particularly in infants. However, if the EMG has not been performed or has been misinterpreted and the infant in fact suffers from a myopathy or muscular dystrophy, those thought to have SMA could be at some increased risk for malignant hyperthermia if triggering agents are used.

REGIONAL ANESTHESIA

Because of the potential complications of neuromuscular blocking agents, a regional technique is preferred over general anesthesia for lower-extremity surgery in infants with SMA. Caudal epidural blockade is the technique of choice in these patients and has been described in detail elsewhere.[12] After application of monitors and placement of an intravenous catheter, 1 mL/kg of 0.25% bupivacaine is injected slowly into the epidural space. Conscious sedation with low concentrations of nitrous oxide administered by mask and/or with a sugar-dipped pacifier may be helpful in keeping the infant comfortable and still during the procedure. An acetaminophen suppository, 15 mg/kg, placed at the conclusion of the procedure will help to supplement analgesia as the effect of the block diminishes.

Blockade of the femoral nerve[12] with 0.3 mL/kg of 1% lidocaine, 0.5% bupivacaine, or a mixture of 0.5% lidocaine and 0.15% tetracaine may also be employed. The surgical site can be infiltrated with a local anesthetic; however, obtaining adequate analgesia without disruption of the muscle architecture is almost impossible.

GENERAL ANESTHESIA

If general anesthesia should be required due to failure of the block, atropine, 0.02 mg/kg, may be given orally, intravenously, or intramuscularly prior to induction. It is particularly useful if the infant has a history of difficulty in swallowing secretions. An inhalation induction is performed and tracheal intubation accomplished with deep halothane anesthesia. The administration of neuromuscular blocking agents is unlikely to be necessary to allow tracheal intubation or prevent laryngospasm. However, deep anesthesia is essential prior to laryngoscopy. Ventilation may be assisted or controlled to prevent fatigue and atelectasis during the operative procedure. At the conclusion of the procedure, infants who maintain adequate oxygen saturation and who are awake and breathing as well as they were preoperatively may be extubated in the operating room.

Positioning difficulties due to the presence of muscle contractures must be considered during any discussion of the anesthetic management of patients with neuromuscular diseases. However, contractures in patients with Werdnig-Hoffmann disease are usually mild[5] and should not be a particular problem during this short procedure.

Fluid administration should include Ringer's lactate solution at a rate sufficient to replace the preexising fluid deficit, 4 mL/kg/hr multiplied by the hours with nothing to eat or drink. Adequate hydration may help prevent inspissation of secretions and decrease the risk of postoperative respiratory complications. An appropriate amount of dextrose should be added, depending on the measured blood glucose.

The risk of a lack of monitoring for postoperative weakness or apnea if the infant is sent home must be balanced against the risk of additional exposure to hospital-acquired respiratory infection. Earlier return to the preoperative level of function as well as postoperative analgesia from the residual block are advantages of regional anesthetic techniques.

An infant presenting for anesthesia for muscle biopsy to confirm a diagnosis of Werdnig-Hoffmann disease has a severe muscle disorder with no sensory deficit. Every effort must be made to keep this infant comfortable during what is likely to be a very brief life.

REFERENCES

1. Melki J, Sheth P, Abdelhak, S, et al: Mapping of acute (type I) spinal muscular atrophy to chromosome 5q12-q14. The French Spinal Muscular Atrophy Investigators. *Lancet* 1990; 336:271–273.
2. Murayama S, Bouldin TW, Suzuki K: Immunocytochemical and ultrastructural studies of Werdnig-Hoffmann disease. *Acta Neuropathol (Berl)* 1991; 81:408–417.
3. Jones HR: EMG evaluation of the floppy infant: Differential diagnosis and technical aspects. *Muscle Nerve* 1990; 13:338–347.
4. Bertini E, Gadisseux JL, Palmieri G, et al: Distal infantile spinal muscular atrophy associated with paralysis of the diaphragm: A variant of infantile spinal muscular atrophy. *Am J Med Genet* 1989; 33:328–335.
5. Dubowitz V: Disorders of the lower motor neurone, in *Major Problems in Clinical Pediatrics: Muscle Disorders in Childhood*. Philadelphia, WB Saunders Co, 1978, pp 146–190.
6. McWilliam RC, Gardner-Medwin D, Doyle D, et al: Diaphragmatic paralysis due to spinal muscular atrophy: An unrecognized cause of respiratory failure in infancy? *Arch Dis Child* 1985; 60:145–149.

7. Azar I: The response of patients with neuromuscular disorders to muscle relaxants: A review. *Anesthesiology* 1984; 61:173–187.
8. Harpey JP, Charpentier C, Paturneau-Jouas M, et al: Secondary metabolic defects in spinal muscular atrophy type II. *Lancet* 1990; 336:629–630.
9. Caro PA, Borden S: Plastic bowing of the ribs in children. *Skeletal Radiol* 1988; 17:255–258.
10. Giacoia GP: Imaging case of the month: Werdnig-Hoffmann disease. *Am J Perinatol* 1987; 4:271–272.
11. Delphin E, Jackson D, Rothstein P: Use of succinylcholine during elective pediatric anesthesia should be reevaluated. *Anesth Analg* 1987; 66:1190–1192.
12. Broadman LM: Regional anesthesia in the pediatric outpatient. *Anesth Clin North Am* 1987; 5:53.

20

Craniosynostosis and Apert Syndrome

A 6-month-old, 9-kg boy with craniosynostosis is scheduled for craniectomy. He also has bilateral syndactyly of the hands. Hemoglobin, 12.2 g/dL; hematocrit, 37%.

Recommendations by Robert E. Creighton, M.D.

Craniosynostosis results from premature fusion of cranial sutures. It may involve single, bilateral, or multiple sutures and may be part of a syndrome involving other anomalies. The bones of the calvarium arise from widely separated centers of ossification that spread centrifugally toward each other. The separation of adjacent bones is a result of expansion of underlying cranial contents and is compensated for by the addition of new bone at the suture edges. Premature fusion results in inhibition of the normal direction of growth of the neurocranial capsule.[1]

The incidence of craniosynostosis is approximately 1 in 2,000.[2] Premature fusion of the sagittal suture is the most common, and males are more often affected than females.[3] Other cranial sutures and multiple sutures are affected in fewer than half the cases.[4]

The incidence of involvement of the individual sutures is[4]:

Sagittal	56%
Single coronal	11%
Bilateral coronal	11%
Metopic	7%
Lambdoid	1%
Three or more	14%

There is a positive family history in as many as 39% of patients with craniosynostosis.[5] In those with both Crouzon syndrome, which consists of craniosynostosis, maxillary hypoplasia, shallow orbits, and proptosis, and Apert syndrome, in which these stigmata occur in association with syndactyly, the pattern of inheritance is autosomal dominant.[6]

Surgery for craniosynostosis is usually carried out in infancy. It may be necessary at a very early age if multiple sutures are involved and produce constriction of the brain. Additional advantages of early correction are that the bone is more malleable and the rapidly growing brain will assist in remodeling.[5] Four percent to 20% of patients will also have hydrocephalus. This complication is seen more commonly in patients with craniofacial syndromes than in those with isolated suture involvement.[7, 8]

Although it is possible that premature fusion of any cranial suture may coexist with bilateral syndactyly, the presence of these two abnormalities strongly suggests a complex syndrome, most likely Apert-type acrocephalosyndactyly.

Acrocephalosyndactyly can be subdivided into five types[4]:

Type I   Apert syndrome
Type II   Vogt cephalodactyly
Type III   Chotzen syndrome
Type IV   Waardenburg syndrome
Type V   Pfeiffer syndrome

Each subdivision has, as a common denominator, varying degrees of syndactyly of the hands and feet and an increase in the vertical diameter of the skull (oxycephaly or acrocephaly). The latter change is due to a progressive sequential combination of fusion of the coronal, sagittal, and lambdoid sutures that leads to a brachycephalic but also an oxycephalic head, a flat occiput and forehead, and hypertelorism. Differences among the types are often subtle. In all probability this child has Apert syndrome, the most common type of acrocephalosyndactyly.

APERT SYNDROME

The skull in patients with Apert syndrome is broad with a prominent, tall, bossed forehead and flat occiput.[9, 10] The supraorbital ridges are prominent, with a transverse groove above them across the forehead. The sinuses are underdeveloped. The eyes show an antimongoloid slant, exophthalmos, and hypertelorism, and the orbits are shallow. Strabismus may be present, as well as optic atrophy secondary to increased intracranial pressure or deformity of the optic canal. The nose is often small, short, broad, and beaked and the nasal bridge depressed. The maxilla is hypoplastic, and as a result, the mandible is relatively prognathic. Facial asymmetry is common. The palate is highly arched and constricted and may have a marked median furrow. The soft palate is excessively long in over half of the patients, and a cleft occurs in 30%. The deformities of the hands and feet are symmetrical. A middigital hand mass with osseous and soft-tissue syndactyly of digits 2, 3, and 4 is always found. Digits 1 and 5 may be joined to digits 2 and 4, respectively, or may be separate. Mental retardation and hydrocephalus may also be present.

ANESTHETIC CONSIDERATIONS

The operative procedure for a 6-month-old child with Apert syndrome consists of multiple craniectomies of fused sutures, forehead advancement, and reshaping of the cranial vault. The major areas of concern for the anesthesiologist are securing and maintaining the airway, preservation of brain function, blood loss and fluid replacement, and temperature homeostasis.

The primary purpose of preoperative assessment is to rule out respiratory infection and the presence of other congenital abnormalities. It is best to omit narcotic and sedative premedication; little can be gained from the psychological point of view, and respiratory depression could be dangerous. Atropine, 0.02 mg/kg, should be given intravenously during induction of anesthesia.

Because of the hypoplastic maxilla, small beaked nose, and long, high, arched palate, the nasal passages of these patients are narrow and often obstructed with secretions. The obstructed nasal passages make inhalation induction difficult until the child is anesthetized sufficiently to tolerate an oropharyngeal airway. On the other hand, the relative prognathism of the mandible is secondary to the hypoplasia of the maxilla and does not present a problem during endotracheal intubation. Therefore, intravenous thiopental, 4 to 5 mg/kg, followed by orotracheal intubation facilitated with succinylcholine, 1.5 mg/kg, is the preferred induction technique.

Either an armored or RAE preformed orotracheal tube should be used. If the child also has hydrocephalus, the administration of barbiturates will reduce the intracranial pressure at this critical time.[11] Lidocaine, 1.5 mg/kg administered intravenously, will attenuate the blood pressure response and protect against increases in intracranial pressure.[12, 13]

The tube position should be checked by auscultation, the lower lip padded with adhesive foam to prevent necrosis, and the tube securely taped in position. Nitrous oxide–oxygen and isoflurane, 1.0 MAC should be administered. The patient should then be mechanically hyperventilated and a large-bore intravenous catheter inserted.

MONITORING

Patient monitoring must be comprehensive.[14] In addition to noninvasive monitoring, an arterial cannula should be placed in a radial or dorsalis pedis artery. A urethral catheter is necessary for measuring urinary output. Arterial blood gas values and hematocrit readings should be determined hourly, serum electrolytes every 2 hours, and a coagulation profile as indicated. A central venous catheter, if suitably positioned, is of value in assessing fluid requirements. Although this operation is performed with the patient supine, there is still a risk of venous air embolism.[15] The precordial Doppler has been shown to be sensitive in detecting air embolism in children.[16] In this study, the incidence of hypotension associated with air embolism was 69% in pediatric patients as compared with only 36% in adults. Unfortunately, the authors also reported that attempts to aspirate air from a right atrial catheter were less successful in children.

MAINTENANCE OF ANESTHESIA

The child is positioned supine in a 10- to 15-degree reverse Trendelenburg position to aid venous return, and the head is placed on a padded Mayfield horseshoe headrest. All potential pressure areas should be padded with adhesive foam because the operation will last between 5 and 6 hours.

Anesthesia should be maintained with nitrous oxide–oxygen, isoflurane, and intermittent fentanyl, 0.002 mg/kg intravenously. A nondepolarizing muscle relaxant is administered, with the dosage being monitored by a nerve stimulator. Isoflurane increases cerebral blood flow at levels in excess of 1.1 MAC, but the increase is less than occurs with halothane,[17] and the intracranial pressure returns to control levels more rapidly after the establishment of hypocapnia.[18] At 1.0 MAC, isoflurane autoregulation appears to be preserved, but at higher concentrations, the cerebral vasculature becomes pressure passive.[19] At higher inspired concentrations, a decrease in cerebral metabolic rate for oxygen ($CMRo_2$) is also seen and may provide some measure of protection against an ischemic insult.[20] In addition, the relatively rapid elimination of isoflurane permits early postoperative neurologic assessment.

PRESERVATION OF BRAIN FUNCTION

The vault of the skull will be removed during surgery, and brain manipulation and retraction are unavoidable. Dexamethasone, 0.2 mg/kg, should be administered since there is evidence that steroid pretreatment reduces cerebral edema.[21] Furosemide, 1.0 mg/kg should be administered intravenously to reduce brain bulk. Controlled hyperventilation to produce an arterial Pco_2 of 25 to 30 mm Hg should be maintained throughout the operation and the level verified with arterial blood gas determinations. Because of the danger of retractor anemia, controlled hypotension should not be employed for this procedure.[22]

HEMOTHERAPY AND FLUID REPLACEMENT

Compared with the older child, the 6-month-old infant has a relatively larger circulating blood volume, a higher cardiac output, and poorer control over his capacitance vessels and peripheral vasoresistance. As a result, he is more dependent on cardiac output to maintain arterial blood pressure. A decrease in the circulating blood volume results in a reduction of systemic blood pressure earlier than it occurs in the older child. My practice is to withhold fluids until the systolic blood pressure falls to 75 to 80 mm Hg or a mean value of 60 to 65 mm Hg. Red blood cells mixed with an equal volume of 5% albumin should then be administered to maintain the arterial pressure at this level during the operation. Prior to closure, enough blood should be administered to return the systemic blood pressure to its preloss level. Ten percent of the estimated blood volume should usually be administered during closure of the scalp.

Urine should be collected and measured continuously. When the urine output equals 10% of the estimated blood volume following furosemide administration, further losses should be replaced with intravenous Ringer's lactate.

TEMPERATURE HOMEOSTASIS

Maintenance of normal body temperature is difficult during this operation. The brain, with 25% of the cardiac output, is continuously exposed to ambient temperature. Ideally the room temperature is kept at 24 to 27°C; however, the surgery is long and arduous. A reasonable compromise is a room temperature of 18 to 21°C. The patient, when exposed during preoperative preparations, should be placed on a covered heating blanket at 40°C and under an infrared heating lamp. A second heating blanket should also be placed over the patient. Inspired gases should be warmed and humidified and a blood warmer utilized.

EMERGENCE FROM ANESTHESIA

Isoflurane should be discontinued during the skin closure. After the dressings are in place, the FIo_2 should be increased to 1, and atropine, 0.025 mg/kg, followed by neostigmine, 0.05 mg/kg, or edrophonium, 1.0 mg/kg, should be administered. The child should be extubated awake.

COMPLICATIONS

The major intraoperative complication is hypotension due to blood loss, which can be avoided with careful monitoring and blood administration. A minor complication is bradycardia when the frontal lobes are retracted. If the cardiac output decreases, intravenous atropine, 0.01 to 0.02 mg/kg, should be administered.

The major postoperative complications are airway obstruction due to nasal obstruction, blood loss into the operative site, and sepsis. The first two require careful nursing care in an intensive care unit. Sepsis is a constant danger and can only be avoided by strict aseptic technique in the operating room.

REFERENCES

1. Moss ML: Functional anatomy of cranial synostosis. *Child Brain* 1975; 1:22.
2. Hockley AD, Wake MJ, Goldin H: Surgical management of craniosynostosis. *Br J Neurosurg* 1988; 2:307.
3. Till K: *Paediatric Neurosurgery*. Oxford, England, Blackwell Scientific Publications, 1975.
4. Harwood-Nash DC, Fitz DR: *Neuroradiology in Infants and Children,* vol 1. St Louis, Mosby–Year Book, 1976.
5. Marchac D, Renier D: Treatment of craniosynostosis in infancy. *Clin Plast Surg* 1987; 14:61.
6. Cohen MM Jr: An etiologic and nosologic overview of craniosynostosis syndromes. *Birth Defects* 1975; 11:137.
7. Golabi M, Edwards MSB, Ousterhout DK: Craniosynostosis and hydrocephalus. *Neurosurgery* 1987; 21:63.
8. Collman H, Sorensen N, Kraub J, et al: Hydrocephalus in craniosynostosis. *Child Nerv Syst* 1988; 4:279.

9. Gorlin RJ, Pindborg JJ, Cohen MM Jr: *Syndromes of the Head and Neck,* ed 2. New York, McGraw-Hill International Book Co, 1976.

10. Aita JA: *Congenital Facial Anomalies with Neurologic Defect.* Springfield, Ill, Charles C Thomas Publishers, 1969.

11. Shapiro HM, Galindo A, Wyte SR, et al: Rapid intraoperative reduction of intracranial pressure with thiopentone. *Br J Anaesth* 1973; 45:1057.

12. Bedford RF, Winn HR, Tyson G, et al: Lidocaine prevents increased ICP after endotracheal intubation, in Shulman K, et al (eds): *Intracranial Pressure,* ed 4. New York, Springer-Verlag NY Inc, 1980.

13. Abou-madi MN, Keszler H, Yacoub JM: Cardiovascular reactions to laryngoscopy and tracheal intubation following small and large intravenous doses of lidocaine. *Can Anaesth Soc J* 1977; 25:12.

14. Davies PRS: *Symposium on Diagnosis and Treatment of Craniofacial Anomalies,* vol 20. St Louis, Mosby–Year Book, 1979.

15. Harris MM, Strafford MA, Rowe RW, et al: Venous air embolism and cardiac arrest during craniectomy in a supine infant. *Anesthesiology* 1986; 65:547.

16. Cucchiara RF, Bowers B: Air embolism in children undergoing suboccipital craniotomy. *Anesthesiology* 1982; 57:338.

17. Eger EI II: Isoflurane: A review. *Anesthesiology* 1981; 55:559.

18. Adams RW, Cucchiara RF, Gronert GA, et al: Isoflurane and cerebrospinal fluid pressure in neurosurgical patients. *Anesthesiology* 1981; 54:97.

19. McPherson RW, Traystman RJ: Effects of isoflurane on cerebral autoregulation in dogs. *Anesthesiology* 1988; 69:493.

20. Newberg LA, Michenfelder JD: Cerebral protection by isoflurane during hypoxemia or ischemia. *Anesthesiology* 1983; 59:29.

21. Eisenberg HM, Barlow CF, Lorenzo AV: Effect of dexamethasone on altered brain vascular permeability. *Arch Neurol* 1970; 23:18.

22. Bennett MA, Albin MS, Bunegin L, et al: Evoked potential changes during brain retraction in dogs. *Stroke* 1977; 8:487.

21

Cystic Hygroma

A 6-month old, 6.2-kg boy is admitted for excision of a large cystic hygroma of the neck. The mass has been present for at least 3 months, but the parents refused to permit surgery. The child is in no respiratory distress despite a mass extending from the right ear to the shoulder (Fig 21–1). Hemoglobin, 12.1 g/dL; hematocrit, 36%.

Recommendations by Jean F. Harrington, M.D.

Cystic hygroma, also called hygroma colli and cystic or cavernous lymphangioma, is a histologically benign congenital tumor of lymphatic origin. Most commonly found in the neck alone, it occurs in other sites corresponding to primitive lymph sac locations such as the axilla, mediastinum, groin, and retroperitoneum. Endothelial membranes sprouting from embryonically sequestered lymph vessels form fibrillae that penetrate into surrounding normal tissues,[1] canalize, and produce large, multiloculated cysts filled with serous secretions.[2, 3]

Antenatal sonograms can alert obstetricians early to a need for cesarean section.[4] Fifty percent of cases are recognized at birth, and 90% appear before the age of 2 years. Showing neither racial nor sexual predilection, the tumor has been reported in association with Turner syndrome. In most instances, these infants appear deceptively asymptomatic despite the unwieldy neck mass.

PREOPERATIVE EVALUATION

The first step in preparing to anesthetize the infant with a cervical hygroma is to learn the extent of the tumor. Even in the absence of respiratory distress, cough, tachypnea, retractions, or stridor,[5] a physical examination should be made for oral and thoracic[6] extension of the tumor. A history of feeding problems or an attenuated cry should lead to inspection of the mouth, tongue, and glottis for distortion of the glottis or for single vocal cord paralysis. To assess mediastinal widening and tra-

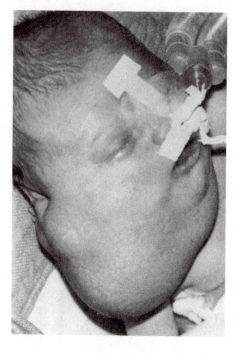

FIG 21–1.
Child with cystic hygroma of the neck. (Courtesy of Charles M.
Myer III, M.D., Department of Otorhinolaryngology, Children's
Hospital Medical Center, Cincinnati.)

cheal narrowing or displacement, a chest radiograph is essential. Should tumor be found in the mediastinum, further delineation is possible with fluoroscopy to check for changes in contour and mobility with respiration. Magnetic resonance imaging (MRI),[7] computerized axial tomography, and
sometimes angiography may aid in defining cardiopulmonary involvement and displacement. Careful evaluation of the trachea and mainstem bronchi is important to determine whether passage of the
endotracheal tube into the distal portion of the trachea or bronchus may be necessary to avoid airway obstruction during surgery.

Only after the extent of the tumor has been as well defined as possible should the child be
brought to the operating room for excision of the tumor. In rare cases, anesthesia for diagnostic
procedures such as MRI or laryngoscopy and bronchoscopy may be necessary. Excisions of combined cervicomediastinal masses are usually staged separately; the cervical approach should be done
first unless respiratory compromise necessitates single-stage excision.[8]

Except in cases of extreme prematurity or debilitation, operative treatment is indicated urgently
but nonemergently, with little merit in delay. There is possible danger in postponement because progressive growth in uninvolved areas decreases chances for complete excision. Infection or hemorrhage into the cyst may cause enlargement, respiratory embarrassment, and increased morbidity in
the previously asymptomatic infant.

ANESTHETIC MANAGEMENT

Induction of anesthesia in each case must be directed toward securing and maintaining the airway.[9] In a 6-month-old, 6-kg, otherwise asymptomatic infant, a controlled inhalation induction us-

ing nitrous oxide–oxygen and halothane following atropine, 0.02 mg/kg administered intramuscularly 45 minutes preoperatively, offers several advantages. Airway maintenance and ease of assisted ventilation can be assessed readily as muscle tone gradually diminishes as the patient falls asleep. An assistant may more easily place two large-bore intravenous catheters in the quiet patient. Spontaneous ventilation can be maintained for laryngeal inspection. Once an intravenous catheter is inserted, oral and then nasal intubation can be accomplished. In cases of glottic and tracheal displacement by tumor, maintenance of spontaneous ventilation is important for unobstructed positioning of the endotracheal tube. A stylet in the endotracheal tube, a lighted stylet, a Bullard laryngoscope, or a fiber-optic bronchoscope may aid the facile anesthesiologist in the rare case of difficult intubation. Tracheostomy is rarely necessary to secure the airway at this stage. The endotracheal tube should be taped securely to withstand changes in head position during the operation.

Tedious dissection of tumor from major blood vessels with the potential for rapid blood loss, constant weeping of fluid from the hygroma complicating the estimation of blood loss, "third-space" losses in the small patient, and possible hampering of gas exchange during the freeing up of the tumor displacing the trachea all dictate the need for placement of an intra-arterial catheter. Serial hematocrits are used to guide blood replacement, and measurement of systemic arterial blood pressure and arterial blood gases is also possible. Other necessary monitors include a pulse oximeter, capnograph, electrocardiograph (ECG), rectal temperature probe, and Foley catheter to collect the desired 1 mL/kg/hr urine output. The ability to heat the operating room itself as well as a thermal blanket beneath the baby on the operating room table helps to maintain the infant's temperature during prolonged cervicothoracic dissection.

Maintenance of spontaneous ventilation with nitrous oxide–oxygen and halothane throughout the operation instantly alerts the anesthesiologist to changes in respiratory compliance with manipulation of the tumor. Vigilant assessment of fluid loss is essential because halothane may contribute to lowering of the blood pressure. Use of muscle relaxants and controlled ventilation should be weighed individually in view of the tumor extent, the patient's reaction to halothane, and the course of the operation. Repeat doses of atropine during a long procedure are warranted to prevent bradycardia associated with surgical manipulation of the carotid sinus or vagus nerve.

The degree of difficulty of tumor resection from the trachea and phrenic, recurrent laryngeal, and superior laryngeal nerves and the overall extent of the tumor dictate postoperative airway management. If the tumor extends into the chest, there is a risk of pneumothorax. Extension into the floor of the mouth or larynx poses another set of airway problems. Awake extubation is possible following easy extirpation of a solitary cyst; but a wait-and-see approach is wise in most cases. Before wound closure in procedures characterized by compromise of the tracheal lumen and precarious endotracheal tube positioning, tracheostomy is indicated. Postoperative care in a recovery room or intensive care setting staffed by personnel competent in handling pediatric respiratory care is mandatory.

POSTOPERATIVE CARE

Attention to maintenance of respiration and adequate hydration to guard against inadvertent hypovolemia are the primary considerations in the first postoperative hours. Patient arm restraints and secure taping of the nasotracheal tube should be ensured early, prior to tissue swelling. A chest x-ray will confirm nasotracheal tube position and rule out intrathoracic operative complications. Tissue edema often contributes to vocal cord and swallowing dysfunctions and to the inability to clear secretions for several days. Prolonged nasotracheal intubation with humidified air or supplemental oxygen, if indicated, is usually well tolerated. The mechanics of respiration should be observed while waiting for tissue edema to diminish; then extubation can be accomplished in a controlled manner by the anesthesiologist. The child should be observed in the intensive care unit for at least 24 hours after extubation.

Since an incompletely excised cystic hygroma may recur,[10] this infant may return for further procedures. In the case of recurrent laryngeal lesions, CO_2 laser excision has been used on a repetitive basis.[11, 12]

REFERENCES

1. Hausamen JE, Stolke D, Trowitzsch E: Diagnostic and therapeutic problems with an unusual congenital cystic hygroma of the orbit. *J Craniomaxillofac Surg* 1988; 16:89–92.
2. Ward PH, Harris PF, Downey W: Surgical approach to cystic hygroma of the neck. *Arch Otolaryngol* 1970; 91:508–514.
3. Goetsche E: Hygroma colli cysticum and hygroma axillare: Pathologic and clinical study and report of twelve cases. *Arch Surg* 1938; 36:394–479.
4. Phillips HE, McGahan JP: Intrauterine fetal cystic hygromas: Sonographic detection. *AJR* 1981; 136:799–802.
5. Maze A, Block E: Stridor in pediatric patients. *Anesthesiology* 1979; 50:132–145.
6. Moore TC, Cobo JC: Massive symptomatic cystic hygroma confined to the thorax in early childhood. *J Thorac Cardiovasc Surg* 1985; 89:459–462.
7. Chisin R, Fabian R, Weber AL, et al: MR imaging of a lymphangioma involving the masseter muscle. *J Comput Assist Tomogr* 1988; 12:690–692.
8. Grosfeld JL, Weber TR, Vane DW: One-stage resection for massive cervicomediastinal hygroma. *Surgery* 1982; 92:693–699.
9. Evans P: Intubation problem in a case of cystic hygroma complicated by a laryngotracheal hemangioma. *Anaesthesia* 1981; 36:696–698.
10. Myer CM III, Bratcher GO: Laryngeal cystic hygroma. *Head Neck Surg* 1983; 6:706–709.
11. Cohen SR, Thompson JW: Lymphangiomas of the larynx in infants and children. A survey of pediatric lymphangioma. *Ann Otol Rhinol Laryngol Suppl* 1986; 127:1–20.
12. Bagwell CE: CO_2 laser excision of pediatric airway lesions. *J Pediatr Surg* 1990; 25:1152–1156.

22

Arthrogryposis

An 8-month-old, 8-kg boy with quadrimelic arthrogryposis (Fig 22–1) is scheduled for a clubfoot repair. Hemoglobin, 13.2 g/dL; hematocrit, 36.5%.

Recommendations by Gopal Krishna, M.D.

The anesthetic care of a child with arthrogryposis is complicated for two reasons: arthrogryposis is a symptom rather than a disease, and there is a paucity of information relating to this entity in the anesthesia literature. In order to develop a logical anesthetic plan for a patient with arthrogryposis it seems reasonable to first provide an overview of arthrogryposis from an anesthesiologist's perspective.

ARTHROGRYPOSIS

Arthrogryposis multiplex congenita, also known as multiple congenital contractures,[1] refers to a physical finding of multiple joint contractures that are present at birth. The condition was first described in 1841,[2] and the term *arthrogryposis* was introduced in 1923.[1] Arthrogryposis is a rare condition with an incidence of 1 in 3,000 live births.[3] It has been found to be associated with more than 150 disease entities, and the list is continually expanding.[4]

On the basis of experimental animal studies and analysis of data from both retrospective and prospective human clinical studies, there is a consensus that arthrogryposis results from any disorder or condition that causes a decrease or failure of fetal movements, i.e., fetal hypokinesia or fetal akinesia, during certain critical periods of growth.[1, 3–5] Although pregnant women do not detect fetal movement until about the 16th to 18th week of gestation, ultrasonographic studies show movement of the head and trunk as early as the 7th week of pregnancy. The fetus moves continuously, and these movements seem to be necessary for normal growth of not only limbs and joints but also other organ systems.[1]

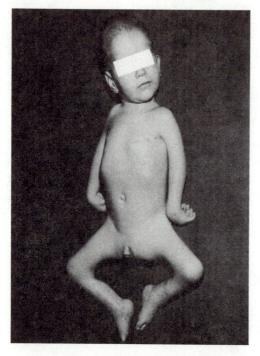

FIG 22–1.
An 8-month-old, 8-kg boy with quadrimelic arthrogryposis.

The majority of disorders that immobilize the developing embryo are neuromuscular in nature. The neuromuscular defect may be located in the central nervous system, peripheral nervous system, motor end plate, or muscle. However, other causes such as decreased intrauterine space have also been reported. The causes of decreased intrauterine fetal movement have been classified into four categories: neuropathic, myopathic, abnormal connective tissue or joints, and restrictive due to decreased space in which the fetus can move.[3]

Most commonly arthrogryposis is neurogenic in origin. In a series of 96 individuals with arthrogryposis, 94% were of neurogenic origin.[5] The neurogenic etiology in these individuals was related to developmental abnormalities such as dysgenesis of the brain and spinal cord with alterations in motor nuclei of the brainstem, anterior horns, and anterior roots. The exact cause for the development of the neurogenic defect is unknown. On the basis of experimental evidence, it is believed that a host of factors such as mitotic abnormalities, infection, mutagenic agents, and toxic chemicals or drugs can produce neuropathic defects.[1] Arthrogryposis of neurogenic origin is frequently associated with other congenital anomalies, with practically every type of congenital anomaly having been reported.[3] Some frequently associated anomalies are micrognathia (39%), congenital heart disease (23%), hypoplastic lungs (19%), cleft palate (11%), and scoliosis (12%).[5] Some of the associated anomalies are a direct result of muscle weakness during fetal life. As an example, since mandibular growth depends on facial movements, weakness of the muscles of mastication results in micrognathia.

Arthrogryposis of myopathic origin is infrequent, and represents only 6% of cases.[5] The disease entities include central core disease, congenital muscular dystrophy, nemaline myopathy, and myotonic dystrophy. Except for micrognathia and scoliosis, associated anomalies are rare. Myopathic defects often exhibit genetic patterns.

Alterations of the motor end plate can also result in arthrogryposis. In one case report, prolonged treatment of maternal tetanus with curare was reported to have resulted in the birth of a baby with arthrogryposis.[6] Experimentally, intravenous administration of curare to chick embryos has consistently resulted in the development of joint contractures.[7] Congenital myasthenia can also result in arthrogryposis.[8]

Finally, immobilization of the fetus that results in arthrogryposis can occur through decreased space such as that due to a bicornuate uterus, twin pregnancy, fibroid tumor, or oligohydramnios.[1] Since beyond 16 weeks of gestation the kidneys make a significant contribution to amniotic fluid, bilateral renal agenesis can cause oligohydramnios with resultant arthrogryposis.

CLINICAL PRESENTATION

The clinical presentation of arthrogryposis may vary from a few joint contractures as the sole abnormality to multiple joint contractures in association with complex congenital anomalies incompatible with life. Prognosis has been related to the type of involvement.[3] Children with limb involvement only generally have good long-term survival and respond well to therapy. These children often require multiple orthopedic surgical procedures and probably constitute the largest group of patients with multiple congenital contractures requiring anesthesia care. The prognosis for patients with involvement of the trunk, craniofacial structures, or viscera is primarily related to the specific diagnosis rather than to joint contractures. In the group with limb involvement and central nervous system dysfunction, 50% of the children do not survive beyond the first year of life.

Since arthrogryposis can be associated with disease entities that are diverse in nature, these patients require extensive clinical and laboratory evaluation to confirm or exclude a specific diagnosis. A team approach is recommended. In addition to a general pediatrician, the team should include a neurologist, geneticist, psychiatrist, pulmonologist, and orthopedic surgeon.[3] Furthermore, since cardiac, otolaryngologic, and ophthalmic involvement are not uncommon, consultation with specialists in these fields may be necessary.

PREOPERATIVE EVALUATION

From the foregoing discussion it is apparent that any patient with arthrogryposis requires very careful evaluation since the myriad of congenital anomalies that are associated with it may profoundly influence anesthesia care. In the absence of a specific diagnosis it must be remembered that arthrogryposis is related to muscle dysfunction and is associated with a high incidence of micrognathia and congenital heart disease,[5] factors that may necessitate modification of the anesthetic technique. Consequently, preanesthetic evaluation must focus on the airway, cardiac function, and neuromuscular status.

EVALUATION OF NEUROMUSCULAR STATUS

In addition to the clinical history and physical examination, the neuromuscular status may be evaluated by measurement of serum creatine kinase (CK) levels, electromyography (EMG), and muscle biopsy. The CK level is elevated in degenerative muscular disorders. The EMG allows differentiation between normal and abnormal muscle and distinguishes between the myopathic form and the neuropathic form of abnormality. Histologic, histochemical, and electron microscopic studies on a muscle biopsy specimen allow a definite diagnosis of muscle disorders.

MUSCLE RELAXANTS AND NEUROMUSCULAR DISEASE

Patients with neuromuscular disorders have an altered response to both depolarizing and nondepolarizing muscle relaxants.[9] Since a number of neuromuscular disorders are associated with malignant hyperthermia (MH), information regarding whether the muscle is normal, neuropathic, or myopathic is significant for anesthesia care.

Histologic studies have demonstrated a deficiency of anterior motor horn cells in a number of patients.[5] It is, however, not known whether the changes in anterior motor horn cells result in denervation injury or upregulation of acetylcholine receptors in muscle. Since hyperkalemia in response to succinylcholine is a known hazard in patients with upper and lower motor neuron disease,[10] it is prudent to avoid succinylcholine administration in patients with arthrogryposis. Muscle relaxation, if required, can be safely accomplished with atracurium, vecuronium, or mivacurium.

In approximately 6% of patients, arthrogryposis has a myopathic etiology. Administration of succinylcholine to patients with myopathies can result in hyperkalemia, contracture, and myoglobinuria; consequently, succinylcholine should be avoided. Patients with myopathies are sensitive to nondepolarizing muscle relaxants, but these drugs, especially atracurium and vecuronium, can be used safely if neuromuscular function is monitored.

ARTHROGRYPOSIS AND MALIGNANT HYPERTHERMIA

MH-like episodes have been reported in patients with a variety of neuromuscular disorders including Duchenne muscular dystrophy, central core disease, King syndrome, myotonia congenita, myotonic dystrophy, fascioscapulohumeral dystrophy, and limb-girdle dystrophy. The strongest correlation in this group is with central core disease, an autosomal dominant myopathy of varying clinical severity.[11, 12] Patients with this disorder have had a high percentage of positive contracture test results for MH susceptibility as well as clinical episodes of MH. These patients should thus be considered MH susceptible. Patients with Duchenne muscular dystrophy have had adverse reactions to anesthesia that have been thought to be MH,[13, 14] and indeed contracture test findings for MH have occasionally been positive.[15, 16] However, a recent report suggests that patients with muscular dystrophy may exhibit false-positive contracture test results due to type I skeletal muscle fiber predominance.[17] Additional evidence against this association comes from a study in which muscle contracture studies for MH were negative in a mouse model of Duchenne muscular dystrophy.[18]

It is not clear whether arthrogryposis per se increases the likelihood of MH. Several reports indicate the association of MH with arthrogryposis.[19-21] However, none of the patients underwent muscle biopsy for confirmation of MH by halothane-caffeine contracture testing. Two recent studies dispute the association of MH and arthrogryposis. In a review of 398 anesthetics that included triggering agents in 67 patients over a 32-year period, no complications were reported.[22] There are two case reports of temperature elevations in children anesthetized with MH triggering agents. In one case the 2-year-old male patient was assumed to have MH and was treated accordingly, and the procedure was canceled. Muscle biopsies were performed in both parents, but they tested negative by the halothane-caffeine contracture test. In the second case treatment with the triggering agent was discontinued, the fever was treated simply by cooling, and the anesthetic was continued with nontriggering agents. After several hours, the patient again developed hyperpyrexia and was again treated by cooling. During a subsequent anesthetic with nontriggering anesthetics 5 months later the patient again developed fever that was treated successfully by cooling. The authors concluded that the hypermetabolic response in patients with arthrogryposis is independent of the type of anesthetic and, unlike MH, it can be treated simply by cooling.[23] On the basis of this information, it would appear that there is no definite evidence for the association of arthrogryposis and MH. However, the possibility of the occurrence of MH or MH-like episodes cannot be completely excluded.

In patients with arthrogryposis, it is reasonable to use volatile anesthetics if indicated. Optimal monitoring to detect signs of development of a hypermetabolic state is essential.

ANESTHETIC MANAGEMENT

It is presumed that the 8-month-old boy with arthrogryposis has some degree of micrognathia but no other associated anomalies. Due to the presence of micrognathia and occasionally temporomandibular joint anomalies,[24] securing the airway with an endotracheal can be a challenge.

Intravenous access, if feasible, should be secured prior to induction of anesthesia. Atropine should be administered to reduce secretions and prevent vagally mediated bradycardia during airway manipulation.

Induction of anesthesia should be accomplished with halothane and oxygen. After attaining a deep level of anesthesia, laryngoscopy is performed and the trachea sprayed with 4% lidocaine (maximum dose, 4 mg/kg or 0.1 mL/kg of 4% lidocaine) to prevent laryngospasm. Halothane anesthesia is continued by mask for several additional minutes to ensure the anesthetizing effect of lidocaine on the vocal cords and trachea. A second laryngoscopy is performed for endotracheal intubation. If, during laryngoscopy for instillation of lidocaine into the trachea, the anesthesiologist is confident that the exposure is easy, endotracheal intubation can be facilitated with atracurium or vecuronium. Succinylcholine should be avoided. An alternate method of securing the airway is with the aid of a small dose of ketamine, 1 mg/kg administered intravenously,[25] and transtracheal block via the cricothyroid membrane with lidocaine. Transtracheal administration of lidocaine can be safely performed even in small infants and children. Finally, intubation can be performed with the aid of a fiber-optic bronchoscope. Other anesthetic considerations in this patient are similar to those for any pediatric patient.

Since patients with arthrogryposis are prone to develop a hypermetabolic state, mostly unrelated to MH, monitoring of end-tidal CO_2 is of special significance. Additional measures include maintenance of the neutral thermal environment and the administration of heated and humidified anesthetic gases. All fluids are administered with the aid of a precision infusion pump. Finally, during positioning, the arthrogrypotic patient should be padded adequately to prevent the occurrence of nerve injuries and fractures.

SUMMARY

Arthrogryposis has a complex heterogeneous etiology. Fetal hypokinesia or akinesia is the common denominator for the development of arthrogryposis. The patients should be carefully evaluated for the existence of associated anomalies. Congenital heart disease, micrognathia, and neuromuscular disease are common problems. Although the development of fever has been frequently observed in these patients, there is no convincing evidence for the association of arthrogryposis and MH. The use of volatile anesthetics is reasonable in patients with arthrogryposis. Adequate monitoring is essential.

REFERENCES

1. Swinyard CA, Bleck EE: The etiology of arthrogryposis (multiple congenital contracture). *Clin Orthop* 1985; 194:15–29.
2. Otto AW: A human monster with inwardly curved extremities. *Clin Orthop* 1985; 194:4–5.
3. Hall JG: Arthrogryposis. *Am Fam Physician* 1989; 39:113–119.
4. Hall JG: Genetic aspects of arthrogryposis. *Clin Orthop* 1985; 194:44–53.
5. Banker BQ: Arthrogryposis multiplex congenita: Spectrum of pathologic changes. *Hum Pathol* 1986; 17:656–672.
6. Jago R: Arthrogryposis following treatment of maternal tetanus with muscle relaxants. *Arch Dis Child* 1970; 45:277–279.
7. Drachman DB, Coulombre AJ: Experimental clubfoot and arthrogryposis multiplex congenita. *Lancet* 1962; 2:523–524.
8. Stoll C, Ehret-Mentre MC, Treisser A, et al: Prenatal diagnosis of congenital myasthenia with arthrogryposis in a myasthenic mother. *Prenat Diagn* 1991; 11:17–22.
9. Ellis FR: Inherited muscle disease. *Br J Anaesth* 1980; 52:153–164.
10. Fung D, White DA, Jones BR, et al: The onset of disuse-related potassium efflux to succinylcholine. *Anesthesiology* 1991; 75:650–653.
11. Brownell AKW: Malignant hyperthermia: Relationship to other diseases. *Br J Anaesth* 1988; 60:303–308.
12. Denborough MA, Dennett X, Anderson R: Central core disease and malignant hyperpyrexia. *Br Med J* 1973; 1:272–273.
13. Miller ED Jr, Sanders DB, Rowlingson JC, et al: Anesthesia-induced rhabdomyolysis in a patient with Duchenne's muscular dystrophy. *Anesthesiology* 1978; 48:146–148.
14. Seay AR, Ziter FA, Thompson JA: Cardiac arrest during induction of anesthesia in Duchenne muscular dystrophy. *J Pediatr* 1978; 93:88–90.
15. Brownell AKW, Paasuke RT, Elash A: Malignant hyperthermia in Duchenne muscular dystrophy. *Anesthesiology* 1983; 58:180–182.
16. Oka S, Igarashi Y, Takagi A, et al: Malignant hyperpyrexia and Duchenne muscular dystrophy: A case report. *Can Anaesth Soc J* 1982; 29:627–629.

17. Mitsumoto H, DeBoer GE, Bunge G, et al: Fiber-type specific caffeine sensitivities in normal human skinned muscle fibers. *Anesthesiology* 1990; 72:50–54.

18. Patel V, Dierdorf SF, Krishna G, et al: Negative halothane-caffeine contracture test in mdx (dystrophin-deficient) mice. *Metabolism* 1991; 40:883–887.

19. Honda N, Konno K, Itohda Y, et al: Malignant hyperthermia and althesin. *Can Anaesth Soc J* 1977; 24:514–521.

20. Oberoi GS, Kaul HL, Gill IS, et al: Anaesthesia in arthrogryposis multiplex congenital: Case report. *Can J Anaesth* 1987; 34:288–290.

21. Relton JE, Creighton RE, Johnston AE, et al: Hyperpyrexia in association with general anaesthesia in children. *Can Anaesth Soc J* 1966; 13:419–424.

22. Baines DB, Douglas ID, Overton JH: Anaesthesia for patients with arthrogryposis multiplex congenita: What is the risk of malignant hyperthermia? *Anaesth Intensive Care* 1986; 14:370–372.

23. Hopkins DM, Ellis FR, Halsall PJ: Hypermetabolism in arthrogryposis multiplex congenita. *Anaesthesia* 1991; 46:374–375.

24. Laureano AN: Severe otolaryngologic manifestations of arthrogryposis multiplex congenita. *Ann Otol Rhinol Laryngol* 1990; 99:94–97.

25. Defalque RJ: Ketamine for blind nasal intubation. *Anesth Analg* 1970; 50:984–986.

23

Prune Belly Syndrome

A 10-kg 10-month-old boy with prune belly syndrome is scheduled for circumcision, cystoscopy, and retrograde pyelography. Hemoglobin, 11 g/dL; hematocrit, 33%; BUN, 50 mg/dL.

Recommendations by J. Michael Badgwell, M.D.

Although the name prune belly syndrome has been given to this constellation of congenital anomalies, the deficient abdominal musculature that gives the "prune belly" appearance is only one manifestation of the primary abnormality: in utero urethral obstruction. Urethral obstruction malformation complex is a more appropriate name to describe the etiology and pathophysiology of this syndrome.[1, 2] Urethral obstruction may cause two significant derangements in utero: bladder distension and the oligohydramnios deformation complex. Bladder distension interferes mechanically with the development of surrounding tissues, producing the other characteristic alterations of prune belly syndrome that may be present in varying degrees: bladder wall hypertrophy, hydroureter (Fig 23–1), and associated renal dysplasia, abdominal distension leading to abdominal muscle deficiency, and excess skin (Fig 23–2), cryptorchidism, persistent urachus, chest deformity, lack of accessory muscles of respiration, colon malrotation, and iliac vessel compression leading to lower limb deficiency.[1, 2]

Because amniotic fluid is essential for pulmonary development,[3] inadequate fetal urinary output secondary to urethral obstruction, and the resultant oligohydramnios can lead to congenital pulmonary hypoplasia.[1] Oligohydramnios may also result in fetal compression causing limb defects and the so-called Potter facies, characterized by micrognathia and malformed ears and nose.[1]

The prune belly syndrome is rare; the incidence is estimated to be 1 in 50,000 births. The mortality rate may approach 50% before age 2 years, depending on the type and severity of abnormalities. Males are affected 20 times more often than females due to transmission by superficial X-link-

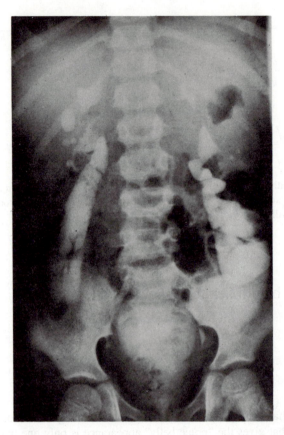

FIG 23–1.
Contrast media accentuates hydroureters in a child with prune-belly syndrome.

age mimicry.[4] Distinguishing features of in utero diagnosis by ultrasound include the presence of fetal ascites, distended bladder, and cystic masses, as well as maternal oligohydramnios.[5, 6] Fetal surgical decompression of urinary tract obstruction has been attempted.[7] While this procedure prevented abdominal wall laxity, it apparently was performed too late to prevent severe pulmonary and renal involvement.[7]

PREOPERATIVE EVALUATION

The anesthetic considerations for children with prune belly syndrome must focus on the renal and pulmonary systems.[8] The weak or absent abdominal muscles, chest deformity, outward flaring of the ribs, and lack of accessory muscles of respiration may lead to atelectasis, recurrent respiratory infection, and reduced expiratory effort. The infant with prune belly syndrome may have little or no ability to cough. Although elective surgery should be rescheduled if the child has a significant pulmonary infection, many of these children are never totally free of respiratory disease. Preoperative antibiotic treatment and chest physiotherapy may be indicated if surgery cannot be delayed.

Evaluation of the child's pulmonary status includes a careful history, physical examination, and

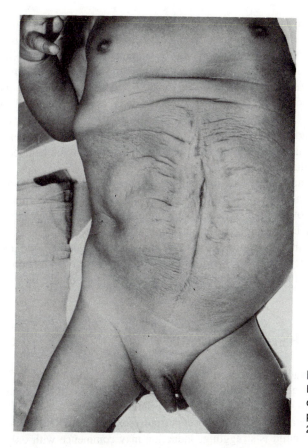

FIG 23–2.
Lax abdominal wall and excess skin producing the characteristic prune-belly appearance in the same child as Figure 23–1.

chest radiographs. Pulmonary function tests would be of limited accuracy and value in this child. The history and physical examination may reveal cyanosis, respiratory distress, fever, nasal flaring, cough, difficulty feeding, and wheezing. The chest radiographs may reveal poor inspiratory effort, changes consistent with a chronic disease such as peribronchiolar thickening, and acute changes indicative of an infectious process.

Preoperative evaluation of renal function will dictate NPO orders (nothing by mouth) and intraoperative fluid and electrolyte management. The BUN concentration of 50 mg/dL may reflect either dehydration or chronic renal insufficiency. Further evaluation of renal function including determination of serum electrolytes, creatinine, and urine specific gravity is indicated. With chronic obstructive nephropathy, the outer cortical nephrons are relatively spared and maintain their glomerular filtration rate, while juxtamedullary nephrons are markedly impaired.[9] As a result, the ability to concentrate urine may be lost and obligate urine flow results. The clinical implications of this type of renal tubular dysfunction and failure to reabsorb water and electrolytes may affect the anesthetic management. A history of polydipsia ("He drinks a lot"), constant voiding ("His diapers are always wet"), and dilute urine would suggest that tubular reabsorption is deficient. If so, the child may be dehydrated and at risk for further dehydration during the NPO interval. If the child is dehydrated, the case should be postponed until appropriate fluid replacement is administered. If the child's state of hydration is adequate, oral intake of clear fluids such as water, apple juice, or Pedialyte should be encouraged until three hours before the scheduled surgery.[10] If the child has renal tubular dysfunction, characterized by obligate urinary loss, IV fluids should be administered during the NPO interval to replace urinary loss and minimize dehydration. A maintenance fluid such as 5% dextrose in .25 normal saline should be administered at a rate of 4 mL/kg/hour. In the absence of renal disease, administration of IV fluids is not needed unless surgery is delayed or IV access is required for antibiotic administration.

A hemoglobin concentration of 11 g/dL with a hematocrit of 33% in a 10-month-old may indicate mild anemia, presumably due to renal disease. If the child is dehydrated, he may be hemoconcentrated and more anemic than these values indicate.

Preoperative sedation has been discouraged by previous authors for fear of respiratory depression.[11] Recently, the use of oral midazolam as a preoperative sedative has gained wide acceptance and is not associated with prolonged recovery or respiratory depression.[12] If this child were a few months older, separation anxiety might be a factor and midazolam, 0.5 mg/kg, could be given orally despite pulmonary involvement. This 10-month-old, however, may be managed appropriately without preoperative sedation. Anticholinergics can be administered IV at the time of induction. If urodynamic studies were planned, anticholinergic agents would be contraindicated because they can interfere with smooth muscle contraction.

ANESTHETIC TECHNIQUE

The ambient temperature in the operating room should be maintained at approximately 25° C and an infrared heating lamp placed 1 m above the child. The child's temperature is further maintained with a heating blanket set to 38° to 40° C and covered with a flannel blanket.

Preinduction monitors should include a precordial stethoscope, pulse oximeter, ECG, and noninvasive blood pressure. However, if the child is struggling, induction may commence with only a precordial stethoscope and the other monitors applied after the child becomes drowsy.

Anesthesia may be induced intravenously with a "butterfly" technique if an intravenous cannula is not in place, or an inhalation induction can be performed. The "butterfly" technique is accomplished using a 25- or 27-gauge butterfly needle inserted into a vein on the dorsum of the hand or the ventral aspect of the wrist. Thiopental, 6 mg/kg, atropine, 0.02 mg/kg, and succinylcholine, 2 mg/kg, are administered in rapid sequence. The child is ventilated briefly with 100% oxygen and then intubated with an endotracheal tube that permits a gas leak at 25 to 30 cm H_2O inspiratory pressure.

A traditional inhalational induction with halothane may be performed, especially if the anesthesiologist is more experienced with this technique. The child is allowed to breathe 70% nitrous oxide and 30% oxygen by mask. Halothane is increased 0.25% every 3 breaths until a concentration of 4% to 5% is inspired. Endotracheal intubation is performed when the depth of anesthesia is appropriate. Succinylcholine should be avoided after halothane because this combination of drugs may produce increased masseter muscle tone[13] and create the dilemma of interpreting masseter muscle rigidity and raise the question of malignant hyperthermia.[14] Either a Mapleson D (Jackson-Rees modification of the Ayre's T-piece or Bain circuit) or pediatric circle breathing system may be used.[15]

Anesthesia is maintained with 65% nitrous oxide with 35% oxygen and isoflurane, 0.5% to 2%, utilizing controlled ventilation. Intraoperative monitoring of airway pressure, tidal volume, end-tidal carbon dioxide (Pco_2) and pulse oximetry are indicated. If aspiration capnography and a Mapleson D circuit are used, gas for analysis of the end-tidal Pco_2 should be sampled from the endotracheal tube for accurate measurement.[16] Measurements of inspired and expired isoflurane are helpful, if available. A heat and moisture exchange device can be used to conserve heat and moisture in lieu of a cascade humidifier system.[17]

Muscle relaxants are not required because the abdominal musculature is lax. Avoiding muscle relaxants eliminates one possibility for postoperative hypoventilation. For the same reason, opioids should not be administered.

Intraoperative fluid management is dependent on fluid and electrolyte status and renal function. In the absence of renal disease or electrolyte imbalance, maintenance fluids can be continued at 4 mL/kg/hr and fluid deficits from the NPO interval replaced in the first hour of surgery.[18] Fluid loss related to surgery should be negligible in this case.

If a combined regional technique and general anesthesia is the clinician's preferred procedure for management of postoperative circumcision pain, it should not be withheld in this patient. An effective alternative to caudal or dorsal penile nerve block is the application of 2% lidocaine gel to the circumcision site.[19]

If this child has absent or minimal pulmonary involvement, he may be extubated at the end of the procedure in the operating room. However, if significant pulmonary pathology was present preoperatively, or if signs of pulmonary disease such as copius secretions, oxyhemoglobin desaturation, or poor compliance were evident intraoperatively, extubation should be delayed until the patient is vigorous and demonstrates adequate ventilatory exchange, both clinically and with pulse oximetry. After extubation, the child should be placed in a humidified hood or croup tent for 24 to 36 hours. If pulmonary involvement is significant, chest physiotherapy may be indicated.

REFERENCES

1. Pagon RA, Smith DW, Shepard TH: Urethral obstruction malformation complex: A cause of abdominal muscle deficiency and the "prune belly." *J Pediatr* 1979; 94:900–906.
2. Pramanik AK, Altshuler G, Light IJ, et al: Prune-belly syndrome associated with Potter (renal nonfunction) syndrome. *Am J Dis Child* 1977; 131:672–674.
3. Inselman LS, Mellins RB: Growth and development of the lung. *J Pediatr* 1981; 98:1–15.
4. Riccardi VM, Grum GM: The prune belly anomaly: Heterogeneity and superficial X-linkage mimicry. *J Med Gen* 1977; 14:266–270.
5. Garrett WJ, Kossof G, Osborn RA: The diagnosis of fetal hydronephrosis, megaureters, and urethral obstruction by ultrasonic echocardiography. *Br J Obstet Gynaecol* 1975; 82:115–120.
6. Bovicelli L, Rizzo N, Orsini LF, et al: Prenatal diagnosis of prune belly syndrome. *Clin Genet* 1980; 18:79–82.
7. Nagayama DK, Harrison MR, Chinn DH, et al: The pathogenesis of prune belly. *Am J Dis Child* 1984; 138:834.
8. Cramolini CM: Diseases of the renal system, in Katz J, Steward DJ (eds): *Anesthesia and Uncommon Pediatric Diseases,* Philadelphia, W.B. Saunders, 1987.
9. Wilson DR: Micropuncture study of chronic obstructive nephropathy before and after release of obstruction. *Kidney Int* 1972; 2:119–130.
10. Splinter WM, Scheffer JD, Zunder IH: Clear fluids three hours before surgery do not affect the gastric fluid contents of children. *Can J Anaesth* 1990; 37:498–501.

11. Hannington-Kiff JG: Prune-belly syndrome and general anesthesia. *Br J Anaesth* 1970; 42:649–652.

12. Feld LH, Negus JB, White PF: Oral midazolam preanesthetic medication in pediatric outpatients. *Anesthesiology* 1990; 73:831–834.

13. Van Der Speck AFL, Fang WB, Ashton-Miller JA, et al: The effects of succinylcholine on mouth opening. *Anesthesiology* 1987; 67:459–465.

14. Rosenberg H, Fletcher JE: Masseter muscle rigidity and malignant hyperthermia susceptibility. *Anesth Analg* 1986; 65:161–164.

15. Fisher DM: Anesthesia Equipment for Pediatrics, in Gregory GA, (ed): *Pediatric Anesthesia,* New York, Churchill Livingston, 1988.

16. Badgwell JM, McLeod ME, Lerman J, et al: End-tidal PCO_2 measurements sampled at the distal and proximal ends of the endotracheal tube in infants and children. *Anesth Analg* 1987; 66:959–964.

17. Bissonnette B, Sessler DI: Passive or active inspired humidification increases thermal steady-state temperature in anesthetized infants. *Anesth Analg* 1989; 69:783–787.

18. Berry FA: Practical Aspects of Fluid and Electrolyte Therapy, in Berry FA, (ed): *Anesthetic Management of Difficult and Routine Pediatric Patients,* New York, Churchill Livingstone, 1990.

19. Tree-Trakarn T, Pirazavaraporn S, Lertakyamanee J: Topical analgesia for relief of post-circumcision pain. *Anesthesiology* 1987; 67:395–399.

24

Radial Clubhand

A 12-month-old, 12-kg boy with bilateral radial clubhands is scheduled for first-stage correction of the right hand. His mother states that he has a heart murmur. Hemoglobin, 13.5 g/dL; hematocrit, 40%.

Recommendations by Richard S. Cartabuke, M.D.

The radial clubhand deformity, first described by Petit in 1733, characterizes the position of the hand as the result of the absence of radial support of the wrist (Fig 24–1). Although complete absence (aplasia) is the most common presentation, some patients exhibit a shortened but fully formed radius (hypoplasia) or a partially formed radius (partial aplasia). Bayne and Klug have classified the radial dysplasias into four categories based on their radiographic appearance (Fig 24–2).[1] The amount of clinical deformity is determined by the extent of the radial defect. Bilateral deformity appears in over 50% of patients who present with radial clubhand. Thumb dyplasias are almost uniformly present and range from hypoplasia to complete aplasia. There are also significant abnormalities of muscles, nerves, and joints that result in varying degrees of functional impairment.

The frequency of this defect is reported to be approximately 1 in 30,000 live births. There are a few examples of genetic transmission, but the condition is generally considered to occur sporadically. It is postulated that the cause of the deformity is a defect in the apical ectodermal ridge during formation of the upper limb buds between the fourth and seventh weeks of gestation.[2] During this time the rudiments of all the major organ systems are laid down, which accounts for the numerous anomalies that are associated with radial clubhand deformities. In Lamb's series, 40% of the cases were related to the use of thalidomide, and approximately 20% were linked to ingestion of some other medication during pregnancy. In the remaining cases no etiologic factor could be identified.[2]

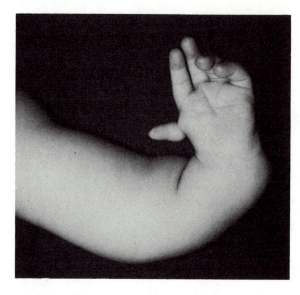

FIG 24–1.
Radial clubhand and deformity of the thumb.

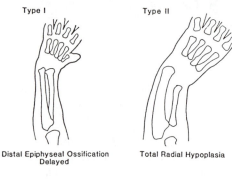

Type I   Type II

Distal Epiphyseal Ossification   Total Radial Hypoplasia
            Delayed

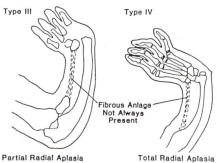

Type III   Type IV

Fibrous Anlage
Not Always
Present

Partial Radial Aplasia   Total Radial Aplasia

FIG 24–2.
Classification system for radial dysplasia. Type I: delayed ossification of the distal end of the radius. Adequate carpal support results in little radial deviation of the hand. Type II: hypoplasia of the entire radius secondary to defects of both the proximal and distal radial epiphyses. The ulna bows radially, and the carpus is unsupported. Type III: complete segmental aplasia of a portion of the radius, usually the distal portion. Type IV: complete radial aplasia. (From Urban MA, Osterman AL: *Hand Clin* 1990; 6:592. Used by permission.)

ASSOCIATED ANOMALIES

Radial clubhand is primarily associated with defects of the cardiovascular and genitourinary systems, but anomalies in virtually all major organ systems have been reported. The frequency and type of associated anomalies differ between patients whose radial defect is the result of thalidomide exposure and those where the etiology is idiopathic. The thalidomide-treated group exhibits a greater number of other limb deficiencies, particularly involving the lower extremities, while the idiopathic group more often has congenital cardiac lesions, including ventricular septal defect, the tetralogy of Fallot, coarctation of the aorta, and patent ductus arteriosus. Other anomalies associated with radial clubhand include renal agenesis, hydronephrosis, esophageal atresia, imperforate anus, encephalocele, hydrocephalus, and idiopathic scoliosis. Carroll and Louis noted that only 19% of their patients with radial deformities had no other defects; the remaining patients averaged 2.4 anomalies per child.[3]

There are four other distinct entities in which radial clubhand is a component: thrombocytopenia with absence of the radius (TAR syndrome), Fanconi anemia, Holt-Oram syndrome, and the VATER association.

TAR Syndrome

The TAR syndrome is a well described combination of amegakaryocytic thrombocytopenia and bilateral absence of the radii. Unlike other presentations, the thumbs and a full complement of digits are present bilaterally, although they may be hypoplastic. Additional abnormalities include those of the lower extremity, cow's milk allergy, eosinophilia, and cardiac defects. The majority of patients demonstrate an autosomal recessive pattern of inheritance.[4]

Thrombocytopenia can vary in severity and is usually precipitated by stress. Anemia in thrombocytopenic patients appears to be secondary to internal blood loss. Platelet transfusions may be required to prevent life-threatening intracranial hemorrhage or gastrointestinal bleeding. Since there is usually a progressive rise in the platelet count with normalization after the first year of life, orthopedic reconstruction should be deferred until the platelet count reaches an acceptable level. Platelet dysfunction and a prolonged bleeding time have been reported in patients with TAR syndrome who have normal platelet counts, but operative procedures have been undertaken with no hemorrhagic complications.

Fanconi Anemia

Chronic progressive pancytopenia (Fanconi anemia) is associated with radial defects. In contrast to the TAR syndrome, in which thrombocytopenia is evident from birth and resolves during the first year of life, hematologic manifestations associated with Fanconi anemia usually present in school-aged children. Patients tolerate their low blood values well but eventually require repeated transfusion as the disease slowly progresses. Therapy with androgenic steroids has proved beneficial; however, such treatment may produce signs of masculinization, and some testosterone preparations can cause hepatic toxicity. Individuals with Fanconi anemia may have associated genitourinary anomalies, microcephaly, microphthalmos, and mental retardation.

Holt-Oram Syndrome

The Holt-Oram, or heart-hand syndrome, is characterized by cardiac defects, primarily of the atrial and ventricular septum, and associated thumb, metacarpal, or radial abnormalities. It has an autosomal dominant pattern of inheritance.

VATER Association

The VATER association comprises vertebral or ventriculoseptal defects (V), imperforate anus (A), tracheoesophageal fistula with esophageal atresia (TE), and renal or radial abnormalities (R). These defects may occur in any combination and usually represent a sporadic pattern of inheritance.

SURGICAL CORRECTION

Bayne and Klug state that the ideal timing for initial surgical repair of the radial club hand is 6 months to 1 year of age. This allows for complete evaluation of other major system abnormalities, assessment of functional impairment, and adequate presurgical soft-tissue stretching.[1] If the reconstruction must be deferred because of underlying medical problems, excellent results can still be obtained if correction is achieved prior to 3 years of age. The major objective is a stable wrist with retention of good wrist motion. A secondary consideration is improvement of the cosmetic appearance of the arm by correcting the deviation of the hand and wrist. This is achieved by centralization of the carpus on the distal end of the ulna with requisite tendon transfers to preserve alignment. Pollicization of the index finger is indicated for aplastic or hypoplastic thumbs to improve grasp and maximize function. This procedure can usually be performed 6 months after centralization is accomplished.

PREOPERATIVE EVALUATION

A carefully conducted preoperative interview should focus on evidence of hematologic, cardiac, genitourinary, and gastrointestinal dysfunction. Important physical findings are pallor, bruising, bleeding, murmurs, and scoliosis. Preoperative assessment of the airway assumes particular importance since micrognathia has been associated with the TAR syndrome with frequencies as high as 60% and cleft lip and/or palate has been reported with Fanconi anemia.[1]

Laboratory evaluation should include a complete blood count, a platelet count, and where indicated, a bleeding time. If any abnormalities are noted, particularly thrombocytopenia or anemia, a preoperative hematology consultation should be obtained. If the child has received multiple transfusions, a blood type and screen are useful to determine the presence of significant antibodies.

The patient who presents at the time of surgery with a known cardiac defect or who has a newly diagnosed heart murmur should have a cardiac consultation prior to surgery. The consultant should describe the defect and its hemodynamic consequences, discuss previous medical therapy and/or surgical intervention as well as anticipated perioperative complications and recommendations for intervention, and finally, suggest orders for the dosage and timing of prophylaxis for bacterial endocarditis.

Other screening laboratory evaluations should be obtained if the history and physical examination suggest additional organ system impairment. For example, if renal problems are suspected, serum electrolyte, blood urea nitrogen (BUN), and creatinine levels should be determined. The presence of scoliosis may indicate the need for preoperative measurement of arterial blood gases and, if warranted, pulmonary function studies.

Preanesthetic medication should consist of an anticholinergic and, at the discretion of the anesthesiologist, a sedative/anxiolytic drug. Oral atropine in a dose of 20 µg/kg is an effective anticholinergic. A host of drugs have been used effectively in the pediatric population for sedation and anxiolysis; the choice should be guided by the preference and experience of the anesthesiologist.

INTRAOPERATIVE MANAGEMENT

The blood pressure cuff should be placed on the lower extremity to avoid potential damage to superficial and aberrant nerves of the upper extremity. If the blood pressure cuff must be placed on the nonoperative upper extremity, the arm should be wrapped with Webril to diminish the risk of compression injury to underlying nerves. Invasive monitoring will be dictated by the child's associated medical problems as well as the anticipated surgical requirements. An indwelling Foley catheter is indicated to help assess fluid management in procedures lasting for more than 2 hours. If invasive arterial monitoring is contemplated, the anesthesiologist must consider the abnormal vascular patterns associated with radial dysplasia: the radial artery is often missing, and blood supply in the hand may be carried entirely by the ulnar or persistent interosseous arteries.[5] Given the uncertainty of adequate collateral circulation, the upper extremity should not be cannulated. Suitable alternative vessels are the dorsalis pedis, posterior tibial, and femoral arteries.

The choice of anesthetic will depend on the presence of other major organ system involvement, particularly congenital heart disease. Significant cardiac compromise is an indication for a narcotic-muscle relaxant-oxygen anesthetic with postoperative mechanical ventilation and possible pharmacologic cardiovascular support. Actually, this scenario represents a very small fraction of patients who undergo radial clubhand correction. An inhalation induction with halothane-nitrous oxide-oxygen is usually satisfactory, although rectal methohexital, 25 mg/kg, is useful if the former approach appears inappropriate. Placement of an oral endotracheal tube is facilitated with the use of intratracheal or intravenous lidocaine and succinylcholine or an intermediate-acting neuromuscular blocking agent. Anesthesia can be maintained with halothane-nitrous oxide-oxygen. The judicious use of intraoperative narcotics toward the termination of the procedure allows a less stormy emergence and provides postoperative analgesia. If muscle relaxants are used, dosing should be guided by the response to train-of-four stimulation to maintain an 80% blockade. This will enable the surgeon to assess the integrity of neural function intraoperatively. Most patients can be extubated at the termination of the procedure and transported to the postanesthesia care unit for recovery.

POSTOPERATIVE CARE

The postoperative course is usually uncomplicated, but the anesthesiologist should be aware of two potential problems: postoperative neuropathy and vascular insufficiency secondary to limited collateral flow.

The median nerve travels along the forearm in an aberrant and unpredictable course, becomes quite superficial in the wrist region,[5] and is easily injured with the initial surgical incision. Since the radial nerve distal to the elbow is absent, its sensory fibers are carried in the median nerve. Therefore, any damage to the median nerve can cause extensive impairment.

Vascular insufficiency may be caused by direct injury to arterial structures or, more commonly, is the result of excessive tension on the vascular bed after transposition of the ulna. Vascular insufficiency may possibly be ameliorated with sympathetic blockade. Audenaert et al. recently reported that an infant who received an axillary block with bupivicaine showed clinical improvement of the ischemic hand.[6] When employed, this procedure should always be performed with a nerve stimulator to guide the location of the needle tip due to the unpredictable course of neurovascular structures in the upper extremity. An additional benefit of axillary blockade is prolonged postoperative analgesia. It remains to be seen whether the use of regional techniques improve operative results.

SUMMARY

There will undoubtedly be refinements in the surgical approach to the correction of radial club-hand. The use of vascularized fibular epiphyseal transfer or limb lengthening with an external fixator device may improve treatment outcomes.[2] An awareness of the myriad number of clinical presentations allows the anesthesiologist to plan appropriate strategies for the care of these often challenging patients.

Acknowledgements

The author would like to thank J. David Martino, M.D., and Louise O. Warner, M.D., for their suggestions in the preparation of this manuscript.

REFERENCES

1. Bayne LG, Klug MS: Long-term review of the surgical treatment of radial deficiencies. *J Hand Surg [Am]* 1987; 12:169–179.
2. Lamb DW: Radial club hand: A continuing study of sixty-eight patients with one hundred and seventeen club hands. *J Bone Joint Surg [Am]* 1977; 59:1–13.
3. Carroll RE, Louis DS: Anomalies associated with radial dysplasia. *J Pediatr* 1974; 84:409–411.
4. Hedberg VA, Lipton JM: Thrombocytopenia with absent radii: A review of 100 cases. *Am J Pediatr Hematol Oncol* 1988; 10:51–64.
5. Urban MA, Osterman AL: Management of radial dysplasia. *Hand Clin* 1990; 6:589–605.
6. Audenaert SM, Vickers H, Burgess RI: Axillary block for vascular insufficiency after repair of radial club hands in an infant. *Anesthesiology* 1991; 74:368–370.

25

Atrioventricular Canal and Trisomy 21

A 10-month-old girl with a complete atrioventricular canal is scheduled for open heart surgery during which profound hypothermia and circulatory arrest will be employed. The child also has Down syndrome. She has had frequent upper respiratory tract infections but appears asymptomatic at this time. Weight, 7 kg; hemoglobin, 16 g/dL; hematocrit, 48%.

Recommendations by Jeffrey P. Morray, M.D.

Trisomy 21, or Down syndrome, is the most common chromosomal abnormality, with an incidence of 1 in every 700 to 1,000 live births.[1] The incidence of congenital heart disease in Down syndrome is approximately 40%,[2] with atrioventricular canal defects accounting for between 40% and 60% of the lesions.[2-4]

ATRIOVENTRICULAR CANAL DEFECTS

Complete atrioventricular canal defects result from failure of fusion of the central portions of the anterior and posterior endocardial cushions (Fig 25–1), and this results in a defect of the central lower portion of the atrial septum, a ventricular septal defect in the posterior portion of the septum, and abnormalities in the development of the mitral and tricuspid valves (Fig 25–2). These defects typically result in shunting of blood in a direction that is determined by the relationship between the outflow resistances of the left and right ventricles. When pulmonary vascular resistance is lower than systemic resistance, left-to-right shunting occurs; the magnitude of the shunt increases as the ratio of pulmonary to systemic vascular resistance decreases. Left-to-right shunting results in an increased volume load to the left ventricle and an increased pressure and volume load to the right

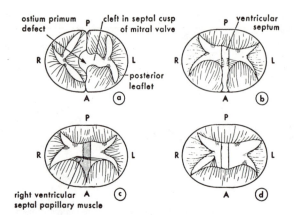

FIG 25—1.
Diagram of atrioventricular valves in different forms of atrioventricular canal defects: **A,** ostium primum defect or partial atrioventricular canal with a cleft in the anterior or septal leaflet of the mitral valve. **B,** complete atrioventricular canal with separation of the anterior endocardial cushion into distinct mitral and tricuspid portions and chordae attached to the upper portion of the ventricular septum. **C,** complete atrioventricular canal with only partial separation of the anterior cushion and chordae extending from the mitral component across the ventricular septal defect to the right ventricular papillary muscle. **D,** complete atrioventricular canal with no separation of the anterior and posterior cushions.

ventricle. Within the first 2 to 3 months of life, signs of congestive heart failure are evident. In those patients with atrioventricular valve dysfunction, symptoms develop early in infancy and are usually severe.

Exposure of the pulmonary vascular bed to high pressure and flow over time results in obliterative pulmonary vascular disease from medial muscular thickening and intimal proliferation. There has been some suggestion that children with Down syndrome have a propensity for early development of pulmonary vascular obstruction.[5, 6] In fact, early pulmonary hypertension has been reported in some children with Down syndrome without significant cardiac lesions.[2, 7] Early corrective surgery is generally recommended to prevent the development of increased pulmonary vascular resistance. In the extreme this is termed the Eisenmenger complex, in which pulmonary vascular resistance exceeds systemic resistance, shunting becomes right to left, and cyanosis ensues. At this point, patients are no longer surgical candidates because closure of the septal defect often results in right ventricular decompensation from pressure overload.

DOWN SYNDROME

Patients with Down syndrome and an atrioventricular canal present significant surgical risk. In one series, the mortality rate was 50% for patients less than 3 months of age and 17% for patients at 12 months.[8] Another group reported a mortality rate of 52% for all patients with Down syndrome and an atrioventricular canal, as compared with 20% for those with a simple ventricular septal defect.[9] In addition, perioperative morbidity appears to be higher in patients with Down syndrome vs. those without Down syndrome who have similar cardiac lesions, including a higher incidence of atelectasis and pulmonary edema and a longer requirement for mechanical ventilation, intensive care, and hospitalization.[10] The reasons for the increased risk for these patients is unclear but may include their higher pulmonary artery pressures,[10] alveolar hypoplasia,[11] and altered cellular immune function.[12] In spite of these perioperative risks, surgical repair is now preferred to long-term medical treatment. In one series, the 20-year survival rate was 69% in patients treated surgically as compared with 31% in the patients treated medically.[4]

Down syndrome is associated with a number of other abnormalities; the most significant from

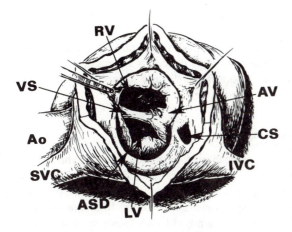

FIG 25–2.
Surgeon's view of the complete atrioventricular canal following incision of the right atrium as though he were looking through the atrioventricular valve *(AV)* into the right and left ventricular cavities *(RV, LV)*, which are separated by the ventricular septum *(VS)*. Also shown are the aorta *(Ao)*, superior vena cava *(SVC)*, ostium primum atrial septal defect *(ASD)*, inferior vena cava *(IVC)*, and coronary sinus *(CS)*.

the perspective of the anesthesiologist relate to airway management. The neck is short, and the tongue is large in relation to the size of the oral cavity. Atlantoaxial instability occurs in approximately 6% of patients.[13]

PREOPERATIVE EVALUATION

The history focuses on signs and symptoms that relate to the physiologic consequences of the cardiac disease. When congestive heart failure (CHF) (Table 25–1) occurs at an early age, especially if the symptoms are severe, the child is likely to be more compromised. The child with CHF may be treated with digitalis and diuretics, so a medication history is elicited. A history of cyanosis is suggestive of increased pulmonary vascular resistance and right-to-left shunting. Severe CHF in infancy is sometimes treated palliatively with a band placed on the pulmonary artery; thus, a question about previous cardiac surgery is appropriate.

It is also important to ask about the child's general medical condition. For example, how frequent have the upper respiratory infections been? Has she ever been hospitalized for an infectious process? When was the most recent episode? Any evidence of an acute upper or lower airway infection should be considered a contraindication to all but the most emergent of procedures. Respi-

TABLE 25–1.

Signs and Symptoms of Congestive Heart Failure

Tachypnea
Grunting
Nasal flaring
Intercostal retractions
Poor feeding, failure to thrive
Pallor, diaphoresis
Irritability

ratory syncytial virus (RSV) infection is potentially lethal in the child recovering from open heart surgery.

The presence of shunting at the atrial or ventricular level places the child at risk for central nervous system embolization, so a question about focal neurologic deficits is appropriate. Questions concerning allergies, previous response to anesthetics, and a family history of problems with anesthesia complete the history.

Physical Examination

Much can be gained from observing the general appearance of the child, including the state of nutrition, respiratory pattern, and skin color. The height, weight, heart rate and rhythm, blood pressure in the right arm and a lower extremity, respiratory rate, and temperature are noted. Appropriate weight for age must be adjusted in the child with Down syndrome. For a normal 10-month-old, 7 kg represents less than the 5th percentile.[13] However, for a 10-month-old with Down syndrome, 7 kg represents the 50th percentile (Developmental Evaluation Clinic, Boston Children's Hospital).

The airway is examined in order to anticipate potential difficulty with intubation; the size of the tongue and configuration of the neck are important.

The chest is auscultated for quality of breath sounds. Rales and wheezing are not uncommon in the child with CHF. The precordium is palpated to detect the point of maximum impulse as well as the presence of thrills. A point of maximum impulse shifted to the left of the midclavicular line suggests left ventricular hypertrophy, while a hyperdynamic epigastric impulse suggests right ventricular hypertrophy. Typical heart sounds in the patient with an atrioventricular canal include a first heart sound accentuated at the upper left sternal border; a loud second heart sound at the upper left sternal border, which may be split if there is a left-to-right atrial shunt; a loud, rough holosystolic murmur at the lower left sternal border that radiates throughout the precordium; and a middiastolic low-frequency murmur at the apex. If atrioventricular valve regurgitation is present, a second holosystolic murmur may be heard at the left sternal border that radiates to the right parasternal region.

The abdomen is palpated, with particular attention to the size of the liver, which is often increased in patients with right heart failure. Careful assessment of distal extremity warmth, color, pulses, and capillary refill yields information about the integrity of peripheral perfusion. Cool, pale extremities with poor pulses and slow capillary refill suggest either depletion of intravascular volume or myocardial failure. The presence of collateral pulses is confirmed in the extremity in which the arterial cannula will be placed. A brief neurologic examination is performed to rule out focal neurologic deficits and establish a preoperative baseline.

Laboratory Evaluation

Marked left-axis deviation is often seen by electrocardiography (ECG), with an axis in the -90 to -150 degree range. A prolongation of atrioventricular conduction is suggested by an increased PR interval. A complete right bundle-branch block may also be present, and varying degrees of both left and right ventricular hypertrophy are common (Fig 25–3). The chest radiograph usually reveals that the heart is enlarged, with both ventricles contributing. The main pulmonary artery segment is large, and pulmonary arterial markings are prominent (Fig 25–4). Right atrial enlargement is common. The vascular markings may be hazy due to pulmonary edema.

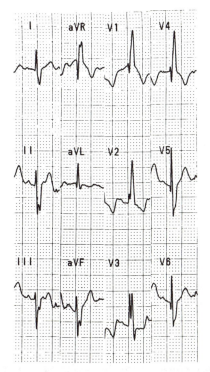

FIG 25–3.
Preoperative electrocardiogram in a 10-month-old child with
Down syndrome and a complete atrioventricular canal. Abnormalities include a superior axis, right bundle-branch
block, and right ventricular hypertrophy.

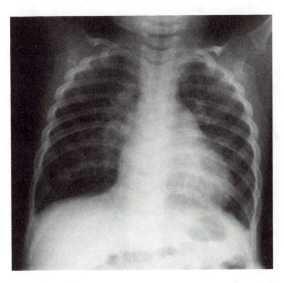

FIG 25–4.
Preoperative frontal chest radiograph in a 10-month-
old with Down syndrome and a complete atrioventricular canal. Abnormal features include mild cardiomegaly, an enlarged pulmonary artery segment, and
prominent pulmonary vasculature bilaterally.

A white blood count and differential are useful to screen for infectious processes. A hematocrit is necessary in order to determine the amount of bank blood required in the cardiopulmonary bypass procedure to reach a bypass hematocrit of approximately 25%. A coagulation profile including platelet count, prothrombin time (PT), and partial thromboplastin time (PTT) establishes a preoperative baseline and identifies patients with unexpected coagulopathies. Serum sodium and potassium values may be abnormal in patients who have been treated with diuretics preoperatively. Blood urea nitrogen and creatinine determinations are useful screening tests for renal function.

All available echocardiographic data should be reviewed, with assistance from the pediatric cardiologist as necessary. Two-dimensional imaging often gives a complete view of the patient's anatomy (Fig 25–5). M mode echocardiography allows measurement of vessel diameter, wall motion, and cardiac function, including estimates of shortening fraction. Doppler echocardiography relies on the receipt of reflected ultrasonic signals from moving red blood cells and can be used to precisely locate areas of disturbed flow. In addition, Doppler echocardiography can generate estimates of cardiac output and pressure gradients and thus allow the echocardiographer to estimate intracardiac pressures. In spite of the increased role of echocardiography in delineating intracardiac anatomy and physiology, cardiac catheterization remains the gold standard for confirming the diagnosis and for delineating the pattern of shunting, the size of the atrial and ventricular septal defects, and the levels of pulmonary arterial pressure and pulmonary vascular resistance.

Catheterization data from a patient with Down syndrome and a complete atrioventricular canal are shown in Table 25–2. The oxygen saturation data reveal a step-up in both the right atrium and the right ventricle, which suggests left-to-right shunts at both levels, although a step-up in the right ventricle can occur with an isolated ostium primum defect from streaming of blood through the adjacent tricuspid valve. The absence of significant pulmonary venous desaturation suggests that there is no pulmonary edema or atelectasis from bronchial compression. Systemic arterial saturation is the same as that in the left ventricle, which suggests that there is no right-to-left shunting through the ductus arteriosus.

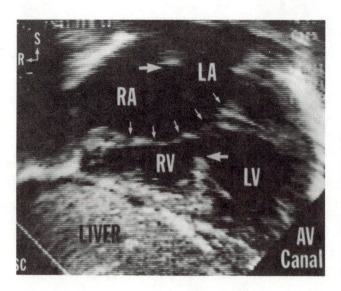

FIG 25–5.
Two-dimension echocardiogram of a complete atrioventricular canal defect from a subcostal view. The *large white arrows* point to the superior and inferior margins of the large atrioventricular septal defect. The *smaller white arrows* point to the anterior bridging leaflet of the common atrioventricular valve.

TABLE 25–2.

Cardiac Catheterization Data

Location	Saturation (%)		Pressure (mm Hg)	
	Room Air	100% O$_2$	Room Air	100% O$_2$
Superior vena cava	64		79	
Right atrium	78	88	7	7
Right ventricle	83	96	55/7	45/7
Main pulmonary artery	82	97	55/23 (mean, 37)	45/15 (mean, 27)
Pulmonary vein	98	100		
Left atrium	98	100	10	10
Left ventricle	98	100	100/10	95/10
Systemic artery	98	100	100/60 (mean, 73)	95/60 (mean, 72)
Flows (L/min/m^2)				
Systemic	3	3.7		
Pulmonary	6.25	10		
Pulmonary/systemic flow	2.2/1	2.7/1		
Resistance (Wood's units)				
Systemic	22	18		
Pulmonary	5.6	2		

Examination of the pressure data reveals normal atrial pressures, and this suggests that there are no ventricular-to-atrial shunts, no significant atrioventricular valve dysfunction, and no ventricular failure. Right ventricular pressure is increased. Pulmonary arterial pressure and resistance are elevated, while systemic pressure and resistance are normal. The increase in pulmonary artery pressure may be secondary to elevated flow or to either dynamic or fixed increases in pulmonary vascular resistance. The fact that pulmonary artery pressure and resistance decrease and pulmonary flow increases when the patient is exposed to 100% oxygen suggests that the pulmonary vascular bed is still reactive, a favorable indicator.

The calculated pulmonary-to-systemic flow ratio suggests a large left-to-right shunt. The reliability of this number is questionable, however. Calculation of systemic flow by the Fick method is unreliable since it is impossible to obtain a true mixed venous sample. Similarly, pulmonary blood flow calculation is subject to error. Often a very narrow arteriovenous oxygen difference is seen. If there is variation in pulmonary venous saturations in different pulmonary veins, the calculation of pulmonary blood flow varies markedly, depending on which pulmonary venous saturation is used. Therefore, the pulmonary-to-systemic flow ratio should be viewed more qualitatively than quantitatively.

The angiograms are reviewed to confirm anatomic lesions and direction of shunting. The left ventricular injection is the most revealing study during systole. Passage of blood into the right ventricle and pulmonary artery, left atrium, or even the right atrium may be seen. During diastole, the classic "gooseneck" deformity may be seen; this is caused by the abnormal attachments of the anterior leaflet of the mitral valve encroaching upon the aortic outflow tract (Fig 25–6). Obstruction to ventricular outflow and patent ductus arteriosus are ruled out. The right ventricular angiogram allows assessment of tricuspid valve function; the levo phase shows the position of pulmonary venous drainage.

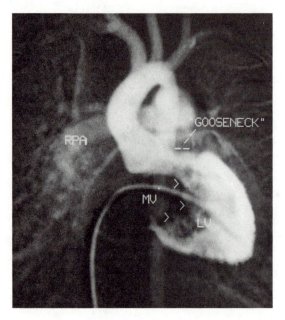

FIG 25–6.
Left ventricular *(LV)* angiogram in a child with Down syndrome and a complete atrioventricular canal. This view of the heart in diastole shows the limits (>) of the abnormally attached mitral valve *(MV)*, which encroaches upon the left ventricular outflow tract and results in a "gooseneck" deformity. The presence of left-to-right shunting through a ventricular septal defect is confirmed by the simultaneous filling of the aorta *(Ao)* and the right pulmonary artery *(RPA)*.

Informed Consent

As our society has become increasingly litiginous, proper informed consent has become a key facet of preoperative care. All anesthesiologists who will be involved in intraoperative management should introduce themselves to both patient and family. The nature and purpose of the proposed procedures must be explained in nontechnical language appropriate for the age of the child. Preoperative feeding orders, premedication, and the anticipated starting time and duration of the operation should be mentioned. Equipment that will be part of the child's postoperative experience such as endotracheal tubes, mechanical ventilators, chest tubes, arterial catheters, and intravenous tubing should be explained in a reassuring way. Risks must be discussed. Most parents understand that there is risk involved; a detailed disclosure of all the possible complications serves only to frighten them. Both child and parents should be given ample opportunity to ask questions. If the child is at particularly high risk or if the parents desire more information concerning risk, a more detailed discussion is warranted, usually in the child's absence. Documentation of the preoperative evaluation is mandatory. This should include a statement relating to informed consent.

Preoperative Team Discussion

A final but very important part of the preoperative process is the anesthesiologist's discussion with the surgeon and cardiologist concerning the details of the planned procedure. Potential complications should be reviewed and contingency plans formulated in an attempt to avoid preventable untoward events.

ANESTHETIC MANAGEMENT

Solids are withheld 6 hours prior to the induction of anesthesia, and clear liquids are given 3 hours prior to induction. Patients who are receiving digitalis and diuretics generally have their medications withheld on the morning of surgery. Premedication is administered according to the needs of the patient. A 10-month-old with Down syndrome can be sedated safely with methohexital or thiopental, 25 mg/kg per rectum, provided that careful attention is paid to the airway as the child goes to sleep.

Four standard limb leads are used to monitor the cardiac rate and rhythm. A V5 precordial lead can be helpful in screening for ischemic changes in ST segments. A printout mode should be available to document baseline QRS conformation as well as significant changes that occur. The blood pressure cuff is placed on an extremity that is free of intravenous catheters or the pulse oximeter probe.

Continuous monitoring of core temperature is critical for the management of hypothermia and rewarming. Both nasopharyngeal and rectal or bladder temperatures are monitored. Nasopharyngeal temperature reflects brain temperature and changes relatively quickly during cooling and rewarming. Rectal or bladder temperatures change more slowly and reflect core temperature in more vessel-poor areas.

Prior to induction, a precordial stethoscope is placed on the left anterior chest wall for continuous monitoring of heart tones and breath sounds. This is replaced by an esophageal stethoscope following induction and intubation. Continuous monitoring of arterial oxygen saturation can alert the anesthesiologist to potentially life-threatening events that result from deterioration in either cardiac or pulmonary function. The device requires a pulsatile vascular bed and thus becomes nonfunctional during nonpulsatile bypass.

Following intubation, the presence of carbon dioxide in the gas sample is corroborative of tube placement within the trachea. Minute ventilation can be adjusted on the basis of end-tidal carbon dioxide readings, provided that such readings are correlated with arterial carbon dioxide tension. A sudden decrease in end-tidal carbon dioxide concentration may signal a ventilator malfunction or a blocked endotracheal tube; alternatively, it might signal an inability to excrete carbon dioxide because of a significant decrease in pulmonary blood flow due to embolism or loss of cardiac output.

Urinary output is a reliable index of renal perfusion and thus is a reflection of circulating blood volume and cardiac output. Adequate urine output is generally considered to be 1 mL/kg/hr. Frequently, urine output falls below this value during nonpulsatile cardiopulmonary bypass but returns to normal values with the re-establishment of pulsatile flow, assuming that blood volume and cardiac output are adequate.

The arterial catheter can be placed percutaneously in most patients following induction. The most commonly used vessels are the radial, ulnar, dorsalis pedis, and posterior tibial arteries, all of which should have good collateral flow as demonstrated by an Allen test or a Doppler device. If these arteries cannot be cannulated percutaneously, the femoral or axillary arteries are reasonable alternatives. Surgical cutdown can be performed if percutaneous attempts fail, although this is rarely necessary. The cannula is connected to a pressure transducer and a constant infusion system containing 1 unit/mL of heparin running at 1 to 3 mL/hr. The transducer is connected to a pressure amplifier and an oscilloscope for continuous display. A stopcock and T-connector are attached to the cannula to facilitate arterial blood sampling. The insertion site must be closely observed intraoperatively and postoperatively. Persistent blanching of the distal end of the extremity or skin discoloration adjacent to the insertion site demands immediate catheter removal to prevent ischemic complications.

A central venous catheter provides a route for rapid volume expansion and for infusion of drugs such as calcium chloride that cause sclerosis or drugs such as dopamine that cause intense local vasoconstriction if administered in a peripheral vein. Central venous pressure (CVP) catheters are also used to measure right ventricular filling pressure, an index of intravascular volume and right ventricular function. Sustained elevation of CVP during cardiopulmonary bypass may indicate superior vena caval obstruction, which, if untreated, could lead to inadequate cerebral perfusion or cerebral edema or hemorrhage. The tip of the catheter is positioned in the cephalad end of the superior vena cava, proximal to the tourniquet placed around the superior vena cava cannula prior to bypass. This can be accomplished in most patients by percutaneous insertion of the CVP catheter into the internal jugular vein following induction of anesthesia. Double-lumen catheters are available and allow simultaneous pressure monitoring and infusion of drugs or fluid. The monitoring port of the catheter is attached to a pressure transducer and a constant infusion system similar to that used for the arterial catheter.

Induction and the Prebypass Period

Surface monitors are placed prior to induction of anesthesia. The child who was premedicated with a rectal barbiturate or other sedative can often have intravenous cannulas inserted prior to induction. Intravenous access facilitates induction since intravenous barbiturates can be used to obtund the child prior to placement of the face mask. Alternatively, an inhalation induction can be performed with oxygen and halothane in the unpremedicated child prior to placement of intravenous catheters. The presence of a large left-to-right shunt may slow the clinical response to intravenous agents but does not affect the speed of an inhalation induction.[14] Theoretically, any agent that reduces systemic vascular resistance might cause reversal of shunting to right to left; however, careful titration of drugs to clinical effect usually prevents this.

A catheter is placed in a peripheral vein for administration of drugs, crystalloid solutions, and blood components. Infusions of Ringer's lactate or normal saline are provided to correct any calculated fluid deficit prior to bypass. It is usually not necessary to provide dextrose intravenously since serum glucose concentrations almost invariably increase during bypass even without exogenous dextrose. Hyperglycemia can cause an osmostic diuresis and potassium depletion. Therefore, serum glucose concentrations are monitored to ensure adequate levels. In children with congenital heart disease, even acyanotic lesions, it is imperative to keep air out of intravenous tubing to prevent systemic air embolization.

High-dose narcotics are used to provide analgesia. Fentanyl is administered by intravenous infusion to achieve a total dose of approximately 25 μg/kg prior to intubation, 50 to 75 μg/kg prior to sternotomy, and 75 to 100 μg/kg prior to bypass. Close attention is paid to the heart rate and blood pressure response throughout the prebypass period. Although fentanyl is usually well tolerated, it can cause bradycardia and hypotension. Tachycardia and hypertension, on the other hand, suggest that additional analgesia is required.

High-dose narcotics also cause sedation but may not obtund the sensorium completely. This can be achieved by supplementing narcotic analgesia with a benzodiazepine such as midazolam, 0.1 mg/kg, or a low concentration of isoflurane.

Nondepolarizing muscle relaxants are required both to prevent the chest wall rigidity associated with high-dose fentanyl and to facilitate intubation. Pancuronium or vecuronium, 0.1 mg/kg, can be used for this purpose. Pancuronium can cause tachycardia but, when combined with fentanyl, usually has little effect on the heart rate. Vecuronium does not affect the heart rate, but is a shorter-acting agent and requires more frequent dosing. Doxacurium is a long-acting agent without chronotropic properties whose major shortcoming at present is cost.

The airway is controlled with mask ventilation as the muscle relaxant takes effect. Because 6% of patients with Down syndrome have atlantoaxial instability, intubation of all such patients is performed with the head and neck in a neutral position and both flexion and extension minimized. Following intubation the endotracheal tube is carefully secured, and mechanical ventilation is begun to achieve satisfactory chest wall expansion and breath sounds, a peak inspiratory pressure of 15 to 25 cm H_2O, and an end-tidal carbon dioxide concentration of 35 to 40 mm Hg. The invasive monitors are then inserted. A nasogastric tube is inserted to remove gastric contents and prevent gastric distension. The patient is positioned on the table, with careful attention to padding of all pressure points, including the occiput, elbows, sacrum, and heels.

For patients who are to undergo profound hypothermia and circulatory arrest, surface cooling before bypass may allow more uniform cooling, particularly in vessel-poor areas. Prebypass surface cooling is achieved with low ambient room temperature and a cooling blanket. Temperatures of 31 to 32° C are usually well tolerated.

Arterial blood gases are measured soon after induction of anesthesia to check the adequacy of oxygenation, ventilation, and acid-base status. Other laboratory parameters assessed at this time include the activated clotting time (ACT), hematocrit, platelet count, and levels of sodium, potassium, glucose, and ionized calcium.

Prior to insertion of arterial and venous cannulas for bypass, heparin, 3 to 4 mg/kg or 300 to 400 units/kg, is administered through the central venous catheter. An ACT of more than 400 seconds is documented before cardiopulmonary bypass is begun. Additional doses of fentanyl and muscle relaxant should be considered prior to bypass. Serum levels of narcotics and muscle relaxants decrease during bypass because of dilution and because of absorption by the Silastic membrane oxygenator. Also, during circulatory arrest, no additional agents can be given.

Cardiopulmonary Bypass

After bypass has begun and the heart has stopped ejecting blood, mechanical ventilation can be discontinued. Intravenous infusions are also stopped. Superior vena cava obstruction is ruled out by close observation of the CVP and the head and neck for plethora and congestion. Perfusion pressure is frequently low after institution of bypass, even at a full calculated flow of about 2.2 L/min/m². Without therapy, pressure usually increases gradually over the first 5 to 10 minutes on bypass before stabilizing. An acceptable perfusion pressure is one that results in normal urine output, no metabolic acidosis, a normal mixed venous oxygen tension, and no loss of blood from the oxygenator to the patient. Perfusion pressures of between 40 and 70 mm Hg are usually adequate. Hypertension during bypass at normal flows usually indicates vasoconstriction, which may result in regions of inadequate perfusion and cooling. If additional doses of narcotic do not remedy the situation, vasodilator therapy with sodium nitroprusside or phentolamine can be employed. Hypotension on bypass at normal flows usually results from low blood viscosity or excessive vasodilation and usually responds to α-adrenergic agents such as phenylephrine, 5 to 10 μg/kg.

After the surgeon administers cold cardioplegia solution into the coronary ostia, the ECG becomes isoelectric. Observed return of electrical activity is communicated to the surgeon so that a decision concerning repeated doses of cardioplegia solution can be made.

During bypass, the perfusionist draws serial blood samples from the pump for determination of arterial blood gases, electrolytes, glucose, hematocrit, platelet count, and ionized calcium. Blood gases are interpreted without temperature correction (alpha-stat),[15] and carbon dioxide is not added to the pump. If bypass lasts for more than 1 hour, a repeat ACT is performed. Heparin is given as necessary to maintain the ACT at more than 400 seconds. The platelet count usually decreases during bypass. If it decreases below 100,000/mm^3, consideration should be given to ordering platelets for the postbypass period, particularly if there are suture lines on the surface of the heart or great vessels.

As the surgical repair is being completed, rewarming is accomplished with the heat exchanger. The warming blanket is turned on, and the ambient temperature is increased. As body temperature increases, spontaneous cardiac rhythm usually returns. As soon as the arterial waveform indicates ejection, mechanical ventilation is begun. Weaning from cardiopulmonary bypass is not attempted until the nasopharyngeal temperature is 36 to 37° C, the rectal temperature is at least 33 to 34° C, the cardiac rate and rhythm are in a normal range, and the mean arterial pressure is at least 50 mm Hg with a CVP of less than 15 mm Hg. Atrial, ventricular, or atrioventricular pacing are used if the spontaneous rate and rhythm are inadequate.

If the mean arterial pressure is low in spite of adequate filling pressure, inotropic support is indicated. If ionized calcium levels are low from citrate-induced chelation, calcium chloride, 10 to 20 mg/kg, is administered slowly into a central vein. Rapid administration of calcium can cause bradyarrhythmias, particularly in digitalized patients. If the arterial pressure remains low, dobutamine is started at a dose of 5 to 10 μg/kg/min and titrated to effect. Dopamine is a pulmonary vasoconstrictor and probably would not be the drug of choice in a patient with pulmonary hypertension. Epinephrine infusions are reserved for patients who do not respond to dobutamine. If there is concern about right ventricular and pulmonary artery pressures, these measurements are made after coming off bypass. If right-sided pressures are high, afterload reduction is indicated; nitroglycerin may be the best agent to achieve this. A useful adjunctive inotrope is amrinone, a phosphodiesterase inhibitor that combines inotropy with afterload reduction in both the systemic and pulmonary vascular bed.[16] A loading dose of 4 to 5 mg/kg[17] is administered, followed by an infusion of 5 to 10 μg/kg/min. If right-sided afterload reduction is to be attempted, pulmonary artery pressures are measured continuously. The surgeon places a transthoracic catheter directly into the pulmonary artery, which is used in the intensive care unit for this purpose.

After removal of bypass cannulas and control of major surgical bleeding, heparin anticoagulation is reversed with protamine sulfate. One milligram of protamine is administered for every milligram of heparin that was given. Protamine is a vasodilator and can cause significant hypotension; thus it is administered slowly once the patient is hemodynamically stable and normovolemic. An ACT is measured after protamine administration to confirm adequate reversal of the heparin effect.

Warmed whole blood is available at the time the patient comes off bypass. Most patients require a postbypass transfusion to replace surgical losses and to maintain normovolemia during vasodilation due to rewarming and protamine infusion. If the bypass has lasted less than 1 hour, the blood that remains in the pump reservoir is used. This has the advantage of not exposing the patient to another unit of blood, a consideration of some importance given the concern over transfusion-related infection. However, pump blood is dilute and partially hemolyzed and contains unreversed heparin. A fresh unit of bank blood is used if the bypass has lasted more than 1 hour or if hemolysis has caused visible hemoglobinuria.

Transesophageal echo-Doppler imaging can be quite useful in assessing the integrity of the surgical repair and identifying residual defects or abnormalities of cardiac function.[18] Use of the echo-Doppler technique requires cooperation between the anesthesia and cardiology personnel since the probe must be placed both prebypass and postbypass in order to interpret the postbypass conditions. Once the practice becomes incorporated into the routine, however, all members of the team, including the surgeons, generally consider the data it provides to be useful and informative, particularly when the heart is not functioning properly following bypass.

TRANSFER TO THE INTENSIVE CARE UNIT

Transfer of the patient to the intensive care unit is done carefully, yet quickly and efficiently. The process is well organized and is not begun until the patient is hemodynamically stable. The anesthesiologist supervises the transfer and maintains continuous monitoring of ECG, arterial blood pressure, and arterial oxygen saturation with a portable monitor. All vasoactive infusions are continued with the use of infusion pumps. The patient is hand-ventilated with 100% oxygen, while breath sounds and heart tones are continuously monitored with an esophageal stethoscope. Upon arrival in the intensive care unit, mechanical ventilation is begun, and monitoring cables are switched from the portable to the intensive care unit monitors. The anesthesiologist gives a full report of pertinent data to the intensive care unit staff, including the diagnosis, allergies, surgical procedure, intraoperative problems, recent laboratory values, fluids and blood administered, urine output, and need for vasoactive drugs or pacing.

INTENSIVE CARE UNIT MANAGEMENT

Postoperative care is a cooperative effort involving surgeons, cardiologists, anesthesiologists, critical care physicians, and nurses. The role of each varies from institution to institution. However, it helps greatly to have a single physician in charge to coordinate care.

Patients with Down syndrome who are recovering from repair of cardiac defects generally require several days of mechanical ventilation.[10] Thus, there seems to be no role for early extubation in this population. A chest radiograph is obtained shortly after admission to the unit. Patients with poor oxygenation are ventilated with positive end-expiratory pressure (PEEP) sufficient to maintain an arterial oxygen tension of 80 to 100 mm Hg in nontoxic oxygen concentrations, i.e., less than 50% to 60%. PEEP is applied judiciously, with the knowledge that excessive levels can increase pulmonary vascular resistance, dead space, and lung water; decrease cardiac output; and cause barotrauma. Tidal volumes of 12 to 15 mL/kg are used, with a breathing frequency necessary to achieve normal arterial carbon dioxide tension. In patients with residual pulmonary hypertension, hyperventilation to achieve a respiratory alkalosis is employed to help control pulmonary artery pressure.[19]

Sedation and analgesia are necessary to facilitate mechanical ventilation and provide relief from pain and anxiety. A combination of a narcotic, usually morphine, 10 to 40 µg/kg/hr, and a benzodiazepine such as midazolam, 100 µg/kg/hr, are administered by infusion. If these are inadequate, a third drug such as droperidol, 0.05 to 0.1 mg/kg given by intravenous bolus every 6 to 8 hours, is helpful. Muscle relaxants are used only if the patient cannot be managed with sedatives and narcotics alone.

Other adjuncts to respiratory care include chest physiotherapy and endotracheal tube suctioning. Chest physiotherapy is usually withheld until the patient is hemodynamically stable and demonstrates a specific problem that might respond to therapy such as isolated lobar atelectasis. Endotracheal tube suctioning is potentially hazardous in the patient with a reactive pulmonary vascular bed. Whether caused by an acute decrease in arterial oxygen tension or by mechanical stimulation of tracheal reflexes, suctioning can cause pulmonary vasospasm, loss of cardiac output, and bradycardia to the point of cardiac arrest. Suctioning is performed after the patient has breathed 100% oxygen for a few minutes, and the catheter should be passed only once. Intratracheal lidocaine or intravenous narcotics can be used to blunt tracheal reflexes.

The duration of mechanical ventilation is determined by a number of factors. Once the patient has minimal blood loss, diminished or no dependence on inotropic drugs, an arterial oxygen tension of 80 to 100 mm Hg with <50% oxygen and <5 cm H_2O PEEP, a clear or improving chest radiograph, and a peak inspiratory pressure of less than 30 cm H_2O with 12- to 15-mL/kg tidal volumes, weaning from mechanical ventilation can begin. Small incremental decreases in ventilator rate and PEEP are performed, with close attention to the arterial blood gases and clinical examination. Tachypnea, dyspnea, and worsening respiratory acidosis suggest that sustained spontaneous ventilation will not be tolerated. If the patient tolerates a respirator frequency of two to four breaths per minute with PEEP of 3 cm H_2O or less and has normal clinical findings and normal arterial blood gases, a trial of extubation is warranted.

REFERENCES

1. Epstein CJ: Genetic disorders and birth defects, in Rudolph AM (ed): *Pediatrics,* ed 17. Englewood Cliffs, NJ, Appleton-Century-Crofts, 1982, pp 243–245.
2. Rowe RD, Uchida IA: Cardiac malformation in mongolism: A prospective study of 184 mongoloid children. *Am J Med* 1961; 20:726.
3. Ferencz C, Neill CA, Boughman JA, et al: Congenital cardiovascular malformations associated with chromosome abnormalities: An epidemiologic study. *J Pediatr* 1989; 114:79.
4. Mathew P, et al: Long term follow-up of children with Down syndrome with cardiac lesions. *Clin Pediatr* 1990; 29:569.
5. Chi TL, Krovetz LJ: The pulmonary vascular bed in children with Down syndrome. *J Pediatr* 1975; 86:533.
6. Shaher RM, Farino MA, Porter IH, et al: Clinical aspects of congenital heart disease in mongolism. *Am J Cardiol* 1972; 29:497.

7. Loughlin GN, Wynne JW, Victorica BE: Sleep apnea as a possible cause of pulmonary hypertension in Down syndrome. *J Pediatr* 1981; 98:435.
8. Berger TJ, Blackstone EH, Kirklin JW, et al: Survival and probability of cure without and with operation in complete atrioventricular canal. *Ann Thorac Surg* 1979; 27:104.
9. Greenwood RD, Nadas AS: The clinical course of cardiac disease in Down syndrome. *Pediatrics* 1976; 58:893.
10. Morray JP, MacGillivray R, Duker G: Increased perioperative risk following repair of congenital heart disease in Down's syndrome. *Anesthesiology* 1986; 65:221.
11. Cooney TP, Thurbeck WM: Pulmonary hypoplasia in Down's syndrome. *N Engl J Med* 1982; 307:1170.
12. Spina CA, Smith D, Korn E, et al: Altered cellular immune functions in patients with Down's syndrome. *Am J Dis Child* 1981; 135:251.
13. Jones KL: Down syndrome, in *Smith's Recognizable Patterns of Human Malformation,* ed 4. Philadelphia, WB Saunders Co, 1988.
14. Tanner GE, Angers DG, Barash PG, et al: Effect of left-to-right, mixed left-to-right, and right-to-left shunts on inhalational anesthetic induction in children: A computer model. *Anesth Analg* 1985; 64:101.
15. Swain JA: Hypothermia and blood pH: A review. *Arch Intern Med* 1988; 148:1643.
16. Coe JY, Olley PM, Vella G, et al: Bipyridine derivatives lower arteriolar resistance and improve left ventricular function in newborn lambs. *Pediatr Res* 1987; 22:422.
17. Lawless S, Burckort G, Diven W, et al: Amrinone in neonates and infants after cardiac surgery. *Crit Care Med* 1989; 17:751.
18. Ungerleider RM, Greeley WJ, Sheikh KH, et al: The use of intraoperative echo with Doppler color flow imaging to predict outcomes following repair of congenital heart defects. *Ann Surg* 1989; 210:526.
19. Morray JP, Lynn AM, Mansfield PB: The effect of pH and P_{CO_2} on pulmonary and systemic hemodynamics following surgery in children with congenital heart disease and pulmonary hypertension. *J Pediatr* 1988; 113:474.

26

Myringotomy and Prior Senning Procedure

A 10-month-old 6-kg boy who had a Senning procedure for transposition of the great vessels at 6 months of age is scheduled for myringotomy and placement of PE tubes. The first surgery was performed in another state and no records are available. Hemoglobin, 15 g/dL; hematocrit, 45%.

Recommendations by M. Lizanne Fox, M.D., and
Paul R. Hickey, M.D.

Transposition of the great arteries (TGA) is a commonly seen cardiac anomaly. In 1980 the New England Regional Infant Cardiac Program reported TGA to be the second most frequently seen form of congenital heart disease, occurring in ten percent of the patients. The frequency of occurrence is reported to be 0.026 per 1,000 live births.[1]

Transposition of the great arteries is defined by anatomic connections between the great arteries and the ventricles. In patients with atrial situs solitus and transposition of the great vessels, the morphological right atrium attaches to the morphological right ventricle and the morphological left atrium attaches to the morphological left ventricle. However, the aorta arises from the morphological right ventricle and the pulmonary artery arises from the morphological left ventricle[2] (Fig 26–1).

In order for TGA to be compatible with life, there must be mixing between these two parallel, separate circuits. Babies with intact ventricular septae usually present early in the newborn period with increasing cyanosis, precipitated by closure of the ductus arteriosus. This terminates mixing and isolates the two circuits. In contrast, babies with ventricular septal defects may have sufficient mixing to allow adequate systemic oxygenation[2] (Fig 26–2).

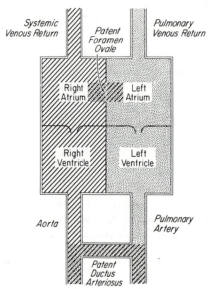

FIG 26–1.
Transposition of the great arteries with an intact ventricular septum. Mixing (shown by the mixed shading) may occur at the level of the patent foramen ovale or at the level of the patent ductus arteriosus. (*Striped areas* represent deoxygenated blood; *stippled areas* represent oxygenated blood; *striped and stippled areas* represent areas of mixing.)

SURGICAL CORRECTION OF TRANSPOSITION OF THE GREAT ARTERIES

Patients with TGA who do not have adequate mixing have a very high mortality unless palliative and/or corrective procedures are performed. The first palliative procedure, described and performed by Blalock and Hanlon in 1948, is the surgical creation of an atrial septal defect (ASD), performed without cardiopulmonary bypass. By creating or enlarging a hole in the atrial septum, mixing of oxygenated and deoxygenated blood can occur between the two circulations. This allows blood from the pulmonary circulation that is more saturated to cross into the morphological right ventricle and perfuse the systemic circulation via the aorta.[2, 3]

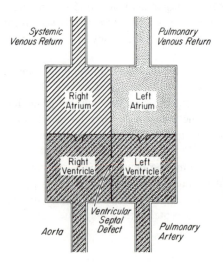

FIG 26–2.
Transposition of the great arteries. Mixing (shown by the mixed shading) occurs at the level of the ventricular septal defect. (*Striped areas* represent deoxygenated blood; *stippled areas* represent oxygenated blood.)

The same principle of enlarging the communication between the two atria was used by Rashkind and Miller in 1966 when they performed the first atrial septostomy in the catheterization laboratory. This procedure has the advantage of eliminating the need for a surgical procedure. The septostomy is performed by entering the heart with a balloon-tip catheter via the femoral vein.[4] Balloon atrial septostomies are routinely performed today in patients with TGA and intact ventricular septa in whom mixing is not adequate.

In 1959, Senning described the first physiological corrective procedure for TGA. He described an intra-atrial baffling procedure and successfully performed this operation in 1960. Senning used flaps of atrial wall and septum to redirect the venous inflow.[5] By redirecting blood flow at the atrial level, he was able to direct the pulmonary venous return, that is, oxygenated blood, to the morphological right ventricle and to direct the blood from the superior and inferior vena cavae, that is, deoxygenated blood, to the morphological left ventricle. This is considered to be a physiologic repair, as oxygenated blood is directed to the systemic circulation and deoxygenated blood is directed to the pulmonary circulation. It is not an *anatomic* corrective procedure, as the morphological right ventricle still functions as the systemic ventricle.

Mustard employed the same principles as Senning, but modified the operation. He used pericardium to create the intra-atrial baffle and reported his first successful repair in 1963[6] (Fig 26–3).

These intra-atrial baffling procedures are not without problems. In a retrospective analysis of patients with TGA who underwent physiologic repair between 1964 and 1985 and who survived at least 30 days, the overall survival rate was 96% at one year, 93% at five years, and 88% at ten years. The majority of nonsurvivors died suddenly, presumably due to dysrhythmias. Based on these findings, aggressive ECG follow-up was instituted to investigate the etiology of the late sudden deaths and Holter monitoring was added in the 1970s. Numerous atrial dysrhythmias were described and pacemakers were placed in patients with signs of high-degree atrioventricular block and in those with significant sinus node dysfunction.[7]

It is understandable that dysrhythmias are the most commonly seen complication after an intra-atrial baffling procedure. There are extensive incisions and suture lines throughout both atria that can interrupt the nutrient arteries to, or the conduction pathways between, the SA and AV nodes.

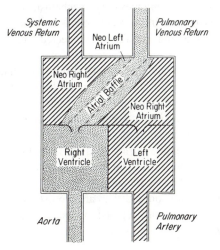

FIG 26–3.
Atrial baffling procedure. Oxygenated blood (stippled shading) is directed from the pulmonary veins to the right ventricle. The right ventricle pumps to the systemic circulation via the aorta. (*Striped areas* represent deoxygenated blood; *stippled areas* represent oxygenated blood.)

Sutures may also be placed in the region of the coronary sinus and these sutures may injure the AV node. It is, however, generally believed that injury to the SA node itself results in most of the rhythm disturbances.[8]

In an eight-year prospective study evaluating the long-term effects on cardiac rhythm of both the Mustard and Senning repairs, only 56% of the Senning patients and 66% of the Mustard patients were found to be in stable sinus rhythm seven years postoperatively.[9] It is clear from long-term follow-up studies that there is a very high incidence of both hemodynamic and electrophysiologic problems documented seven to nine years postoperatively, even in children who are asymptomatic.[10, 11]

These and other problems led surgeons to pursue the idea of an arterial switch technique. In this procedure it is the great vessels, that is, the aorta and pulmonary artery, that are dissected and reimplanted.[12] The first successful arterial switch procedure was reported in 1975 by Jatene. An advantage of the technique is that there are no extensive intra-atrial suture lines; therefore, the incidence of dysrhythmias is much lower. Also, the arterial switch is an anatomic correction and therefore the morphological left ventricle becomes the new functioning systemic ventricle.[13, 14]

Although dysrhythmias are most common, other complications can occur after an atrial repair. These include baffle leaks, systemic and pulmonary venous obstruction, and right ventricular dysfunction.

PREOPERATIVE CONSIDERATIONS

Myringotomy with placement of PE tubes is a commonly-performed, simple surgical procedure usually lasting no longer than ten minutes. The standard anesthetic in a fasting healthy patient consists of halothane, nitrous oxide and oxygen administered by mask.

In this particular case, the patient is a ten-month-old child who at four months of age underwent a Senning procedure. There is no information available to us except that his hematocrit is 45%. This is higher than normal for a 10-month-old child.

During the history and physical examination, the anesthesiologist should look specifically for signs of desaturation because the elevated hematocrit suggests a compensatory mechanism to increase oxygen-carrying capacity. A period of pulse oximetry monitoring is recommended. If there is evidence of desaturation, a baffle-leak with right-to-left shunting should be suspected and an echocardiogram performed.

An ECG and 24-hour Holter monitoring would be useful in evaluating the stability of the sinus mechanism. In the presence of sick-sinus syndrome or high degrees of atrioventricular block, a prophylactic pacemaker might be considered. However, these problems most often occur later than six months after the Senning or Mustard procedure. At a minimum, an isoproterenol infusion should be available and an external pacemaker is advisable if there is any question of sinus dysfunction.

If there are signs of heart failure, such as poor feeding, sweating during feedings, rapid respiratory rate, failure to thrive, or an enlarged liver, echocardiography should be performed to evaluate ventricular function. If the ventricular function is markedly depressed, the anesthetic risk is greater and the urgency of the procedure must be discussed with the surgeon and the cardiologist. Again, failure of a right, systemic ventricle *early* after a Senning or Mustard repair is unusual, whereas mild degrees of depression of right ventricular function would not be unusual.

ANESTHETIC MANAGEMENT

The management of this patient is discussed assuming four different scenarios.

Scenario 1: Normal ECG, Holter Monitoring, Arterial Saturation, and Echocardiogram.—A *well* conducted mask anesthetic utilizing halothane, nitrous oxide and oxygen would be safe. The sensitivity to halothane[15, 16, 17] in the immature heart of a 10-month-old and the mild dysfunction of the right ventricle that can be demonstrated in these patients when they are stressed should be appreciated. High concentrations of halothane should thus be avoided and a slow induction with low halothane concentrations should be planned. Use of prophylactic atropine to attenuate the cardiovascular depression associated with halothane induction in infants should be carefully considered.[18, 19]

Scenario 2: Abnormal Rhythm Demonstrated by ECG and Holter Monitoring.—Consideration should be given to insertion of a prophylactic pacemaker. If a pacemaker is deemed unnecessary, halothane should probably be avoided as it is a myocardial depressant and also depresses the conduction system in the heart. An isoproterenol infusion should be immediately available. It would also be wise to have an external pacemaker available. Ketamine would be a safe anesthetic choice in this setting.

Scenario 3: Desaturation Evident by Oximetry.—If the echocardiogram confirmed a baffle leak and the decision was made to go ahead with the myringotomy, the anesthetic technique must preserve the ratio of systemic vascular resistance (SVR) to pulmonary vascular resistance (PVR) to minimize shunting of deoxygenated blood across to the oxygenated side of the circulation. The ratio of SVR to PVR is, however, of somewhat less importance with an atrial level shunt than with a ventricular level shunt. The PVR should be kept low and the SVR maintained at a normal level. Conditions that may precipitate high pulmonary vascular resistance including airway obstruction, acidosis and hypothermia, must be avoided. Effective measures for lowering PVR include hyperventilation which induces alkalosis, and the administration of 100% oxygen. If the SVR falls below normal, an alpha-agonist such as phenylephrine should be effective in increasing arterial oxygen saturation by elevating SVR in ventricular level right-to-left shunts.[20, 21] Efficacy of the drug with atrial level right-to-left shunts is less certain.

In this setting, both intravenous and inhalation anesthetics can be used if carefully titrated and monitored. In the presence of a known intracardiac right-to-left shunt, air filters should be placed on intravenous infusions to minimize the risk of systemic air emboli resulting from air in venous lines. Airway obstruction must be avoided even if it necessitates endotracheal intubation.

Scenario 4: Cardiac Failure.—In the presence of cardiac failure, the severity of the recurrent infection must override the increased risk due to anesthesia. The case should at least be cancelled until the child's cardiac status is completely reevaluated with an echocardiogram and cardiac catheterization so that the etiology of the congestive heart failure and the appropriate treatment can be determined. If, at that point the child's physician still wishes to go ahead with the procedure, ketamine may be the agent of choice because it will preserve hemodynamic function in the presence of moderate heart failure. If the myocardium is severely depressed, a narcotic-relaxant technique may be preferred. At the very least, an inotrope should be immediately available in case the circulation deteriorates.

REFERENCES

1. Fyler DC: Report of the New England Regional Infant Care Program. *Pediatrics* 1980; 65:375.
2. Trusler GA, Freedom RM: Complete Transposition of the Great Arteries, in: Arciniegas E, (ed) *Pediatric Cardiac Surgery*. Chicago, Year Book Medical Publishers, Inc, 1985, pp 257–283.
3. Blalock A, Hanlon CR: The surgical treatment of complete transposition of the aorta and pulmonary artery. *Surg Gynecol Obstet* 1950; 90:1.
4. Rashkind WJ, Miller WW. Creation of an atrial septal defect without thoracotomy: A palliative approach. *JAMA* 1966; 196:991.
5. Senning A: Surgical correction of transposition of the great vessels. *Surgery* 1959; 45:966.
6. Mustard WT: Successful two stage correction of transposition of the great vessels. *Surgery* 1964; 55:469.
7. Turina M, Siebenmann R, Nussbaumer P, et al: Long-term outlook after atrial correction of transposition of great arteries. *J Thorac Cardiovasc Surg* 1988; 95:828–35.
8. Gillette PC, Kugler JD, Garson A Jr, et al. Mechanisms of cardiac arrhythmias after the Mustard operation for transposition of the great arteries. *Am J Cardiol* 1980; 45:1225.
9. Deanfield J, Camm J, McCartney F, et al: Arrhythmia and late mortality after Mustard and Senning operation for transposition of the great arteries. *J Thorac Cardiovasc Surg* 1988; 96:569–76.
10. Bink-Boelkens MT, Bergstra A, Cromme-Dijkhuis AH, et al: The asymptomatic child a long time after the Mustard Operation for transposition of the great arteries. *Ann Thorac Surg* 1989; 47:45.
11. Gewillig M, Cullen S, Mertens B, et al: Risk factors for arrhythmia and death after Mustard operation for simple transposition of the great arteries. *Circulation* 1991; 84(suppl 3):187, 1991.
12. Idriss FS, Ilbawi MN, DeLeon SY, et al. Arterial switch in simple and complex transposition of the great arteries. *J Thorac Cardiovasc Surg* 1988; 95:29.
13. Jatene AD, Fontes VF, Souza LC, et al. Anatomic correction of transposition of the great arteries. *J Thorac Cardiovasc Surg* 1982; 83:20.
14. Quaequebeur J, Rohmen J, Ottenkamp J, et al. The arterial switch operation (An eight-year experience). *J Cardiovasc Surg* 1986; 92:361–384.
15. Krane EJ, Su JY. Comparison of the effects of halothane on newborn and adult rabbit myocardium. *Anesth Analg* 1987; 66:1240–1244.
16. Rao CC, Boyer MS, Krishna G, et al: Increased sensitivity of the isometric contraction of the neonatal isolated rat atria to halothane, isoflurane and enflurane. *Anesthesiology* 1986; 64:13–18.
17. Murat I, Hoerter J, Ventura-Clapier R. Developmental changes in effects of halothane and isoflurane on contractile properties of rabbit cardiac skinned fibers. *Anesthesiology* 1991; 71:103–109.
18. Cartabuke RS, Davidson PJ, Warner LO. Is premedication with oral glycopyrolate as effective as oral atropine in attenuating cardiovascular depression in infants receiving halothane for induction of anesthesia? *Anesth Analg* 1991; 73:271–274.
19. Palmisano BW, Setlock MA, Brown MP, et al: Dose-response for atropine and heart rate in infants and children anesthetized with halothane and nitrous oxide. *Anesthesiology* 1991; 75:238–242.
20. Shaddy RE, Viney J, Judd VE, et al: Continuous intravenous phenylephrine infusion for treatment of hypoxemic spells in tetralogy of Fallot. *J Pediatrics* 1989; 114:468–470.
21. Nudel D, Berman N, Talmer N. Effects of acutely increasing systemic vascular resistance on arterial oxygen tension in tetralogy of Fallot. *Pediatrics* 1976; 58:248–251.

27

Liver Transplantation

A 10-month-old girl is scheduled for orthotopic liver transplantation. She had a Kasai procedure as an infant for biliary cirrhosis. On physical examination she is jaundiced, has splenomegaly and is underweight for her age (6 kg). Hemoglobin, 8 g/dL; hematocrit, 24%; bilirubin, 20 mg/dL.

Recommendations by D. Ryan Cook, M.D.

Biliary atresia is a disease of the intrahepatic and extrahepatic bile ducts.[1] Microscopic biliary ductules that communicate with the intrahepatic biliary tree are present in the grossly occluded duct early in the disease. As these structures gradually sclerose and disappear during the first several months of life, the infant becomes progressively more jaundiced. The sclerotic process is panductal and affects both the intrahepatic tree and the extrahepatic system.

SURGICAL TREATMENT OF BILIARY ATRESIA

Biliary atresia is surgically addressable in about 50% of the infants by a Roux-en-Y intestinal anastomosis to the proximal bile duct or by a hepatic portoenterostomy, the Kasai procedure. With this procedure, the fibrotic extrahepatic ductal structures are removed and bile drainage established by anastomosis of an intestinal conduit to the transected porta hepatis. Operative success depends on the continued presence of microscopic biliary structures at the liver hilus that allow autoanastomosis between the intestinal and patent ductal epithelial elements. Biliary drainage can be sluggish for several weeks after operation and jaundice may not significantly resolve for several months. The long-term prognosis following a Kasai procedure varies from 20% to 45% and cholangitis is a common complication. Portal hypertension and poor absorption of fat-soluble vitamins are common sequelae to biliary atresia with or without the Kasai procedure.

Orthotopic liver transplantation is currently an accepted therapeutic option for treatment of a variety of children in hepatic failure, for selected children with hepatomas and biliary tract tumors, and for hepatic replacement in certain inherited metabolic disorders. Three groups of infants with biliary atresia may be candidates for liver transplantation: (1) patients in whom a Kasai procedure is impossible; (2) those who had a Kasai procedure but in whom bile flow was never established; and (3) children who achieve bile drainage but who, because of the severity of the underlying liver damage and intrahepatic ductal disease, remain or become moderately jaundiced, fail to thrive, have severe growth retardation, and develop clinical manifestations of portal hypertension.[2-5] Previous operations, the young age and small size of the recipient, portal vein size and patency, and associated malformations increase the complexity of liver transplantations in these infants. Advances in surgical and anesthetic techniques, introduction of better immunosuppressive agents, establishment of brain-death criteria, and increased public awareness of organ donation have allowed transplantation in small infants.[6, 7] Reduction or split liver harvesting techniques from cadavers or living-related donors, better preservation techniques, and piggyback implantation techniques have minimized perioperative problems.[8]

PREOPERATIVE ASSESSMENT

The emergency nature of this surgery rarely allows time to completely correct preoperative abnormalities in the patient's laboratory values. Use of so-called UW (University of Wisconsin) preservative fluid prolongs the cold ischemia time of the donor liver for at least 12 to 16 hours, allowing many procedures to be performed during the day and more time for preoperative preparation. Often patients are anemic as a result of nutritional deficiencies, coagulation abnormalities, or upper gastrointestinal tract bleeding. Coagulation profiles are often abnormal: the prothrombin time is frequently elevated, partial thromboplastin time abnormal, and the platelet count low. Moderate to massive ascites is usually present and has been treated with loop diuretics with oral replacement of potassium. Fortunately, serum electrolyte disturbances occur infrequently, although serum potassium concentrations may occasionally be depressed. Previous renal tubular injury, inadequate renal preload, and hepatorenal syndrome may contribute to renal dysfunction and failure, which may be treated preoperatively with peritoneal dialysis.

Patients in liver failure may have a restrictive lung defect as the result of simple lung compression due to chronic ascites. More significantly, an increased alveolar-arterial oxygen difference may result from diffuse pulmonary arteriovenous shunting. Preexisting right-to-left shunts in the pulmonary bed increase the risk of systemic air embolization when the vascular anastomoses are performed intraoperatively.

ANESTHETIC AND INTRAOPERATIVE CARE

Because coagulation may be abnormal preoperatively, it may not be prudent to premedicate a liver transplant patient by intramuscular injection. If coagulation is normal, standard medications are not contraindicated. A rapid-sequence anesthetic induction is prudent if the patient has a full stomach. Nasotracheal intubation, if possible, provides greater endotracheal tube stability during the long intraoperative and postoperative period. However, the child's coagulation status determines if this approach is appropriate. A radial artery catheter, double- or triple-lumen central venous catheter, and urinary catheter are inserted. If necessary, a femoral arterial catheter can be used. Several large intravenous catheters are inserted in the upper extremities. The extremities and all pressure points, including the head, should be padded.

Isoflurane-nitrogen-oxygen relaxant is currently the most frequently used anesthetic. The isoflurane can be reinforced by fentanyl. We prefer high-dose vecuronium, 0.3 to 0.4 mg/kg, or a combination of metocurine, 0.4 mg/kg, and pancuronium, 0.15 to 0.2 mg/kg. The combination of isoflurane and pancuronium can cause significant tachycardia and mask useful signs of hypovolemia or inadequate analgesia. The massive bleeding and transfusions required during liver transplantation lead to hemodilution, which in turn increases the required dose of intravenous narcotics and relaxants. Nitrous oxide, if used for induction of anesthesia, is usually discontinued to reduce bowel distension and the consequences of air embolization. It may be desirable to administer intravenous amnesic agents such as diazepam or midazolam if isoflurane is not tolerated.

Although patients with diseased livers are presumed to have disturbances in pseudocholinesterase production, prolongation of the action of succinylcholine is not a clinical problem because of the duration of surgery and the occurrence of multiple blood volume exchanges with fresh frozen plasma. Since hepatic and renal routes of pancuronium, vecuronium, and metocurine elimination are also frequently impaired, the duration of neuromuscular blockade may be significantly prolonged. This can be a positive feature, since postoperative ventilation is usually required.

The results of arterial blood gas tensions and pH, hemoglobin, hematocrit, colloid osmotic pressure, and serum concentrations of sodium, potassium, and ionized calcium, should be available from the laboratory within 10 minutes of the time samples are drawn. Serum concentrations of glucose, as well as platelet counts, prothrombin, and partial thromboplastin times should be obtainable from the laboratory within an hour of the time a sample is drawn. An intraoperative thromboelastogram may be useful in determining blood component therapy.[9] When the clinical situation requires immediate estimation of serum glucose, Dextrostix analysis of whole blood may be used in the operating suite.

Surgical Technique

To increase the availability of donor organs for small infants it is possible to reduce or split the liver from older, larger donors.[8] A transparenchymal ex vivo right hepatectomy or lobectomy is performed on the so-called back table. This procedure takes about 2 hours. A choice is made between the two variants according to the amount of tissue to be removed to have a residual liver of appropriate size to fit the recipient's liver fossa. Liver fragments from donors 3 to 4 times larger than the recipient or even greater can be made to fit if the appropriate size reduction procedure is selected. The resected portion usually is discarded. Transplantation of liver fragments is thought to be associated with a lower incidence of hepatic artery thrombosis because of the larger size of the donor artery.

The first stage of a liver transplantation procedure itself is the preanhepatic phase.[9] After the transplant recipient has been anesthetized and positioned, a wide subcostal incision with cephalad extension to the xyphoid is made bilaterally, and the xyphoid process is removed without entering the thorax. The recipient's liver is then dissected to its vascular pedicle.

The next stage of the surgical procedure is referred to as the anhepatic phase. After clamping of the suprahepatic inferior vena cava, the infrahepatic inferior vena cava, the portal vein, and the hepatic artery, the diseased liver is removed. Revascularization of the donor liver begins with the

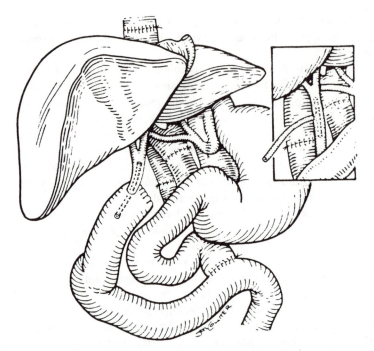

FIG 27–1.
Orthotopic liver transplantation. Biliary reconstruction can be accomplished through choledochojejunostomy or duct-to-duct anastomosis *(inset).*

anastomosis of the suprahepatic inferior vena cava and preparation for anastomosis of the infrahepatic inferior vena cava, although the latter anastomosis is not completed at this time. The donor liver is then flushed via the portal vein with 200 to 300 mL of Ringer's lactate solution, which is allowed to drain from the incomplete infrahepatic inferior vena cava anastomosis. This removes the transport infusate, which is rich in potassium, and clears the liver vasculature of entrapped air. The infrahepatic inferior vena cava and portal vein anastomosis are then completed, but clamps are left in place.

In the third or neonepatic stage the donor liver is incorporated into the recipient's circulatory system by releasing, in sequence, clamps on the portal vein, the infrahepatic inferior vena cava, and the suprahepatic inferior vena cava. The hepatic artery anastomosis is performed, and after adequate hemostasis has been achieved, the bile duct is reconstructed (Fig 27–1). If the patient has a normal extrahepatic ductal system, a duct-to-duct anastomosis with a T-tube or indwelling stent is performed. If the extrahepatic bile ducts are abnormal, a Roux-en-Y choledochojejunostomy is performed. Finally, an intraoperative cholangiogram is obtained to assess the patency of the biliary drainage system.

Intraoperative Complications

Preservation of intravascular volume and myocardial stability are the anesthesiologist's greatest challenges in these infants.[6] Blood loss may vary from 0.5 to 30.0 blood volume replacements. Correction of abnormal coagulation as determined by hourly measurement of prothrombin and partial thromboplastin time often requires the administration of at least 1 mL fresh frozen plasma for each 1 mL of red blood cells. Preexisting and/or dilutional thrombocytopenia almost always occurs.

A platelet count must be obtained hourly to monitor this condition, and transfusion of platelets is usually necessary. Minimal quantities of crystalloid should be infused, both to allow for the infusion of adequate amounts of blood components and to reduce the risk of pulmonary edema from fluid overload. The infusions of crystalloid and fresh frozen plasma should be carefully titrated using central venous pressures to minimize the incidence of intraoperative pulmonary edema.

Intraoperative hypotension occurs because of inadequate replacement of massive amounts of fluid and blood lost during the procedure; cardiac dysfunction resulting from decreased serum concentration of ionized calcium, presumably the result of increased citrate concentration after massive transfusion with red blood cells; surgical manipulations that disturb preload, including occlusion of the inferior vena cava during the anhepatic phase; life-threatening arrhythmias; and preexisting myocardial disease.

Blood salvage and rapid-infusion devices and venovenous bypass are not practical alternatives for limiting blood loss and maintaining hemodynamic stability in infants. The cardiopulmonary profiles of older patients who receive venovenous bypass include no change in heart rate or cardiac filling pressures, with a decreased cardiac index and increased systemic vascular resistance. The decrease in cardiac index has been attributed to reduced whole body oxygen consumption caused by removal of the liver, an organ with high metabolic activity, and reduction of the core temperature. Venovenous bypass maintains near-normal cardiovascular physiology. Bypass is also reported to reduce surgical blood loss, improve 30-day survival rate, and prevent increases in hydrostatic pressure in the portal and systemic venous beds, which otherwise would aggravate preexisting portal hypertension, decreasing perfusion of the kidneys, bowel, and pancreas.

Citrate intoxication with ensuing myocardial dysfunction from hypocalcemia may occur as a result of massive blood transfusion in hypothermic and anhepatic patients. Moderate hypothermia is almost an inevitable feature of liver transplantation despite the use of warming blankets, heated humidified gases, and warmed blood components and crystalloid solutions. Calcium chloride or calcium gluconate is administered by bolus or constant infusion to normalize ionized calcium levels. Although calcium gluconate is reported to be metabolized in the liver, an almost immediate increase in serum ionized calcium concentration is seen following bolus injection of calcium gluconate in anhepatic animals and in patients.

Significant cardiovascular changes during liver transplantation occur at the time of vascular clamping and reanastomosis. When the inferior vena cava is clamped at the onset of the anhepatic phase, preload to the heart decreases precipitously. The presence of collateral circulation resulting from portal hypertension modulates this decrease in preload from the infradiaphragmatic portion of the body. During revascularization, the infrahepatic inferior vena cava is opened first, and the intravascular volume enlarges to include the donor liver. The suprahepatic inferior vena cava is opened immediately thereafter. A transient decrease in the systolic and diastolic arterial pressures (30 to 50 mm Hg), often occurs at this time, despite volume preloading. Changes in blood pressure are associated with a decreased heart rate, cardiac index, systemic vascular resistance, and mixed venous oxygen saturation. Myocardial contractility may decrease as a result of perfusion of the heart with acidotic blood because the pH decreases an average of 0.15 when vessels are unclamped after completion of the vascular anastomosis. Serum potassium increases transiently and may produce systemic vasodilation. However, even when pH and serum potassium values remain stable, hypotension is observed. This may be due to the release of unknown vasodilating agents from the gut. This hypotension should be treated by administration of crystalloid or colloid infusion, a bolus dose of calcium chloride, and dopamine, 10 to 15 μg/kg/minute.

Hypertension is a frequent occurrence in the operating room after revascularization and the administration of cyclosporin and steroids. It is associated with a decrease in vasopressin levels, an increase in atrial natriuretic factor and plasma renin, and a negative water clearance.[10] Use of large volumes of fresh frozen plasma may significantly contribute to hypertension. Control of hypertension frequently requires multiple antihypertensive agents.

Acute hyperkalemia may also occur when the vessels are unclamped, causing life-threatening arrhythmias. Even though cold Ringer's lactate solution infused before transport is washed out of the donor liver before the infrahepatic inferior vena cava anastomosis is completed, "potassium cardioplegia" can lead to cardiac arrest when the vessels are unclamped. During the revascularization period, potassium is taken up by the donor liver and by all cells because of the intracellular shift of potassium resulting from metabolic alkalosis. Supplemental potassium is usually required during this phase.

Preexisting myocardial disease and the effects of profound metabolic derangements, especially decreased ionized calcium, on cardiac output as well as the requirement for infusion of massive quantities of fluids almost invariably result in cardiac dysfunction during liver transplantation. However, intraoperative measurements of central venous pressure and pulmonary artery wedge pressures have rarely shown right-to-left heart dissociation. Therefore, pulmonary artery catheters are rarely needed for the clinical management of infants during the postoperative period.

Early clinical experiences with hepatic transplantation indicated that intraoperative hypoglycemia occurred frequently. However, this has not been found in our series. Administration of blood components may be responsible for the marked increase in serum glucose concentration. Neither limiting nor eliminating crystalloid solutions containing glucose or administering regular insulin by intravenous bolus or infusion had any effect during this period of hyperglycemia, which peaks within 1 hour of the end of the anhepatic phase. After revascularization of the donor liver is complete, serum glucose decreases spontaneously, and may be hastened by administration of insulin.

Despite the osmotic diuretic effects of glucose and adequate renal preload, it is difficult to maintain adequate urine output. Furosemide or dopamine, 5 µg/kg/minute, may be administered. Renal output usually improves markedly after hepatic revascularization.

Hypernatremia may occur intraoperatively and is usually a result of the administration of sodium bicarbonate. Characteristically, patients have an increasing metabolic acidosis intraoperatively until the beginning of revascularization. This metabolic acidosis should be treated conservatively, based on determinations of arterial blood gas tension and pH, as moderate to severe metabolic alkalosis is observed soon after completion of orthotopic liver transplantation and persists for days to weeks. This occurs as a result of the metabolism of exogenously administered citrate, and the vigorous use of furosemide throughout the postoperative period.

Many children undergoing liver transplantation have preexisting arterial-to-alveolar oxygen gradient abnormalities including intrapulmonary arteriovenous shunting and atelectasis from massive ascites. Intraoperative arterial-to-alveolar oxygen gradient abnormalities occur because of profound cephalad displacement of the right diaphragm as a result of surgical traction, pulmonary air embolization at the time of revascularization, or pulmonary edema as a result of abnormal intravascular-extracellular osmotic pressure gradients or fluid overload. Arterial blood gases are usually maintained with conventional ventilation, although high-frequency ventilation is occasionally required. Other complications noted in our series were barotrauma from either surgical dissection, internal jugular cannula insertion, or high-peak airway pressure, and inability to close the abdomen due to bowel distension or the use of an oversized donor liver in a child. In the latter cases, the abdomen was closed temporarily with a Silastic silo similar to that used to repair a large omphalocele. With the advent of newer surgical techniques that involve splitting the donor liver into fragments, inability to close the abdomen has not been a problem. In general most patients remain intubated for at least 24 hours postoperatively. The intensive care stay has averaged 2 to 3 days.

REFERENCES

1. Lilly JR: Biliary atresia: The jaundiced infant, in Welch KJ, et al (eds): *Pediatric Surgery,* Chicago, Year Book Medical Publishers, Inc, 1986, pp 1047–1054.
2. Falchetti D, deCarvalho B, Clapuyt P, et al: Liver transplantation in children with biliary atresia and polysplenia syndrome. *J Pediatr Surg* 1991; 26:528–531.
3. Kasai M, Mochizuki I, Ohkohchi N, et al: Surgical limitation for biliary atresia indication for liver transplantation. *J Pediatr Surg* 1989; 24:851–854.
4. Lloyd-Still JD: Impact of orthotopic liver transplantation on mortality from pediatric liver disease. *J Pediatr Gastroenterol Nutr* 1991; 12:305–309.
5. Starzl TE, Iwatsuki S, Shaw BW: Liver transplantation, in Welch KJ, et al. (eds): *Pediatric Surgery,* Chicago, Year Book Medical Publishers, Inc, 1986, pp 373–382.
6. Borland LM, Roule M, Cook DR: Anesthesia for pediatric orthotopic liver transplantation. *Anesth Analg* 1985; 64:117–124.
7. Robertson KM, Cook DR: Perioperative management of the multiorgan donor. *Anesth Analg* 1990; 70:546–556.
8. Otte JB, deVille de Goyet J, Sokal E, et al: Size reduction of the donor liver is a safe way to alleviate the shortage of size-matched organs in pediatric liver transplantation. *Ann Surg* 1990; 221:146–157.
9. Kang YG, Martin DJ, Marquez J, et al: Intraoperative changes in blood coagulation and thromboelastographic monitoring in liver transplantation. *Anesth Analg* 1985; 64:888–896.
10. Lawless S, Ellis D, Thompson A, et al: Mechanisms of hypertension during and after orthotopic liver transplantation in children. *J Pediatr* 1989; 115:372–379.

28

Neuroblastoma

An 11-month-old, 12-kg girl with a large abdominal mass is scheduled for exploratory laparotomy. Radiographic studies indicate that the mass is extrarenal, most likely a neuroblastoma. Her blood pressure since admission has ranged from 130/90 to 170/120. Temperature, 37° C; pulse, 110; respirations, 22; hemoglobin, 8.6 g/dL; hematocrit, 26%.

Recommendations by Charles M. Haberkern, M.D.

Neuroblastoma is the most common solid tumor occurring in infancy and the third most common malignancy in children, preceded in frequency only by leukemias and brain tumors.[1] About one fourth of neuroblastomas are congenital, and over half are diagnosed by 2 years of age. The tumor occurs more frequently in boys (2:1) and has a reported incidence of 1:10,000 live births. Cases of neuroblastoma have been associated with Hirschsprung disease and other neurocristopathies, fetal alcohol and hydantoin syndromes, and subtle chromosomal abnormalities.

Neuroblastoma, along with the related tumors ganglioneuroblastoma and ganglioneuroma, is an embryonal tumor of neural crest origin that may arise at any site in the sympathetic nervous system. The distribution of site of origin is neck, 3%; mediastinum, 20%; pelvis, 3%; adrenal medulla, 50%; and paraspinal sympathetic ganglia, 24%. Metastases are present in over half of the children at the time of diagnosis, particularly in bone cortex, bone marrow, and lymph nodes. For the purposes of clinical description, treatment, and prognosis, neuroblastomas are categorized as follows: stage I, tumor confined to the structure of origin; stage II, tumor extension beyond the structure of origin but not across the midline; stage III, tumor extension beyond the midline, possibly with bilateral regional lymph node involvement; stage IV, metastatic disease to bone, organs, soft tissues, and distant lymph nodes; and stage IVS, stage I or II with remote disease in the liver, skin, and/or bone marrow.

CLINICAL PRESENTATION

The clinical presentation of the tumor varies widely, depending on the age of the patient, the site of origin of the mass, and the presence of associated clinical findings. In the newborn, the diagnosis may be made in an otherwise healthy-appearing infant by palpation of an abdominal mass on routine examination. It may also be suspected on the basis of abnormal fetal ultrasound findings. Older infants and children often appear chronically ill with fever, weight loss, pallor, and gastrointestinal disturbances. Other presenting signs and symptoms may indicate specific tumor location: respiratory distress with mediastinal tumors, Horner syndrome with tumors of the stellate ganglion, proptosis or bilateral orbital ecchymoses with tumors metastatic to the orbits, paraplegia with extradural extension of tumor, and impaired walking with long-bone metastases. A newborn may present with blue-red cutaneous metastases that look like blueberries (the "blueberry muffin baby" syndrome), and a child may present with rapidly alternating eye movements and myoclonic jerks (the "myoclonus-opsoclonus" syndrome). The release of vasoactive intestinal peptide (VIP) can cause watery diarrhea with resultant dehydration and electrolyte imbalance. The release of catecholamines is reported to produce fever, sweating, flushing, or hypertension in up to 35% of children,[1, 2] although these signs are usually not as prominent as they are with pheochromocytoma. In our review of 108 children with neuroblastoma coming to the operating room for resection over a period of 20 years, only 8% had signs or symptoms indicative of excessive VIP or catecholamine secretion at the time of diagnosis.

The clinical diagnosis of neuroblastoma can be confirmed by radiologic and chemical studies. Plain roentgenograms often show stippled calcifications of the tumor. Intravenous pyelography usually delineates the tumor when it is suprarenal and can help distinguish it from a Wilms tumor by its displacement rather than intrinsic distortion of the kidney. Computed tomography and magnetic resonance imaging can further characterize the tumor and its local extension. Long-bone roentgenograms and isotope bone scans demonstrate the presence of bone cortex metastases. About 80% to 90% of patients with neuroblastoma will have elevated levels of the urinary catecholamines norepinephrine and epinephrine as well as their metabolites vannillylmandelic acid and homovanillic acid. Bone marrow aspirates may show foci of tumor cells containing the specific oncogene N-*myc*. In addition, serum ferritin and neuron-specific enolase (NSE) levels may be elevated in patients with neuroblastoma.

The prognosis for children with neuroblastoma has remained relatively unchanged in recent years despite the changing modalities of treatment. For children under 2 years of age or those with stage I, II, or IVS disease, the expected survival rate is over 75%; for those over 2 years of age or those with stage III or IV disease, the expected survival rate is less than 40%. Children with primary tumors of the retroperitoneum have a relatively poor prognosis. Interestingly, about 1% to 2% of tumors undergo spontaneous regression for reasons that are not well understood.

TREATMENT

Treatment for children with stage I and many with stage II disease is surgical removal of the tumor alone. Treatment for many children with stage III and most with stage IV disease entails chemotherapy prior to delayed primary tumor resection; irradiation may be used as adjunctive therapy before or after surgery. Those with IVS disease are generally managed conservatively, but surgery, chemotherapy, and/or radiation therapy may also be employed as supportive measures. An additional therapeutic regimen now utilized for children with extensive disease is total-body irradiation and high-dose chemotherapy, followed by bone marrow transplantation.

PREOPERATIVE ASSESSMENT

The child under consideration here has many of the previously described problems associated with neuroblastoma, and these problems should be addressed in all aspects of perioperative care of this patient by the anesthesiologist.[3] If the child has stage III or IV disease by initial evaluation or by staging at the time of surgical exploration, she will probably not undergo removal of the tumor at this time. For purposes of discussion, it will be assumed that she has stage I or II disease that is appropriate for primary surgical excision.

Evaluation for metastatic disease, including a skeletal survey and bone scan, should be performed prior to laparotomy. The presence of anemia may indicate chronicity of the process, bleeding within the tumor, or bone marrow involvement. The latter is appropriately assessed with a bone marrow aspiration performed at the time of laparotomy. In any case, at least 2 units of red blood cells should be crossmatched for expected transfusion during the operation. A history of diarrhea should prompt a determination of serum electrolytes and assessment of intravascular volume status. The presumed diagnosis of neuroblastoma warrants a 24-hour urine collection for catecholamines, particularly in the presence of hypertension, since these values are followed postoperatively as an index of disease recurrence.

Management of the child's severe hypertension is an important aspect of preoperative care. First, high blood pressure may pose a danger to the patient before and during the surgical procedure and necessitate medical management. Hypertensive crises can be precipitated by almost any stress and even by contrast radiographic studies in patients with catecholamine-secreting tumors.[4] Second, in this patient with chronic hypertension, depletion of intravascular volume is to be expected. As the blood pressure is normalized in preparation for surgery, the intravascular volume should be restored with crystalloid fluid and, perhaps, with red blood cells since the hematocrit is expected to decrease with volume repletion.

For control of high blood pressure in this patient, oral antihypertensive agents should be administered for a period of 10 to 14 days prior to surgery. Phenoxybenzamine, a long-acting α_1- and α_2-blocking agent, is the most effective antihypertensive. The dose is 0.2 to 1.2 mg/kg/day administered in two to three divided doses. Prazosin, a shorter-acting α_1-blocking agent, has also been used (5 to 25 μg/kg administered every 6 hours). The initial dose of either agent should be low and then subsequently increased incrementally over several days. The most common side effect is postural hypotension, which may be difficult to assess in a small child. β-Adrenergic blockade is occasionally needed to control secondary tachycardia and tachydysrhythmias once α-blockade is established. The end point of treatment is control of blood pressure and alleviation of sweating and other symptoms. On occasion, acute hypertensive crises mandate more aggressive therapy such as parenteral administration of phentolamine (0.1 mg/kg by intravenous bolus or 1 to 7 μg/kg/min by continuous intravenous infusion) or sodium nitroprusside.

INTRAOPERATIVE MANAGEMENT

The child will probably arrive in the induction area with an intravenous catheter already in place for fluid administration. In order to minimize stress and fear, which can induce catecholamine secretion, it is appropriate to administer sedation before separating the child from her parents if there is no contraindication. Thiamylal, 2 to 3 mg/kg, or midazolam, 0.5 to 1.0 mg/kg, is effective. If there is, in fact, no functioning intravenous catheter in place at the time of induction, rectal thiamylal, 22 mg/kg, can be administered for sedation prior to removing her from the induction area.

In the operating room, all noninvasive monitors are placed, and anesthesia is induced with a parenteral barbiturate or, in the absence of intravenous access, with an inhalation agent, usually halothane. It is important to achieve a deep level of anesthesia prior to laryngoscopy and tracheal intubation in order to prevent a surge of catecholamine release. Once the child is asleep, two large-bore intravenous catheters should be inserted, preferably in the upper extremities in case removal of the tumor leads to obstruction or disruption of the inferior vena cava. A peripheral arterial catheter should be placed for monitoring of blood pressure. A urinary catheter is indicated for assessing urine output. Placement of a central venous catheter is usually not necessary unless peripheral venous access is poor or the intravascular volume status remains tenuous.

Anesthesia is maintained with a volatile anesthetic; isoflurane is probably a better agent than halothane since the latter may sensitize the myocardium to circulating catecholamines. Judicious administration of a potent opioid such as fentanyl permits the use of lower concentrations of the volatile agent and may thereby alleviate fluctuations in blood pressure that often accompany tumor removal. In anticipation of wide surgical exposure, a nondepolarizing neuromuscular blocking agent is administered, preferably an agent such as vecuronium or doxacurium that does not cause significant tachycardia or histamine release. Finally, in the absence of an underlying coagulopathy and persistent depletion of intravascular volume, placement of a caudal epidural catheter and administration of a local anesthetic prior to the incision should be considered to provide regional anesthesia as a complement to other anesthetic agents. However, one must be prepared to recognize and treat hypotension caused by sympathectomy in this child with chronic hypertension. A loading dose of bupivacaine (0.25%, 1.0 mL/kg) should be administered slowly to provide a sensory level appropriate for laparotomy. No epinephrine is used, except for the test dose.

Management of fluid and blood replacement is a critical aspect of the patient's care. As previously noted, the intravascular volume may be depleted due to chronic hypertension. Ideally, the child is rendered euvolemic prior to induction of anesthesia. Any fluid deficits should be replaced early in the procedure in anticipation of fluid and blood losses during tumor removal. In addition, the maintenance fluid requirement (approximately 4 mL/kg/hr) as well as replacement for third-space losses associated with intra-abdominal procedures (approximately 10 to 12 mL/kg/hr) should be administered. A urine output of 1 to 2 mL/kg/hr is a good indication of adequate intravascular volume. In the face of high levels of circulating catecholamines, blood glucose levels are usually elevated. The blood glucose content should be measured before dextrose is added to intravenous fluids since excessive dextrose administration can lead to hyperglycemia and secondary osmotic diuresis, further compromising intravascular volume. This chronically anemic child can probably tolerate a hematocrit near 20%. However, the low baseline hematocrit, which is probably below 26% once volume repletion is achieved, and expected blood losses with surgery will necessitate blood transfusion.

Marked fluctuations in blood pressure can be expected during surgical removal of the tumor. Manipulation of the tumor may induce the release of catecholamines and sudden elevations in blood pressure, which can be effectively treated by deepening anesthesia or by administering a vasodilating agent such as phentolamine or sodium nitroprusside. However, a more common event in our experience is hypotension during and after removal of the tumor. Fluid and blood loss may contribute to hypotension, but the primary cause appears to be mechanical: interference with venous return by intra-abdominal surgical retraction and manipulation. In anticipation of these changes, maintenance of adequate intravascular volume with crystalloid fluid and/or red blood cells before surgical removal of the tumor is important. In addition, as the tumor is isolated from the circulation, there is the potential for sudden hypotension as the catecholamine infusion from the tumor is withdrawn. On occasion, pharmacologic support of the blood pressure with vasopressors such as phenylephrine or dopamine is necessary.

POSTOPERATIVE MANAGEMENT

Once the tumor is removed and the surgical procedure is being completed, plans for postoperative care should be made. Whether or not she should be awakened and extubated after surgical wound closure depends on the condition of the child, including oxygenation, metabolic and fluid status, the presence or absence of coagulopathy resulting from massive blood replacement and the extent of residual neuromuscular blockade. If the child's condition is good, there is no specific contraindication to prompt emergence and tracheal extubation. Attention in the postanesthesia care unit and on the hospital ward should be directed to the intravascular volume status and blood pressure, although hypertension usually resolves with tumor removal.

Postoperative pain control is an important consideration. The presence of a caudal epidural catheter permits epidural morphine administration. However, there is evidence to suggest that respiratory depression due to epidural opioids is more common in infants less than 1 year of age, particularly if they have received intraoperative parenteral opioids.[5] Therefore, alternative approaches to postoperative pain control should be considered. These include bolus dosing of the epidural catheter with local anesthetic; continuous infusion of local anesthetic through the epidural catheter (e.g., bupivacaine, 0.0625% to 0.125%, 3 to 4 mL/hr); bolus dosing with intravenous morphine (0.05 to 0.1 mg/kg) as needed; and continuous intravenous infusion of morphine (10 to 30 μg/kg/hr). Whichever method of pain control is used, it is essential that the nursing staff be familiar with the method employed and that the child be closely monitored for respiratory depression. Supplemental oxygen should be administered postoperatively because of the adverse effects of the surgical incision, postoperative pain, and the method of pain control on gas exchange.

REFERENCES

1. Grosfeld JL: Neuroblastoma: A 1990 review. *Pediatr Surg Int* 1991; 6:9–13.
2. Weinblatt ME, Heisel MA, Siegal SE: Hypertension in children with neurogenic tumors. *Pediatrics* 1983; 71:947–951.

3. Farman JV: Neuroblastomas and anaesthesia. *Br J Anaesth* 1965; 37:866–870.
4. Raisanen J, Shapiro B, Glaser GM, et al: Plasma catecholamines in pheochromocytoma: Effect of urographic contrast media. *AJR* 1984; 143:43–46.
5. Valley RD, Bailey AG: Caudal morphine for postoperative analgesia in infants and children: A report of 138 cases. *Anesth Analg* 1991; 72:120–124.

29

Cleft Palate

A 13-month-old girl is admitted for cleft palate repair. She is "chubby" and weighs 14 kg. Hemoglobin, 11 g/dL; hematocrit, 33.2%.

Recommendations by Jon-Bruce Chopyk, M.D.

Cleft lip and palate are the most common of the craniofacial anomalies, with an incidence of 1 in 800 live births.[1] Fifty percent of patients have both cleft lip and palate. This discussion will focus on isolated cleft palate, which occurs about a third as often as cleft lip and palate. Seventy percent of isolated cleft palates occur in females.

Embryologically, there is a primary and secondary palate with the point of division being the incisive foramen.[2] The secondary palate lies posterior to the incisive foramen and includes the hard and soft palate. During the 7th to 12th gestational weeks, the lateral palantine shelves of the maxilla fuse in the midline. Failure of such fusion produces clefting of the palate.

ASSOCIATED ANOMALIES

Over 154 syndromes have been associated with cleft lip and palate.[3] Isolated cleft palate is associated with half of these syndromes. The most common syndrome, the Pierre Robin anomalad, includes micrognathia and glossoptosis. Approximately 33% of children born with cleft palate have other congenital defects, including umbilical hernia, clubfoot, cervical spine anomalies, and limb and ear deformities. There is also an increased incidence of congenital heart disease. However, the exact incidence is unknown due to inadequate reporting and the early death of the sickest of infants. In one series of 150 consecutive patients with cleft lip and/or palate, the incidence of congenital heart malformation was 1.3%.[4] This in all probability is due to the fact that the embryologic timetables for the formation of the heart and the lip/palate are different.

The child presenting with cleft palate may have several associated problems. Deglutition may be impaired with resultant poor feeding and anemia. Children with cleft palate often weigh less than normal; however, this difference is not statistically significant. Aspiration and frequent upper respiratory infections may complicate their course, as does the almost universal occurrence of middle-ear disease.[5] Hearing loss is not uncommon. Speech and language development may be affected prior to surgical correction.

SURGICAL REPAIR

Cleft palates are usually corrected at 12 to 18 months of age to allow for normal speech development and early growth of the maxilla.[6] A palatoplasty is performed by mobilizing the tissues of the hard and soft palate and closure of the midline defect. The duration of this procedure approximates 60 to 120 minutes. During a push-back palatoplasty, a local soft-tissue flap is taken to add length to the soft palate. In 25% to 30% of patients having cleft palate repair, velopharyngeal incompetence occurs and is manifested by speech hypernasality and nasal regurgitation.[7] A pharyngeal flap procedure is performed to correct this velopharyngeal incompetence by taking a mucosal/muscle flap from the posterior pharyngeal wall and attaching it to the velum. It is important to recall that a nasal intubation should never be attempted in a child who has undergone a pharyngeal flap procedure.

The simultaneous repair of cleft lip and palate between the ages of 3 and 4 months has been reported.[8] The preliminary results showed normal maxillary growth and function, normal speech development, and a lesser incidence of middle-ear infections. However, this is not as yet standard surgical practice in the United States.

PREOPERATIVE PREPARATION

The child presenting for cleft palate repair may undergo several operations throughout life. The anesthesiologist should be aware of this and attempt to minimize the psychic trauma associated with disfigurement and repeated surgery.

The parents are instructed not to feed the child formula or breast milk after midnight. Should the child awaken during the night, apple juice or water may be offered. Clear liquids may be offered up to 3 hours prior to surgery. Premedication is usually not necessary in children presenting for palatoplasty. However, anesthesiologists have their own personal preference regarding premedication. A preoperative hemoglobin/hematocrit determination may be useful since these children may be anemic secondary to feeding difficulties. Surgery should not be delayed if these values are not obtained as long as the history and physical examination are normal.

ANESTHETIC MANAGEMENT

The author prefers a volatile agent for induction of anesthesia and a loading dose of narcotic followed by narcotic infusion for maintenance.[9] Induction is with increasing concentrations of halothane administered by mask. Nitrous oxide and oxygen are utilized as carrier agents. Once consciousness is lost, monitors are applied. At this point, manual control of ventilation is attempted. If the depth of anesthesia is adequate, the control of respiration can be easily attained in the child with cleft palate. An oral airway or cleft gauze packing may be necessary should the tongue become lodged in the cleft and cause upper airway obstruction.

Intravenous access in any child is often fraught with difficulty, and multiple attempts are frequently required. In the overweight child with no visible veins, my greatest success is with the saphenous vein at the level of the medial malleolus. In most instances the vein cannot be seen but can be palpated on the superior aspect of the medial malleolus.

Once the intravenous catheter is in place, halothane and nitrous oxide administration is discontinued and the patient is ventilated with 100% oxygen to provide maximal time for placement of the endotracheal tube. Prior to intubation an anticholinergic agent, an intermediate-acting nondepolarizing muscle relaxant, and a loading dose of narcotic are administered. Glycopyrrolate, 0.01 mg/kg, is a better drying agent and produces less tachycardia at half the dose of atropine. Either atracurium or vecuronium at two times the 95% effective dose (ED_{95}) may be used for intubation. A loading dose of fentanyl, 5 to 7 μg/kg, or alfentanil, 100 to 125 μg/kg, is appropriate.

An appropriate laryngoscope blade for intubation is the Miller 1 or the Wis-Hipple 1.5. The blade may slip into the cleft and make visualization of the vocal cords impossible, in which case the cleft is packed with moist or petrolatum-coated gauze. Use of an oral RAE tube is suggested. Breath sounds should be auscultated prior to taping the tube in the midline under the chin. Some surgeons prefer to suture the endotracheal tube to the gum to prevent accidental dislodgement. Because accidental dislodgement is an ever-present danger during the course of the procedure, continuous monitoring with a precordial stethoscope, end-tidal CO_2, and pulse oximetry are recommended, as is hand-controlled ventilation. Prior to turning the child over to the surgeon, her eyes should be taped and the stomach emptied.

Anesthesia is maintained with a continuous narcotic infusion, a muscle relaxant, and nitrous oxide–oxygen. Sixty percent nitrous oxide will provide amnesia. Atracurium or vecuronium administration should be continued to prevent inadvertent movement during the surgical procedure. Continuous infusion of fentanyl or alfentanil may be instituted immediately after the loading dose or shortly thereafter at rates of 0.05 and 3.0 μg/kg/min, respectively. Infusion rates are titrated to heart rate and blood pressure response.

Positioning of the patient for cleft palate repair requires that the child's head be at the top of the operating table with the neck in moderate hyperextension and a 15-degree Trendelenburg tilt. The table is usually rotated 90 degrees from the anesthesiologist. After the child is draped, only about 5% of the total-body surface area remains exposed. However, most anesthesiologists use a warming blanket and a heated humidifier.

A Dingman mouth gag is inserted to provide surgical exposure. Malposition of the gag may cause partial or total occlusion of the endotracheal tube. Often a surgical pack is inserted to prevent the aspiration of blood. The pack insertion and removal should be noted on the anesthesia record. Blood loss during the repair is usually minimal to moderate and should be replaced with crystalloid solution.

Epinephrine-containing solutions are infiltrated into the operative site prior to incision to provide hemostasis. For unknown reasons, children are less sensitive to the development of cardiac dysrhythmias than are adults. It is generally agreed that a mean dose of 7 to 10 μg/kg of epinephrine can safely be used for this procedure in patients anesthetized with halothane.[10, 11] Interestingly, trigeminal nerve irritation appears to be responsible for the dysrhythmias rather than the exogenous administration of epinephrine. In all probability, higher concentrations can be used with a narcotic-based technique. Usually the total amount of lidocaine with epinephrine that the surgeon desires to use is well within the accepted dosage since greater volumes may cause distortion of the anatomy.

Fifteen to 20 minutes prior to completion of surgery, the fentanyl infusion is discontinued. Because of the shorter elimination half-life for alfentanil, its use should be discontinued 5 to 10 minutes prior to the planned time of awakening the child. The patient should remain paralyzed but "reversible" for the remainder of the procedure. At the conclusion of surgery, the muscle relaxant is reversed with atropine, 0.01 mg/kg followed by edrophonium, 0.5 to 1.0 mg/kg. The patient is ventilated with 100% oxygen for 3 to 5 minutes before spontaneous ventilation or awakening occurs. Once awake, the patient may be safely extubated. With this technique airway reflexes will be present, and the child will respond appropriately to external stimuli and be comfortable when not disturbed.

COMPLICATIONS

Five life-threatening cases of airway obstruction in the early postoperative period have been described.[12-14] In all instances, a Dingman retractor was used to provide surgical exposure, and all cases lasted in excess of 3.5 hours. One author has shown that the incidence of postoperative airway obstruction increased tenfold if the duration of the procedure was more than 2 hours.[15] Thus, the development of macroglossia appears to be clearly related to the duration of the surgical repair of the cleft palate. All children developed massive lingual and sublingual edema in the immediate postoperative period, and reintubation was required for a period of 1 to 11 days. In one case reintubation was extremely difficult, and the patient sustained a cardiac arrest. In order to avoid this complication, the lingual surface of the tongue should be examined for evidence of edema prior to extubation. If lingual edema is present, it may be prudent to leave the child intubated in the pediatric intensive care unit for continued observation.

REFERENCES

1. Steward RE: Craniofacial malformations—clinical and genetic considerations. *Pediatr Clin North Am* 1978; 25:485.
2. Johnston MC, Hassel JR, Brown KS: The embryology of cleft lip and palate. *Clin Plast Surg* 1975; 2:195.
3. Cohen MM: Syndromes with cleft lip and palate. *Cleft Palate J* 1978; 15:306.
4. Shah CV, Pruzansky S, Morris W: Cardiac malformations with facial clefts. *Am J Dis Child* 1970; 119:238.
5. Paradise JL, Bluestone CD, Felder H: The unreversality of otitis media in 50 infants with cleft palate. *Pediatrics* 1969; 44:35.
6. Millard DR: *Cleft Craft: The Evolution of Its Surgery,* vol 3. Boston, Little, Brown & Co Inc, 1980.
7. Serafin D, Riski JE: The velopharyngeal portal: Anatomy, physiology, and the management of incompetence, in Serafin D, Georgiade NG (eds): *Pediatric Plastic Surgery.* St Louis, Mosby–Year Book, 1984, p 301.

8. Kaplan I, Dresner J: The simultaneous repair of cleft lip and palate in early infancy. *Br J Plast Surg* 1974; 27:134.

9. Cook DR, Chopyk J: Infusion of narcotics and relaxants as an adjunct to nitrous oxide–oxygen anesthesia. *Semin Anesth* 1988; 7:226.

10. Ueda W, Hirakawa M, Mae O: Appraisal of epinephrine administration to patients under halothane anesthesia for closure of cleft palate. *Anesthesiology* 1983; 58:574.

11. Karl HW, Swedlow DB, Lee KW, et al: Epinephrine-halothane interactions in children. *Anesthesiology* 1983; 58:142.

12. Patane PS, White SE: Macroglossia causing airway obstruction following cleft palate repair. *Anesthesiology* 1989; 71:995.

13. Bell C, Oh TH, Loeffler JR: Massive macroglossia and airway obstruction after cleft palate repair. *Anesth Analg* 1988; 67:71.

14. Lee JT, Kingston HGG: Airway obstruction due to massive lingual oedema following cleft palate surgery. *Can Anaesth Soc J* 1985; 32:265.

15. Schettler D: Intra- and post-operative complications in surgical repair of clefts in infancy. *J Maxillofac Surg* 1973; 1:40.

30

Stridor in the Recovery Room

A 2-year-old, 12-kg boy who had an uneventful anesthetic for removal of a nevus from his face develops stridor in the recovery room approximately 15 minutes following extubation. He is tachypneic, and sternal retraction is evident. Oxygen saturation, 92%.

Recommendations by Robert B. Mesrobian, M.D.

Stridor is a clinical diagnosis defined as high-pitched, noisy respiration and is a sign of respiratory obstruction, especially in the trachea or larynx. Inspiratory stridor implies *extra*thoracic airway obstruction; expiratory stridor is associated with *intra*thoracic causes. In this child, it is assumed that inspiratory stridor is present. In the postoperative child who is alert, the most common cause of an extrathoracic airway problem is postextubation subglottic edema (PESE).

POSTEXTUBATION SUBGLOTTIC EDEMA

A recognized entity since airways have been secured by intubation, PESE is also referred to as postintubation, or extubation, croup. It can be one of the most serious immediate postoperative complications of endotracheal intubation. The incidence of stridor after *short*-term intubation in children has been reported to be 1% to 6%,[1-4] with an incidence of up to 40% with long-term intubation.[5]

Pediatric patients are more prone to develop PESE than are adults due to both anatomic and physiologic differences. The narrowest portion of the young child's airway is at the level of the cricoid cartilage due to incomplete development of the thyroid and cricoid cartilages.[6] The adult larynx is described as cylindrical, whereas the pediatric larynx is "funnel" shaped. This invites internal tracheal injuries in children since an endotracheal tube can easily pass through the vocal cords and become snug in the subglottic area. Small degrees of swelling will dramatically increase airway resistance: 1 mm of circumferential edema at the level of the cricoid can reduce the lumen from 4 to 2 mm, a 75% reduction in cross-sectional area. Resistance, which is proportional to the fourth power of the radius, will increase by a factor of 16. Stridor is produced by turbulent airflow. This nonlaminar flow further adds to resistance and varies by the fifth power of the radius.

As subglottic edema develops, extrathoracic airway resistance increases. A child's skeleton is highly elastic due to its cartilaginous nature. The trachea is particularly prone to dynamic airway collapse with upper airway obstruction. Even though the cricoid ring has a constant size, the trachea will collapse distal to the subglottic obstruction in the extrathoracic region on inspiration. This further increases airway resistance, markedly increasing the work of breathing by requiring the child to generate forceful intrathoracic pressures. Crying aggravates the obstruction by promoting dynamic airway collapse, increases oxygen consumption, and raises the demand for more alveolar ventilation.

The very compliant chest wall of small children further adds to this vicious cycle by poorly maintaining an adequate tidal volume. As suprasternal and intercostal retractions develop, the respiratory rate increases. Airflow becomes more turbulent at higher respiratory rates since peak airflow must increase. Respiratory work increases dramatically, the child becomes restless and sweaty, and eventually respiratory failure occurs. These effects are most pronounced in the youngest children with the smallest airways and most elastic skeletons.

Hypoxemia can develop in several ways. Baseline oxygen consumption in children is high, 5 to 6 cc O_2/kg/min in infants, and when combined with an increased need for alveolar ventilation due to increased respiratory work and crying, leads to hypoxia. Normal functional residual capacity in children is lower at rest than it is in the adult, 30 cc/kg vs. 34 cc/kg, due to an increased elastic recoil. This further decreases with extrathoracic airway obstruction. Acute pulmonary edema can develop with either acute or chronic airway obstruction. Acute pulmonary edema has been associated with many causes of upper airway obstruction, including croup, epiglottitis, laryngospasm, laryngeal edema,[7, 8] and foreign bodies. The etiology is unclear, but acute pulmonary edema can occur both before and after relief of airway obstruction.[9] Pulmonary secretions, poorly cleared because of the inability to take large tidal volumes, accumulate. This is a more serious problem with infectious croup since it involves the bronchial tree.

The severity of PESE is primarily assessed visually. Numerous scoring systems have been devised[10-12] and rely on clinical parameters, including the character of inspiratory sounds, stridor, cough, retractions, cyanosis, and mental status. The ability to compare various therapeutic regimens has often been criticized for the lack of a standard scoring system.

PREDICTORS OF POSTEXTUBATION SUBGLOTTIC EDEMA

What children are at risk of developing PESE? This is a difficult question to answer since most studies are flawed by design. A landmark prospective study published in 1977 defined several risk factors.[2] Age is important. Children between the ages of 1 and 4 years had a higher incidence of PESE than did those less than 1 year of age. Other studies[1, 13] support this age-related increased incidence, although a few show no difference.[14]

Trauma related to intubation is also important. Defining difficult intubation as more than one attempt at intubation, the author found a positive correlation with the development of stridor. Finally, endotracheal tube size has long been suspected as being a factor in the development of PESE. There is a correlation with the absence of an air leak around the endotracheal tube. Some investigators recommend replacement of the endotracheal tube if there is no leak with airway pressures above 20 to 25 cm H_2O. One author has reported that there was no correlation with leak pressure and stridor on extubation unless a prior history of infectious or postintubation croup existed,[15] but the study size was small and of questionable design. Marked variability in airway pressures at which a leak occurs, depending on patient position and neuromuscular blockade status, has been shown.[16] The air leak was much higher when the child's head was turned to the side than when the head was midline. It was also greater when neuromuscular blocking agents were not used.

The development of PESE is not reliably predictable from the size of the tube as determined by the presence of an air leak. Whether this relates to the technique of measurement or other variables is unclear. At present it seems prudent to use an endotracheal tube with an air leak at airway pressures above 20 to 25 cm H_2O.

The development of stridor is also related to head position and movement. In one series, changing the head position while the child was intubated was associated with a 25% incidence of stridor, whereas the incidence was less than 2% when the head was not moved. There is not as strong a relationship between the site of surgery and PESE, although one group reported that most children who developed stridor had surgery of the head and neck or dental surgery.[1] Tonsillectomies, which should have a higher incidence of stridor on extubation, were not found to have a higher association with PESE.[1] Coughing may also increase the incidence of stridor.[2] While it appears that changing head position contributes strongly to stridor on extubation, the mechanism is unclear.

Prolonged intubation may contribute to the development of PESE. While one group reported an increased incidence if intubation lasted longer than 1 hour, this is not supported by other studies[5, 14] from pediatric intensive care units (ICUs) unless intubation extended beyond 5 days.

In summary, it appears that the development of PESE cannot be predicted reliably. The majority of studies and surveys imply that children are at more risk if

1. An endotracheal tube without an air leak at airway pressures greater than 25 cm H_2O is used, although the presence of a leak will depend on head position and neuromuscular blockade status.
2. The head position is changed during the operative procedure while the patient is intubated.
3. There is a previous history of croup, PESE, or prior intubation.
4. The child is between 1 and 3 years of age.

There does not appear to be any correlation with patient sex or coexisting upper respiratory infection (URI). Of historical interest is the increased incidence of damage to the trachea due to toxic substances created when γ-ray–sterilized polyvinyl endotracheal tubes were resterilized with ethylene oxide.[17] Currently, endotracheal tubes used in this country all carry the marking "I.T.," which indicates that the manufacturer has tested a device from each lot, either by implantation in rabbits or by cell culture.

Both congenital subglottic stenosis,[18–20] with an incidence of 1/1,000,[21] and acquired stenosis have been implicated in the development of PESE. In particular, premature infants with a history of multiple intubations may have acquired subglottic stenosis. This may be asymptomatic and unrecognized preoperatively.[14, 20] Previous intubation for infectious croup is also associated with a higher rate of complications.[14] Children with Trisomy 21 are reported to have an incidence of stridor on extubation as high as 38%.[22] Cutaneous hemangiomas have a slight association with subglottic hemangiomas, and these patients have been reported to develop stridor.[18]

THERAPY

The clinical course of PESE is highly variable and unpredictable. After extubation, stridor typically develops within 1 to 2 hours, but severe respiratory obstruction can occur almost immediately. Most of the children develop stridor by 1 hour and the severity peaks by 4 to 6 hours. A very small percentage will proceed to respiratory failure despite therapy.

For mild stridor, cool humidification of inspired oxygen may soothe irritated airways and prevent drying of secretions. In animal studies, droplet deposition in the upper airways may reflexly alter the pattern of breathing and improve flow rates.[11] Oxygen administration is indicated due to the factors promoting hypoxemia in small children. Delivery of mist and oxygen is difficult in a preschool child arousing from an anesthetic when a quiet state is desired. Face masks and head boxes are usually poorly tolerated, and "blow-by" mist, unless constantly directed at the child's face, is of little benefit. The child's parents can often keep him calm so that a face mask is tolerated. A scoring system should be used if symptoms are not improved by 1 hour.

Racemic epinephrine has been used to treat croup and PESE for more than 30 years. When introduced, racemic epinephrine was controversial but has proved valuable in the management of subglottic edema.[1, 23-25] Racemic epinephrine is most effective when delivered by intermittent positive-pressure breathing (IPPB).[26] IPPB may improve delivery of the epinephrine by preventing tracheal collapse on inspiration. Even so, racemic epinephrine is not routinely administered by IPPB. Instead, 0.5 mL of 2.25% racemic epinephrine in 2 to 4 mL normal saline is delivered by nebulization. It should be used no more frequently than every 30 minutes. Children will usually become more calm as airway edema decreases. The need for increasing treatments and a worsening score may indicate the need for an artificial airway. Patients with dynamic obstruction to left ventricular outflow, that is, idiopathic hypertrophic subaortic stenosis and the tetralogy of Fallot, may not tolerate epinephrine.

"Racemic" epinephrine was initially used instead of epinephrine because it was thought to have less rebound vasodilation and other undesirable systemic effects.[27] Racemic epinephrine is a mixture of l- and d-isomers of epinephrine, with the l-isomer 15 to 20 times more active. Since it is an equal mixture of both isomers, it is therefore equivalent to half-strength epinephrine, all l-isomer. Racemic epinephrine has the same adverse effects as epinephrine. However, since it has become firmly established in the literature, the use of the racemic mixture is unlikely to be dislodged.

Rebound edema may occur, and in the past children were routinely admitted after treatment with racemic epinephrine. There is still controversy, but most are discharged home if symptoms are diminished after 2 hours.

Steroids administered just prior to or after extubation are commonly believed to minimize airway edema. Animal studies[28-30] show that steroids reduce edema or stenosis after induced subglottic damage. The authors of a 1980 review of steroid use in croup could not reach a conclusion after analyzing nine studies since all studies had major inadequacies in clinical trial design.[31] A 1989 meta-analysis of ten randomized studies does support the use of steroids in croup.[32] It was found that dexamethasone in a dose of 0.5 to 1 mg/kg intravenously was the most effective. There is no support for multiple doses beyond 12 to 24 hours. The issue is still unresolved. In ICU patients, dexamethasone, 0.5 mg/kg, was not of benefit in the prevention of PESE in uncomplicated airway management.[5] Unless there is a contraindication, most practitioners think that steroids should be used. Onset is generally in 45 minutes, and duration is between 4 and 8 hours.

Heliox is a mixture of helium and oxygen and has 33% of the density of room air. This decreases turbulence, improves airflow through a narrow orifice, and is very effective in PESE.[33-35] Heliox decreases the work of breathing and buys time for inflammation to subside. It must therefore be administered in as high a concentration as possible. A prior oxygen requirement may limit the concentration used. Helium is expensive and must be efficiently administered with a mask or small head box.

Respiratory failure can occur despite all therapy. Intubation should be performed in as controlled a fashion as possible by utilizing an approach similar to an epiglottitis protocol. An endotracheal tube one size smaller than calculated is used.

OTHER CAUSES OF POSTOPERATIVE STRIDOR

Not all patients with inspiratory stridor have subglottic edema. Injury to the recurrent laryngeal nerve from surgery or excessive stretch can result in unilateral vocal cord paralysis. Vocal cord damage is also reported with local compression from an endotracheal tube. Arytenoid dislocation can result from traumatic intubation or extubation. Indirect laryngoscopy is useful in differential diagnosis.

Foreign bodies in the oropharynx, especially with nose, throat, and dental cases, can lead to stridor. Retained small sponges or other appliances lead to varying degrees of obstruction. The author has personally found a small oral airway deep in the posterior portion of the pharynx in a 6-month-old neurosurgical patient on the fourth postoperative day when progressive airway stridor required reintubation. Severe posterior pharyngeal edema is uncommon but has been reported after intraoral surgery when mouth "gags" were used. Swelling required reintubation for several days.

Laryngospasm and edema of the upper airway may occur with severe allergic reactions. Patients with undisclosed angioneurotic edema and a deficiency of C_1 esterase inhibitor can develop massive facial and oral edema with only minimal trauma.

Extrapulmonary air associated with pneumothorax or pneumomediastinum may be difficult to distinguish initially from subglottic edema. A chest radiograph may be required.

SUMMARY

When a 2-year-old child presents postoperatively with signs of upper airway obstruction, the following is the appropriate clinical course:

1. Suction and clear the upper airway of all secretions.

2. If subglottic edema is suspected, administer humidity and oxygen. Consider intravenous administration of 0.5 to 1 mg/kg dexamethasone if symptoms are severe or progressive.

3. Administer 0.5 mL of 2.25% racemic epinephrine in 2 to 4 mL normal saline by nebulization, with IPPB if available. Consider other causes if deterioration continues. Obtain a chest radiograph, and consider the administration of heliox. If reintubation is required, it should be performed under controlled conditions in the operating room.

REFERENCES

1. Jordan WS, Graves CL, Elwyn RA: New therapy for postintubation laryngeal edema and tracheitis in children. *JAMA* 1970; 212:585–588.
2. Koka BV, Jeon IS, Andre JM, et al: Postintubation croup in children. *Anesth Analg* 1977; 56:501–505.
3. Pender JW: Endotracheal anesthesia in children: Advantages and disadvantages. *Anesthesiology* 1954; 15:495–506.
4. Super DM, Cortelli NA, Brooks LJ, et al: A prospective randomized double-blind study to evaluate the effect of dexamethasone in acute laryngotracheitis. *J Pediatr* 1989; 115:323–329.
5. Tellez DW, Golvis AG, Sturgion SA, et al: Dexamethasone in the prevention of postextubation stridor in children. *J Pediatr* 1991; 118:289–294.
6. Butz RO: Length and cross-section growth patterns in the human trachea. *Pediatrics* 1968; 42:336–341.
7. Lee KW, Downes JJ: Pulmonary edema secondary to laryngospasm in children. *Anesthesiology* 1983; 59:347–349.
8. Weissman C, Damask MC, Yang J: Noncardiogenic pulmonary edema following laryngeal obstruction. *Anesthesiology* 1984; 60:163.
9. Kanter RK, Weiner LB: Pediatric life threatening infections, in Shoemaker WES, Thompson WL, Holbrook PR (eds): *Textbook of Critical Care*. Philadelphia, WB Saunders Co, 1984.
10. Downs JJ, Raphaely R: Pediatric intensive care. *Anesthesiology* 1975; 43:242–250.
11. Hen J: Current management of upper airway obstruction. *Pediatr Ann* 1986; 15:274–294.
12. Taussig LM, Castro O, Beandry PH: Treatment of laryngotracheobronchitis (croup): Use of intermittent positive pressure breathing and racemic epinephrine. *Am J Dis Child* 1975; 129:700–793.
13. Hallowell P: Endotracheal intubation of infants and children. *Int Anesthesiol Clin* 1962; 1:135–153.
14. McEniery J, et al: Review of intubation in severe laryngotracheobronchitis. *Pediatrics* 1991; 87:847–853.
15. Lee KW, Templeton JJ, Dougal RM: Tracheal tube size and post-intubation croup in children. *Anesthesiology* 1980; 53:A325.
16. Finholt DA, Henry DB, Raphaely RC: The "leak" test—a standard method for assessing tracheal tube fit in pediatric patients. *Anesthesiology* 1984; 61:A450.
17. Stetson JB, Wallace LG: Causes of damage to tissues by polymers and elastomers used in the fabrication of tracheal devices. *Anesthesiology* 1970; 33:635–652.
18. Friedman EM, Vastula AP, McGill TJ, et al: Chronic pediatric stridor: Etiology and outcome. *Laryngoscope* 1990; 100:277–280.
19. Holinger PH, Kutnick SL, Schid JA, et al: Subglottic stenosis in infants and children. *Ann Otol Rhinol Laryngol* 1976; 85:591–599.
20. Otherson HB: Intubation injuries of the trachea in children. *Ann Surg* 1979; 189:601–606.
21. Phillips JJ, Sansome AJ: Acute infective airway obstruction associated with subglottic stenosis. *Anaesthesia* 1990; 45:34–35.
22. Sherry KM: Post-extubation stridor in Down's syndrome. *Br J Anaesth* 1983; 55:53–55.

23. Davis HW, Gartner JC, Galvis AG, et al: Acute upper airway obstruction: Croup and epiglottitis. *Pediatr Clin North Am* 1981; 28:859–880.

24. Ferrara TB, et al: Routine use of dexamethasone for the prevention of postextubation respiratory distress. *J Perinatol* 1989; 9:287–290.

25. Westley CR, Cotton EK, Brooks JG: Nebulized racemic epinephrine by IPPB for the treatment of croup. *Am J Dis Child* 1978; 132:484–487.

26. Gardner HG, et al: The evaluation of racemic epinephrine in treatment of infectious croup. *Pediatrics* 1974; 52:52–55.

27. Ellis EF, Taylor JC, Lefkowitz MS: Letter to the editor. *Pediatrics* 1974; 53:291.

28. Biller HF, Harvey JE, Bone RC, et al: Laryngeal edema: An experimental study. *Ann Otol Rhinol Laryngol* 1970; 79:1084–1087.

29. Croft C, Zub K, Borowiecki B: Therapy of iatrogenic subglottic stenosis: A steroid antibiotic regimen. *Laryngoscope* 1979; 89:482–487.

30. Woods CW, et al: Effects of dexamethasone and oxymetazoline on "post intubation croup": A ferret model. *Otolaryngol Head Neck Surg* 1986; 96:554–558.

31. Tunnessen WW, Feinstein AR: The steroid-croup controversy: An analytic review of methodologic problems. *J Pediatr* 1980; 96:751–756.

32. Kairys SW, Olmstead BA, O'Connor GT: Steroid treatment of laryngotracheitis: A meta-analysis of the evidence from randomized trials. *Pediatrics* 1989; 83:683–693.

33. Duncan PG: Efficacy of helium-oxygen mixtures in the management of severe viral and post-intubation croup. *Can Anaesth Soc J* 1979; 26:206–212.

34. Kemper KJ, Izenberg S, Marvin JA, et al: Treatment of postextubation stridor in a pediatric patient with burns: The role of heliox. *J Burn Care Rehabil* 1990; 11:337–339.

35. Kemper KJ, et al: Helium-oxygen mixture in the treatment of postextubation stridor in pediatric trauma patients. *Crit Care Med* 1991; 19:356–359.

31

Circumcision

A healthy 2-year-old boy is scheduled for circumcision on an outpatient basis. The procedure is scheduled for 11 A.M.

Recommendations by Linda Jo Rice, M.D., and Mary Ann Pudimat, M.D.

This otherwise healthy toddler presents two special challenges: What is the appropriate period with nothing to eat or drink in a healthy outpatient, and what options are there for postoperative analgesia?

NOTHING TO EAT OR DRINK (NPO) AFTER MIDNIGHT?

Recent studies have questioned the traditional 8-hour fasting requirement prior to anesthesia in healthy children undergoing elective surgery. One group studied 64 healthy children with a mean age of 5.6 years who had nothing to eat or drink after midnight and a group of 57 similar children who received no food after midnight but were allowed free access to clear fluids until 3 hours prior to surgery.[1] The mean duration of fasting of the first group was 14 hours, while the mean amount of liquid ingested by the second group was 203 mL (range, 30 to 605 mL). The investigators found that the volume and pH of the gastric contents were no different between the two groups. The same study also examined the effects of different volumes of apple juice administered 2.5 hours prior to surgery in children 5 to 10 years of age.[2] Volumes of 0, 6, and 10 mL/kg were administered. Gastric pH averaged 1.7 to 1.8 in all three groups, while gastric volume was 0.45 ± 0.31 mL/kg in the fasting group, 0.66 ± 0.79 mL/kg in the group that received 6 mL/kg of apple juice, and 0.71 ± 0.76 mL/kg in the group that received 10 mL/kg of apple juice. Children who drank 6 mL/kg of apple juice had decreased thirst and were less irritable prior to anesthesia than were those who fasted.

These and other studies would indicate that starving healthy children for 8 hours prior to elective surgery does not reduce the risk of aspiration and may make children less comfortable.[3, 4] Of importance is the fact that all children were healthy, were taking no medications, and were allowed only clear fluids—not milk, formula, or solid foods. Based on these studies, a period with nothing to eat or drink for 2 to 3 hours for clear liquids seems sufficient. These studies did not address the issue of hypoglycemia, a problem that has been reported in children fasted for 12 to 18 hours.

It would seem reasonable to notify this child's parents that their son should have no food, milk, or milk products after midnight the night prior to surgery. He should be allowed to drink sugared clear liquids (such as Kool-Aid or apple or nonparticulate orange juice) until 7 to 8 A.M. The prudent anesthesiologist may slightly increase the period for eating or drinking nothing in order to allow some flexibility for rescheduling cases.

ANESTHETIC MANAGEMENT

Circumcision is one of the most common pediatric surgical procedures performed in the United States. If circumcisions in the newborn nursery are included, it is *the* most common surgical procedure. No adult male would tolerate this procedure without anesthesia; however, most newborn circumcisions are performed on restrained patients with no analgesia.

In this patient, as in all patients, optimal management includes not only a surgical anesthetic but also a continuum of analgesia extending into the postoperative period. One of the most frequent reasons for admission of outpatients is pain management.

This child could receive any combination of premedication to facilitate separation from parents, followed by mask or intravenous induction, and any number of different general anesthetic techniques. Regional anesthesia combined with a light general anesthetic would provide excellent analgesia extending well into the postoperative period; blockade of noxious reflexes, particularly upon clamping the foreskin; and a quicker wake-up due to the decreased requirement for general anesthesia.

Having decided to use a combined technique, we would choose halothane, nitrous oxide, and oxygen as the general anesthetic agents and plan to have the child spontaneously ventilating via a mask throughout the procedure. The regional anesthetic will be administered following induction of general anesthesia but prior to the beginning of surgery. There are several regional anesthetic options.

Penile Block

Block of the dorsal nerves of the penis provides effective analgesia for hypospadias repair as well as circumcision. The distal two thirds of the penis is innervated by the dorsal nerves, which are bilateral and adjacent to the midline. The dorsal nerves are distal twigs of the pudendal nerves. They are covered by Buck's fascia and lay alongside other midline structures of the penis: the single dorsal artery and paired dorsal veins. The base and proximal part of the penis are innervated by the genitofemoral and ilioinguinal nerves.

The simplest penile block technique is a ring block of the penis, where a circumferential subcutaneous skin wheal is performed by using a few milliliters of 0.25% bupivacaine *without epinephrine*.[5] This block will provide analgesia for up to 8 hours. Since the penis is an end organ, it is important not to add epinephrine to any penile block technique.

Topical lidocaine has also been found useful once the foreskin is amputated and the mucous membranes exposed, and it can even be used for several days for additional postoperative analgesia.[6, 7] Once 1% lidocaine is dripped onto the exposed mucous membranes following amputation of the foreskin, halothane use can often be discontinued completely for the remainder of the procedure.[6] A decreased volatile agent requirement allows faster wake-up at the end of surgery.

This block also provides excellent analgesia for newborns undergoing circumcision. One milliliter of the local anesthetic is employed.

Caudal Block

Caudal analgesia is useful, simple to perform, and easily adaptable to modern anesthesia practice. Because of the loose areolar fat in the young patient, it is easier to achieve higher levels of neuroblockade than in the adult. Since prepubertal children have not yet developed the presacral fat pad, it is often easier to perform a caudal block than it is to place an intravenous catheter in a toddler. Caudal blockade is also excellent for surgery and extends into the lower thoracic dermatomes. It is particularly effective for sacral segment surgery since the sacral nerves are most accessible with this approach to the epidural space.

Caudal blockade combined with light general anesthesia reduces the intraoperative requirement for potent inhalation agents and ensures excellent postoperative pain relief.[8, 9] In addition, caudal analgesia results in a lower minute ventilation and respiratory rate and therefore improves ventilatory efficiency in spontaneously breathing children anesthetized with halothane. Caudal blocks provide longer postoperative analgesia for sacral segment surgery than for operations in higher dermatomes. In addition, in short procedures, there is no difference in the duration of postoperative analgesia in pediatric ambulatory patients whether the block is placed at the beginning or the end of the surgical procedure.[10] Therefore, placing the block following induction of anesthesia but prior to the beginning of surgery will decrease the need for volatile anesthetics while not depriving the child of analgesic time.

It is important to consult major references for a more complete description before performing any new block for the first time.[11] The anatomy of the lumbosacral epidural canal in infants and small children is different from that in adults. The infant's sacrum is a triangular bone formed by fusion of the five sacral vertebrae. This ossification is incomplete at birth and occurs over the ensuing 8 years of life. The sacral hiatus, due to the nonfusion of the fifth sacral vertebral arch, is easily identified in young children. The cornua are large bony processes on each side of the arch. The coccyx lies immediately caudal to the sacral hiatus, and the hiatus is covered by the sacrococcygeal membrane.

In addition to the dural and arachnoid sacs, the sacral canal contains nerves, blood vessels, lymphatics, and alveolar tissue. Whereas the dural and arachnoid sacs usually terminate at the level of the second sacral vertebra in adults, they may extend to the third or fourth sacral levels in infants. Also, the distance between the sacral hiatus and the end of the dural sac in the small child is relatively short.

With the child in the lateral position, the sacral hiatus is identified by palpating the tip of the coccyx with the left index finger. The palpating finger advances in a cephalad direction while moving from side to side. The first pair of bony protuberances encountered are the sacral cornua that surround the sacral hiatus. They should be marked with a fingernail. After careful skin preparation, the sacral hiatus is again identified. Asepsis *must* be maintained by wearing sterile gloves or palpating over a sterile alcohol sponge.

Once the sacral hiatus has been identified, the caudal space is entered by using a 1-in. 23-gauge needle attached to a syringe containing the appropriate volume of local anesthetic solution. The needle must be placed exactly in the midline and inserted at a 60-degree angle to the coronal plane, perpendicular to all other planes. The bevel of the needle should be facing anteriorly, that is, toward the feet, to minimize the chance of piercing the anterior sacral wall or digging a trough in the periosteum. The needle is advanced until a distinct "pop" is felt as the sacrococcygeal membrane is pierced. The needle is then lowered to an angle of 20 degrees and advanced an additional 2 to 3 mm to make sure that all of the beveled surface is in the caudal space. Further advancement of the needle is not necessary and will increase the chance of dural puncture. After aspiration has demonstrated the absence of blood or cerebrospinal fluid, 0.5 mL/kg of 0.25% bupivacaine is injected, and the child is placed in the supine position.

Placement of local anesthetic in the caudal epidural space can provide a block well into the upper thoracic area. Because the initial dose must be large enough to produce the required level of analgesia, it is important to utilize an adequate volume of local anesthetic. It is even more important to avoid overdoses of local anesthetic agents; one must therefore calculate not only the volume of local anesthetic but also the dose that will be employed. Lower concentrations of bupivacaine will avoid the troubling issue of motor blockade of sacral segment fibers. It should be recalled that the sciatic nerve arises from the sacral plexus and that high concentrations of bupivacaine will cause motor blockade of the legs and delayed ambulation. In terms of both intraoperative analgesia[12] and postoperative pain relief,[13] 0.125% bupivacaine is equivalent to 0.25% bupivacaine. Since syringe swaps are the most common anesthetic mishap, meticulous attention to detail is required when diluting local anesthetics with preservative-free normal saline. Experience with the commercially available 0.25% concentration of bupivacaine indicates that although motor weakness, particularly on standing, may be apparent 1 hour after the block was placed, it will resolve by 3 hours. Numerous studies indicate no delay in discharge due to an inability to ambulate; therefore we continue to employ the more concentrated solution and avoid the risk of inappropriate dilution.

Although micturition may be delayed due to the site of surgery, it has been demonstrated that children undergoing genital surgery will micturate by about 8 hours following surgery. This is true whether the child received regional analgesia or parenteral narcotics for postoperative analgesia. Caudal blockade does not delay micturition; thus there is no need to delay discharge from the ambulatory surgery unit until the child has voided.

Caudal blocks are relatively easy to perform in children less than 7 years of age. A success rate of 96% has been reported when the block was performed by experienced practitioners.[13] However, several attempts were necessary in 25% of children. Most failures occurred in children older than 7 years of age. Although infection is frequently listed among the complications of caudal block, it has not been reported in pediatric patients. However, the possibility of intraosseous injection must always be considered when caudal blocks are performed in children. The cancellous mass of sacral bone is covered by a wafer-thin brittle layer of cortex that can easily be damaged. Unfortunately, unlike adult epidural anesthesia, there is no reliable "test dose" that is effective in children; the addition of epinephrine will not reliably detect an intravascular injection, although it may slightly prolong the duration of the block.

SUMMARY

This toddler will benefit by an enlightened approach to the subject of fasting. He and his parents will be more comfortable if he is allowed to have sugared, clear liquids up to 3 hours prior to surgery. His vital signs will probably be more stable with this improved hydration. However, neither this nor improvement in blood glucose due to this shortened period of starvation have been studied.

He will also benefit from a combined general and regional anesthetic. Light general anesthesia and a regional block will allow better acceptance of the block by the patient, his parents, and the surgeon. Regional anesthesia will allow use of less volatile anesthetic and an earlier discharge.

The choice is between penile block and caudal block, both of which are efficacious, have a high safety record, and do not delay ambulation, voiding, or discharge from the outpatient unit. In addition, the parents may be given some topical anesthetic to apply to the surgical site for the first few postoperative days. This is truly a "balanced anesthetic" as originally described by George Crile in the early 1900s.

REFERENCES

1. Splinter WM, Schaefer JD, Zunder IH: Clear fluids three hours before surgery do not affect the gastric fluid contents of children. *Can J Anaesth* 1990; 37:498–501.
2. Splinter WM, Stewart JA, Muir JG: Large volumes of apple juice preoperatively do not affect gastric pH and volume in children. *Can J Anaesth* 1990; 37:36–39.
3. Coté CJ: NPO after midnight for children—a reappraisal. *Anesthesiology* 1990; 72:589–592.
4. Miller DC: Why are children starved? *Br J Anaesth* 1990; 64:409–410.
5. Broadman LM, Hannallah RS, Belman AB, et al: Post-circumcision analgesia—a prospective evaluation of subcutaneous ring block of the penis. *Anesthesiology* 1987; 67:399–402.
6. Andersen KH: A new method of analgesia for relief of circumcision pain. *Anaesthesia* 1989; 44:118–120.
7. Tree-Trakarn T, Pirayavaraporn S, Lertakyamanee J: Topical analgesia for relief of post-circumcision pain. *Anesthesiology* 1987; 67:395–399.
8. Hannallah RS, Broadman LM, Belman AB, et al: Comparison of caudal and ilioinguinal/iliohypogastric nerve blocks for control of post-orchiopexy pain in pediatric ambulatory surgery. *Anesthesiology* 1987; 66:832–834.
9. Blaise G, Roy WL: Postoperative pain relief after hypospadias repair in pediatric patients: Regional analgesia versus systemic analgesics. *Anesthesiology* 1986; 65:84–86.
10. Rice LJ, Pudimat MA, Hannallah RS: Timing of caudal block placement in relation to surgery does not affect duration of postoperative analgesia in pediatric ambulatory patients. *Can J Anaesth* 1990; 37:429.

11. Rice LJ, Hannallah RS: Local and regional anesthesia, in Motoyama EK, Davis PJ (eds): *Smith's Anesthesia for Infants and Children*. St Louis, Mosby–Year Book, 1990.

12. Dalens B, Hasnaoui A: Caudal anesthesia in pediatric surgery: Success rate and adverse effects in 750 consecutive patients. *Anesth Analg* 1989; 68:83–89.

13. Wolf AR, Valley RD, Fear DW, et al: Bupivacaine for caudal analgesia in infants and children: The optimal effective concentration. *Anesthesiology* 1988; 69:102–106.

32

Bronchoscopy for a Foreign Body

A 2-year-old, 13-kg boy is scheduled for bronchoscopy and removal of a screw lodged in the right mainstem bronchus. Hemoglobin, 12.1 g/dL; hematocrit, 36%.

Recommendations by Thomas P. Keon, M.D.

Foreign-body aspiration is a leading cause of death in children under 1 year of age and occurs most often between the ages of 7 months and 4 years. Symptoms include cough, dyspnea, and cyanosis at the time of aspiration. Physical findings are decreased breath sounds, tachypnea, stridor, wheezing, and fever. These symptoms and signs indicate the presence of an obstructive-inflammatory process affecting the airways. Radiographic abnormalities are air trapping, infiltrates, and atelectasis, alone or in combination. The most frequent site of foreign-body enlodgement is a main bronchus, with the right bronchus being slightly more common than the left.[1] Food particles are the most common type of foreign body, but beads, pins, tacks, and toy parts are not unusual. Vegetable objects are troublesome because they expand with moisture and can fragment into multiple small pieces, oil-containing substances such as peanuts produce chemical inflammation, and sharp objects can cause bleeding.

PREOPERATIVE ASSESSMENT

The patient's previous medical history, allergies, medications, prior anesthetic experiences, and last oral intake should be determined. Preoperative physical examination should emphasize airway examination, uniformity of breath sounds, detection of bronchospasm, and signs of arterial desaturation.

The most recent chest roentgenogram should be examined for the location of the foreign body and for evidence of secondary pathologic changes (Fig 32–1). Abnormal radiographic changes that

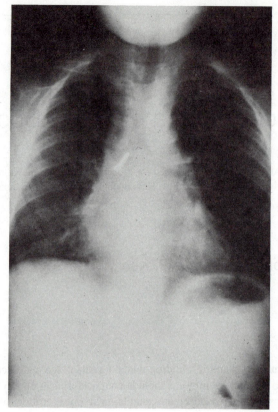

FIG 32–1.
Radiograph illustrating a screw lodged in the right mainstem bronchus.

could be encountered include unilateral hyperaeration as a result of obstructive emphysema, localized atelectasis or pneumonia, and loss of patency in air bronchograms.[2]

Premedication with atropine, 0.02 mg/kg, administered orally or intravenously 45 minutes preoperatively will reduce troublesome tracheobronchial secretions. Heavy premedication should be avoided because active protective airway reflexes may be necessary to maintain respiratory function both prior to bronchoscopy and at the end of the procedure.

INDUCTION OF ANESTHESIA

The majority of patients should be managed with precautions taken for a "full stomach." If the endoscopist insists on the maintenance of spontaneous ventilation during bronchoscopy, then the patient should not have consumed solids for at least 8 hours, and the operation should be delayed if the patient is stable.

The patient should be monitored with a precordial stethoscope, noninvasive blood pressure apparatus, electrocardiograph, temperature probe, pulse oximeter, and capnograph. Bilateral auscultation of the chest for baseline air entry prior to induction will allow the anesthesiologist to detect changes that may occur during the procedure.

A rapid-sequence induction consisting of preoxygenation with 100% oxygen, rapid administration of thiopental, 5 mg/kg, and succinylcholine, 2 mg/kg, application of cricoid pressure, and placement of a 4.5-mm endotracheal tube is recommended. A large-bore gastric tube should be inserted to aspirate stomach contents and the eyes taped closed to prevent injury. The endoscopist can easily follow the endotracheal tube to the glottis, and the bronchoscope can be inserted immediately upon removal of the endotracheal tube.

INTRAOPERATIVE MANAGEMENT

Successful management of this child requires clear communication and cooperation between the endoscopist and the anesthesiologist. When spontaneous ventilation is requested, the depth of anesthesia must be increased. Topical instillation of lidocaine, 3 mg/kg, into the tracheobronchial tree will reduce airway reactivity. During insertion of the bronchoscope and removal of the foreign body, 100% oxygen should be administered.

Controlled ventilation with neuromuscular blockade has the advantage of reducing the incidence of hypercarbia, intermittent coughing, and bronchospasm. Neuromuscular blockade may be continued with a nondepolarizing intermediate-acting agent or a succinylcholine infusion. Halothane or isoflurane with 100% oxygen should be administered in concentrations that result in stable cardiovascular parameters.

A ventilating bronchoscope equipped with a 15-mm side port allows oxygen and anesthetic gases to be delivered into the lumen of the bronchoscope. The proximal end of the bronchoscope can be occluded by a removable window. When a telescope is placed in the bronchoscope, it partially occludes the lumen. This is especially significant with small bronchoscopes because of the exponential influence of tube cross-sectional area on gas flow. Resistance to airflow imposed by the 3.5-mm bronchoscope with the standard telescope is approximately five times the normal upper airway resistance of infants. The passive elastic recoil of the lungs and chest wall, which provides the driving pressure for deflation of the lungs, may be insufficient to overcome the expiratory resistance of the bronchoscope/telescope apparatus. Periodic withdrawal of the telescope from the bronchoscope is necessary to re-establish a low-resistance airway and reduce the risk of air trapping.[3]

Ventilation should be monitored by observing chest movement and bilateral auscultation for air entry. Capnography is frequently inaccurate because exhaled gas leaks around the bronchoscope and therefore inaccurately low end-tidal carbon dioxide measurements are obtained. When ventilation is judged to be inadequate, the distal end of the bronchoscope should be placed above the carina, the telescope removed, and 3 to 4 minutes of ventilation completed before continuing with the procedure. Removal of the screw may be difficult, and complete relaxation of the vocal cords may be necessary to allow passage through the glottis. If the screw is manipulated into the trachea and complete obstruction occurs, then it must be removed immediately or displaced into a main bronchus to continue ventilation and oxygenation. The screw may be removed "en bloc" with the bronchoscope, and the anesthesiologist must be prepared to ventilate the patient by mask prior to reinsertion of the bronchoscope.

The removal of organic foreign bodies may be difficult because mucosal edema develops and traps the fragments. The administration of extremely dilute racemic epinephrine through the bronchoscope can facilitate removal of organic matter such as impacted peanut fragments with minimal associated cardiovascular changes.[4]

PROBLEMS TO ANTICIPATE

Intraoperative complications that can occur include bronchospasm, cardiac arrhythmias, hypoxemia, hypercarbia, laryngospasm, pneumothorax, and postoperative croup. Premature ventricular contractions are most common and are caused by hypoventilation, hypoxia, or an ill-defined pulmonary reflex mechanism. Inadequate ventilation caused by a large leak around the bronchoscope at the larynx should be managed by gentle pressure in the cricoid area or by changing the bronchoscope to a larger size. Ventilation is also impeded when the telescope is in place and the bronchoscope is deeply inserted in the bronchus. Hyperventilation and correction of hypercarbia can be accomplished by placement of the bronchoscope above the carina, removal of the telescope, and administration of large tidal volume breaths for 3 to 4 minutes. Increasing ventilation usually results in a return to sinus rhythm, and antiarrhythmic treatment with lidocaine or other drugs is rarely necessary.

Bronchospasm may be severe and impede ventilation. Treatment with increasing depths of anesthesia, nebulized albuterol, or intravenous aminophylline may be necessary. Pneumothorax is rare, but must be suspected if acute deterioration occurs during the procedure.

At the end of the procedure a 4.5-mm endotracheal tube should be inserted when the bronchoscope is removed. Tracheobronchial suctioning is frequently necessary. Criteria for extubation are a regular respiratory pattern, full neuromuscular strength, and eye opening. Extubation during the excitement stage of anesthesia may result in laryngospasm. Dexamethasone, 0.5 mg/kg, may be administered intraoperatively to reduce airway edema associated with prolonged and traumatic instrumentations. Bronchoscopy with an oversized bronchoscope may result in inflammation and edema of the larynx and subglottic area.[5] Postoperative croup may require treatment with humidified oxygen and nebulized racemic epinephrine.

REFERENCES

1. Laks Y, Barzilay Z: Foreign body aspiration in childhood. *Pediatr Emerg Care* 1988; 4:102.
2. Esclamado RM, Richardson MA: Laryngotracheal foreign bodies in children. *Am J Dis Child* 1987; 141:259.
3. Woods AM, Gal TJ: Decreasing airflow resistance during infant and pediatric bronchoscopy. *Anesth Analg* 1987; 66:457.
4. Bready LL, Orr MD, Petty C, et al: Bronchscopic administration of nebulized racemic epinephrine to facilitate removal of aspirated peanut fragments in pediatric patients. *Anesthesiology* 1986; 65:523.
5. Lockhart CH, Elliot JL: Potential hazards of pediatric rigid bronchoscopy. *J Pediatr Surg* 1984; 19:239.

33

Burn Debridement

A 2-year-old boy is transferred to the burn unit 4 hours after sustaining a 50% third-degree burn in a house fire. His trunk, both hands, and one leg are involved. He received 500 mL of Ringer's lactate solution, 100 mL of 5% albumin, and 250 mL of red blood cells prior to transfer. His weight is estimated to be 15 kg; blood pressure, 76/38; pulse, 130; respirations, 42; hemoglobin, 12.9 g/dL; hematocrit, 42%. The surgeon would like to proceed with debridement as soon as you feel the child is prepared.

Recommendations by Charles J. Coté, M.D.

The anesthetic management of the pediatric burn patient begins at the time the patient first arrives in the emergency room and does not end for many years thereafter because of the multiple plastic surgery repairs required to restore function and cosmesis. In this child with an extensive injury, the immediate response was appropriately directed toward volume resuscitation; however, blood components are rarely required on the day of injury.

AIRWAY MANAGEMENT

The child should have had the adequacy of his ventilation secured with an endotracheal tube. He was burned in a closed space and most likely has sustained a severe pulmonary inhalation injury as well as a heat injury and carbon monoxide poisoning. Pulmonary injury secondary to smoke inhalation and carbon monoxide poisoning account for 50% to 60% of the 12,000 fire-related deaths in the United States annually.

Carbon monoxide itself does not cause direct injury to the lung. It binds to hemoglobin with an affinity 200 times greater than oxygen; the net result is cellular hypoxia. In addition, there is a left shift of the oxygen-hemoglobin dissociation curve, which also prevents what normal oxygen there is from being released.[1] Looking for cherry-red mucous membranes is not very helpful because the mucous membranes may have been damaged by noxious fumes resulting in the same clinical picture. Blood gas analysis is not of great value either because the color of the blood will be red and the Pao_2 normal. Pulse oximetry will be inaccurate since carboxyhemoglobin is interpreted as oxyhemoglobin.[2] The diagnosis of carbon monoxide poisoning must be made by the history and direct measurement of carboxyhemoglobin. In room air, the half-life of carboxyhemoglobin is 4 hours.[1, 3] However, with 100% oxygen this can be reduced to less than 1 hour. The influence of hyperbaric oxygenation on patient survival remains controversial.[4] The patient in this case should have received 100% oxygen as soon as he arrived in the emergency room and should continue to receive a high inspired oxygen concentration until carboxyhemoglobin levels have fallen to less than 10%.

Heat-related injury is primarily limited to the upper airway and larynx because the nose and mouth are excellent absorbers of heat. Thus, the majority of the energy spent on heat absorption results in damage to the upper airway structures. If a patient is burned in a closed space such as a car or house or has carbonaceous material on the nares or soot in the mouth, careful assessment of the airway must be made.[1, 3, 5–12] It is mandatory that the trachea be intubated if there is any suspicion of an upper airway burn. A facial burn in a closed space is an example of such a situation. If the airway is not secured soon after injury, within 2 to 4 hours it may not be possible to intubate the patient because the airway has become so distorted. The endotracheal tube should not be secured with adhesive tape because damaged tissue exudes protein, which will loosen the tape. To avoid accidental advancement or extubation, the endotracheal tube should be fastened with cloth "tracheostomy tape" and a mark placed with indelible ink at a point even with the nares or alveolar ridge. These patients should receive 100% oxygen acutely and the need for further therapy titrated. Tracheostomies should be strenuously avoided if possible because they increase the morbidity and mortality significantly, which in some series reach 100%.[13] In children, it is often necessary to maintain nasal intubation for prolonged periods, sometimes several months.

This child should be intubated immediately because of carbon monoxide poisoning and, more important, because he probably has a burn of the upper airway with impending airway obstruction. The intubation should be attempted only by a person skilled in airway management. The problems anticipated are analogous to those encountered with acute epiglottitis, laryngotracheobronchitis, and macroglossia combined. Therefore, muscle relaxants should not be used. He should be breathing spontaneously at all times. Gentle assisted ventilation may help. The combative child may require general anesthesia or ketamine. This should be undertaken only after adequate vascular access has been established.

Noxious fumes and carbonaceous materials may damage the airway at all levels because toxic gases and smoke are carried deep into the lungs. Sulfur dioxide, NO_2, and other fumes combine with water to form corrosive acid and alkali, which burn the mucosa far down into the tracheobronchial tree. Combustion of man-made products, especially plastics, results in the formation of hydrogen cyanide, hydrochloric acid, sulfuric acid, and other toxic fumes that may result in chemical burn of the distal airways. Aldehydes produced by cotton and wool combustion may cause pulmonary edema. The pathology that results is defective or lost mucociliary transport, edema, loss of capillary integrity, destruction of surfactant, peribronchial cuffing, the formation of hyaline membranes, mucopurulent bronchitis, and bronchospasm.[1, 3, 5, 8–12, 14, 15]

Many patients have normal chest x-ray findings soon after injury but exhibit severe bronchospasm. This bronchospastic component often responds to bronchodilator therapy. A necrotizing bronchitis develops later and progresses in most cases to bronchopneumonia. It is not unusual to suction "casts" of the tracheobronchial tree due to sloughing of the mucosal layer. Bronchoscopy has been advocated to assess the severity of the pulmonary injury. Steroids are contraindicated because they may promote the spread of infection.

This child's circumferential chest burns also affect airway management. When skin is burned, it shrinks in size. Tissue shrinkage combined with the rapid onset of edema may result in a tourniquet effect on the chest and inadequate ventilation.[5, 6, 16] Most patients will demonstrate abdominal breathing. Immediate escharotomy in both the anterior and posterior axillary lines may be required to restore normal respiratory mechanics (Fig 33–1).

VOLUME RESUSCITATION

Volume resuscitation must begin simultaneously with management of the airway. Massive fluid shifts and loss of plasma into burned tissues rapidly result in systemic hypotension. To accomplish resuscitation safely, insertion of a urinary catheter, arterial cannula, and central venous pressure catheter is essential. There is still considerable debate about the most appropriate fluids, and many formulas have been derived.[17–20] In general, crystalloid is utilized for the first 18 to 24 hours and is followed by colloid administration. Glucose-containing solutions should be avoided since endogenous responses to stress generally result in elevated blood glucose values.[21, 22] It probably makes little difference which fluid is initially utilized so long as close attention is paid to urinary output,

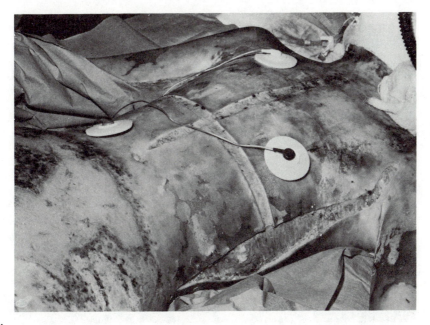

FIG 33–1.
Escharotomy of the chest in both the anterior and posterior axillary lines may be required to relieve the tourniquet effect on the chest to restore normal breathing mechanics.

oxygenation, and cardiac filling pressures. Standard burn wound resuscitation formulas such as the Brooke or Parkland formulas will underestimate fluid requirements in children 10 kg or less.

The arterial catheter may be inserted percutaneously in any available nonburned area or, if necessary, in the femoral artery. The preferred method of inserting a femoral artery cannula and central venous catheter is the Seldinger technique, which minimizes the chance of significant injury and hematoma formation.

This child presented with a blood pressure of 76/38 and a pulse of 130. If his central venous pressure is in the range of 12 to 15 cm H_2O and the systemic blood pressure remains low, it must be suspected that myocardial depressant factor of burns is present and the use of an inotropic agent such as dopamine may be indicated.[23] If the cardiac filling pressure is low, additional volume should be administered prior to administration of an inotrope.[20, 24]

ASSOCIATED PROBLEMS

After initial volume resuscitation and control of the airway, a careful physical examination and history are mandatory. It is not unusual for a fire victim to have sustained an associated head injury or organ rupture. Emergency escharotomy of extremities and digits, if carried out soon after injury (Fig 33–2), may preserve function. Other problems that may be manifested during the acute injury period along with signs, appropriate diagnostic tests, and treatment are presented in Table 33–1.

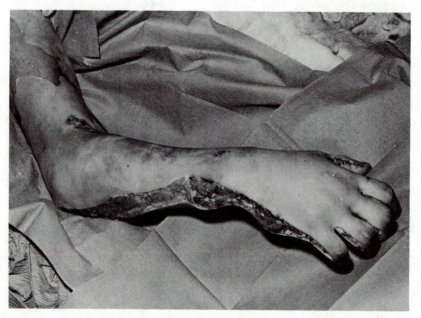

FIG 33–2.
Escharotomy of the limbs and digits may preserve blood flow and diminish the need for amputation.

TABLE 33–1.

Problems Associated With Major Burn Injury

Problem	Diagnostic Tests or Signs	Treatment
Carbon monoxide poisoning	Carboxyhemoglobin level	Oxygen administration
Noxious gas inhalation	Bronchoscopy, chest x-ray, blood gas analysis, widening A-a gradient	Bronchodilators, ventilation
Combined restrictive and obstructive pulmonary disease	Blood gases, high inflation pressures	Mechanical ventilation, oxygen, positive end-expiratory pressure
Cerebral toxicity	Seizures	Phenobarbital, phenytoin, (Dilantin), respiratory support
Acute gastric dilatation	Physical examination	Nasogastric drainage
Hyperkalemia	Serum potassium, ECG	Diuresis, polystyrene sulfonate (Kayexalate), glucose, insulin therapy
Hemolytic anemia	Blood smear, frequent hematocrits	RBC transfusion
Cardiac arrhythmias secondary to hyperkalemia or electrical injury	ECG, rhythm strip	Reduction in potassium, antiarrhythmic pharmacology, treatment of hyperkalemia
Hypothermia	Frequent temperature measurement	Warmed environment, radiant heaters, warming blankets, heated humidified inspired gases
Tetanus		Tetanus toxoid booster
Disseminated intravascular coagulopathy	Clotting studies	Appropriate factor support
Thrombocytopenia	Platelet levels	Platelet concentrates if clinical bleeding
Hypocalcemia	Total and ionized calcium, ECG	Calcium chloride or calcium gluconate
Myoglobinuria	Urinary myoglobin, urinary color	Forced diuresis, mannitol, furosemide
Hemoglobinuria	Urinary hemoglobin, urinary color	Forced diuresis, mannitol, furosemide
Pain	Agitation, tachycardia, hypertension	Continuous narcotic infusion, intermittent bolus for dressing changes

ANESTHETIC CONSIDERATIONS

The immediate preoperative evaluation of the acutely burned patient should include a bleeding profile consisting of a platelet count, prothrombin time (PT), and partial thromboplastin time (PTT); determinations of hematocrit, electrolytes, blood urea nitrogen (BUN), glucose, ionized calcium, and total protein; electrocardiogram (ECG) in the case of electrical burns; urinalysis for myoglobin and hemoglobin; arterial blood gas analysis; and chest x-ray. A careful physical examination is important, with particular attention paid to the face, oropharynx, and adequacy of air exchange in order to anticipate the rapidly compromised airway. Evaluating the level of consciousness is important in assessing central toxicity. Finally, the appropriate monitors for evaluating the adequacy of volume status must be in place prior to beginning anesthesia.

General endotracheal anesthesia should be undertaken only after all metabolic parameters have been normalized or at least partially corrected. If there is any question of a compromised airway, muscle paralysis is contraindicated, even in the presence of a full stomach. In this situation, either awake intubation or intubation with halothane or ketamine anesthesia and spontaneous respiration is preferable. If there is no airway compromise, a muscle relaxant can be used. We do not recommend the use of succinylcholine, even during the first postburn day, because of the possibility of acute hyperkalemia.[25, 26] Instead, rapid-sequence induction following preoxygenation would be performed, and vecuronium, 0.15 to 0.20 mg/kg, would be administered 30 seconds prior to thiopental, 4 to 6 mg/kg. Ketamine, 2 mg/kg, should be used in place of thiopental if there is the possibility of hypovolemia. With this technique, adequate muscle relaxation occurs within 60 to 90 seconds. If there is no pulmonary damage, a nitrous oxide-narcotic-relaxant technique could be used. There is, however, no objection to repeated halothane anesthesia. Some burned children are highly susceptible to the myocardial depressant effects of halothane, and its dose must be carefully titrated.

So that all possible complications can be anticipated and treated immediately, it is important to have a variety of anesthetic masks, airways, laryngoscope blades, and a full retinue of resuscitation equipment available. When dealing with the pediatric patient, it is particularly important to know the weight and estimated blood volume. An appropriate volume of blood components and intravenous solutions must be immediately available.

PHYSIOLOGIC CONSIDERATIONS

Early after burn injury there may be a marked decrease in cardiac output with a low peripheral vascular resistance (PVR). However, some patients have a high PVR in addition to the low cardiac output. The decrease in cardiac output is greater than would be expected by fluid shifts and has been attributed to a circulating myocardial depressant factor.[27]

In adults, right ventricular dysfunction and increased pulmonary vascular resistance often make central venous pressure monitoring inaccurate.[24] There are no data regarding the pediatric patient. Children usually have healthy hearts with equal right and left ventricular pressures. We have, however, had several with right-sided dysfunction who did require pulmonary artery catheters to be properly treated with inotropic agents or vasodilators.

Five to 7 days following the injury, the cardiovascular system becomes hyperdynamic, with cardiac output doubling or tripling. This persists for several months after the injury and may, in part, be catecholamine mediated.[14] In addition, children have a significant incidence of hypertension that is multifactorial in origin. It is both episodic and persistent and, if left untreated, may progress to hypertensive encephalopathy.[28, 29]

Careful assessment of baseline arterial blood gas values and the chest x-ray is important. In addition to upper and lower airway obstructive lesions, if there is a circumferential chest burn, significant restrictive disease may be present.[6] It is common for the patient to require a high inspired oxygen concentration and elevated inflation pressures.[1, 5, 7] Because of metabolic alterations, an increase in minute ventilation is necessary to maintain a normal $Paco_2$.[3, 22] Children with long-term nasotracheal intubation are susceptible to all the problems associated with artificial airways, including subglottic stenosis, granuloma formation, erosion of the trachea, tracheal–innominate artery fistula, and tracheomalacia. It is important to maintain careful records of endotracheal tube size and use high-volume, low-pressure cuffed tubes. Uncuffed endotracheal tubes should be used whenever possible. If the child requires progressively smaller endotracheal tubes after repeated anesthetics, bronchoscopic evaluation should be considered for suspected tracheal damage.

Initially, there is the possibility of renal damage secondary to myoglobinuria, hemoglobinuria, and hypotension. After this acute phase, however, glomerular filtration increases markedly, which may reduce the half-life of drugs excreted by glomerular filtration.[25, 26, 30, 31] This is especially true of antibiotics.

There is some evidence to suggest that burn patients have reduced liver function that may result in a prolonged half-life of drugs with hepatic excretion.[25] Conversely, the polypharmacy to which these patients are exposed may induce hepatic enzyme function. The increased hepatic blood flow may also result in increased hepatic drug excretion. Because of multiple transfusions, the possibility of hepatitis is ever present.

With extensive burn injury, there is major damage to capillary integrity that results in localized edema and pulmonary edema.[9, 12, 14, 15] In addition to abnormal capillary integrity, altered protein metabolism and content may result in a variable volume of distribution of drugs as well as in differences in protein binding.[25] The marked increase in the requirements for nondepolarizing muscle relaxants in burn patients is well recognized.[25, 26] Burn patients can demonstrate adequate air exchange although serum levels of d-tubocurarine are well above the ED_{95} of normal patients. That is, 95% of individuals would have been completely paralyzed with the serum levels at which these patients function normally. This is a striking demonstration of altered pharmacodynamic response, due in part to altered protein binding and altered drug receptors.[32, 33] The response of burn patients to many drugs may be quite variable from day to day or from patient to patient.[34]

The skin is responsible for protection from the environment. When the skin is damaged, there is a tremendous alteration in its ability to conserve heat and to protect against evaporative water and electrolyte losses. It is important that burn patients be covered, particularly the head, and maintained in a thermal- and humidity-controlled environment so that they do not waste calories needed for tissue repair in maintaining temperature.

There are marked alterations in metabolism following thermal injury,[21, 22] including increases in gluconeogenesis, protein degradation, and fat utilization. Increased oxygen consumption and carbon dioxide production are always associated with thermal injury, as is increased heat production secondary to increased metabolism. For these reasons, it is mandatory that a vigorous feeding schedule be initiated shortly after injury. Intravenous alimentation is usually required. Intraoperative monitoring of blood glucose levels is important in patients receiving hyperalimentation.

Increased oxygen consumption and carbon dioxide production must be considered when calculating ventilatory requirements. If one would normally choose 150 mL/kg/min, it may be more appropriate to choose 225 to 300 mL/kg/min initially and check the blood gases frequently. End-tidal carbon dioxide determination will be helpful as a trend monitor. However, in the presence of severe pulmonary injury or pulmonary edema, the end-tidal CO_2 value may be 10 to 15 mm Hg less than $Paco_2$ due to ventilation-perfusion mismatch.

Hypocalcemia is present in the majority of burned patients for the first 7 weeks following injury.[35] We have observed electrical mechanical dissociation with severe hypotension during or shortly following the rapid transfusion of fresh frozen plasma (FFP). Citrate toxicity with resultant hypocalcemia is perhaps the most common complication during rapid administration of FFP or whole blood to these patients. However, in a prospective study, we were unable to demonstrate a dose-response effect (Fig 33–3).[36] When we examined the clinical data more carefully, we realized that the majority of patients who had an adverse cardiovascular event were anesthetized with halothane in a concentration of 1.0% or greater, whereas the study patients were not. An animal study demonstrated more severe hypotension and a greater reduction in ionized calcium levels during a deeper vs. a lighter plane of halothane anesthesia.[37] A follow-up study using an isolated rat heart model demonstrated dose-related myocardial depression with increasing halothane concentrations or decreasing ionized calcium levels.[38] The combination of halothane and ionized hypocalcemia resulted in potentiation of this myocardial depression. If these data can be applied to the pediatric patient, it suggests that if FFP must be administered at a rate of 1.0 mL/kg/min or more and if the patient is anesthetized with halothane, or probably with any potent inhalation agent that has calcium

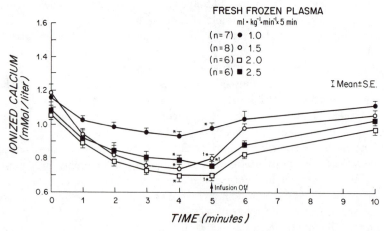

FIG 33–3.

Changes in ionized calcium levels in children with severe thermal injuries during the infusion of FFP. Note the dangerous although transient decrease in ionized calcium levels. Exogenous calcium should be administered whenever FFP is rapidly infused (≥1.0 mL/kg/min). (From Coté CJ, Drop LJ, Hoaglin DJ, et al: *Anesth Analg* 1988; 67:152–160. Used by permission.)

channel blocking properties, then exogenous calcium should be administered *during* the FFP infusion. Calcium chloride or calcium gluconate should be available at all times.[39]

ANESTHETIC CONSIDERATIONS WITH BURN DEBRIDEMENT

It has been demonstrated that the more rapidly burn wounds are closed, the shorter the hospital stay and the greater the chances for survival.[16] It is not unusual for children to come to the operating room every 2 to 4 days for major wound debridement. Each of these debridement procedures may involve a one to three blood volume loss.

Preparation for such a major physiologic insult should include proper psychological support and adequate analgesia prior to transport to the operating room. Adequate monitoring preoperatively and prior to starting major debridement is essential. At least one and preferably two intravenous cannulas, one of which is centrally located, are indicated. The patient must be carefully positioned and the eyes protected. Nasogastric drainage is initiated or continued. All operating room staff must wear gloves. Blood pressure cuffs, endotracheal tubes, laryngoscope blades, and masks must be sterilized. Maintenance of body temperature is critical. The operating room is occasionally warmed as high as 37°C. Heated humidified inspired gases, overhead radiant warmers, warming blankets, and blood warmers are used. Sterilized plastic bags can be wrapped around each extremity and the head wrapped.

When the debridement procedure begins, we usually initiate volume resuscitation to avoid hypovolemia. Since blood loss is difficult to quantitate and evaporative losses are great, close attention should be paid to maintaining a constant central venous pressure.

If blood loss is one blood volume or less, the need for FFP is minimal, however if blood loss will exceed one blood volume, then FFP will likely be required. Because burn trauma patients are chronically hypocalcemic and highly susceptible to hypocalcemia from the citrate in FFP or whole blood,[35] we routinely administer calcium chloride during FFP transfusion. It cannot be overemphasized that calcium should be drawn up and ready for use in addition to its prophylactic administration. If there is evidence of hypovolemia, we ask the surgeons to stop and compress the open areas until we are able to catch up. A team approach is extremely important.

The need for platelet transfusion depends upon the baseline platelet count and the volume of blood shed. Patients with burns of 50% of their body surface area (BSA) or less and who are not septic will generally have a thrombocytosis after the fifth postburn day and will also have elevated levels of factors *V, VIII, VII,* and fibrinogen. Patients with greater than a 50% BSA burn or who are septic may have multiple clotting factor deficiencies and thrombocytopenia. Blood replacement is therefore based upon a knowledge of baseline coagulation profiles, platelet count, volume of blood shed, and frequent intraoperative coagulation profile determinations. We monitor arterial blood gases for acid-base status and oxygenation as well as hematocrit, glucose, potassium, ionized calcium, and total protein every 45 to 60 minutes, or more frequently if indicated during each surgical procedure. It is not unusual for significant alterations in the alveolar-to-arterial oxygen and carbon dioxide gradient to occur, which are detected by blood gas analysis, pulse oximetry, and capnography, long before life-threatening complications such as hypoxia are evident. In patients with extensive burn injury, we have found that a pulse oximeter applied to the tongue will provide a reasonable alternative means of monitoring oxygen saturation in patients who have no peripheral pulses.[40]

Tangential excisions are much more bloody than full-thickness skin excision. All the problems of massive blood transfusion should be anticipated. Frequent assessment of clotting parameters must be coupled with judicious use of FFP and platelet concentrates.

Postoperatively, we are often able to extubate patients who are without an artificial airway pre-operatively. However, the adequacy of ventilation must be assessed on an individual basis for each procedure. After major wound debridement procedures, it is not unusual for the patient to require overnight ventilation.

SUMMARY

The anesthetic management of burn trauma patients must include an understanding of the altered physiology and pharmacology associated with even small burns. Proper psychological support for the family and patient can be greatly facilitated by thoughtful, considerate anesthetic care. The anesthesiologist is often the friend of such patients if he or she provides periods free of pain, including the time of transport from the intensive care unit to the operating room. It is important to remember that a normal personality resides in that devastatingly injured body, and we must remain sympathetic and supportive at all times and under all circumstances.

REFERENCES

1. Fein A, Left A, Hopewell PC: Pathophysiology and management of complications resulting from fire and the inhaled products of combustion: Review of the literature. *Crit Care Med* 1980; 8:94–98.
2. Barker SJ, Tremper KK: The effect of carbon monoxide inhalation on pulse oximetry and transcutaneous PO_2. *Anesthesiology* 1987; 66:677–679.
3. Trunkey DD: Inhalation injury. *Surg Clin North Am* 1978; 58:1133–1140.
4. Grim PS, Gottlieb LJ, Boddie A, et al: Hyperbaric oxygen therapy. *JAMA* 1990; 263:2216–2220.
5. Demling RH: Postgraduate course: Respiratory injury. Part III: Pulmonary dysfunction in the burn patient. *J Burn Care Rehabil* 1986; 7:277–284.
6. Garzon AA, Seltzer B, Song IC, et al: Respiratory mechanics in patients with inhalation burns. *J Trauma* 1970; 10:57–62.
7. Mellins RB, Park S: Respiratory complications of smoke inhalation in victims of fire. *J Pediatr* 1979; 87:1–7.
8. Nieman GF, Clark WR, Wax SO, et al: The effect of smoke inhalation on pulmonary surfactant. *Ann Surg* 1980; 191:171–181.
9. Nieman GF, Clark WR Jr, Goyette D, et al: Wood smoke inhalation increases pulmonary microvascular permeability. *Surgery* 1989; 105:481–487.
10. Silverman SH, Purdue GF, Hunt JL, et al: Cyanide toxicity in burned patients. *J Trauma* 1988; 28:171–176.
11. Stothert JC Jr, Herndon DN, Lubbesmeyer HJ, et al: Airway acid injury following smoke inhalation. *Prog Clin Biol Res* 1988; 264:409–413.
12. Zikria BA, Ferrer JM, Floch HF: The chemical factors contributing to pulmonary damage in "smoke poisoning." *Surgery* 1972; 71:704–709.
13. Eckhauser FE, Billote J, Burke JF, et al: Tracheostomy complicating massive burn injury. *Am J Surg* 1979; 127:418–423.

14. Herndon DN, Barrow RE, Traber DL, et al: Extravascular lung water changes following smoke inhalation and massive burn injury. *Surgery* 1987; 102:341–349.
15. Pitt RM, Parker JC, Jurkovich GJ, et al: Analysis of altered capillary pressure and permeability after thermal injury. *J Surg Res* 1987; 42:693–702.
16. Burke JF, Quinby WC Jr, Bondoc CC: Primary excision and prompt grafting as routine therapy for the treatment of thermal burns in children. *Surg Clin North Am* 1976; 56:477–494.
17. Baxter C, Burke JF, Jelenko C, et al: Fluid resuscitation, burn percentage, and physiologic age. *J Trauma* 1979; 19:864–877.
18. Bowser-Wallace BH, Caldwell FT Jr: A prospective analysis of hypertonic lactated saline vs. Ringer's lactate–colloid for the resuscitation of severely burned children. *Burns* 1986; 12:402–409.
19. Bowser-Wallace BH, Caldwell FT Jr: Fluid requirements of severely burned children up to 3 years old: Hypertonic lactated saline vs. Ringer's lactate–colloid. *Burns* 1986; 12:549–555.
20. Mueller M, Sartorelli K, DeMeules JE, et al: Effects of fluid resuscitation on cardiac dysfunction following thermal injury. *J Surg Res* 1988; 44:745–753.
21. Burke JF, Wolfe RR, Mullany CJ, et al: Glucose requirements following burn injury. *Ann Surg* 1979; 190:274–285.
22. Wolfe RR, Herndon DN, Jahoor F, et al: Effect of severe burn injury on substrate cycling by glucose and fatty acids. *N Engl J Med* 1987; 317:403–408.
23. Moati F, Sepulchre C, Miskulin M, et al: Biochemical and pharmacological properties of a cardiotoxic factor isolated from the blood serum of burned patients. *J Pathol* 1979; 127:147–156.
24. Martyn J, Wilson RS, Burke JF: Right ventricular function and pulmonary hemodynamics during dopamine infusion in burned patients. *Chest* 1986; 89:357–360.
25. Martyn J: Clinical pharmacology and drug therapy in the burned patient. *Anesthesiology* 1986; 65:67–75.
26. Martyn J, Goldhill DR, Goudsouzian NG: Clinical pharmacology of muscle relaxants in patients with burns. *J Clin Pharmacol* 1986; 26:680–685.
27. Mooti F, Sepulchre C, Miskulin M, et al: Biochemical and pharmalogical properties of a cardiotoxic factor isolated from the blood serum of burned patients. *J Pathol* 1979; 127:147–156.
28. Falkner B, Roven S, DeClement FA, et al: Hypertension in children with burns. *J Trauma* 1978; 8:213–217.
29. Krami A, Falkner B, Bould AB, et al: Plasma renin and occurrence of hypertension in children with burn injuries. *J Trauma* 1980; 20:130–134.
30. Ciaccio EI, Fruncillo FJ: Urinary excretion of D-glucaric acid by severely burned patients. *Clin Pharmacol Ther* 1979; 25:340–344.
31. Loirat P, Rohan J, Baillet A, et al: Increased glomerular filtration rate in patients with major burns and its effect on the pharmacokinetics of tobramycin. *N Engl J Med* 1978; 299:915–919.
32. Kim C, Martyn J, Fuke N: Burn injury to trunk of rat causes denervation-like responses in the gastrocnemius muscle. *J Appl Physiol* 1988; 65:1745–1751.
33. Martyn JAJ, Abernethy DR, Greenblatt DJ: Plasma protein binding of drugs after severe burn injury. *Clin Pharmacol Ther* 1984; 35:535–539.
34. Bonate PL: Pathophysiology and pharmacokinetics following burn injury. *Clin Pharmacokinet* 1990; 18:118–130.
35. Szyfelbein SK, Drop LJ, Martyn JAJ: Persistent ionized hypocalcemia in patients during resuscitation and recovery phases of body burns. *Crit Care Med* 1981; 9:454–458.
36. Coté CJ, Drop LJ, Hoaglin DC, et al: Ionized hypocalcemia after fresh frozen plasma administration to thermally injured children: Effects of infusion rate, duration, and treatment with calcium chloride. *Anesth Analg* 1988; 67:152–160.

37. Coté CJ: Depth of halothane anesthesia potentiates citrate-induced ionized hypocalcemia and adverse cardiovascular events in dogs. *Anesthesiology* 1987; 67:676–680.
38. Brussel T, Coté CJ, Stanford GG, et al: Dose response to calcium and halothane in the isolated rat heart preparation. *Anesthesiology* 1989; 71:A166.
39. Coté CJ, Drop LJ, Daniels AL, et al: Calcium chloride versus calcium gluconate: Comparison of ionization and cardiovascular effects in children and dogs. *Anesthesiology* 1987; 66:465–470.
40. Coté CJ, Daniels A, Connolly M, et al: Tongue oximetry in children with extensive thermal injury: Comparison with peripheral oximetry. *Can J Anaesth* 1992; 39:454–457.

34

Hyperthermia During Osteotomy

A 7-year-old, 22-kg boy was scheduled for an innominate osteotomy. He was premedicated with oral midazolam, 11 mg, 15 minutes before surgery. Anesthesia was induced by mask with halothane, nitrous oxide, and oxygen. After tracheal intubation without a muscle relaxant, anesthesia was maintained with halothane and nitrous oxide via a Mapleson D circuit. Ventilation was spontaneous at a rate of 50 breaths per minute. One hour after induction of anesthesia, his axillary temperature had increased from 36 to 39°C, his pulse had increased from 110 to 150 beats/min, the end-tidal P_{CO_2} had risen from 48 to 66 mm Hg, and the blood in the surgical field was dark.

Recommendations by Jerrold Lerman, M.D., F.R.C.P.C.

This constellation of signs must immediately alert the anesthesiologist that the patient may be experiencing an episode of malignant hyperthermia (MH). Early diagnosis and treatment are essential.

THE DISEASE

MH is a rare, but potentially fatal pharmacogenetic defect in intracellular calcium regulation. The systemic manifestations are attributable to a massive increase in skeletal muscle activity and include respiratory and metabolic acidosis, fever, muscle rigidity, and serum electrolyte abnormalities.[1] These manifestations provide the diagnostic clues necessary to detect an acute MH reaction in evolution and to follow the resolution of a reaction during therapy.

The incidence of MH is approximately 1:15,000 children and 1:50,000 adults.[2] Acute MH reactions have been reported in patients of all ages, from infants to the elderly. Many patients give histories of multiple exposures to known triggering agents of MH without sequelae before the acute event. The explanation for this observation remains unclear. In the past three decades, many families have been identified as MH susceptible either by confirmed reactions to triggering agents or by positive muscle biopsies. Notwithstanding the infrequency of this disorder, the seriousness of an MH reaction cannot be overstated.

A new entity, isolated masseter muscle rigidity (MMR), has been identified as a relatively common clinical conundrum. MMR is reported in several studies to occur in 1% of children anesthetized with halothane and succinylcholine. Fifty percent of these children have tested positive for MH on the basis of halothane-caffeine contracture testing. This incidence of MH susceptibility (0.5%) exceeds the incidence of MH reported in the population by a factor of 100- to 200-fold. It is not surprising, therefore, that most instances of MMR do not progress to overt MH reactions even in the presence of known MH triggers.[3] Recent data suggest that in some instances, false-positive muscle biopsy findings may explain the high incidence of MMR.[4] If such is the case, it might also explain the difficulty in cosegregating the genetic defect in MH with the muscle biopsy results.

An acute MH reaction may be triggered by two groups of agents used during anesthesia: the depolarizing muscle relaxant succinylcholine and the potent inhalation anesthetics halothane, isoflurane, enflurane, methoxyflurane, desflurane, and sevoflurane.[2] An MH reaction is more likely to occur if succinylcholine is administered concurrently with an inhalation anesthetic. However, if succinylcholine is not used, an inhalation anesthetic itself may trigger an MH reaction. Sporadic MH reactions have also been reported in the absence of any known trigger and have presumably been caused by stress alone.

The temporal relationship between administration of the triggering agents and evidence of the reaction is variable. Acute MH reactions can occur at any time after induction of anesthesia, including the postoperative period. The severity of the reaction may vary from mild and poorly defined to fatal. The progression of the acute reaction is also unpredictable. Overt acute MH reactions may occur precipitously and evolve over several minutes, or may progress slowly as smouldering reactions over a period of several hours.

The mortality from an acute MH reaction continues to be a matter of serious concern. In the 1960s, more than 80% of patients with acute MH reactions succumbed during the event. Since then, the mortality rate from MH has decreased to less than 10%. This decrease has been attributed to three causes:

1. Increased awareness of MH
2. More frequent monitoring of temperature and end-tidal carbon dioxide tensions
3. The use of intravenous dantrolene

Despite improved management of these reactions, episodes of reversible MH still escape early diagnosis and result in permanent brain damage and death.

MH is inherited in an autosomal dominant pattern with variable penetrance and expression. Recent evidence suggests that it is caused by a defect in the ryanodine receptor on chromosome 19.[5] In pigs with porcine stress syndrome, the swine equivalent to MH in humans, a similar defect has been identified on chromosome 6. Research into the mysteries of the MH gene defect in humans continues, and a blood test may soon be available to detect susceptibility.

Successful resolution of an acute MH reaction requires early recognition of the signs and prompt and decisive therapy. While signs that herald the onset of an acute reaction vary when a reaction occurs, the signs are unmistakable: a sudden increase in the end-tidal P_{CO_2}, hyperventilation in the spontaneously breathing patient, tachycardia and/or arrhythmias, rapid increase in temperature, arterial oxygen desaturation, and muscle rigidity. When a majority of these signs occur together, MH is the presumed diagnosis. However, MH is a rare disorder, and more common causes for these signs should also be sought.

END-TIDAL P_{CO_2}

The differential diagnosis of an increase in end-tidal P_{CO_2}, the earliest sign of MH, may be attributed to an increase in the inspired partial pressure of carbon dioxide, an increase in the production of carbon dioxide, or a decrease in alveolar ventilation. Increases in the inspired carbon dioxide partial pressure are most likely due to a failure of the expiratory valve in a circle circuit or an inadequate fresh gas flow. Increases in the production of carbon dioxide may be attributed to one of the causes of a hypermetabolic rate (Table 34–1). If the increase in end-tidal carbon dioxide tension is due to MH, spontaneous respiration will be rapid and deep, and the carbon dioxide absorber, if present, will be hot. Decreases in the alveolar ventilation are the result of inadequate clearing of carbon dioxide from the lungs due to a decrease in tidal volume or respiratory rate or an increase in dead space.

FEVER

The temperature of every patient should be monitored continuously during anesthesia. MH should be first on the differential diagnosis when fever occurs during anesthesia, although other

TABLE 34–1.

Fever Under Anesthesia*

Malignant hyperthermia
Iatrogenic fever (environmental, external heat sources)
Endocrinopathies
  Thyroid storm
  Pheochromocytoma
  Hypothalamic dysfunction
Sepsis
  Bacterial (respiratory, urinary, endocardial, abscess)
  Viral (hepatitis)
  Fungal
Malignancy
Drugs (cocaine overdose, monoamine oxidase inhibitors
  and meperidine, atropine)
Allergic reactions (blood transfusion, drugs)
Miscellaneous (fat embolism)

*From Lerman J, Relton JES: Anaesthesia for malignant hyperthermia susceptible patients, in Britt BA (ed): *Malignant Hyperthermia*. Boston, Martinus Nijhoff Publishing, 1987, p 382. Used by permission)

causes such as iatrogenic or environmental overheating are far more common in infants and children. The latter causes include an overheated operating theater, humidifier, or heating blanket. Another common cause of fever is an underlying focus of infection in the respiratory tract, middle ear, or intestine. Additional causes for fever during anesthesia are listed in Table 34–1.

How rapidly has the temperature increased? In the case of an acute MH reaction, the temperature may increase 1°C every few minutes until a temperature of 46°C is reached. Several sites may be used to monitor the temperature: central (rectal or tympanic), superficial (skin), or areas of major muscle groups (axilla). The normal limits for temperature in a child vary with the site of the probe: the upper limit for rectal temperature is 38.5°C, and for axillary temperature it is 37.5°C. Temperature measurements in the axilla reflect changes in the metabolism of large shoulder muscle groups long before there is evidence of increases in the central or core temperature. For this reason, the axilla is the preferred site to monitor temperature in children >10 kg. If, however, central temperature is monitored, an increase in temperature may be a late sign of an acute MH reaction.

LABORATORY EVALUATION

Laboratory evidence of an acute MH reaction is quite valuable.[1] Analysis of a mixed or free-flowing venous or an arterial blood sample will indicate a mixed respiratory and metabolic acidosis. Electrolyte disturbances early in the acute reaction include hyperkalemia and hypercalcemia or hypocalcemia. Creatine phosphokinase (CPK) levels increase, but not during the immediate phase of the acute reaction. Peak CPK blood levels up to 100,000 IU/L occur 12 to 18 hours after onset of the reaction. Myoglobinemia and myoglobinuria are commonly present. Thrombocytopenia as well as decreased concentrations of factor VIII and fibrinogen may result in coagulopathy as a late manifestation of an MH reaction.

DIFFERENTIAL DIAGNOSIS

Few clinical syndromes present with the combination of increased end-tidal Pco_2, fever, and tachycardia. These signs point to a hypermetabolic state that is similar but not identical to that observed in thyroid storm. The latter, a rarity, differs from MH in that the degree of metabolic and respiratory acidosis is not as severe, peak temperatures are lower, and the CPK level is not increased to the same extent. Perhaps most importantly, thyroid storm is treated symptomatically during the acute reaction, whereas an MH reaction is reversible if treatment with dantrolene is instituted early. Neuroleptic malignant syndrome may also present as an MH-like reaction but differs in that it evolves over an extended period of time and there is usually a history of phenothiazine or butyrophenone ingestion. Monoamine oxidase inhibitors, type A, when combined with the narcotic meperidine, may present a picture that is very similar to that of an acute MH reaction. The diagnosis in this situation is also clear from the drug history. Pheochromocytoma has also been confused with MH. However, patients with pheochromocytoma usually present with hemodynamic instability and, to a lesser extent, metabolic and respiratory disturbances. These differences, together with an increased concentration of 3-methoxy, 4-hydroxy mandelic acid in the urine, usually make the diagnosis of pheochromocytoma easy to distinguish from MH.

TREATMENT

Early diagnosis and immediate treatment with intravenous dantrolene are the keys to a successful outcome. Every operating and recovery room should have a copy of a protocol for the treatment of an MH reaction. Treatment begins with the immediate discontinuation of anesthesia and surgery. The use of all triggering drugs should be discontinued, 100% oxygen administered, and positive-pressure ventilation instituted to restore adequate oxygenation and decrease the P_{CO_2}.

Assistance should be sought. An MH cart that contains a clean anesthetic circuit, dantrolene for intravenous administration, the antiarrhythmic agents procainamide, lidocaine, and bretylium, 50% dextrose in water, and sodium bicarbonate, together with an arterial catheterization kit, blood gas syringes, a Foley catheter, and urometer is required. All local anesthetics, including the amide local anesthetic lidocaine, are safe for use in MH.

It is essential that a sufficient supply of dantrolene be available in every institution to treat an acute MH reaction. A stock of 36 ampules, corresponding to a dose of 10 mg/kg for a 70-kg adult, should be immediately available. Many institutions stock sufficient dantrolene to administer 2.5 to 5.0 mg/kg to an adult and share the remainder of the recommended dose of dantrolene among local institutions. At The Hospital for Sick Children, we stock 10 ampules in the operating room area and a further 26 in the pharmacy. The local supply of dantrolene should provide approximately 2.5 to 5.0 mg/kg for the average adult in the immediate vicinity of the operating rooms, and the remainder, up to 10 or more mg/kg, should be in a readily accessible location.

The MH cart should contain a clean anesthetic circuit to replace all rubber and soft plastic equipment. Since most modern anesthetic machines contain little or no rubber components, it is no longer necessary to replace the anesthetic machine with one that is free of inhalation anesthetic agents. It is, however, prudent to flush the anesthetic machine with an air-oxygen mixture at 12 L/min fresh gas flow for at least 6 minutes to reduce the concentration of potent inhalation agent to less than 1 ppm.[6] While the anesthetic machine is being purged, a freestanding oxygen tank can be used as a fresh gas source for positive-pressure ventilation. If anesthesia must be continued, then a narcotic, sedative, muscle relaxant, and nitrous oxide anesthetic should be used. All narcotics and sedatives are safe to use. Propofol also appears to be safe. All nondepolarizing muscle relaxants appear safe. In the past, *d*-tubocurare was alleged to be a triggering agent, but there is little evidence to support this notion.

A large-bore intravenous catheter should be inserted to administer medications such as dantrolene and fluids. Ringer's lactate solution should be administered at a rapid flow rate to maintain a urine output of 1 to 2 mL/kg/hr in order to prevent renal damage from precipitation of myoglobin in the renal tubules. Since dantrolene contains mannitol, administration of dantrolene itself should maintain the diuresis. A Foley catheter is essential for monitoring the urine output, and a urine sample should be sent for myoglobin determination.

An arterial catheter should be inserted to provide access for multiple blood gas analyses. Blood gas analysis and electrolyte and glucose determinations should be performed frequently during the acute reaction to monitor the severity of the acidosis and the response to dantrolene. Administration of bicarbonate, 2 mEq/kg, at the time of diagnosis serves two purposes: first, it attenuates the severity of acidosis, and second, it decreases the serum potassium level. Glucose (50%) may be required if hyperkalemia persists. Hyperkalemia refractory to glucose alone can be treated with insulin plus glucose, i.e., 1 mL/kg 50% dextrose with 0.1 units of regular insulin per kilogram infused over a period of 10 to 30 minutes.

Continuous electrocardiographic monitoring is essential during the reaction. Tachycardia may deteriorate to ventricular arrhythmias if the treatment of acidosis, hyperkalemia, and hypercapnia is inadequate. Treatment strategies must include the administration of sodium bicarbonate, dantrolene, other pharmacologic agents aimed at reducing the serum potassium concentration, and antiarrhythmics. Lidocaine, 1.5 mg/kg administered slowly intravenously, procainamide, 15-mg/kg loading dose intravenously over a period of 15 to 30 minutes followed by 15 to 30 μg/kg/min, or bretylium, 5 mg/kg, are the drugs of choice for treating arrhythmias. Calcium channel blocking drugs have no specific role in either the treatment of arrhythmias or treatment of the MH reaction itself. Moreover, the combination of calcium channel blocking drugs and dantrolene may result in hypotension and asystole.[7]

The use of inotropic drugs to augment cardiac output in MH-susceptible individuals has received little attention. In most instances, these measures are not required but may be necessary during severe cardiac decompensation. α-Agonists induce MH reactions in swine, possibly on the basis of intense vasoconstriction, and are generally not recommended for use in MH-susceptible individuals. β-Agonists cause tachycardia and may obscure an important sign of an MH reaction. The effects of dopaminergic drugs on the course of MH reactions have not been fully elucidated. Digoxin and intravenous calcium do not trigger MH reactions in susceptible swine, although their use in MH-susceptible humans has not been generally accepted.

Although some clinicians recommend insertion of a central venous catheter, such a blanket policy is not recommended. Most MH reactions in children do not require a central venous catheter for monitoring or for venous access. Insertion of the catheter might distract the anesthesiologist from the more important role of monitoring the patient during the acute phase. In addition, many clinicians are inexperienced at inserting these catheters in young children, and complications may occur. Only in the presence of cardiac failure should a central venous or pulmonary artery catheter be inserted. Since cardiac failure is likely to be biventricular in children, a central venous catheter may provide as much information as a pulmonary artery catheter.

Is there a role for ice, ice baths, and iced intravenous solutions during an acute MH reaction? Since the availability of intravenous dantrolene, the role of ice in the treatment of an acute MH reaction has become a moot point. Dantrolene, not cold temperature, reverses an MH reaction. Furthermore, it has been suggested that surface cooling may actually increase the severity of the cutaneous vasoconstriction and muscle acidosis and paradoxically increase core body temperature.

Management of an MH reaction should continue until the patient is stable. Once there is evidence that the reaction is abating, the patient may be transferred to an area of constant observation where invasive monitoring and mechanical ventilation, if required, are available. A recrudesence of the reaction may occur hours later and must be anticipated. If recrudesence of the reaction is detected, additional intravenous dantrolene must be administered. Late complications include disseminated intravascular coagulopathy, cardiac failure, renal failure, and neurologic deficits. Muscle pain and stiffness may continue for several hours. Persistent pain or stiffness is an indication for additional dantrolene therapy.

DANTROLENE PHARMACOLOGY

Dantrolene, a hydantoin derivative, has been and continues to be the mainstay treatment of an MH reaction. Dantrolene is not a new medication; indeed, it has been used for many years in an oral formulation for the treatment of spasticity. The intravenous preparation of dantrolene has been available for only 15 years. Its effectiveness in arresting acute MH reactions has been demonstrated in both MH-susceptible pigs and humans. Dantrolene blocks calcium ion flux within cells, thereby attenuating the hypermetabolic signs of the acute MH reaction, including metabolic, respiratory, sympathetic, electrolyte, and neurohumoral disturbances. The parenteral formulation of dantrolene is available as a lyophylized powder 20 mg/ampule, that includes 6 g of sodium carbonate and 3 g of mannitol in a 70-mL glass ampule. Sodium carbonate is added to the preparation to increase the pH of the mixture in order to facilitate dissolution of the dantrolene. When 2.5 mg/kg of dantrolene is administered intravenously, approximately 0.4 g/kg mannitol is also administered. The parenteral formulation of dantrolene has a 3-year shelf-life and costs approximately $2.00 per milligram. It is reconstituted with 60 mL of sterile water per ampule to yield a concentration of 0.33 mg of dantrolene per mL of water. Since the initial treatment of an MH reaction requires 2.5 mg/kg, a 22-kg child requires 3 ampules of dantrolene, and a 70-kg adult requires approximately 9. Although the contents of each ampule dissolve in water within 90 seconds, it takes several minutes to dissolve the contents of 9 ampules. To speed up preparation of a large volume, some clinicians combine the powdered contents of a large number of ampules with the appropriate volume of sterile water in a sterile basin and dissolve the dantrolene en masse. This latter approach may be useful for the large child or adult.

Intravenous dantrolene 2.5 mg/kg should be administered into a large vein as a rapid intravenous infusion over a period of 10 to 15 minutes. In children, it may be infused into a saphenous or antecubital vein with little risk of thrombophlebitis. If the MH reaction does not begin to abate within 5 to 10 minutes, repeated doses, 1 mg/kg, should be administered every 5 minutes until the reaction begins to subside. There is no maximum dose of dantrolene, although it is suggested that the total dose not exceed 10 mg/kg. The side effects of dantrolene are usually minor when it is administered acutely. These include weakness of the respiratory muscles and local thrombophlebitis after prolonged infusion. Hypotension and asystole can occur after dantrolene administration in patients with congestive heart failure or if calcium channel blockers are also administered. Most patients do not develop evidence of respiratory distress after a single intravenous dose of 2.5 mg/kg dantrolene. However, in the presence of partial neuromuscular blockade, respiratory depressants, or chronic respiratory failure, signs of acute respiratory decompensation may ensue.

The pharmacokinetics of intravenous dantrolene have been studied in children 3 to 12 years of age and they are very similar to those reported in adults (Fig 34–1).[8] Following the administration of 2.5 mg/kg in children, plasma levels exceed 3.0 μg/mL, which is believed to be the treatment threshold for MH, for approximately 6.5 hours and then decrease with a half-life of 10 hours. If a second dose of dantrolene is required to maintain blood levels above 3.0 μg/mL, it should be administered within 6 hours of the first dose. This should maintain the blood level above the therapeutic threshold for a total of 18 hours.

Continuous axillary plus nasopharyngeal or rectal temperature monitoring and monitoring of end-tidal P_{CO_2}, the electrocardiogram, and blood pressure are mandatory throughout an acute MH

DANTROLENE

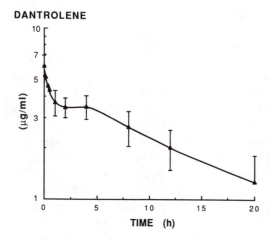

FIG 34–1.
Pharmacokinetics of intravenous dantrolene in children.
(From Lerman J, Strong HA, McLeod ME: *Anesthesiology* 1989; 70:627. Used by permission.)

reaction. The end-tidal P_{CO_2} and temperature should provide continuous evidence of the efficacy of treatment.

FAMILY COUNSELING

As soon as the MH reaction subsides and the child is stabilized, the anesthesiologist should explain the events surrounding the MH reaction and its implications to the parents. Information on lay support groups, including the Malignant Hyperthermia Association of the United States (MHAUS) and the Malignant Hyperthermia Association (MHA) of Canada, should be provided. A Medic-Alert bracelet for the child and family members is strongly recommended.

A family history of unusual reactions to anesthesia or unexplained fever or death during anesthesia in blood relatives should also be sought. This may help to determine which, if either, parent carries the MH gene. In most instances, the family history does not clarify the inheritance pattern, and all blood relatives should be notified of the risk of an MH reaction should they undergo general anesthesia. The parents should be counseled regarding the need for a muscle biopsy to identify the family source of the MH gene. There has been a noticeable shift away from performing muscle biopsies in children. This change in attitude may be attributed in part to the paucity of control biopsies from normal healthy children and to the identification of a candidate for the gene defect in MH, the ryanodine receptor on chromosome 19. It is hoped that in the near future a commercial blood test for MH based on identification of the gene defect will be available and will replace the invasive muscle biopsy.

I do not recommend that children who are MH susceptible limit either their activity or diet. Children will set their own limits and learn to live within these limits. Most children who are MH susceptible will avoid overstrenuous activity in the hot summer period and overindulgence in caffeine-containing foods, including chocolate, if they develop evidence of sensitivity such as muscle aches and pains. The most important information that the anesthesiologist can offer these families is his address and phone number for continued advice and support.

REFERENCES

1. Steward DJ, O'Connor GAR: Malignant hyperthermia—The acute crisis, in Britt BA (ed): *Malignant Hyperthermia*. Boston, Martinus Nijhoff Publishing, 1987, pp 1–10.
2. Britt BA: Malignant hyperthermia. *Can Anaesth Soc J* 1985; 32:666–677.
3. Littleford JA, Patel LR, Bose D, et al: Masseter muscle spasm in children: Implications of continuing the triggering anesthetic. *Anesth Analg* 1991; 72:151–160.
4. Larach MG, Landis JR: Sources of variation in false positive diagnostic rates of malignant hyperthermia using the North American protocol for caffeine halothane contracture testing. *J Neurol Sci* 1990; 98:521.
5. MacLennan DH, Duff C, Zorzato F, et al: Ryanodine receptor gene is a candidate for predisposition to malignant hyperthermia. *Nature* 1990; 343:559–561.
6. McGraw TT, Keon TP: Malignant hyperthermia and the clean machine. *Can J Anaesth* 1989; 36:530–532.
7. Rubin AS, Zablocki MD: Hyperkalemia, verapamil, and dantrolene. *Anesthesiology* 1987; 66:246–249.
8. Lerman J, Strong HA, McLeod ME: Pharmacokinetics of intravenous dantrolene in children. *Anesthesiology* 1989; 70:625–629.

35

Strabismus

A 2 1/2-year-old, 11-kg girl is scheduled for correction of strabismus as an outpatient. She is otherwise healthy. Hemoglobin, 11.5 g/dL; hematocrit, 34.5%.

Recommendations by Michael D. Abramowitz, M.D.

Strabismus is a deviation of the eyes that cannot be voluntarily corrected. The visual axes assume an abnormal position in relation to one another. Extensive terminology has been applied to strabismus, and various prefixes are attached to the word "tropia." Although the child may have an isolated strabismus, it may be part of a syndrome necessitating thorough preoperative evaluation.

Usually these children are in good health, and the procedure is performed on an outpatient or ambulatory basis. The younger ones may not understand the need for surgery because there is no pain or gross physical abnormality. The prospect of hospitalization may produce fear and anxiety. To alleviate the anxiety, preparation for the hospital visit should include counseling of the parents and a visit to the hospital for an orientation program. A puppet show, films, or other audiovisual techniques are commonly used in children's and larger community hospitals.

HISTORY AND PHYSICAL EXAMINATION

A full and meticulous history should be obtained from the parents, who should be assured that the morbidity and mortality for ophthalmic surgery in a major medical center is extremely low.[1, 2] There is a reported association of strabismus and malignant hyperpyrexia. A greater incidence of masseter spasm in strabismus patients receiving halothane-succinylcholine for induction has been cited.[3] While the author was at Children's Hospital National Medical Center in Washington, DC, where 750 to 1,000 strabismus procedures are performed annually, there was only one possible case of malignant hyperpyrexia in this group of patients between 1978 and 1985.

When obtaining the history, possible etiologies of the strabismus should be elicited. Infrequent causes include previous removal of an intracranial tumor or meningitis. Occasionally patients are encountered who have developed strabismus following head trauma.

There is a correlation between motion sickness, vomiting, and strabismus surgery. Therefore, the anesthesiologist should ask whether the child is subject to motion sickness. In our experience, nearly all children subject to motion sickness will have postoperative vomiting and should receive antiemetic prophylaxis with droperidol. This prophylaxis will control vomiting in 50% of motion sickness–prone patients.[4]

Although this patient is said to be normal, the anesthesiologist must be aware of syndromes with strabismus as a component. These include Apert, Crouzon, and Pfeiffer syndromes.[5] Children who have had cytomegalovirus infection in infancy and central nervous system disease may have strabismus. Those with a history of prematurity and associated respiratory distress syndrome may have pseudostrabismus.

During the elicitation of a drug history, the anesthesiologist must be aware that phospholine iodide, which is occasionally given to patients for treatment of fluctuating, variable, or inconsistent strabismus, inhibits pseudocholinesterase and prolongs the action of succinylcholine.

Physical examination of the patient may reveal a head tilt in the case of an oblique type of eye muscle palsy. This head tilt is functional and should present no airway management problem once the child is anesthetized.

PREMEDICATION

The approach to premedication varies among institutions and also depends on the personal preference of the anesthesiologist. Parents may be allowed in the induction room, depending on the policy of the institution. However, many anesthesiologists, especially those who work less frequently with children, prefer to use premedication. No specific premedicant is contraindicated, and the choice should be based on the physician's knowledge of the drug's mode of action, duration of onset, and side effects. The use of midazolam has radically changed the preoperative management of children. Midazolam can be administered orally. The usual dosage range is 0.25 to 0.75 mg/kg.[6] However, up to 1 mg/kg can be employed. With surgery lasting up to about 2 hours there is no prolongation of recovery. The problem with midazolam is the taste, so it is usually mixed in apple juice or fruit-flavored syrup. Premedication may be given up to 1 hour prior to induction of anesthesia. Some surgeons prefer to make a brief examination of the extraocular muscles prior to surgery in a cooperative, awake patient. If so, narcotic premedication is contraindicated.

THE OCULOCARDIAC REFLEX

The role of anticholinergics in attenuating the oculocardiac reflex is controversial. This reflex originates in the short and long ciliary nerves. The efferent impulse then travels via the branches of the ophthalmic division of the fifth cranial nerve, and the efferent impulse travels through the tenth cranial nerve, the vagus, to the heart. The end response of this reflex may be junctional rhythm, atrioventricular block, or asystolic cardiac arrest. Hypercapnia and hypoxia may cause the oculocardiac reflex to occur at a lower threshold.

In one series, traction on extraocular muscles caused slowing of the heart rate in 80% of patients, one third of whom developed cardiac arrhythmias.[7] It has been postulated that premedication with atropine, 0.01 mg/kg, will provide protection from this reflex for 30 minutes.[8] An adequate depth of anesthesia combined with assisted or controlled ventilation to avoid hypercardia plays an important role in reducing the frequency of the oculocardiac reflex. Retrobulbar blockade will also block the reflex; however, this technique is not commonly used in pediatric patients.[9] The muscle relaxant employed may also be important. One group has reported the indication for atropine administration was significantly greater in children who received atracurium than in those who received pancuronium.[10]

Occasionally adjustable sutures are used and manipulated in the postanesthesia recovery area. The anesthesiologist must be aware that the oculocardiac reflex can occur during manipulation of the sutures.[11]

The authors of one study compared the effects of atropine, glycopyrrolate, and a saline placebo in patients undergoing strabismus surgery and concluded that the incidence of bradycardia during strabismus surgery was great enough to justify the use of anticholinergic drugs.[12] Atropine and glycopyrrolate were found to be effective in preventing the oculocardiac reflex if administered intravenously prior to the start of surgery. The patients were also premedicated with droperidol, 0.1 mg/kg, which may have influenced the findings because droperidol has a membrane-stabilizing effect.

Initiation of the oculocardiac reflex usually occurs with initial traction of the muscle after incision of Tenon's capsule. The sequence in the surgical procedure where this is most likely to occur is shown in Figure 35–1. If slowing of the pulse does occur, the anesthesiologist should ask the surgeon to release the traction on the eye muscle (Fig 35–2). The medial rectus is said to be involved more frequently than other muscles, and the lateral rectus the least often involved. Repeated episodes of traction on the muscles may fatigue the reflex so that no further cardiac rhythm disturbance occurs.

INDUCTION OF ANESTHESIA

Inhalation induction is initiated with nitrous oxide–oxygen, and halothane is added slowly. When the child is asleep, the parents are accompanied to the waiting room by a hospital playroom volunteer if they were allowed to be present during induction of anesthesia. From the onset of induction the patient is monitored with a precordial stethoscope. In addition, a blood pressure cuff, pulse oximeter, axillary temperature probe, and electrocardiogram (ECG) are used. The ophthalmologist may perform a forced duction test for eye mobility prior to surgery; therefore depolarizing muscle relaxants are not employed. However, the effect of succinylcholine on this test lasts no more than 30 minutes, and it should be administered if indicated to manage an acute airway problem such as laryngospasm. Patients are usually intubated under deep halothane anesthesia. Intravenous access is important should the oculocardiac reflex occur and treatment be required. Gastric contents are aspirated after endotracheal intubation.

Anesthesia is usually maintained with nitrous oxide–oxygen and halothane, and ventilation is assisted intermittently. The anesthesia circuit is chosen on the basis of the child's age. The Jackson Rees modification of the Ayre T-piece is appropriate for children weighing up to 20 kg. In larger

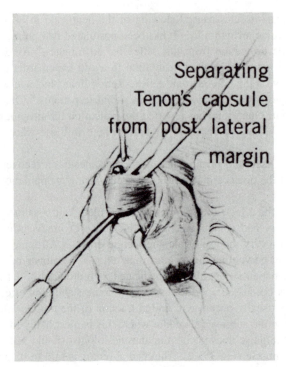

FIG 35–1.
Traction on the inferior rectus muscle during correction of strabismus.

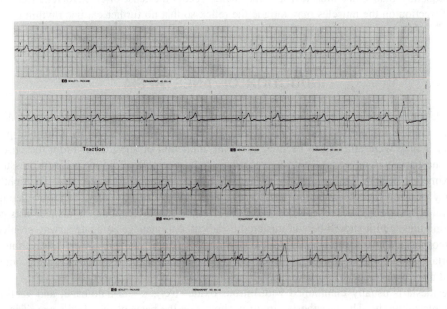

FIG 35–2.
Electrocardiographic tracing illustrating bradycardia initiated by traction on the eye muscles.

patients, a semiclosed circle system is used. A Bain system may also be used. A preformed curved endotracheal tube may be used to facilitate positioning of the breathing system.

The increased availability of infusion pumps makes total intravenous anesthesia and analgesia easier, and the popularity of the new intravenous agent propofol may result in greater use of this technique during strabismus surgery.[13] The effects of propofol on the incidence of vomiting following strabismus surgery in pediatric outpatients has been studied.[14] Propofol, with and without nitrous oxide (N_2O) and droperidol, was compared with halothane-N_2O and droperidol. These authors concluded that maintenance of anesthesia with a total intravenous regimen using propofol resulted in more rapid recovery and less postoperative emesis than when halothane-N_2O plus droperidol were administered. They also noted a higher incidence of the oculocardiac reflex with propofol infusion. The addition of N_2O to propofol increased the incidence of emesis.

ANTIEMETIC PROPHYLAXIS

The antiemetic agents most frequently used are droperidol and metoclopramide. The original extensive study evaluating the antiemetic effect of droperidol following outpatient strabismus surgery evaluated dose-response curves of droperidol, the incidence of nausea and vomiting, and the length of postoperative hospital stay.[14] It was concluded that droperidol is very effective in decreasing the incidence and severity of vomiting without significantly delaying discharge when administered prophylactically in a dose of 75 µg/kg. Lower doses of the drug are also effective.[15–17] Oral droperidol has also been evaluated and reported to be associated with a lower incidence of postoperative vomiting when compared with diazepam, meperidine and atropine administered orally.[18] A disadvantage of droperidol is the occasional occurrence of extrapyramidal side effects.[19] The groups that evaluated intravenous lidocaine to reduce the incidence of vomiting in children after surgery to correct strabismus had favorable results.[20] However, droperidol is significantly more effective than lidocaine. Metoclopramide also reduces the incidence of vomiting following strabismus surgery and does not produce the drowsiness of droperidol.[21]

POSTANESTHESIA CARE

Vital signs are taken as soon as the patient is admitted to the recovery room and at regular intervals thereafter. Pain is minimal, but photophobia is distressing, so patients are kept in subdued lighting. The major factor postponing discharge of short-stay strabismus patients is postoperative nausea and vomiting. It is also the most frequent reason for hospital admission.[22, 23]

Anesthetic management of pediatric patients for strabismus surgery presents a variety of subtle challenges. The child feels well prior to surgery, is generally healthy, and yet is subjected to an operation. The anesthesiologist must deal with a child who may have fears and is reluctant to cooperate. Recognition of the oculocardiac reflex, its prophylaxis, and its treatment is essential.

REFERENCES

1. Romano P, Robinson T: General anesthesia morbidity and mortality in eye surgery in a children's hospital. *J Pediatr Ophthalmol Strabismus* 1981; 18:17–26.
2. Cooper J, Medow N, Dibble C: Mortality rate in strabismus surgery. *J Am Optom Assoc* 1982; 53:82.
3. Carroll JB: Increased incidence of masseter spasm in children with strabismus anesthetised with halothane and succinylcholine. *Anesthesiology* 1987; 67:559–561.
4. Abramowitz MT, Oh TH, Epstein BS, et al: The antiemetic effect of droperidol following outpatient strabismus surgery in children. *Anesthesiology* 1983; 59:579–583.
5. Carruthers JD: Strabismus in craniofacial dysostosis. *Graefes Arch Clin Exp Ophthalmol* 1988; 226:230–234.
6. Feld LH, Negus JB, White PF: Oral midazolam preanesthetic medication in pediatric outpatients. *Anesthesiology* 1990; 73:831–834.
7. Bosomworth PP, Ziegler CH, Jacoby J: The oculocardiac reflex in eye muscle surgery. *Anesthesiology* 1958; 19:7–10.
8. Jacoby J: Pediatric cardiac arrest in strabismus surgery. *JAMA* 1971; 217:87–88.
9. Szmyd S: Retrobulbar block in strabismus surgery. *Arch Ophthalmol* 1985; 103:809–810.
10. Loewinger J, Friedmann-Neiger I, Cohen M, et al: Effect of atracurium and pancuronium on the oculocardiac reflex in children *Anesth Analg* 1991; 73:25–28.
11. Vrabec MP, Preslan MW, Kushner BJ: Occulocardiac reflex during manipulation of adjustable sutures after strabismus surgery. *Am J Opthalmol* 1987; 4:61–63.
12. Meyers EF, Tomeldan SA: Glycopyrrolate compared with atropine in the prevention of the oculocardiac reflex during eye-muscle surgery. *Anesthesiology* 1979; 51:350–352.
13. Hannallah RS, Baker SB, Casey W, et al: Propofol; effective dose and induction characteristics in unpremedicated children. *Anesthesiology* 1991; 74:217–219.
14. Watcha MF, Simeon RM, White PF, et al: Effect of propofol on the incidence of postoperative vomiting after strabismus surgery in pediatric outpatients. *Anesthesiology* 1991; 75:204–209.
15. Lin DM, Furst SR, Rodarte AA: Double-blinded comparison of metoclopramide and droperidol for prevention of emesis following strabismus surgery. *Anesthesiology* 1992; 76:357–361.
16. Fassoulaki A, Galanaki E: The anti-emetic effects of droperidol: Is it dose dependent? *Acta Anaesth Belg* 1989; 40:179–182.
17. Lerman J, Eustis S, Smith DR: Effect of droperidol pretreatment on postanesthetic vomiting in children undergoing strabismus. *Anesthesiology* 1986; 65:322–325.
18. Nicholson SC, Kaya KM, Betts E: The effect of preoperative oral droperidol on the incidence of postoperative emesis after paediatric strabismus surgery. *Can J Anaesth* 1988; 35:364–367.
19. Goal DG, Rice LJ, Hannallah RS: Droperidol induced extrapyramidal symptoms in an adolescent following strabismus surgery. *Middle East J Anesthesiol* 1990; 10:102.
20. Warner LL, et al: Intravenous lidocaine reduces the incidence of vomiting in children after surgery to correct strabismus. *Anesthesiology* 1988; 68:618–621.
21. Broadman LM, Hannallah R, DeLeon E, et al: Metoclopramide reduces the incidence of vomiting following strabismus surgery in children. *Anesthesiology* 1990; 72:245–248.
22. Isenberg SJ, et al: Overnight admission of outpatient strabismus patients. *Opthalmic Surg* 1990; 21:540–543.
23. Patel RI, Hannallah RS: Anesthetic complications following pediatric ambulatory surgery: A 3 year study. *Anesthesiology* 1988; 69:1004–1012.

36

Hypospadias and von Willebrand Disease

A 3-year-old, 14-kg boy with von Willebrand disease is scheduled for hypospadias repair. The bleeding time (Ivy) is 16 minutes; hemoglobin, 11.6 g/dL; hematocrit, 34.5%.

Recommendations by Catherine E. Wood, M.B., Ch.B, and Gerald V. Goresky, F.C. Anaes., M.D.C.M., F.R.C.P.C.

The two special anesthetic considerations for hypospadias repair in a child with von Willebrand disease are (1) the risk of hemorrhage in association with surgery in a highly vascular area such as the foreskin and (2) the provision of adequate analgesia during and after what is a very painful procedure. If the coagulation abnormality associated with von Willebrand disease is identified and corrected, special alterations in anesthetic technique may not be needed.

VON WILLEBRAND DISEASE

Von Willebrand disease is an inherited disorder of coagulation that is most frequently transmitted as an autosomal dominant trait with variable penetrance. A wide range of clinical variants are seen that result in a mild to moderately severe defect of hemostasis. In any one individual, the severity of the clinical picture may fluctuate, with a tendency to improve into adulthood. The features of von Willebrand disease are primarily those of mucocutaneous hemorrhage: spontaneous epistaxis, bruising following minor trauma, prolonged bleeding after dental extractions, gastrointestinal bleeding, and menorrhagia.[1]

The underlying abnormality in von Willebrand disease is a deficiency of or defect in a glyco-protein known as Von Willebrand factor (vWF). vWF is synthesized by endothelial cells and mega-karyocytes and is found in platelets, plasma, and subendothelial cells. vWF has recognized functions as a mediator of platelet adhesion to damaged vascular endothelium and as a carrier protein for coagulation factor VIII (VIII:c).[2]

The laboratory abnormalities in von Willebrand disease reflect decreased platelet adhesiveness, which leads to delayed formation of the primary platelet plug; reduced vWF activity; and impairment of the intrinsic pathway of the coagulation cascade due to reduced levels of circulating VIII:c. Platelet adhesiveness is assessed by the bleeding time, which is prolonged in the presence of a normal platelet count. vWF activity can be measured either directly or indirectly. When assayed directly, vWF levels generally correlate with the severity of the clinical picture. vWF activity is assessed indirectly by using the ristocetin aggregation test. This test is based on the observation that the plasma of patients with von Willebrand disease does not support the aggregation of washed platelets in the presence of the antibiotic ristocetin. Because vWF acts as a carrier protein for factor VIII:c, factor VIII:c is also reduced in moderate to severe cases of von Willebrand disease, although it may be normal in milder cases. The activated partial thromboplastin time, a measure of the integrity of the intrinsic pathway and therefore of VIII:c activity, may also be prolonged. Because the results of coagulation studies may fluctuate in a given individual, they are occasionally within the normal range. For some patients, therefore, serial testing may be required to establish both the presence of the disease and the severity of the coagulopathy.[2]

During a potential or actual bleeding episode, levels of functioning vWF must be restored to allow effective hemostasis. This may be accomplished either by stimulation of the patient's intrinsic vWF with 1-desamino-8-D-arginine vasopressin (DDAVP) or by replacement therapy in the form of cryoprecipitate.

DDAVP is a synthetic analogue of antidiuretic hormone. It stimulates the release of stored vWF from platelets and subendothelial cells. This results in a transient threefold to fourfold increase in circulating levels of vWF. DDAVP may be administered either intranasally or by intravenous infusion in a dose of 0.3 μg/kg. A response is usually seen within 30 minutes and persists for about 6 hours. Tachyphylaxis may develop if repeated doses of DDAVP are given within a short time, probably the result of the depletion of available vWF stores. The main side effects are flushing due to cutaneous vasodilation and, occasionally, fluid retention leading to hyponatremia.[3] Although the response to DDAVP is consistent for an individual, DDAVP is not effective in all variants of von Willebrand disease, and it corrects the bleeding time in only about 62% of affected subjects.[4] In some variants of the disease, it may be contraindicated.[1] If the bleeding time and levels of vWF and factor VIII:c are measured before and after the administration of DDAVP, a subject may then be characterized as a "responder" or a "nonresponder". DDAVP has been used successfully for patients undergoing surgical procedures, in many cases as the sole therapy.[5, 6]

Cryoprecipitate is the treatment of choice for replacement of vWF and correction of the bleeding time for nonresponders to DDAVP. As with other blood components, the possible transmission of transfusion-related infections remains the primary concern associated with its use. The dose is usually on the order of 1 unit/5 kg, but will depend on the patient's weight and initial vWF level. This dose should correct the coagulopathy for up to 12 hours, but the effect may be abbreviated during an acute bleeding episode.

PREOPERATIVE MANAGEMENT

A child with von Willebrand disease presenting for elective surgery should be assessed in conjunction with a hematologist. The subtype of von Willebrand disease and the severity of the coagulopathy are determined from the history and the coagulation studies. In light of the unpredictable fluctuations in laboratory abnormalities that may occur in von Willebrand disease, it is particularly important that a careful history be taken regarding previous bleeding manifestations in order to characterize the nature of the bleeding disorder. The aim is to correct the underlying coagulopathy during the immediate perioperative period. In order to plan the most appropriate management, the child must be identified as a responder or nonresponder to DDAVP well in advance of elective surgery.

A child with von Willebrand disease should be admitted to a hospital preoperatively. In addition to the routine preparation for surgery, blood should be crossmatched and cryoprecipitate prepared. Intravenous access is required prior to surgery. For those patients who have been demonstrated to be responders to DDAVP, a dose of 0.3 μg/kg is infused in normal saline over a period of 15 minutes, half an hour prior to surgery. For nonresponders to DDAVP, the appropriate dose of cryoprecipitate is given. Following infusion of either agent, the bleeding time should be checked prior to the start of surgery to ensure that clotting has returned to normal.

ANESTHETIC MANAGEMENT

Premedication is not essential but may be helpful to sedate the child during the infusion and while the bleeding time is being measured. The choice of induction technique will depend on the psychological state of the child and the personal preference of the anesthesiologist. Either an inhalation induction using nitrous oxide, oxygen, and halothane or an intravenous induction with thiopental via the previously inserted intravenous infusion is appropriate.

Monitoring requirements are straightforward. A precordial stethoscope, noninvasive blood pressure device, electrocardiograph, and pulse oximeter should be used. The inspired oxygen concentration should be monitored and a ventilator disconnection alarm and capnography utilized if ventilation is controlled.

The provision of adequate analgesia during the procedure is essential. Although regional techniques have traditionally been contraindicated in patients with coagulopathies, epidural analgesia has recently been used successfully in adults with von Willebrand disease whose vWF and VIII:c levels were temporarily raised to normal as a result of pregnancy.[7, 8] Therefore, in a child whose bleeding time has been restored to normal by the administration of DDAVP or cryoprecipitate, the caudal administration of a local anesthetic agent can be undertaken without undue risk of epidural hematoma. The use of a longer-acting agent such as 0.25% bupivacaine with adrenaline, 0.5 mL/kg, will provide effective analgesia during surgery and the early postoperative period.

A caudal block will reduce requirements for other anesthetic agents and should eliminate the need for intraoperative opiates. Nitrous oxide, oxygen, and a low concentration of a volatile agent delivered via either a mask or a laryngeal mask-airway to a spontaneously breathing child should be well tolerated and provide good operating conditions. If it is anticipated that the surgery will be protracted, then endotracheal intubation and controlled ventilation following the administration of a muscle relaxant may be preferred.

During the surgery, the fluid deficit from the period of preoperative fasting must be replaced and maintenance fluids administered. The need for intraoperative transfusion during this surgery would be unusual, but the anesthesiologist should be prepared to transfuse the child with red blood cells if excessive bleeding were to occur.

POSTOPERATIVE MANAGEMENT

It is essential to maintain normal clotting into the early postoperative period, and further DDAVP or cryoprecipitate will be needed. DDAVP responders should mount a second response if the initial dose is repeated after 6 hours. However, oozing from the surgical site may herald the early development of tachyphylaxis, in which case cryoprecipitate must be administered. In those children who received cryoprecipitate originally, a repeated bleeding time is indicated after 6 to 8 hours to assess further requirements. Ideally, the bleeding time should be monitored regularly. In practice, this is distressing to the child and technically difficult. For this reason, it is appropriate to observe the child in the hospital for signs of bleeding and to monitor vWF and VIII:c levels daily as a guide to further management.

The child will need further analgesia once the caudal block has worn off. Intramuscular injections and nonsteroidal anti-inflammatory drugs, which adversely affect platelet adhesion, are contraindicated. A loading dose of intravenous morphine, 0.1 mg/kg, followed by an infusion, 10 to 20µg/kg/hr, should provide adequate pain relief if indicated. Alternatively, oral medications such as codeine phosphate, 1 mg/kg, and/or acetaminophen, 15 mg/kg, may be sufficient.

SUMMARY

Any child with von Willebrand disease who requires surgery presents potential problems. Careful planning by surgical, anesthetic, and hematology staff will enable the coagulopathy to be controlled so that surgery can proceed without the need for unusual intraoperative intervention and with a minimum of risk to the child.

REFERENCES

1. Ruggeri ZM: Structure and function of von Willebrand factor: Relationship to von Willebrand's disease. *Mayo Clin Proc* 1991; 66:847–861.
2. Williams WJ, Beutler E, Erslev AJ, et al: *Hematology,* ed 4. New York, McGraw-Hill International Book Co, 1990.
3. Aledort LM: Treatment of von Willebrand's disease. *Mayo Clin Proc* 1991; 66:841–846.
4. Rose EH, Aledort LM: Nasal spray desmopressin (DDAVP) for mild hemophilia A and von Willebrand disease. *Ann Intern Med* 1991; 114:563–569.

5. Blombäck M, et al: Surgery in patients with von Willebrand's disease. *Br J Surg* 1989; 76:398–400.

6. Petrover MG, Cohen CI: The use of desmopressin in the management of two patients with von Willebrand's disease undergoing periodontal surgery, 2 case reports. *J Periodontol* 1990; 61:239–242.

7. Cohen S, et al: Epidural analgesia for labor and delivery in a patient with von Willebrand's disease. *Reg Anaesth* 1989; 14:95–97.

8. Milaskiewicz RM, Holdcroft A, Letsky E: Epidural anaesthesia and von Willebrand's disease. *Anaesthesia* 1990; 45:462–464.

37

Myringotomy and Atrial Septal Defect

A 3-year-old, 12-kg girl with recurrent otitis media is scheduled for bilateral myringotomy and insertion of tympanostomy tubes. She is known to have an atrial septal defect (ASD) and will "probably" require surgical correction of the defect. She is normally active for her age. Hemoglobin, 13.5 g/dL; hematocrit, 40%. The surgeon would prefer to perform the procedure on an outpatient basis.

Recommendations by Burton S. Epstein, M.D.

Two major factors must be considered when assessing the feasibility of scheduling a surgical procedure on an outpatient basis. These are (1) the operative procedure and (2) the patient. Bilateral myringotomy is an ideal operation for an outpatient. It is short and associated with minimal bleeding and minor physiologic derangements. Minimal or no postoperative complications should be anticipated, and the recovery period is not usually prolonged as a result of extensive vomiting or intense pain. In most geographic areas of the country, a myringotomy *must* be performed on an outpatient basis; otherwise, there is no reimbursement for hospitalization by the insurance carrier. Obviously, there can be extenuating circumstances that make hospitalization safer and, indeed, a requirement. One of these is the physical condition of the patient.

Most outpatient facilities will accept a patient who is free of disease or in whom a systemic disease is well controlled. A 3-year-old patient with an ASD, normally active for her age and in whom no complications exist or are anticipated because of the disease or the surgical procedure, is usually a reasonable candidate for outpatient surgery. A patient with an ASD is characteristically asymptomatic and rarely goes into cardiac failure. Development of marked pulmonary hypertension with reversal of shunt flow is a late phenomenon and is very rare in the pediatric age range. Noncardiac anomalies, however, appear in 25% of patients with congenital heart disease. Particular attention should be paid to associated diseases in other major organ systems. In addition, the patient must be in optimal condition and free of acute disease such as upper respiratory infection. With this preamble, what then are the usual areas that must be dealt with in this patient once she is scheduled for outpatient surgery?

PREOPERATIVE EVALUATION AND MEDICAL PREPARATION

In advance of the procedure, the patient should be evaluated by the pediatrician and noted to be free of acute disease. In addition, a cardiology consultation is required and must include a written, precise evaluation of the disease and the supporting data that confirm the diagnosis, for example, electrocardiograph (ECG), chest x-ray, echocardiograph, and cardiac catheterization, if performed. Recommendations for subacute bacterial endocarditis (SBE) prophylaxis must be included.

The recommendations of the American Heart Association (AHA) for prevention of bacterial endocarditis are somewhat confusing.[1] The decision to recommend SBE prophylaxis is based largely on the type of congenital heart defect and the proposed surgical procedure. Although endocarditis prophylaxis is recommended for children with "most congenital malformations," it is not for those with an "isolated secundum atrial septal defect." Moreover, endocarditis prophylaxis is not recommended for "tympanotomy tube insertion." Since studies that define the risk of bacteremia are not available, many cardiologists prefer to be conservative and recommend prophylaxis, regardless of the official AHA recommendations.

If therapy is instituted and there is no known allergy, an acceptable regimen is amoxicillin, 50 mg/kg orally 1 hour before the procedure and 25 mg/kg orally 6 hours after the initial dose. In some facilities, the first dose is given intravenously if a catheter is inserted during induction of anesthesia. The complete article on the subject should be displayed prominently in every outpatient facility.

PREOPERATIVE EVALUATION AND PREPARATION FOR ANESTHESIA

If any questions exist regarding the physical condition of the patient and recommendations by the family physician and/or consultants, the latter should be consulted and the issues clarified. The child and parents are best interviewed in advance of the day of surgery so that anxiety can be minimized. A preoperative tour of the facility and an animated demonstration of anesthesia and surgery (puppet show, movie, and so on) are frequently utilized and are highly recommended. In a well-prepared patient, premedication is rarely needed or is limited to an oral medication such as diazepam, 0.1 mg/kg, 1 1/2 hours prior to induction of anesthesia. Although not endorsed by the manufacturer, oral midazolam (0.5 to 0.75 mg/kg) or nasal midazolam (0.2 mg/kg) is being used successfully. Onset is rapid and duration reasonably short, usually less than 60 minutes. It is hoped that a well-adjusted, carefully oriented child will be able to undergo an inhalation or intravenous induction with few surprises.

Orders for nothing to eat or drink should be clearly written and understood by the parents. No milk or solids should be given after midnight. Although the protocol in many facilities restricts ingestion of clear liquids to 6 to 8 hours before surgery, there are data indicating that on the average, clear liquids are emptied from the stomach in 2 to 3 hours.[2, 3]

INDUCTION AND MAINTENANCE OF ANESTHESIA

If inhalation induction is selected, nitrous oxide–oxygen and halothane are usually administered and titrated slowly until the child is asleep. Otherwise, thiopental, 4 to 5 mg/kg, with 0.2 mg atropine can be given intravenously through a 25-gauge needle, followed by inhalation anesthesia. Lesions with increased pulmonary blood flow as a result of left-to-right shunting of blood, such as ASD, cause rapid uptake of inhalation agents from the alveoli, and this results in rapid induction of anesthesia. This same defect leads to a slower induction with intravenous agents owing to recirculation of blood in the pulmonary vascular bed. In the event that the child decompensates mentally prior to induction and preoperative preparation is for naught, rectal methohexital, 25 mg/kg of a 10% solution, can be used.[4] Maintenance of anesthesia should be achieved with the above inhalation agents and no less that 50% oxygen. Halothane should be titrated to effect, i.e., no movement or reaction to surgical stimuli. If hypotension cannot be avoided with the concentration of halothane required, supplementation with 1 µg/kg fentanyl intravenously is useful and enables the concentration of halothane to be reduced. Endotracheal intubation is rarely needed and is reserved for situations in which an anesthetic cannot be administered by mask. These situations include persistent airway obstruction unrelieved by insertion of an oropharyngeal airway, laryngospasm, or poor mask fit.

OTHER CONSIDERATIONS

Routine monitoring for this patient includes a precordial stethoscope, ECG, blood pressure cuff with or without a Doppler device, pulse oximetry, and measurement of the inspired oxygen concentration.[5] Monitoring of axillary temperature is also encouraged. Intravenous fluids such as 5% dextrose in one-third normal saline at a rate of 45 mL/h should be infused. If an attempt is made to replace the intake deficit, it should not be accomplished in less than a 4-hour period, should surgery and recovery last that long. Although an intravenous infusion is frequently not started in many healthy patients scheduled for myringotomy, it is recommended when one is dealing with a patient who may require therapy in addition to hydration.

RECOVERY

Monitoring of blood pressure and oxygen saturation by pulse oximetry should be continued in the recovery period.[6] Monitoring of the ECG should be considered since an arrhythmia may occur during recovery from anesthesia. Oxygen should be administered by mask until the child is fully recovered. Discharge criteria include stability of vital signs; the presence of swallowing, cough, and gag reflexes; the absence of vomiting; the ability to tolerate oral fluids; the ability to ambulate; the absence of respiratory distress; and an alert and oriented state of consciousness. In an uncomplicated procedure, full recovery usually occurs within 1 to 1 1/2 hours following termination of anesthesia.

COMPLICATIONS

A child with an ASD is not expected to develop congestive heart failure or a shift in the intracardiac shunt. However, serious atrial arrhythmias such as atrial flutter or supraventricular tachycardia may occur, may require treatment, and could be serious. These can be seen with induction or maintenance of anesthesia or in the recovery period. A serious, persistent arrhythmia or one that requires treatment mandates hospitalization and careful observation during this period. As a result, it is possible that a patient with this potential problem might be better scheduled for outpatient surgery in a hospital-based facility rather than one that is "freestanding." Obviously, a freestanding unit in close proximity to a hospital where transfer can be accomplished quickly and safely is perfectly satisfactory.

REFERENCES

1. Dajani AS, Bisno AL, Chung KJ, et al: Prevention of bacterial endocarditis. Recommendation of the American Heart Association. *JAMA* 1990; 264:2919.
2. Cote CJ: NPO after midnight for children— a reappraisal. *Anesthesiology* 1990; 72:589–591.
3. Shreiner MD, Triebwasser A, Keon TP: Ingestion of liquids compared with preoperative fasting in pediatric outpatients. *Anesthesiology* 1990; 72:593–597.
4. Goresky GV, Steward DJ: Rectal methohexitone for induction of anesthesia in children. *Can Anaesth Soc J* 1979; 26:213–215.
5. American Society of Anesthesiologists: *Standards for Basic Intra-operative Monitoring*. Park Ridge, Ill, American Society of Anesthesiologists, 1991.
6. American Society of Anesthesiologists: *Standards for Postanesthesia Care*. Park Ridge, Ill, American Society of Anesthesiologists, 1991.

38

Magnetic Resonance Imaging

A 4-year-old, 18-kg hyperactive boy with a seizure disorder is scheduled for magnetic resonance imaging (MRI). The seizures have become more frequent in the last 2 months, and the child complains of headaches. Current medications are phenobarbital and valproic acid. Hemoglobin, 12.8 g/dL; hematocrit, 35%.

Recommendations by Robert B. Forbes, M.D., F.R.C.P.C.

A 4-year-old child with a history of increasing seizure activity and headaches who is scheduled for MRI presents two major anesthetic considerations that must be confronted. The first concern is common to any patient who requires anesthesia for an MRI scan, and it is related to the powerful magnetic field and radio frequency (RF) waves generated by the scanner and the inaccessibility of the patient during the scanning process. The second concern, specific to this child, is the possible presence of increased intracranial pressure (ICP) suggested by his history of headaches and the increasing frequency of his seizures. Each of these considerations must be carefully evaluated if serious anesthetic complications are to be avoided. The problems associated with providing anesthesia in an MRI unit require interdepartmental planning and organization prior to the day of the procedure. The problems associated with providing anesthesia in the face of potentially increased ICP can be minimized by careful selection of an appropriate anesthetic technique. Each of these concerns will be discussed in turn.

PRINCIPLES OF MRI

MRI has become increasingly important in the clinical diagnosis of a wide variety of conditions because it produces high-resolution, multiplane cross-sectional images of the body by using the magnetic properties of atomic nuclei (Fig 38–1) and avoids the use of ionizing radiation.[1] Each atomic nucleus possesses an intrinsic "spin" due to rotation of its protons or neutrons and is surrounded by a magnetic field. Normally these small magnetic fields are randomly oriented, but when

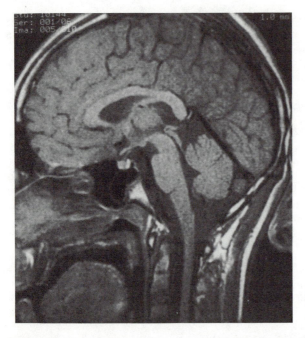

FIG 38–1.
A normal parasagittal T1-weighted magnetic resonance image of a 12-year-old child.

placed within the larger, stronger magnetic field produced by the MRI scanner, the magnetic fields surrounding each nucleus become aligned in parallel to the MRI scanner's static magnetic field. MRI makes use of this phenomenon by placing the patient into a large cylindrical magnet. Within this magnetic tube is an RF transmitter coil that surrounds the patient and emits RF pulses that displace the nuclear magnetic fields aligned parallel to the static magnetic field. When the RF pulse is terminated, the magnetic fields return to their parallel alignment. It takes a known amount of time for the realignment to occur, during which time a signal is emitted by each nucleus and detected by a receiver coil. These signals are used to produce the magnetic resonance image. Because recovery times are determined in part by inherent tissue properties, they can be used to differentiate normal and abnormal tissue. In addition, specific atomic nuclei will only respond to certain radio frequencies, and the response is proportional to the strength of the static magnetic field. By placing the patient in a gradient magnetic field, a specific radio frequency can be used to define a certain distance along the body. This allows a patient to be scanned in successive cuts, similar to computed tomographic (CT) scans, and the final image is constructed by computer from the signals that are received. Resolution of the image depends upon the strength of the magnetic field (most units are 0.5 to 1.5 Tesla). It is the great strength of the magnetic field and the RF pulses emitted by the magnetic resonance imager that introduce many of the problems and hazards confronting an anesthesiologist when caring for children during MRI.

INDICATIONS FOR ANESTHESIA

Although MRI is not painful, the pounding noise generated by the scanner, the claustrophobic sensation many children experience when placed within the enclosed tunnel of an MRI unit, and the requirement that they remain motionless during the long period of time required to complete the scan are the primary reasons that anesthesiologists become involved in the care of these patients. In addition, contrast material is frequently required to augment the image obtained, and gaining intravenous access in anxious, uncooperative children can be difficult. In adults and older children adequate sedation can usually be achieved with oral medication given prior to the examination, but in younger children effective sedation using oral medication may be difficult to achieve, unpredictable in duration, and associated with unpleasant or life-threatening side effects. As a result, only very deep sedation using intravenous medications or general anesthesia can ensure that the child remains absolutely still while the scan is being performed.[2, 3] General anesthesia may also be required for patients who are mentally impaired or who have movement disorders or painful conditions that prevent them from lying still for prolonged periods of time. In addition, anesthesiologists may become involved in the care of children with serious medical diseases or traumatic injuries who require intense monitoring during an MRI scan.

FUNDAMENTALS OF ANESTHETIC CARE DURING MRI

Providing anesthesia care for MRI often makes anesthesiologists uncomfortable for several reasons. The MRI suite is rarely designed with the needs of the anesthesiologist in mind and is usually located far away from the main operating suite. It may lack pipeline oxygen, nitrous oxide, and suction and gas evacuation lines, and electrical outlets are often inadequate in number, location, or grounding. The anesthesia equipment and supplies required in the MRI unit often must be transported from the operating room, and MRI personnel are less familiar with the needs of the anesthetized patient than are operating room personnel. As a result, they may have difficulty providing the support and assistance required during a medical emergency. Finally, the size and design of the magnetic resonance imager makes access to the patient difficult. Therefore, before embarking on an anesthetic adventure in the MRI unit, the anesthesiologist must be familiar with the procedure to be performed, including the patient's position, the need for contrast material, and the constraints placed upon the use of common anesthesia equipment and monitoring techniques by the powerful magnetic field that is generated in the magnetic resonance imager.

It is important that the evaluation and management of these children be discussed and coordinated with everyone involved in their medical care so that an organized approach to scheduling, preanesthetic evaluation, informed consent, and postanesthesia recovery can be established. When organizing anesthesia services for children who require general anesthesia for MRI, it is essential that they receive the same preanesthetic evaluation as patients undergoing surgical procedures. Basic intraoperative monitoring during the scan, although often complicated or difficult to achieve, should include an assessment of oxygenation, ventilation, circulation, and temperature. Postanesthesia recovery may take place in the MRI unit, or the child may be transported back to the main recovery area. Appropriate monitoring must be continued during transport, and supplemental oxygen, airway equipment, and resuscitative drugs should accompany the patient. Finally, the same criteria for discharge from the recovery area that are used for surgical patients also apply to children sedated or anesthetized for MRI. By anticipating and planning for all the potential problems that may be encountered when anesthetizing a child in an unfamiliar location the unnecessary delays and compromise of patient care that can occur when these types of problems must be dealt with at the last minute will be avoided, and the anesthesiologist's full attention can be focused on care of the individual child.

There are three major problems related to the powerful magnetic field and RF pulses emitted by the scanner that are encountered during anesthesia in the MRI unit. First, any ferromagnetic material brought into the scanner, and this includes much of our anesthesia equipment such as laryngoscopes, stethoscopes, Magill forceps, gas cylinders, and anesthesia machines, will be attracted by the magnetic field and can literally fly across the room and injure the patient or other people in the room. Second, most electronic monitoring equipment does not function properly when brought near the MRI scanner, so monitors must be shielded or alternate monitoring techniques employed. Third, metal objects or electronic monitors placed near the MRI scanner can emit RF waves that interfere with the image generated and result in a degraded, nondiagnostic scan. In addition, image artifacts will occur if the patient does not remain still during the period of time required to make each cut. With current MRI technology individual cuts take up to 15 minutes to complete, and depending upon the anatomic area to be evaluated, the total scanning period may last from 30 minutes to 3 hours. Any significant movement during an individual cut may require that it be repeated. Adults are generally able to tolerate remaining still for this period of time, but many young children cannot, and these are the children who will require sedation or general anesthesia to ensure that a high-quality diagnostic scan is obtained.

SEDATION FOR MRI

In an attempt to avoid general anesthesia, radiologists will frequently request a sedation regimen that can be used for all pediatric patients. Although many different "recipes" for sedation have been advocated, at present there is no drug or combination of drugs that will safely and reliably sedate all children. All of these techniques have significant failure rates, and all have been associated with serious complications.[4–7] Infants less than 6 months of age can often be adequately immobilized without the use of drugs by simply bundling them snugly in a blanket. Toddlers and young children, up to about 5 years of age, often require some type of pharmacologic intervention. Older school-age children and adolescents almost always do well with simple oral sedation and reassurance given prior to the procedure.

Chloral hydrate is a time-honored and safe sedative for pediatric patients, but during MRI supplemental sedation is often required. Prolonged sedation and delayed discharge from the hospital following an MRI scan can be a problem following large doses of chloral hydrate as well as other sedatives. Various combinations of drugs have been used for sedation prior to radiologic scans, including narcotics, barbiturates, anticholinergics, major tranquilizers, and benzodiazepines. These "lytic cocktails" have varying degrees of success and numerous adverse reactions. Thompson et al.[4] found that the time required to achieve sedation with a combination of intramuscular atropine, meperidine, promethazine, and secobarbital was almost an hour; more than 10% of the children required additional sedation; and 12% of the scans were technically unsatisfactory. Burchart et al.[5] reported that 14% of scans were unsatisfactory when children received a combination of chlorpromazine, promethazine, and meperidine and the duration of sedation exceeded 7 hours. Mitchell et al.[6] identified serious adverse reactions following various types of premedication given for CT in 13 of 106 pediatric patients aged 5 months to 16 years, with life-threatening cardiorespiratory depression occurring in 4 children. Sedation with intramuscular methohexital for children undergoing CT scanning has been shown to be safe and effective. Varner et al.[7] reported sleep onset at 3.3 minutes following intramuscular methohexital, 10 mg/kg. Although 4 of 50 children required supplemental medication because of movement during the scan, no complications except pain on injection were noted, and the children were awake and alert within 90 minutes. Rectal methohexital is also safe and effective for anesthetizing children having diagnostic scans because it is easily administered, is relatively rapid in onset, and has an appropriate duration of action and minimal effect on cardiorespiratory function, although apnea can occur. However, methohexital has little analgesic effect, and patients may move during placement of an intravenous catheter, during injection of contrast material, or during other manipulations, and this can necessitate small supplemental doses of intravenous methohexital to maintain an adequate level of sedation. The monitoring standards are the same whether a child receives sedation or general anesthesia for magnetic imaging, and appropriate equipment to control the airway and maintain adequate oxygenation and ventilation during sedation must be immediately available.

ANESTHETIC MANAGEMENT

General anesthesia is preferred to deep sedation in this 4-year-old child for a number of reasons. In the presence of increased intracranial pressure, sedation may be associated with respiratory depression and hypercarbia, which could worsen intracranial hypertension. In addition, this child is hyperactive and is in an age group that is most likely to become upset when separated from his parents, placed in the extremely confining imaging unit, and exposed to the loud pounding that occurs during the MRI. Therefore, it is unlikely that any type of sedation would adequately control him for the period of time necessary to obtain the MRI.

An appropriate anesthetic induction technique in a child with clearly increased ICP includes intravenous sodium thiopental, nitrous oxide, and a narcotic such as fentanyl. Hyperventilation should be established immediately following induction and maintained throughout the procedure. In addition, appropriate therapy to reduce ICP prior to inducing anesthesia should be considered. This approach assumes that intravenous access will be easily and quickly accomplished. If attempts to place an intravenous catheter result in vigorous resistance with struggling and crying, this in itself may significantly raise the ICP.

In this child the presence of increased ICP is less certain, and an inhalation induction with nitrous oxide and a volatile agent would be a reasonable alternative to an intravenous barbiturate induction. Although there are some theoretic advantages to the use of isoflurane for patients with increased ICP, halothane, which causes less coughing, breath holding, and laryngospasm, provides a smoother induction and would be preferred over isoflurane. Once the child has lost consciousness, ventilation should be assisted, then controlled, and the inspired concentration of halothane decreased. An intravenous catheter can then be placed and the airway secured with an endotracheal tube. Anesthesia could be maintained with a low concentration of halothane, or if appropriate, halothane could be discontinued and replaced with an infusion of narcotic, barbiturate, or propofol.

Anesthesia should be induced outside of the room containing the magnetic resonance imager, with all the standard monitors used and the parents present to comfort and reassure the child. This eliminates the effects of the strong magnetic field on anesthesia equipment and monitors and allows induction and intubation to be completed without concern that the MRI magnetic field will interfere with function of the anesthesia equipment during this critical period. For example, although most laryngoscopes are not magnetic, the batteries inside the handle are, and if intubation is attempted near the scanner, the magnetic attraction of the batteries can make the laryngoscope impossible to control. Once the child loses consciousness, the parents are asked to leave, intravenous access is established, and the airway is secured. The use of succinylcholine for intubation is best avoided, in part because it can cause a transient increase in ICP but more importantly because of the relatively high incidence of masseter muscle spasm that occurs following the combination of halothane and succinylcholine in children. Intubation is best facilitated with a nondepolarizing muscle relaxant with an appropriate duration of action and minimal tendency to release histamine. Following induction and intubation the child and an MRI-compatible anesthesia machine are transferred into the scanning room. The child is positioned on the sliding platform and then advanced into the imaging unit. Once in the scanner, the patient is out of reach of the anesthesiologist and almost completely hidden from view. Extended tubing using either a circle system or a Mapleson D circuit will be required to reach the patient's endotracheal tube. In this child, ventilation should be controlled to maintain the P_{CO_2} at an appropriate level.

To as great an extent as possible, all the basic monitors used in the operating room must also be used during anesthesia for MRI. However, because of interference from the magnetic field and the RF waves generated by the scanner, some ingenuity and flexibility may be required to ensure that adequate monitoring is maintained throughout the procedure. In addition to a pulse oximeter, some of which are MRI compatible, heart and breath sounds should be monitored using an esophageal or precordial stethoscope. The electrocardiogram is frequently distorted during MRI because the chest leads pass through the varying magnetic field and are exposed to the RF waves generated by the scanner. Although the interference can be reduced by using RF filters and telemetry, this is rarely entirely successful. Blood pressure can be monitored using a sphygmomanometer, which contains little metal and is kept as far away from the scanner as is possible. An automated blood pressure machine can also be used in some MRI units if it is carefully situated within the scanning room. To protect the computer, MRI suites are air-conditioned, and infants and small children cool rapidly when exposed to this environment. However, once the scanning process begins, the changing magnetic and RF fields can produce sufficient heating to significantly increase a child's body temperature. Therefore, temperature should be monitored throughout the procedure. With the child virtually out of sight during the scan, adequate monitoring is imperative, and the value of pulse oximetry cannot be overestimated. Also, an end-tidal carbon dioxide analyzer with an extended sampling tube can be used to effectively assess ventilation in both anesthetized and sedated patients. In the absence of painful stimulation, anesthesia can be maintained with a very low concentration of volatile agent. In this child, if the ICP is clearly elevated, a continuous infusion of thiopental or propofol would also be appropriate. Because methohexital and enflurane have been associated with seizures in susceptible patients, they should be avoided. For most children undergoing MRI the specific drugs used to provide anesthesia are not as critical to a successful outcome as is careful, yet flexible organization and meticulous monitoring.

OTHER HAZARDS

In addition to the anesthetic problems encountered during MRI, there are other potential hazards of MRI that can affect not only the patient but also anyone working near the scanner. Although there have been no apparent adverse effects on healthy people exposed to static magnetic fields below 2 Tesla, for people with implanted metallic devices such as cerebrovascular clips or cardiac pacemakers, substantial risk exists. Many vascular clips are magnetic, and the force exerted upon them by the MRI may be sufficient to cause displacement or dislodgement. Demand pacemakers may be converted to the asynchronous mode if placed within the static magnetic field, and older stainless steel pacemakers may be displaced or the leads fractured. The RF waves generated by the scanner may be interpreted by the pacemaker as cardiac activity and result in inhibition of a demand pacemaker. The changing magnetic fields can also cause localized heating of metal objects such as an orthopedic prosthesis or external wire leads and produce severe burns. Finally, of little medical concern but of some practical importance is the damage done to pocket calculators, watches, paging devices, and magnetic strips on credit cards when they are exposed to the magnetic field of an MRI machine.

CONTRAST MEDIA

As with other radiologic procedures, the images produced by magnetic resonance can often be enhanced by the administration of contrast media (Fig 38–2). Although useful in defining the pathology, these drugs are associated with significant physiologic side effects and a relatively high incidence of adverse reactions. The majority of reactions are mild and require no treatment; however, severe and fatal reactions can occur. The two types of problems seen are those due to physiologic changes associated with the administration of a large osmotic load and unpredictable, idiosyncratic anaphylactoid reactions.

There is a significant increase in intravascular volume and osmolality leading to a transient hy-

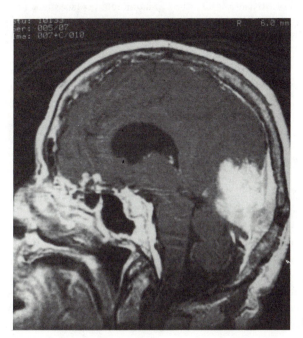

FIG 38–2.
A parasagittal postcontrast image in a 73-year-old patient demonstrates a meningioma.

pertensive response following the injection of hypertonic contrast media. Over a matter of minutes the osmolality and intravascular volume return toward normal as the contrast material is excreted by the kidneys. The diuresis that follows administration of the osmotic load can lead to relative hypovolemia and acute bladder distension. Contrast material can also cause dysrhythmias, ischemia, and myocardial depression, even in healthy patients. Other important side effects include competition with other medications for protein binding sites and interference with the complement and coagulation systems.

Also of concern, whenever contrast material is used, are the unpredictable allergic reactions that occur in some patients and range from relatively minor nausea and vomiting to severe hypotension, bronchospasm, airway edema, and anaphylaxis. The initial reaction often appears to be benign and is frequently short-lived, but it may also be a prodromal sign of a severe anaphylactoid reaction. It is therefore important that these initial, minor signs, which may include chills, fever, and nausea, do not pass unnoticed. Patients who have had previous reactions to contrast material or significant allergic disease are at higher risk of having a severe reaction. Mild reactions to contrast media are easily treated with fluid, observation, and reassurance of the patient. More severe anaphylactoid reactions, including hypotension, bronchospasm or anaphylaxis, require aggressive treatment with oxygen, epinephrine, antihistamines, and steroids.[8]

POSTANESTHESIA CARE

Following completion of the MRI, this child requires the same postanesthesia care that every child in the operating room receives. Appropriate equipment and personnel must always be immediately available to ensure that the recovery period is uncomplicated. Recovery may occur in the MRI suite, but in many hospitals patients from MRI are transferred to a suitable postanesthesia care unit, and this may involve traveling long distances through hospital corridors and elevators. Oxygen and equipment to control the airway as well as an emergency drug kit must accompany the child, and monitoring with an electrocardiogram and pulse oximeter should be continued during the transfer. If it is anticipated that recovery will be prolonged, the patient can be transported to the postanesthesia care unit while still anesthetized and intubated. Recovery and extubation can then be accomplished in the postanesthesia care unit. The same discharge criteria used for surgical patients should be applied to children undergoing MRI.

CONCLUSION

Typically, when sedation or general anesthesia is requested for a patient having a diagnostic procedure such as an MRI scan, the request occurs because the patient is a young, uncooperative child or because a medical or behavioral disorder prevents the study from being completed in the standard fashion. Almost invariably MRI studies are done far from the anesthesiologist's familiar operating room environment with equipment and personnel that may also be unfamiliar. When patient care is provided in these anesthesia "outposts," the basic principles of good anesthesia care apply. The anesthesiologist must ensure that facilities, anesthesia equipment, monitors, and personnel are adequate to provide the care required, and the patient must receive the same quality of preoperative evaluation, anesthesia care, transportation, and postanesthesia recovery provided to patients in the operating room. Because services such as the MRI unit may only occasionally require the assistance of an anesthesiologist, it cannot be expected that the personnel will understand the problems and requirements of the anesthesiologist without advance in-service education, careful planning, and a cooperative approach to problem solving.

REFERENCES

1. Council on Scientific Affairs: Fundamentals of magnetic resonance imaging. *JAMA* 1987; 258:3417–3423.
2. American Academy of Pediatrics Committee on Drugs, Section on Anesthesiology: Guidelines for the elective use of conscious sedation, deep sedation and general anesthesia in pediatric patients. *Pediatrics* 1985; 76:317–321.
3. Keeter S, Benator RM, Weinberg SM, et al: Sedation in pediatric CT: National survey of current practice. *Radiology* 1990; 175:745–752.
4. Thompson JR, Schneider S, Ashwal S, et al: The choice of sedation for computed tomography in children: A prospective evaluation. *Radiology* 1982; 143:475–479.
5. Burchart GJ, White TJ III, Siegle RL, et al: Rectal thiopental versus an intramuscular cocktail for sedating children before computerized tomography. *Am J Hosp Pharm* 1980; 37:222–224.
6. Mitchell AA, Louik C, Lacouture P, et al: Risks to children from computed tomographic scan premedication. *JAMA* 1982; 247:2385–2388.
7. Varner PD, Ebert JP, McKay RD, et al: Methohexital sedation for children undergoing CT scan. *Anesth Analg* 1985; 64:643–645.
8. Goldberg M: Systemic reactions to intravascular contrast media. *Anesthesiology* 1984; 60:45–56.

39

Broviac Catheter Placement

A 4-year-old, 18-kg, boy with acute lymphoblastic leukemia is scheduled for replacement of a nonfunctioning Broviac catheter. He is being treated with vincristine, prednisone, and L-asparaginase. Hemoglobin, 7 g/dL; hematocrit, 21%; platelet count, $30,000 \times 10^9$/L.

Recommendations by David J. Murray, M.D.

Every year in North America, one child in 10,000 develops a malignancy. Leukemia, the most prevalent childhood malignancy, accounts for 30% of the malignancies. Acute lymphoblastic leukemia (ALL) is the most common form of childhood leukemia. Carefully designed international treatment protocols, newer chemotherapeutic agents, and a better understanding of requirements to achieve remission have decreased the frequency of recurrence and the long-term survival of children with ALL. Defining cure in a childhood malignancy is difficult, but the current therapy has been successful in achieving long-term remission of lymphoblastic leukemia in greater than 70% of afflicted children. A variety of prognostic factors, such as age, sex, initial cell count and hematocrit, and preliminary response to therapy can be used to define subsets of patients with a better overall survival.

Treatment protocols and an enhanced chemotherapeutic armamentarium have defined therapy associated with a rapid remission, a lower incidence of recurrence, and less severe side effects for many children with malignancies. Ancillary management measures, in particular "permanent" indwelling central venous catheters, have an essential role in patient management and have contributed in a variety of ways to improved survival. This 4-year-old boy's chemotherapeutic medications suggest that he is in the active induction phase of treatment for ALL. The period from diagnosis to complete remission is characterized by administration of sequential pulses of antineoplastic agents, which in combination provide maximum cytotoxic effect on tumor cells for a period of four weeks. The intensive treatments are spaced to allow partial recovery of hematologic elements between administration of drugs. However, as is evident in this patient, anemia and thrombocytopenia are common. Following induction, a chemotherapeutic maintenance regimen is continued for three to five years in an attempt to maintain long-term remission.

CENTRAL VENOUS CANNULATION

Silastic venous catheters provide vascular access for administration of sclerotic antineoplastic drugs, for obtaining blood samples to monitor the effects of chemotherapeutic agents on tumor cells and the formed elements of blood, and for administration of blood components, fluids, and parenteral nutrition.

Peripheral intravenous (IV) catheters of polyvinylchloride, polyethylene, and teflon provide short term vascular access. Thrombosis and infectious complications, such as cellulitis and septic thrombophlebitis, increase in a logarithmic fashion as the duration of cannulation increases. A variety of long-term IV devices have been used to overcome many of the problems with IV catheters.[1, 2]

Originally described by Broviac in 1973, the silicone catheter was used to provide parental nutrition. In 1979, Hickman introduced a larger-lumen catheter for the care of bone marrow recipients.[2] Access to a large central vein such as the external or internal jugular, subclavian, or cephalic vein generally requires a cutdown. The silicone catheter, which is impregnated with barium, is inserted into the vein, and a portion of the catheter is tunneled to an exit site on the lower chest (Fig 39–1). The two most common late complications following insertion of an indwelling central catheter are thrombosis and infection, which occur in 10% of patients.[3] Superior vena cava obstruction from thrombosis, atrial thrombus, and catheter perforation have also been reported. Even with meticulous aseptic technique and frequent irrigation with heparinized flush solutions, the high incidence of thrombosis and infection remain a significant problem. Unlike peripheral IV catheters, infectious and thrombotic complications with silicone catheters do not increase in a logarithmic fash-

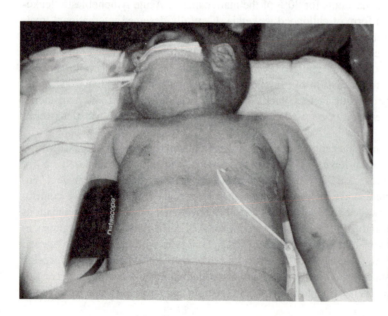

FIG 39–1.
Broviac catheter in situ. Note incision in neck and catheter, which has been tunneled beneath skin to exit site on anterior chest wall.

ion with increased time of cannulation. Despite the infectious and thrombotic complications, the diagnostic and therapeutic benefits of the indwelling central catheter far outweigh the complications. When thrombosis occurs, a concentrated heparin solution or thrombolytic agent such as urokinase may help reestablish its patency. When this fails, catheter replacement is necessary.

Prior to placement of the central venous catheter, many children have endured multiple phlebotomies and administration of sclerotic drugs via peripheral IV catheters. The thrombosis of the central catheter represents a setback to the treatment regimen, both from a medical and psychological standpoint. The patient, family, and oncologist are often anxious to have the Broviac catheter rapidly replaced. While the procedure is elective, there is a degree of urgency to reestablishing central venous access. Nevertheless, there is ample time for a complete history and physical examination.

ANEMIA

The answers to a number of questions will help determine the most appropriate approach to perioperative management of the patient's anemia. The child's intravascular volume status must also be taken into account. Do the measured hematocrit and hemoglobin levels reflect the red cell mass? Since induction chemotherapy for leukemia is frequently associated with renal complications due to rapid lysis and excretion of cellular byproducts, diuresis is often induced by administration of large volumes of fluid, orally and intravenously, to facilitate excretion and minimize the potential for renal damage. Thus, the hematocrit may be lower than the actual red cell mass due to a dilutional effect.

How long has the anemia been present, and is it stable? Is blood loss contributing to the anemia, is it related to chemotherapy, or is it secondary to marrow infiltration with leukemic cells? Does recovery of red cell mass occur between pulses of chemotherapy? Assessment of the child's activity level is important in determining how the anemia has influenced his cardiorespiratory status. Is he still active despite the anemia?

If the patient has received red blood cells (RBCs) in the past, the frequency of administration and the indications for therapy should be ascertained. What RBC preparations were administered? Since cytomegalovirus (CMV) infection can be very serious in immunocompromised patients, CMV-negative blood components are often administered. Alternatively, if CMV-positive blood is used, leukocyte-depletion filters will effectively remove most of the leukocytes that harbor the virus. Transfusion-associated graft-vs.-host disease can occur in immunocompromised patients when viable donor lymphocytes are infused. This complication can be prevented by irradiation of blood components prior to transfusion. The anesthesiologist must be familiar with the types of blood components previously administered so that the same type of components can be requested if transfusion is indicated intraoperatively.

If the child's hemoglobin level has remained stable throughout the hospitalization, the decision to treat the anemia prior to anesthesia and surgery must be based on some expectation that anesthesia, surgery, or physiologic alterations occurring in the perioperative period will adversely alter oxygen reserve or oxygen demand.[4] The anticipated intraoperative and postoperative course of this child is unlikely to be associated with a prolonged catabolic period or an increased oxygen demand. The incisions are small, postoperative pain mild, and recovery rapid. In addition, further decrements in oxygen supply that might occur with markedly altered perioperative pulmonary function or significant blood loss are not usually associated with the operation. While hemorrhage is a cited complication of the procedure, the incidence of this complication is reported to be less than 1%. In the author's experience, blood loss greater than 5% of the child's blood volume has not been encountered in more than 500 such operations. For these reasons, RBC transfusion does not appear necessary. If this is a stable, diagnosed anemia that has not compromised the child's cardiorespiratory reserve, then transfusion is not required.

If the child receives frequent RBC transfusions to treat progressive declines in hematocrit due to chemotherapy, then transfusion should be accomplished electively in the preoperative period. The hematocrit of RBCs is between 60% and 70%; therefore, 10 mL of RBCs contains 6 to 7 mL of red cells. If 10 mL of RBCs is administered for each kilogram of body weight, assuming a blood volume of 70 mL/kg, the anticipated increase in hematocrit would be 10%. A unit of RBCs has a volume of approximately 225 mL and would increase this 18-kg patient's hematocrit from 21% to approximately 35%.

THROMBOCYTOPENIA

In determining whether platelet transfusion is indicated, the anesthesiologist must inquire about the patient's bleeding history. What bleeding problems have been encountered and at what platelet level? Patients with chronic thrombocytopenia of malignancy frequently tolerate platelet counts of $10,000 \times 10^9$/L without clinical signs of bleeding or blood loss. Spontaneous bleeding, such as epistaxis or melena, in patients with hematologic malignancies becomes an increasing problem as the platelet count decreases below $10,000 \times 10^9$/L. This observation, as well as the problems associated with development of platelet alloantibodies, is the basis for not routinely maintaining higher platelet counts in patients with hematologic malignancies.[5]

Coagulation factors, platelets, and the vasculature are interrelated in achieving surgical hemostasis. Even a minor operative procedure tests the integrity of hemostasis. In this child, pharmacologic doses of prednisone will contribute to fragility of the microvasculature. Thrombocytopenia, steroid use, and the antineoplastic therapy will also lead to more frequent wound complications,[6] including delayed healing, infection, and wound hematoma.

While this patient has an acceptable platelet count to prevent spontaneous bleeding during daily activities, it is not adequate to prevent bleeding complications during surgery. For minor surgical procedures, an increase in the platelet count to a level greater than $50,000 \times 10^9$/L for a 24-hour period would seem a reasonable approach. With major operations such as craniotomy, thoracotomy, or intra-abdominal procedures, achieving a higher platelet count and maintaining it for a longer perioperative period is recommended. The half-life of transfused platelets is reduced in patients who receive multiple platelet transfusions. The etiology of the decreased survival is not clear; however, the half-life may be only 24 hours.

One unit of platelets per 10 kg of body weight will produce a platelet count increment of approximately $50,000 \times 10^9$/L. A single platelet unit derived from an adult whole blood donor unit contains 5 to 7×10^{10}/L platelets. While transfused platelets distribute primarily in the intravascular space, they are also sequestered in the spleen, adding to the volume of distribution. Assuming an intravascular volume of 70 mL/kg, a total volume of distribution of 100 mL/kg would be a reasonable estimate. In this 18-kg child, the platelet distribution volume would be 1800 mL and the anticipated increase in platelet count from a single platelet unit would be as follows:

$$\frac{5 \text{ to } 7 \times 10^{10} \text{ platelets}}{1800 \text{ mL}} = 30,000 \times 10^9 \text{ platelets}$$

Two units of platelets would thus raise the platelet count by approximately $60,000 \times 10^9$/L.

Under ideal circumstances, platelet transfusion should precede the operation by about two hours so a one-hour posttransfusion platelet count can be performed to ensure that an increase in platelet count occurred. In a patient who has had multiple prior platelet transfusions, the first sign of clinically significant platelet alloantibodies is failure of the platelet count to increase following transfusion. When this occurs, a larger platelet dose may be adequate or HLA-matched platelets may be required. Preoperative platelet administration would be ideal. However, if obtaining vascular access is difficult, the transfusion could be delayed until IV access is achieved following inhalation induction of anesthesia.

ADVERSE EFFECTS OF CHEMOTHERAPEUTIC AGENTS

In addition to concerns regarding anemia and thrombocytopenia, additional specific side effects of chemotherapeutic agents must be considered. Vincristine not only has hematologic side effects, but an autonomic and peripheral neuropathy may occur.[6, 8] Early satiety and abdominal fullness, as well as nausea and vomiting, which are also common with antineoplastics, suggest the presence of this complication. This information is important in determining whether a significant risk of aspiration exists and, therefore, whether special precautions should be taken during induction of anesthesia.

Pharmacologic doses of steroids will undoubtedly lead to evidence of iatrogenic Cushing's syndrome from steroid excess.[6] Hypokalemia, hyperglycemia, petechiae, and ecchymosis are common side effects of steroids. In addition, the phenotypic changes associated with steroid use, such as moon facies and excess adipose tissue, may make what usually is an easy mask fit in this age group more difficult (Fig 39–2).

L-Asparinase acts to deplete extracellular reserves of L-asparagine, an essential amino acid. Tumor cells without the intracellular enzyme, L-asparaginase are unable to incorporate this amino acid and are prevented from growth and mitotic activity.[6] Anaphylactic reactions, pancreatitis, and neurologic depression are side effects of this antineoplastic agent.

Acute lymphocytic leukemia is primarily a hematologic malignancy, but involvement of the meninges and CNS can lead to signs and symptoms of increased intracranial pressure. CNS involvement is unusual as a presenting problem with ALL, but frequently occurs with relapse.

PREMEDICATION AND ANESTHESIA INDUCTION

The child's prior experiences with anesthesia and surgery and his attitude toward the impending operation will be the primary determinants of how he responds to anesthesia induction. At this age, he may be able to understand the benefits of the planned procedure and cooperate, if time is invested in a preoperative visit to explain the anticipated events. There are a number of clues in predicting whether the child will be cooperative. The child's response to prior events of hospitalization,

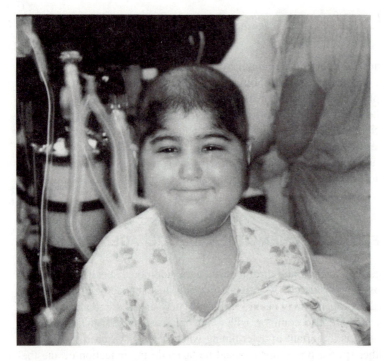

FIG 39–2.
Cushingoid appearance of child who has received steroid therapy. Securing a tight mask fit may be difficult in such a patient.

behavior during the last anesthetic induction, and response to other procedures are helpful guides. If, based on this information, he needs sedation, a rapid-acting drug can be administered IV on arrival in the preanesthetic care unit.

If parental presence decreases the child's apprehension, the parents could be present during induction. Most children hospitalized with malignancies establish rapport with one of the nurses who might be encouraged to come to the operating room with the child if parental presence is not an option.

INDUCTION OF ANESTHESIA

At one extreme, a 4-year-old child can be the most cooperative and calm patient encountered by the anesthesiologist in the operating room. At the other extreme, the mere mention of another operative procedure is fraught with terror and panic, which may become manifest when the child enters the presurgical area. For this reason, the plan for induction needs to be flexible, since IV, rectal, or inhalation induction are all acceptable alternatives, depending on the child. If the child is frightened and panic-stricken, a small IV dose of midazolam, 0.02 mg/kg, or thiopental, 1 mg/kg, may be administered in the preanesthetic area, if appropriate airway equipment and oxygen are readily available. The sedated child can be transported to the operating room where additional monitors can be applied and anesthesia induced with supplemental IV doses of thiopental, 3 to 4 mg/kg. If no IV access has been established and placement appears difficult, an inhalation induction with N_2O and halothane would be most appropriate. Rectal methohexital, 25 mg/kg, rectal midazolam, 0.3 mg/kg, or nasal midazolam, 0.2 mg/kg, may be rapidly effective in sedating the extremely apprehensive child enough for an inhalation induction.[9]

Fortunately, nausea and vomiting are generally short-term side effects of antineoplastic agents, lasting only about 24 hours. If chemotherapy has not been administered in the preceding 24-hour period, a rapid induction technique does not seem warranted in this child unless there is evidence of gastroparesis.[7]

ANESTHESIA MAINTENANCE

After establishing a patent airway, nitrous oxide and either isoflurane or halothane would be added to maintain anesthesia. Even though halothane hepatitis is a distinctly unlikely occurrence in any pediatric patient, the diagnosis is difficult to differentiate from other more common causes of liver dysfunction. This 4-year-old is at increased risk of developing liver dysfunction from either chemotherapeutic agents or a virus. To avoid this potential diagnostic problem, isoflurane anesthesia would be preferred. Endotracheal intubation would be facilitated using a dose of an intermediate-acting muscle relaxant, such as vecuronium, 1.0 mg, or atracurium, 5 mg. Endotracheal intubation performed with adequate anesthesia and neuromuscular blockade will minimize the possibility of upper airway trauma and bleeding. A lubricated 5.0-mm endotracheal tube will probably provide the best fit based on formulae estimating approximate tube size. The key to tube fit is to assure a tube large enough to provide controlled ventilation, yet small enough to minimize the likelihood of cricoid edema and postintubation croup caused by a tightly fitting endotracheal tube. Proper depth is best accomplished by visualizing passage of the tube beyond the glottis. An inhalation anesthetic rather than a nitrous oxide-narcotic technique is preferable, as it is less likely to be associated with prolonged periods of nausea and vomiting, which might prevent the child from rapidly returning to normal activity and nutrition.

SURGICAL REQUIREMENTS AND COMPLICATIONS

Access to the central circulation may be obtained by cannulating a number of large veins using a small incision at the base of the neck. The external jugular or internal jugular vein can be exposed via a right or left neck incision, providing access to the central circulation. The catheter's passage to the junction of the superior vena cava and right atrium is confirmed by fluoroscopy. The operative procedure may last from 15 to 60 minutes or more. Complications include bleeding, arrhythmias, and perforation of a central vein. Supraventricular tachycardia and premature ventricular contractions may occur during catheter passage, but are usually self-limited in the child with a healthy cardiovascular system.

The catheter is tunneled to an exit site on the chest. A dacron sleeve prevents extrusion of the catheter and serves as a nidus for fibrosis to maintain a secure catheter position for months, or possibly years, if required. The rigid stent used to tunnel the catheter in the subcutaneous tissue during the operation can briefly limit excursion of the child's compliant chest wall and lead to a transient period of decreased ventilation and a fall in Po_2 and oxygen saturation if the stent is left in place more than a brief period. The stent has been reported to cause pneumothorax if tunneled under the chest wall. The Broviac catheter is ready for use as soon as placed in a central vein and may be used intraoperatively if necessary.

At the conclusion of the operation, residual neuromuscular blockade is reversed and after the return of airway reflexes, extubated is performed. The goal is to have the patient return to normal nutrition and the chemotherapeutic treatment program as rapidly as possible in the postoperative period.

REFERENCES

1. Broviac JW, Jole JJ, Scribner BH: A silicone rubber atrial catheter for prolonged parenteral nutrition. *Surg Gynecol Obstet* 1973; 136:602–606.
2. Hickman RO, Buckner CD, Clift RA, et al: A modified right atrial catheter for access to the venous system in marrow transplanted recipients. *Surg Gynecol Obstet* 1979; 148:874–875.
3. Nelson TR, West KW, Grosfield JL: Broviac central venous catheterization in infants and children. *Am J Surg* 1983; 145:202–204.
4. Zauder HL: Preoperative hemoglobin requirements. *Anesth Clin North Am* 1990; 8:471–480.
5. Gaydos LA, Freirich EJ, Mantel N: The quantitative relationship between platelet count and hemorrhage in patients with acute leukemia. *N Engl J Med* 1962; 266:905.
6. Selvin BL: Cancer chemotherapy: Implications for the anesthesiologist. *Anesth Analg* 1981; 60:425–434.
7. Cote CJ, Liu LMP, Szyfelbein SK, et al: Changes in platelet counts following massive blood transfusion in pediatric patients. *Anesthesiology* 1985; 62:197–201.
8. Rosenthal S, Kaufman S: Vincristine neurotoxicity. *Ann Intern Med* 1974; 80:733–737.
9. Wilton NCT, Leigh J, Rosen DR: Preanesthetic sedation of preschool children using intranasal midazolam. *Anesthesiology* 1988; 69:972–975.

40

Ventriculoperitoneal Shunt Revision

A 4-year-old, 15-kg girl is admitted for revision of a ventriculoperitoneal shunt. She is lethargic and has been vomiting. Despite repeated attempts, the pediatrician was unable to insert an intravenous catheter. The neurosurgeon feels that immediate surgical intervention is necessary. No laboratory data are available.

Recommendations by Masao Yamashita, M.D.

This child presents several problems. She is a 4-year-old child with increased intracranial pressure (ICP) due to shunt malfunction, probable dehydration and electrolyte imbalance due to vomiting possible retention of gastric contents, and difficult venous access. In addition, she requires "urgent" surgical intervention. These problems are compounded by the lack of laboratory data. This is an unwelcome case resulting from poor follow-up by the pediatrician or neurosurgeon.

HYDROCEPHALUS

Hydrocephalus can be caused by excessive production of cerebrospinal fluid (CSF), obstruction to CSF flow, or a defect in absorption of CSF. The most common cause is obstruction of CSF flow; thus CSF shunting procedures are indicated to decompress the ventricular system. Ventriculoperitoneal shunting is the preferred method for infants at the present time because of its benign nature and ease of revision. A ventriculoatrial shunt is seldom performed because of potential complications including septicemia, bacterial endocarditis, pulmonary embolism, and pulmonary hypertension. CSF shunting, including shunt revision, for hydrocephalus is the most commonly performed pediatric neurosurgical procedure. The revision rate averages 2.6 operations per patient.[1]

It has been reported[2] that replacement of the entire shunt system, including the ventricular catheter, valve, and abdominal catheter, was required in 36% of ventriculoperitoneal shunt revisions. The abdominal catheter alone was replaced in 24%, and the ventricular catheter alone was replaced in 20%. Valve replacement alone was also required in 7% and valve and abdominal catheter replacement in only 3%.[2]

The etiology of the hydrocephalus is related to the patency time of the shunt. Hydrocephalus caused by neoplasm has the shortest patency time and requires revision most frequently.[1]

The number of ex–premature infants with hydrocephalus secondary to intraventricular hemorrhage during the perinatal period is increasing. The infection rate is high in these patients, and shunt revision is frequent.[1] Shunt survival is also limited in patients weighing less than 3,000 g.[2] Ex–premature infants tend to have residual multisystem problems including bronchopulmonary dysplasia, cerebral palsy, epilepsy, poor neural integration, and language deficits. Child abuse or neglect must also be considered in patients who require CSF shunting procedures.

Hydrocephalus is commonly associated with multisystem congenital defects, and congenital anomalies should be carefully sought. Many infants with hydrocephalus have associated meningomyelocele with partial or complete paraplegia. These children are prone to urinary tract infection and impaired renal function. A careful history should be obtained, and such laboratory tests as blood urea nitrogen and serum creatinine ordered.

PREOPERATIVE MANAGEMENT

During a careful preanesthetic assessment, the degree of dehydration should be assessed by checking tissue turgor, whether the eyes are sunken, and urine output and specific gravity. If available, the recorded body weight can be used to calculate any recent acute weight loss. If dehydration is severe, rapid rehydration must be considered before the induction of anesthesia. Despite the fact that a pediatrician was unable to insert an intravenous catheter, a pediatric anesthesiologist should look carefully at the possibility of cannulating a peripheral vein. If this is not possible, rehydration must be achieved by using one of several other routes: saphenous vein cutdown; central vein catheterization via the femoral, jugular, or subclavian route; or indirect intravenous infusion via the intraosseous method.[3] Performing a cutdown is a time-consuming technique, especially since cutdowns are infrequently performed today. Central venous catheterization via the femoral vein should be attempted as the first choice since the success rate in this age group is high. Central venous catheterization of the internal jugular vein is difficult in unanesthetized children. In addition, positioning the child head down with the head rotated would interfere with cerebral venous return, thus aggravating the elevated ICP.

Catheterization of a subclavian vein is an alternative, but the position of the shunt catheter must be considered. If the catheter is on the right side, an attempt may be made on the left. However, in the event that revision is required, it may be necessary to place the new shunt on that side. As a final resort, the intraosseous route may be chosen. A needle is inserted into the bone marrow in the midline of the medial flat surface of the anterior aspect of the tibia 1 to 3 cm below the tibial tuberosity.[3] This technique has been rediscovered as a means of emergency treatment of infants and children. After restoration of the circulating blood volume, it becomes much easier to insert a peripheral or central venous catheter. After venous access is established, the intraosseous infusion should be discontinued to avoid infection.

No sedative premedication should be ordered since it may cause a further rise in ICP. Intravenous administration of atropine at induction is preferred to other routes. A blood sample for determination of serum electrolytes and a complete blood count (CBC) should be sent to the laboratory, but the unavailability of the results should not delay the induction of anesthesia.

In the critical situation of respiratory arrest due to raised ICP and tonsillar herniation, the child's trachea should be intubated immediately and the patient hyperventilated with 100% oxygen. A ventricular tap must then be performed without delay.

ANESTHETIC MANAGEMENT

The anesthetic requirements in this case are a rapid-sequence induction to prevent aspiration, maintenance of anesthesia with stable cerebral and systemic hemodynamics, and rapid emergence. Thiopental decreases ICP and is the intravenous agent of choice. However, careful titration is the golden rule in the potentially hypovolemic patient. Ketamine is contraindicated in the presence of increased ICP. Struggling and coughing increases ICP, thus contraindicating awake intubation.

In this age group, succinylcholine rarely causes fasciculation and does not increase intragastric pressure, which makes it possible to rapidly secure the airway by endotracheal intubation. Atropine is administered prior to succinylcholine to prevent succinylcholine-induced bradycardia. In the presence of conditions that contraindicate the use of succinylcholine such as paraplegia, muscular dystrophies, etc., excellent intubating conditions can be obtained with vecuronium, 0.4 mg/kg, almost as rapidly as with succinylcholine.[4] It is a reasonable alternative to succinylcholine for rapid-sequence induction in children because it lacks any adverse effects on cerebral and systemic hemodynamics.[5] Thus it would be useful for intubation and/or maintenance of muscle relaxation in this patient. A large intubating dose of pancuronium is not appropriate for this relatively short operation. The effects of endotracheal intubation on ICP may be minimized by intravenous lidocaine, 1.5 mg/kg, 2 to 3 minutes prior to induction.

Low concentrations of volatile inhalation agents are convenient since they are easily controllable and recovery from anesthesia is usually rapid and predictable. All inhalation agents increase intracranial blood flow and ICP; however, the use of low concentrations together with mild hyperventilation minimizes the increase in ICP.[6] While the difference in effects on cerebral blood flow between halothane and isoflurane are probably insignificant, the latter agent is preferred by many neurosurgical anesthesiologists.

After application of the standard monitors, the patient is preoxygenated. A functional suction should be at hand. If a nasogastric tube is in place, it should be aspirated prior to induction. If the tube is not in place, one should not be inserted since the maneuver may increase ICP.

Intravenous induction is preferred. Lidocaine, 1.5 mg/kg, and atropine, 0.01 to 0.02 mg/kg, are administered prior to thiopental. The usual induction dose of thiopental is 4 to 5 mg/kg, but the dose must be carefully titrated in the potentially hypovolemic patient. As soon as the patient loses consciousness, cricoid pressure is applied. Oral endotracheal intubation is facilitated by a full paralyzing dose of succinylcholine, 2 mg/kg, or vecuronium, 0.4 mg/kg. A small dose of a short-acting narcotic such as fentanyl or alfentanil may also be administered. After the patient is positioned for the shunt revision, the position of the endotracheal tube is checked by auscultation of both lungs. Extension of the neck tends to pull the endotracheal tube back, so accidental extubation may occur. If a nasogastric tube was not in place before induction, one should be inserted at this time to aspirate gas or gastric fluid. During the procedure, it is kept open for drainage.

Anesthesia can be maintained with low concentrations of halothane or isoflurane in nitrous oxide and oxygen. Vecuronium or atracurium can be used for neuromuscular blockade. The lungs are mildly hyperventilated to avoid an increase in cerebral blood flow and ICP secondary to the accumulation of CO_2.

A sudden decrease in ICP as a result of the surgical intervention may lead to systemic hypotension. If this occurs, use of the potent volatile agents should be discontinued until the systemic blood pressure returns to an acceptable level.

Although surgery is usually of short duration, catheterization of the urinary bladder is useful in assessing the degree of rehydration. Ringer's lactate solution is infused at a rate of 50 mL/h until the serum electrolyte results are available. If the child is hypokalemic, administration of potassium may be indicated. Blood transfusion is not usually necessary.

At the end of surgery, anesthesia with the volatile agent and nitrous oxide is discontinued, and the lungs are ventilated with 100% oxygen or an air-oxygen mixture. Residual neuromuscular blockade is reversed with atropine, 0.025 mg/kg, and neostigmine, 0.05 mg/kg. Alternatively, if the muscle blockade is not intense, a mixture of edrophonium, 1 mg/kg, and scopolamine, 0.4 mg/kg, can be administered. Advantages of this mixture are rapid reversal with minimal fluctuation of the heart rate and no central cholinergic action.[7] In the recovery room, the patient is cared for in a slight head-up position to facilitate CSF drainage. Potent narcotic analgesic drugs are usually unnecessary. Codeine, 1.0 to 1.5 mg/kg administered intramuscularly, will suffice.

REFERENCES

1. Serlo W, Fernell E, Heikkinen E, et al: Functions and complications of shunts in different etiologies of childhood hydrocephalus. *Child Nerv Syst* 1990; 6:92–94.
2. Liptak GS, McDonald JV: Ventriculoperitoneal shunts in children: Factors affecting shunt survival. *Pediatr Neurosci* 1985; 12:289–293.
3. Fiser DH: Intraosseous infusion. *N Engl J Med* 1990; 322:1579–1581.
4. Sloan MH, Lerman J, Bissonette B: Pharmacodynamics of high-dose vecuronium in children during balanced anesthesia. *Anesthesiology* 1991; 74:656–659.
5. Rosa G, Sanfilippo M, Vilardi V, et al: Effects of vecuronium bromide on intracranial pressure and cerebral perfusion pressure. A preliminary report. *Br J Anaesth* 1986; 58:437–440.
6. Gordon E, Lagerkranser M, Rudehill A, et al: The effect of isoflurane on cerebrospinal fluid pressure in patients undergoing neurosurgery. *Acta Anaesthesiol Scand* 1988; 32:108–112.
7. Yamashita M, Tajima K: Edrophonium–hyoscine butylbromide mixture for reversal of neuromuscular blockade: Heart rate changes in infants and children. *Anaesthesia* 1988; 43:591–593.

41

Hernia Repair and Hurler Syndrome

A 4-year-old, 20-kg boy with Hurler syndrome and a very large umbilical hernia is scheduled for umbilical herniorrhaphy. He is severely retarded and known to have a heart murmur. Hemoglobin, 12.5 g/dL; hematocrit, 37.5%.

Recommendations by James H. Diaz, M.D.

Hurler syndrome is the prototype disorder of the hereditary mucopolysaccharidoses (MPS). Children with these disorders have multisystem disease and present significant challenges for the anesthesiologist.

THE MUCOPOLYSACCHARIDOSES

The MPS are connective tissue diseases caused by an insufficiency or absence of key enzymes catalyzing metabolism of the major mucopolysaccharide substrates of connective tissue: dermatan sulfate, heparan sulfate, and keratan sulfate. As a result of enzyme deficiency, these substrates cannot be biotransformed and accumulate excessively in the skin, brain, heart, bone, liver, and spleen. MPS are true inborn errors of metabolism and should not be confused with such primary connective tissue disorders as Marfan syndrome, Ehlers-Danlos syndrome, osteogenesis imperfecta, and fibrodysplasia ossificans progressiva. These primary connective tissue disorders can be easily differentiated from MPS by skin biopsy, urinalysis, and serum analyses and present significantly different problems for the anesthesiologist.

The diagnosis of MPS can now be made prenatally by amniotic fluid analysis for missing enzymes or accumulating substrates. After birth, MPS are suspected by the unique appearance of affected infants (Fig 41–1) and confirmed by skin biopsy, serum enzyme analysis, and urinary muco-

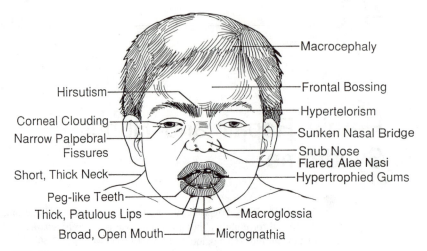

Macrocephaly

Frontal Bossing

Hypertelorism

Sunken Nasal Bridge

Snub Nose
Flared Alae Nasi
Hypertrophied Gums

Hirsutism

Corneal Clouding

Narrow Palpebral
Fissures

Short, Thick Neck

Peg-like Teeth

Thick, Patulous Lips

Broad, Open Mouth

Macroglossia

Micrognathia

FIG 41–1.
The typical facies of a 4-year-old boy with Hurler syndrome.

polysaccharide screening. The MPS are classified into eight recognized types, each with its own eponym, isolated enzyme defect, and characteristic findings on urinalysis (Table 41–1). Fresh human amnion implants have been performed in children with MPS in an attempt to supply missing enzymes. There is, however, no definitive therapy.

Hurler syndrome, MPS type IH, occurs with an incidence of 1 in 40,000 live births and is characterized by increased production, accumulation, and excretion of two mucopolysaccharides, dermatan sulfate and heparan sulfate. The deficient or absent enzyme for mucopolysaccharide biotransformation in Hurler syndrome is α-L-iduronidase. All forms of MPS, including Hurler syndrome, are characterized by progressive craniofacial, joint, and skeletal deformities; progressive cardiac involvement; and early demise from pulmonary or cardiac failure. Patients with Morquio syndrome (MPS IV A and B) and, to a lesser extent, Hurler syndrome may exhibit odontoid hypoplasia with a predisposition to atlantoaxial subluxation and brain stem compression during cervical hyperextension for endotracheal intubation.[1] Quadriplegia and cardiac arrest have been reported following cervical subluxation in such patients.[1]

Common clinical manifestations of Hurler syndrome include mouth breathing with tongue protrusion, frequent upper respiratory infections, adenotonsillar hypertrophy, acquired laryngotracheobronchomalacia, and mucopolysaccharide deposition throughout the upper and lower airways (Fig 41–2). Smith has characterized Hurler syndrome as presenting "the worst airway problems in pediatric anesthesia."[2]

Cardiovascular changes in Hurler syndrome include mitral valvular thickening and insufficiency, widespread coronary occlusive disease often without angina or myocardial infarction, congestive heart failure, and cardiomyopathy. Cardiorespiratory failure commonly causes death before 10 years of age. Pulmonary hypertension from combinations of chronic hypoxia, mitral insufficiency, and recurrent pulmonary infection is common. Hepatosplenomegaly with little functional impairment, inguinal hernia, diastasis recti, umbilical hernia, joint contractures, corneal clouding,

TABLE 41–1.

Current Classification of the Mucopolysaccharidoses (MPS)

MPS Type	Eponym Syndrome	Mental Performance	Progressive Craniofacial Deformities	Progressive Joint and Skeletal Deformities	Progressive Cardiac Involvement
IH	Hurler	Retarded	Macrocephaly, coarse facies, macroglossia, micrognathia	Stiff joints, thoracolumbar kyphosis, possible odontoid hypoplasia, short neck, short stature	Coronary intimal and valvular thickening, mitral regurgitation, cardiomegaly
IS	Scheie	Normal	Mild coarse facies, macroglossia, prognathia	Short neck, normal stature	Aortic regurgitation
IH/S	Hurler-Scheie	Mildly retarded to normal	Macrocephaly, coarse facies, macroglossia, micrognathia	Diffuse joint limitation, short neck, short stature	Mitral and aortic valvular thickening and regurgitation
II	Hunter	Normal	Macrocephaly, coarse facies	Diffuse joint limitation, short neck, short stature	Coronary intimal thickening, ischemic cardiomyopathy
III (A–D)	San Filippo	Retarded	Mild coarse facies	Mild stiff joints, lumbar vertebral dysplasia, short stature	Minimal to none
IV (A,B)	Morquio	Normal	Mild coarse facies	Joint laxity, severe kyphoscoliosis, odontoid hypoplasia, short neck, subluxation possible, short stature	Aortic regurgitation
VI	Maroteaux-Lamy	Normal	Macrocephaly, coarse facies, macroglossia	Mild joint stiffness, kyphoscoliosis, odontoid hypoplasia possible, short stature	Mitral and aortic valvular thickening and regurgitation
VII	Sly	Retarded	Macrocephaly, coarse facies	Joint flexion contractures, thoracolumbar gibbus, hip dysplasia, odontoid dysplasia possible, short stature	Mitral and aortic valvular thickening and regurgitation.

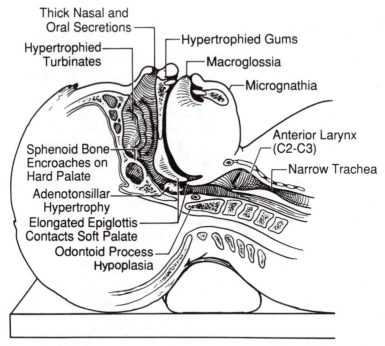

Thick Nasal and
Oral Secretions

Hypertrophied
Turbinates

Hypertrophied Gums

Macroglossia

Micrognathia

Sphenoid Bone
Encroaches on
Hard Palate

Anterior Larynx
(C2-C3)

Narrow Trachea

Adenotonsillar
Hypertrophy

Elongated Epiglottis
Contacts Soft Palate

Odontoid Process
Hypoplasia

FIG 41–2.
Supine sagittal view of a 4-year-old boy with Hurler syndrome. The anatomic features shown predispose this patient to intra-anesthetic upper airway obstruction at the nasopharyngeal, oropharyngeal, laryngeal, and subglottic levels.

nerve deafness, and generalized hirsutism are also common. Mental retardation with failure of intellectual advancement beyond 2 to 5 years of age always occurs. Behavior ranges from uncooperative and totally unmanageable to placid, malleable, and lovable. Communicating hydrocephalus is possible, but rare.

PREOPERATIVE EVALUATION

A number of general considerations may be applied to the anesthetic management of any child with hereditary MPS. Such considerations include the anticipation of difficult upper airway and ventilatory management; severe mental retardation with uncooperative, often belligerent behavior; and most importantly, the significance of associated heart disease.

The selection of anesthetic agents and techniques for a 4-year-old boy with Hurler syndrome depends on the personality and behavior of the patient and the site and extent of surgery. Premedication cannot be counted on to produce a sedated or malleable patient because of the dangers of upper airway obstruction, respiratory depression, hypercarbia, and cardiorespiratory arrest. Intraperitoneal procedures such as umbilical herniorrhaphy carry the potential for bowel manipulation or entry and require general endotracheal anesthesia to prevent pulmonary aspiration and permit controlled ventilation during neuromuscular paralysis. Inhalation induction is preferred for patients with anticipated or previously demonstrated difficult intubation but is difficult in an uncooperative retarded patient. Intravenous induction with ketamine or thiopental may prove more satisfactory in a retarded patient as long as spontaneous ventilation can be maintained until the upper airway is secured by tracheal intubation. The ability to maintain a patent airway during spontaneous or assisted ventilation by mask does not necessarily mean that such ventilatory control will continue after the administration of muscle relaxants. Regional anesthesia may therefore offer a valuable and safe alternative for children with MPS who are having lower abdominal, perineal, or extremity surgery without need of neuromuscular paralysis.

Preoperative preparation should include a careful history from the parents, a swift precise physical examination of the patient, specific laboratory analyses, an electrocardiogram, a chest x-ray, and often other diagnostic investigations such as cervical spine x-ray films or tomograms and precordial echocardiography. The history, chest auscultation, and chest x-ray findings will rule out pre-existing pneumonia and atelectasis requiring preoperative antibiotic and respiratory therapy. Commonly occurring otitis media and nasal stuffiness can be differentiated from acute infections by history, physical examination, temperature patterns, ear, nose, and throat (ENT) examination; and the presence of leukocytosis with a differential shift toward immature leukocytes. Lateral cervical spine films, tomograms, or computed tomography or magnetic resonance imaging will identify odontoid hypoplasia in rare infants predisposed to atlantoaxial subluxation during cervical hyperextension for endotracheal intubation. The diameter of the subglottic trachea may also be assessed by chest x-ray to assist in the selection of appropriately sized endotracheal tubes, always smaller than would be predicted on the basis of age.

Cardiomegaly and pulmonary venous engorgement detected on chest x-ray suggest cardiomyopathy or mitral insufficiency and should prompt further evaluation by real-time precordial echocardiography before elective surgery. A preoperative electrocardiogram will rule out right ventricular hypertrophy with strain, interventricular conduction block, left atrial enlargement, and tachydysrhythmias. Systolic murmurs are common in patients with MPS, especially those with Hurler syndrome. Angina pectoris or congestive heart failure will dictate more invasive diagnostic procedures such as angiography for precise diagnosis and preoperative treatment with coronary vasodilators or diuretics and inotropes.

In addition to chest x-rays, further pulmonary investigations may include arterial blood gas analysis and pulmonary function testing. Chronic hypoxemia and compensatory respiratory alkalosis are common. Vital capacity, functional residual capacity, and total lung capacity are often reduced by kyphoscoliosis, pectus excavatum or carinatum, and lung parenchymal loss from chronic lobar collapse. Lung function must be optimized preoperatively by energetic physiotherapy and pulmonary toilet.

In addition to the hemogram, other preoperative laboratory tests should include serum electrolyte determinations, especially for children receiving digoxin or diuretic therapy, and liver function tests for patients with massive hepatomegaly. Bleeding times are often prolonged in patients with hereditary MPS, due primarily to the inability of transected blood vessels to vasoconstrict amidst poor support offered by loosely surrounding connective tissue. Acquired clotting factor deficiencies secondary to hepatic disease are uncommon.

PREMEDICATION

The premedication of patients with MPS has been widely discussed but remains controversial. Narcotics and barbiturates are best avoided if airway problems are anticipated. Full preoperative atropinization was formerly recommended but recently challenged because atropine thickens secretions and thus increases the possibility of inspissation and plugging of small airways in the postoperative period.[3] Thin, watery secretions may be controlled preoperatively with intramuscular or intravenous scopolamine or glycopyrrolate. Thick secretions remain a problem, however, and dictate the requirement for readily accessible suction apparatus at the bedside as well as in the operating room.

Severely retarded patients, particularly those with joint flexion contractures, may be lightly sedated and even relaxed with low intramuscular or intravenous dosages of short- or intermediate-acting benzodiazepines such as midazolam and lorazepam. Diphenhydramine, frequently underutilized as a premedicant in children, offers a combination of anticholinergic, antiemetic, and light sedative effects. Children with gross hepatosplenomegaly or large umbilical hernias may in addition receive oral nonparticulate antacids such as 0.3M sodium bicitrate or a parenteral H_2 antagonist, either cimetidine or ranitidine. Metaclopramide may be administered intravenously immediately before induction to further decrease the danger of regurgitation and aspiration of gastric contents in children with delayed gastric emptying from hepatosplenomegaly or intermittently obstructing umbilical or inguinal hernias.

I would premedicate an uncooperative, severely retarded, 20-kg 4-year-old child with Hurler syndrome with 20 mg diphendydramine, 2 mg midazolam, and 0.1 mg scopolamine intramuscularly 30 to 60 minutes before establishing an intravenous infusion for bacterial endocarditis prophylaxis. Additional intravenous anticholinergic medication may be indicated to control watery oral secretions promoted by airway manipulations or ketamine anesthesia. Intravenous narcotics, barbiturates, or benzodiazepines should not be administered if constant observation by an anesthesiologist is not possible.

Preinduction of anesthesia, a new concept in pediatric anesthesia, has unique applications in children with hereditary MPS, particularly a severely retarded child with Hurler syndrome. Preinduction describes a period of further pharmacologic preparation before the induction of anesthesia. Preinduction agents are administered between pharmacologic premedication, if any, and the actual induction of inhalation, intravenous, or regional anesthesia. It is often best to establish intravenous access in the presence of parents capable of calming their child. This can be facilitated if an accessible vein, usually the antecubital or saphenous, is selected during the preoperative interview and covered with an adhesive bandage to keep phlebotomists from using the vein. In the preoperative staging area, the patient or the parents can uncover the vein. Following a topical or intradermal local anesthetic, swift venipuncture is performed while the child is gently distracted and restrained. Intravenous preinduction of the patient may then commence with incrementally titrated dosages of midazolam, 0.1 to 0.2 mg/kg, or ketamine, 0.5 to 1.0 mg/kg.

ANESTHETIC MANAGEMENT

Any child with hereditary MPS should be fully monitored prior to induction of anesthesia. Electrocardiographic leads II and V_{1-4} are preferred for P wave and right ventricular conduction-axis monitoring, respectively. Automated blood pressure, pulse oximetry, skin temperature, and end-tidal carbon dioxide analysis are also recommended. Additional monitoring that may prove useful includes mass spectometry for continuous analysis of inspired and expired gases, measurement of airway temperature, airway manometery, and neuromuscular blockade monitoring. An additional intravenous catheter and arterial cannula for perioperative blood gas determinations may be inserted after induction of anesthesia.

In addition to establishing hemodynamic, ventilatory, and thermal monitoring before induction, a number of instruments and drugs should be assembled before anesthesia is administered to a patient with Hurler syndrome. Useful instruments include an assortment of face masks, endotracheal tubes, laryngoscope blades and handles, as well as a pediatric fiber-optic endoscope with cold fiber-optic light source, a high-pressure compressed oxygen source for transtracheal or translaryngeal insufflation, a pediatric ventilator, Magill forceps in pediatric and adult sizes, sterile towel clamps, a short needle holder, and 1-0 or 2-0 black silk sutures with cutting needles for tongue sutures (Fig 41–3). A variety of endotracheal tubes should be available since age-adjusted and anatomic formulas for endotracheal tube selection do not apply to patients with MPS because of the unique configurations of the laryngeal inlet and the narrow subglottic trachea.[4] Special instruments that may prove useful in establishing a tracheal airway in this patient are a short-handled laryngoscope and laryngoscope blades with gas-insufflating ports.[5]

Because of the shape of the face in patients with Hurler syndrome, standard pediatric face masks may not offer a secure fit over a face with a patulous mouth, protruding tongue, and broad nose. In such cases, an air-cushioned pediatric face mask can be applied upside down with the broad chin edge of the mask over the patient's brow and nose and the narrow nasal bridge of the mask over the open mouth and protruding tongue. The air cushion on the facial aspect of the mask may be inflated or deflated, as indicated by fit, with an air-containing syringe. As with the best vein, the best mask fit should be determined before induction of anesthesia.

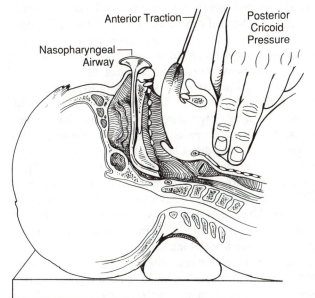

FIG 41–3.
Supine sagittal view of a 4-year-old with Hurler syndrome. A sterile towel clamp or tongue suture placed in the midline anterior aspect of the tongue for gentle anterior traction combined with a soft nasopharyngeal airway and posterior cricoid pressure often relieves upper airway obstruction and facilitates orotracheal intubation by rigid or fiber-optic techniques.

Although emergency tracheostomy is rarely indicated, it may become necessary. A surgeon fully experienced in the techniques of difficult pediatric tracheostomy should be available in the operating suite in the event that tracheal intubation is impossible or swift airway access is indicated for cardiopulmonary resuscitation. Tracheostomy may be extremely difficult in children with hereditary MPS, and in one patient with Hunter syndrome, tracheostomy was impossible both during life and at postmortem examination.[6]

Direct laryngoscopy for awake orotracheal intubation will be difficult in a severely retarded patient with Hurler syndrome. Blind nasotracheal intubation techniques utilizing airflow sounds have been reported but are not recommended because of adenotonsillar hypertrophy, the elongated epiglottis, and easily traumatized hyperemic upper airway mucosa (see Fig 41–2). The sharp tip of a blindly advancing nasotracheal tube may skewer adenoidal tissue, precipitate nasopharyngeal bleeding, trigger laryngospasm or aspiration of blood, and potentially deliver an obstructing pellet of adenoidal tissue into the lungs.

Nasopharyngeal and oral airways should be available, but avoided if possible. Soft nasopharyngeal airways, like nasotracheal tubes, can cause adenoidal hemorrhage but may offer better airway patency than oral airways, which may contact the long epiglottis and cause laryngospasm or buckle the posterior third of a long tongue and cause airway obstruction (Fig 41–3). A sterile towel clamp or, preferably, a silk tongue suture placed in the midline anterior third of the tongue for gentle forward traction can often re-establish an obstructed upper airway. This maneuver may also simplify orotracheal intubation by either rigid or fiber-optic techniques, especially when combined with cricoid pressure (Fig 41–3).

Airway manipulations are easier to perform in consciously sedated or anesthetized patients with Hurler syndrome. Spontaneous breathing may offer the best airway such patients will have prior to tracheal intubation. In addition, spontaneous breathing often provides the sights (air bubbles near the glottis) and sounds (airflow noises as the endotracheal tube tip approaches the glottis) necessary to direct tracheal intubation under conditions of poor visibility, heavy secretions, edematous oropharyngeal mucosa, and a glottis that cannot be easily suspended or visualized by direct laryngoscopy. A soft cervical collar and an assistant to stabilize the neck and prevent extension are necessary during airway manipulations in patients with odontoid hypoplasia. A knowledgeable assistant can also provide suction, cricoid pressure, jaw thrust, and additional anesthetic equipment when necessary.

Anesthetic doses of narcotics or barbiturates should not be administered prior to tracheal intubation unless it can be demonstrated that the patient can be easily ventilated by mask. This also applies to neuromuscular blocking agents. For this patient, I would recommend intravenous induction with glycopyrrolate, 0.2 mg, and ketamine in 10-mg increments supplemented with topical 4% lidocaine spray to the tongue, oropharynx, and larynx during direct laryngoscopy. Such a technique maintains spontaneous ventilation, provides intact vocal cord reflexes to prevent aspiration, and permits quick diagnostic direct laryngoscopy to assess the difficulty of tracheal intubation. Spontaneous ventilation should be supplemented with 100% inspired oxygen. A carefully titrated intravenous induction permits more flexibility in switching from intravenous to inhalation techniques, in aborting the anesthetic and coming back on another day, or in performing preliminary diagnostic laryngoscopy to select either rigid or fiber-optic laryngoscopy for tracheal intubation.

Tracheal intubation techniques include, in order of preference, direct laryngoscopy for antegrade tracheal intubation, flexible fiber-optic intubation, retrograde catheter-guided tracheal intubation, and tracheostomy. As noted, blind nasotracheal intubation and tracheostomy carry significant hazards in patients with MPS and should be employed only in emergencies by experienced clinicians, or as dictated by the nature of the surgical procedure.[6] Following tracheal intubation, the stomach and small bowel may be decompressed with an orogastric tube. Some surgeons will perform a temporary gastrostomy to provide early enteral alimentation and avoid oral or nasogastric tubes in patients who may need prolonged postoperative ventilation.

Once the upper airway has been secured, a light plane of general anesthesia may be maintained with 1.5 MAC or less of isoflurane or halothane in humidified 100% oxygen. Since MPS are central nervous system storage disorders and not hereditary muscle disorders, malignant hyperthermia is not a risk. Like ether, enflurane may promote more tracheobronchial secretions. Nitrous oxide can distend bowel incarcerated in the umbilical hernia sac, aggravate pulmonary hypertension, depress the myocardium when combined with narcotics and other adjuvants, and dilute the inspired oxygen concentration. Isoflurane permits generous supplementation of the anesthetic by infiltration of the surgical wound with an epinephrine-containing local anesthetic. Bupivacaine provides longer postoperative analgesia of incisional pain than lidocaine but presents greater risk of myocardial depression on unrecognized intravascular injection. Theoretically a risk in patients with coronary occlusion, ketamine- and epinephrine-induced tachydysrhythmias and isoflurane-induced intracoronary steal pose less risk to patients with MPS than do acute increases in systemic and pulmonary vascular resistance or direct depression of a dilated myocardium by high inspired concentrations of inhaled anesthetics.

Neuromuscular paralysis with a short-acting nondepolarizing muscle relaxant such as vecuronium or atracurium is recommended for controlled ventilation, hernia reduction and repair, and ease of reversal during skin closure with the anticholinesterases edrophonium or neostigmine. Intravenous anesthetic adjuvants may be added incrementally to the balanced anesthetic technique. The short-acting, reversible narcotics alfentanil, fentanyl, and sufentanil are preferable to additional doses of the intermediate-acting benzodiazepines midazolam and lorazepam.

At the completion of surgery, the following criteria should be met for tracheal extubation: full reversal of neuromuscular blockade, naloxone reversal of any narcotic-induced apnea, tidal volume ≥ 5 to 10 mL/kg, oxygen saturation greater than 95%, ability to generate a negative inspiratory force of -15 to -20 cm H_2O or more and thus ensure a forceful cough reflex, return of the gag reflex, and the ability to sustain head lift. Renarcotization is possible even after naloxone reversal of narcotic adjuvants and may contraindicate early tracheal extubation. To question the safety of early tracheal extubation in this case is reason enough to leave the patient's trachea intubated until all extubation criteria are met, documented, and sustained.

The airflow resistance presented by a small-caliber endotracheal tube may predispose an awakening child, struggling to breath through a straw, to negative pressure pulmonary edema. Such patients will require positive-pressure mechanical ventilation and often sedation with benzodiazepines if prolonged mechanical ventilation is indicated.

Multiple traumatic attempts at tracheal intubation intraoperatively or multiple reintubations postoperatively will predispose a patient with Hurler syndrome to symptomatic glottic and subglottic edema. Such iatrogenic conditions are difficult to treat due to the progressive narrowing of the tracheal lumen by mucopolysaccharide deposits. A dose of dexamethasone, 0.5 mg/kg, can be administered intravenously 30 minutes prior to planned tracheal extubation. A nebulized racemic epinephrine treatment can also be administered following extubation to ameliorate postextubation sublglottic mucosal edema.

POSTOPERATIVE CARE

Intravenous fluids and antibiotic prophylaxis for endocarditis, pneumonia, and wound infection should be continued postoperatively until oral feeding and antibiotics are resumed. Humidified oxygen, chest physiotherapy, and postural drainage should also be continued until the patient is ambulatory and able to handle excessive tracheobronchial secretions.

Although skilled in coping with uncooperative behavior and a difficult daily routine, the parents of a child with Hurler syndrome also suffer postoperatively from witnessing their child's needed restraints, multiple vascular punctures, and intensive respiratory care. Parents appreciate the attention paid to them and their child in the immediate postoperative period. As is usually the case, anesthesiologists often develop considerable expertise at managing patients with MPS by reanesthetizing a small group of such patients for multiple operations over their shortened lifetimes. The development of such technical expertise will inevitably prepare the anesthesiologist to handle the most difficult airway encounters in patients of any age and underscore Smith's early warning that Hurler syndrome presents the most difficult airway in our specialty.[2]

REFERENCES

1. Brill CB, Rose JS, Godmilow L, et al: Spastic quadriparesis due to C1–C2 subluxation in Hurler syndrome. *J Pediatr* 1978; 92:441.
2. Smith RM: *Anesthesia for Infants and Children,* ed 4. St Louis, Mosby–Year Book, 1980, p 533.
3. Sjøgren P, Pedersen T, Steinmetz H: Mucopolysaccharidoses and anaesthetic risks. *Acta Anaesthesiol Scand* 1987; 31:214.
4. Wilder RT, Belani KG: Fiberoptic intubation complicated by pulmonary edema in a 12-year-old child with Hurler syndrome. *Anesthesiology* 1990; 72:205.
5. Diaz JH: Further modifications of the Miller blade for difficult pediatric laryngoscopy. *Anesthesiology* 1984; 60:612.
6. Hopkins R, Watson JA, Jones JH, et al: Two cases of Hunter's syndrome—the anesthetic and operative difficulties in oral surgery. *Br J Oral Surg* 1973; 10:286.

42

Epiglottitis

A 5-year-old girl is brought to the emergency room by her parents who state that she was well when put to bed the night before but awoke with a fever and sore throat. The child is sitting up and anxious and refuses to talk. The presumed diagnosis is epiglottitis. Her color is normal. Respiration, shallow at a rate of 40; pulse, 130.

Recommendations by Raafat S. Hannallah, M.D.

Acute epiglottitis is a clinical and pathologic entity that should more correctly be called supraglottitis because the arytenoids and aryepiglottic folds as well as the epiglottis itself are usually affected. All structures become swollen and stiffened by inflammatory edema. The causative organism is usually *Haemophilus influenzae* type B.[1] Although the main focus of infection is in the supraglottic structures, the disease produces a generalized toxemia. Epiglottitis is notorious because it can produce sudden and complete airway obstruction and can be fatal if the airway is not secured.[2]

CLINICAL PRESENTATION

Epiglottitis is most common between the ages of 3 and 5 years but can occur at any age. The onset of the disease is usually abrupt, with a brief history of high fever, severe sore throat, and difficulty swallowing. The history is seldom more than 10 to 12 hours in duration. Stridor, if present, is usually inspiratory, and since the subglottic structures are usually unaffected, there is little or no hoarseness. The clinical appearance of the child is classic and, when combined with the history, diagnostic. The child appears ill and, in an attempt to improve airflow past the swollen epiglottis, insists on sitting up and leaning forward in the sniffing position. The mouth is open, with the tongue protruding. The child frequently drools because of difficulty and pain on swallowing.

In addition to high fever, other signs of toxemia may include tachycardia, a flushed face, and prostration. The respiratory pattern, unlike that of croup patients, is usually slow and quiet to allow more peripheral air entry (Table 42–1). If respiratory obstruction increases, hypoxia, hypercapnia, and acidosis result.

When epiglottitis occurs in young infants, the symptoms may include cough and coryzal illness.[3] Infants may not be able to assume the sitting position typically seen in older children. A high index of suspicion should be maintained in infants who have respiratory distress associated with fever, irritability, and drooling.

TABLE 42–1.
Differential Diagnosis of Croup and Epiglottitis*

Variable	Croup	Epiglottitis
Incidence	More common	Less common
Obstruction	Subglottic	Supraglottic
Age	Younger (<3 yr)	Older (3–6 yr)
Etiology	Viral	Bacterial
Recurrence	Possible (5%)	Rare
Clinical features		
Onset	Gradual (days)	Sudden (hours)
Fever	Low grade	High
Dysphagia	None	Marked
Drooling	None	Present
Posture	Recumbent	Sitting
Toxemia	None	Present
Cough	Barking	Usually none
Voice	Hoarse	Clear to muffled
Respiratory rate	Rapid	Normal
Larynx palpation	Not tender	Tender
Leukocytosis	+ (Lymphocytic)	+++ (Polymorphonuclear cells)
Neck x-rays	Anteroposterior: steeple sign	Lateral: thumb-like mass
Clinical course	Longer	Shorter
Treatment		
Primary therapy	Medical and supportive	Secure airway first
O_2 and humidity	Essential	Usually desirable
Hydration	Oral or IV	Intravenous
Racemic epinephrine	Usually effective	No value
Steroids	Controversial	Not indicated
Antibiotics	Not indicated	Effective
Airway support	Occasionally needed (<3%)	Always indicated (100%)
Preferred airway	Nasotracheal Tracheostomy	Nasotracheal
Extubation	4–7 days	1–3 days

*Foreign bodies in the airway should also be considered.

DIAGNOSIS

Acute epiglottitis is a clinical diagnosis. However, in some early cases, the clinical presentation alone may not be conclusive. If so, there are two ways of confirming the diagnosis: (1) lateral x-ray of the neck and (2) direct laryngoscopy.

In patients with epiglottitis, the radiograph will usually show the swollen epiglottis and aryepiglottic folds (Fig 42–1). The vallecula may be obliterated, but subglottic structures are usually clear. It is important that x-ray films be ordered only to establish the diagnosis if it cannot be made on clinical grounds. They should be taken with the patient in the sitting position. A physician capable of establishing an airway should always be in attendance since total airway obstruction can develop during the time necessary to complete the x-ray procedure.

Although direct laryngoscopy will confirm the diagnosis, it should only be attempted in the operating room, with adequate staff and equipment prepared to intervene should upper airway obstruction develop. Examination of the larynx or pharynx should not be attempted without these preparations because complete, instantaneous airway obstruction and fatal asphyxiation may be provoked by the manipulation.

PRINCIPLES OF MANAGEMENT

The safest, most conservative approach to management of epiglottitis is to establish an artificial airway as soon as the diagnosis is made and, then, with the airway secured, to proceed with appropriate antibiotic and supportive therapy. Since management of these patients is a team effort, a detailed interdisciplinary protocol is necessary. The basic steps can be summarized as follows:

A child suspected of having acute epiglottitis should be immediately transported to the intensive

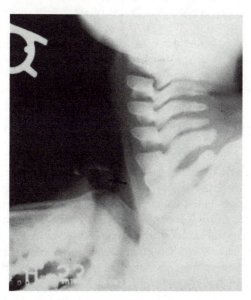

FIG 42–1.
Radiograph indicating a swollen epiglottis and aryepiglottic folds.

care unit or operating room by a physician capable of and equipped for establishing an airway. No attempts to examine the larynx or to start an intravenous infusion should be made in the emergency room. Oxygen can be administered if the child appears hypoxic. There is no indication, however, to check arterial blood gases at this stage. The child should remain sitting at all times and never be forced to lie on her back.

The designated team of pediatrician, otolaryngologist, respiratory therapist, and anesthesiologist should be notified. The operating room staff should be alerted to set up for direct laryngoscopy and to have equipment for rigid bronchoscopy and tracheostomy or cricothyrotomy immediately at hand.

Any radiologic examination needed to confirm a nontypical presentation should be performed with portable equipment, with the child still sitting up. If the diagnosis is confirmed or if epiglottitis cannot be ruled out, the child should be taken to the operating room for direct laryngoscopy.

In the operating room, a precordial stethoscope, cardioscope, pulse oximeter, and blood pressure cuff should be attached before any manipulations are initiated. Unless the child is moribund—in which case awake intubation is preferred—general inhalational anesthesia is induced with oxygen and halothane and the child maintained in the sitting position. Intravenous induction agents or muscle relaxants should be avoided at this time. When the child gets sleepy, she is gently positioned on her back. Signs of airway obstruction are usually increased in that position, but gentle manual assisting of inspiration should improve air exchange. This must be confirmed by the precordial stethoscope.

An intravenous cannula can now be inserted, and blood cultures should be drawn. When the surgical stage of anesthesia is achieved, direct laryngoscopy, which will confirm the diagnosis, is performed. The larynx is then sprayed with 1 mL of 4% lidocaine. Ventilation is assisted for a few more moments, after which an orotracheal tube of appropriate size is inserted. The endotracheal tube used should be one or two sizes smaller than usually recommended for a child of this age. A larger tube is not necessary and may contribute to the development of serious laryngeal complications. The child should be able to breathe around the tube as well as through it.

If the epiglottis is very swollen, visualization of the vocal cords may be impossible. In such cases it is often helpful to bend the tube acutely at the distal end with a stylet in order to direct it below the central epiglottic raphae. Since most of the edema in epiglottitis accumulates in the lingual surface of the epiglottis, the median raphe is usually present regardless of the amount of swelling. One can often identify bubbles that exude from the larynx during exhalation. Gentle pressure on the chest may increase the air bubbles and facilitate identification of the glottic opening as a method of locating the laryngeal opening.

With the oral tube in place and while the child remains in the surgical stage of anesthesia, the stomach contents are aspirated with a catheter. A decision is then made to proceed with nasotracheal intubation or with elective tracheostomy. Once the airway is secured, aggressive medical therapy should be started. Intravenous antibiotics are essential. Ampicillin is usually prescribed in a dose of 200 mg/kg/day administered in divided doses every 6 hours. Because resistance to ampicillin is now quite common, it is better to use a cephalosporin such as ceftriaxone, 50 mg/kg per dose. The duration of treatment is controversial, but at least 3 to 5 days of intravenous antibiotics followed by oral therapy is usually the minimum. Supportive measures include intravenous hydration, airway care, sedation as necessary, and acetaminophen for high fever.

The child is usually ready for extubation in 24 to 48 hours. The best clinical indication is resolution of toxemia, even if the epiglottis is still slightly swollen. Direct laryngoscopy can be performed in the intensive care unit to visualize the epiglottis prior to extubation. The size of the epiglottis and the degree of inflammation are noted and compared with the findings at the time of intubation.

CARE OF THE AIRWAY

Both tracheostomy and endotracheal intubation have been advocated to control the airway in children with croup or epiglottitis. The safety of intubation and the absence of residual laryngeal damage have been established; however, selection of the narrowest tube that ensures a quiet airway at rest is critical.

To prevent accumulation and crusting of secretions in the tube, inspired gas must be humidified. Secretions should be suctioned whenever necessary. Sterile saline solution may be used to facilitate aspiration of tenacious secretions. Accidental extubation must be prevented in patients with an artificial airway. Meticulous attention to details in fixing the tube and the use of waterproof tape are essential. The child should be sedated until she becomes accustomed to the airway. The arms should be splinted to prevent flexion at the elbows and reaching for the tube. Equipment and expert personnel necessary to re-establish the airway must be immediately available.

ASSOCIATED ILLNESSES AND OUTCOME

Other forms of *Haemophilus* infection can be present in the same patient.[4] One should look specifically for meningitis or otitis media. There have been occasional reports of pulmonary edema developing in children with severe epiglottitis.[5] The exact mechanism is not clear, but it may be related to increased negative intra-alveolar pressure and hypoxia resulting from upper airway obstruction. The edema has a benign course and can be controlled by simple increases in airway pressure (positive end-expiratory pressure [PEEP])

Epiglottitis does not recur. With the airway always secured as described, the life-threatening potential of epiglottitis is eliminated.

REFERENCES

1. Hannallah RS, Rosales JK: Acute epiglottitis: Current management and review. *Can Anaesth Soc J* 1978; 25:84–91.
2. Crysdale WS, Sendi K: Evolution in the management of acute epiglottitis: A 10-year experience with 242 children. *Int Anesthesiol Clin* 1988; 26:32–38.
3. Blackstock D, Adderley RJ, Steward DJ: Epiglottitis in young infants. *Anesthesiology* 1987; 67:97–100.
4. Molteni RA: Epiglottitis—incidence of extraepiglottic infection. *Pediatrics* 1976; 58:526.
5. Bonadio WA, Losek JD: The characteristics of children with epiglottitis who develop the complication of pulmonary edema. *Arch Otolaryngol Head Neck Surg* 1991; 117:205.

43

Adenoidectomy and Upper Respiratory Tract Infection

A 5-year old girl, 24 kg, with recurrent otitis media, is scheduled on an outpatient basis for bilateral myringotomy with insertion of PE tubes and adenoidectomy. On physical examination she is noted to have a "runny nose." The pharynx is clear, and auscultation of the chest reveals no abnormalities. The mother states the child has had no fever or cough. However, she thinks she may be "getting a cold." When the possibility of postponing surgery is mentioned, the mother becomes upset because she has hired a babysitter for her other children and has taken a vacation day to be with the patient. She asks why a 20-minute operation needs to be canceled because her daughter may be getting a cold. Temperature, 37°C; pulse, 88; respirations, 22.

Recommendations by Willis Alexander McGill, M.D.

This case illustrates one of the most common dilemmas faced by the anesthesiologist who cares for pediatric patients. In our hospital, the presence of an upper respiratory tract infection (URI) remains one of the most frequent medical reasons for cancellation of elective surgery. Whether or not to cancel surgery because of URI symptoms remains controversial. There is often confusion regarding the etiology of the respiratory symptoms which may be due to infectious or noninfectious causes. Furthermore, some authorities suggest that an uncomplicated URI poses no significant additional risk of complications if the surgical procedure is minor.[1, 2] Medical cost containment concerns, as well as social and practical considerations, add pressure to proceed as scheduled. Because upper respiratory illness is so prevalent and generally so benign and self-limited in the otherwise healthy child, reluctance to postpone surgery is frequently voiced not only by parents but by surgeons as well. It is not uncommon for parents to assert that the examining pediatrician, the day prior to hospitalization, thought the "cold" would not affect the outcome of surgery.

Three fundamental questions must be answered in this situation: (1) What is the etiology of the rhinorrhea? (2) Should elective surgery be delayed, and if so how long? (3) How can complications be minimized when a child with a URI must be anesthetized?

DIFFERENTIAL DIAGNOSIS

Because the symptom, rhinorrhea, is so ubiquitous it may be difficult, especially in a preschool-aged child, to assign an etiology. Rhinorrhea can represent either a benign process such as allergic or vasomotor rhinitis, or a developing or incompletely resolved infectious illness due to viral or bacterial agents.

Allergic rhinitis can occur at any age and may be seasonal or perennial. Perennial rhinitis is frequently associated with low-grade infection and purulent secretions. Both varieties can be accompanied by eustachian tube obstruction and recurrent otitis media, causing frequent febrile episodes.

Another cause of rhinorrhea is vasomotor rhinitis which can be triggered by a number of factors. It is seen in the crying small child who has been subjected to the pain and upset of the hospital admission process. In addition, teething is a frequent trigger. Such apparently inconsequential factors as changes in temperature and humidity may provoke rhinorrhea in some children.

Of greater concern during the preoperative assessment are symptoms of infectious origin. Viral nasopharyngitis, or the "common cold", is the most frequent cause of infectious rhinorrhea, and is caused by a variety of viral agents.[3] The course is generally benign, but may be complicated by secondary bacterial infection. More serious illnesses which cause upper respiratory symptoms are contagious diseases of childhood; including measles and chicken pox, and acute bacterial infections such as epiglottitis and streptococcal pharyngitis. Because of the potentially more serious nature of complications associated with these contagious diseases, differential diagnosis is essential.

History

A child's history provides the most important clues in defining the etiology of respiratory symptoms. The child in the presentation above exhibits rhinorrhea but mother denies cough and fever. While the symptom is insufficient to sustain a diagnosis of URI, the mother's intuition that her daughter may be "getting a cold" should be taken seriously and a history of other symptoms should be sought. A positive history of an outbreak of respiratory illness among other family members, day care center playmates or classmates helps to confirm a suspicion of URI.

In the child who is normally symptom-free, sneezing and rhinorrhea suggest the onset of respiratory infection. Though these signs may be the earliest clinical manifestations of a cold, they are nonspecific and other symptoms are necessary to corroborate the diagnosis. Recent studies indicate that at least two of the following symptoms should be present to sustain the diagnosis: sore throat, sneezing, rhinorrhea, congestion, malaise, nonproductive cough, and low-grade fever.[2, 4] In addition, they suggest that certain combinations of symptoms require that a third symptom also be present.

Identifying or ruling out an infectious etiology is particularly difficult in the child with chronic respiratory symptoms due to allergic or other causes. In assessing these children, it is important to get the parent's opinion as to whether the exhibited symptoms represent the child's usual state or whether they represent a new active process. Some parents may initially minimize the significance of the new symptoms if they sense that surgery may be canceled. Therefore, they deserve a careful explanation of the significance of a URI if it exists. Virtually all appreciate a sympathetic explanation of why postponement of surgery is in the best interest of their child.

Physical Examination

Positive findings during the physical examination are valuable. However, negative findings do not rule out a URI. A child's temperature pattern may be helpful, but in outpatient surgery only one temperature observation is usually recorded during the short preoperative assessment period. If the temperature is above 38°C orally or rectally, a URI is presumed to be present. However, a temperature between 37.5°C and 37.9°C requires critical evaluation. A slightly dehydrated child, who is agitated and upset by the admission procedures, can develop a mildly elevated temperature in the absence of disease. In younger children, teething can contribute to both fever and airway secretions. Clear nasal secretions, nasal obstruction and tearing may be signs of respiratory infection, vasomotor rhinitis or allergy. While the presence of purulent nasal secretions, pharyngeal infection, and fever suggests an infectious etiology, their absence does not rule out the possibility of infection. Signs of allergic rhinitis include boggy, pale, or slightly blue nasal mucous membranes, cobblestone appearance of the conjunctiva, and flattened malar eminence.

Examination of the chest is important but usually negative. Rhonchi auscultated over the lung fields represent transmitted upper airway sounds from increased secretions and are commonly encountered during teething, in the crying child, as well as in allergic or infectious rhinitis. Wheezing associated with URI symptoms is heard infrequently but, when present, is an indication of bronchiolitis or the onset of an asthmatic attack. Elective surgery should definitely be postponed when wheezing is present. More rarely absence of breath sounds may be encountered over a lung field and may result from a bronchial mucous plug.[5, 6]

Laboratory Studies

In patients with overt signs of a bacterial infection or contagious disease the blood count is confirmatory. When viral nasopharyngitis is present, the white blood cell count may be low, but it is frequently normal. Eosinophilia is indicative of an allergic condition but does not rule out a simultaneous infection. Chest x-ray is considered of little value in the preoperative screening of children.[7] Though our experience has been that positive radiologic findings are more frequent in these selected patients, x-rays can also be negative in children with the most severe symptoms. Furthermore, we and others have found that children with normal preoperative chest x-rays can develop atelectasis following induction of anesthesia.[5, 6] No combination of history, physical findings and laboratory results can distinguish unequivocally between infectious and noninfectious etiologies for upper respiratory symptoms. Even viral culture may be falsely negative[2] and culture is neither practical nor cost-effective as a screening test. Consequently, misdiagnosis can occur from time to time. Occasionally a child will be canceled needlessly, while, on the other hand, a child with an apparently mild URI can develop complications intraoperatively or postoperatively. Parents should be given an explanation of risks and benefits of whatever course is chosen, and as suggested by Berry,[5] they should be included in the decision-making process.

ANESTHETIC COMPLICATIONS ASSOCIATED WITH URI

In deciding whether to proceed with surgery, the anesthesiologist is concerned with whether the interaction of the viral illness and respiratory effects of anesthesia will increase the incidence of complications. A number of reports have addressed the issue. In 1978, we reported on the nature of intraoperative pulmonary complications in children giving a history of URI during the month preceding scheduled surgery. The findings included coarse breath sounds and persistent tracheal secretions, cyanosis, unequal breath sounds, asymmetrical chest wall expansion, alveolar-arterial gradients of more than 300 mm Hg, and atelectasis on portable chest x-ray (Fig 43–1).

In contrast, others have demonstrated no increased incidence of anesthetic complications among children with active but uncomplicated URI symptoms.[1] However, they did find a three-fold increase in respiratory complications among asymptomatic children who had experienced URI symptoms during the previous two weeks. In a prospective study, these authors demonstrated no increased incidence of intraoperative adverse respiratory events among 1- to 12-year-old children with symptoms of uncomplicated URI.[2] In this series, surgery was the placement of tympanostomy tubes, lasted less than 20 minutes per patient, and patients were not intubated. Interestingly, the authors noted an amelioration of the subsequent course of respiratory symptoms in children who had anesthesia and surgery compared to those who did not. They concluded that uncomplicated URI need not delay anesthesia for brief superficial surgery in otherwise healthy children in whom the trachea was not intubated.

In a prospective study comparing postoperative oxygen saturations in children 1 to 4 years of age who were symptomatic or asymptomatic for URI at the time they presented for scheduled surgery, one group of investigators discovered a 20% incidence of transient hypoxemia during postan-

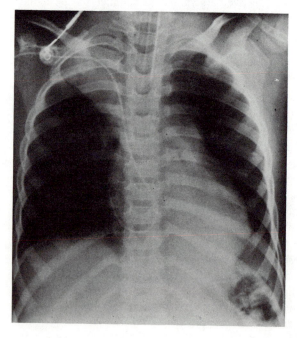

FIG 43–1.
Intra-anesthetic chest x-ray demonstrating right upper lobe atelectasis.

esthetic recovery in the symptomatic group but no hypoxemia in the children without URI symptoms.[4] No children experienced intraoperative complications and postanesthetic transient hypoxemia was unrelated to intraoperative tracheal intubation. The authors concluded that children with upper respiratory infection are at increased risk for postoperative hypoxemia.

Other investigators have confirmed that URI increases the incidence of anesthetic complications. Infants with URI symptoms experience significantly more "critical incidents" during induction of anesthesia and are more likely to develop postintubation croup.[8] There appears to be not only an overall increased risk of anesthetic complications in children with URI symptoms, but tracheal intubation further increases the incidence of complications.[8]

SCHEDULING SURGERY

While it may be preferable to avoid anesthetizing a child with a cold, dogmatic insistence on cancellation may not be in the best interest of the child or family. Each situation must be evaluated individually, assessing the child's present and past condition, as well as the urgency and nature of the surgery. The following conclusions appear to be supported by the available evidence:

1. Children older than 1 year with an uncomplicated URI who are having superficial surgery with halothane administered by mask appear to be at minimal risk for significant complications.[2]

2. Infants younger than 1 year are at highest risk for airway obstruction and postintubation croup.[8, 9]

3. Children older than 5 years have less risk of respiratory complications than those younger than 5 years.[8]

Choosing the right interval for rescheduling surgery following URI presents another dilemma. Respiratory complications appear to be related to the interaction of pulmonary effects of anesthesia and subclinical viral pneumonitis.[9, 10] However, pulmonary function abnormalities can persist for more than four weeks following URI.[10, 11] Therefore, the commonly recommended two-week interval may be inadequate. On the other hand, waiting for longer periods may be impractical for many patients. Since 25% of children have three to eight URIs in the course of a year, this leaves very little time when pulmonary function is absolutely normal.

It is not uncommon for a child to be scheduled repeatedly for elective surgery, only to be canceled because of persistent or recurrent respiratory symptoms. This is particularly common among children who need otolaryngologic procedures. Arriving at a decision in these circumstances is difficult. The anesthesiologist, in consultation with the surgeon and pediatric colleagues, as well as parents, must select an interval during which it seems likely the symptoms will recede. In spite of careful planning and assessment, intraoperative complications may develop.

ANESTHETIC MANAGEMENT

Anesthetic management of the child with a URI is directed toward minimizing the occurrence of intraoperative and postoperative complications. The preoperative goal is reduction of respiratory

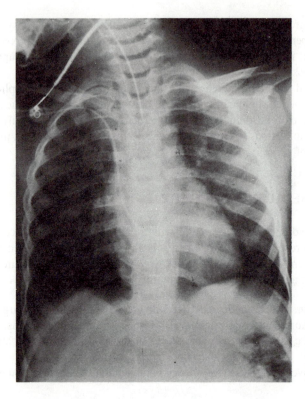

FIG 43–2.
Chest x-ray of the same patient following tracheobronchial toilet and chest percussion prior to awakening and removal of endotracheal tube.

symptoms using decongestants and antibiotic therapy if indicated by bacterial colonization of secretions. Premedication should include an anticholinergic. Atropine not only reduces secretions by its antisialogogue effect, but also blocks vagal reflexes which play a role in the airway hyperactivity that is associated with viral respiratory infections.[10, 12]

Anesthetic induction should be achieved without provoking excessive crying in order to minimize airway secretions. Thus, any of the commonly used induction techniques is acceptable. We most commonly use an inhalation induction with halothane as it causes less airway irritation than either enflurane or isoflurane. Inspired concentrations are increased gradually to avoid airway stimulation and coughing. However, inserting oral or nasopharyngeal airways and pharyngeal suctioning should be delayed until surgical levels of anesthesia have been achieved. Unfortunately, the irritability of the airway in these children often makes earlier intervention necessary.

An intravenous catheter is inserted as soon as feasible following induction. Laryngospasm during induction occurs frequently and it is important to be able to administer succinylcholine quickly to overcome laryngospasm that does not respond to mechanical airway support. If an intravenous route is not readily available, succinylcholine, 4 mg/kg, administered intramuscularly, permits positive pressure ventilation by mask within 1 minute and tracheal intubation within 2 to 3 minutes.

For procedures of one-half hour or less, maintaining anesthesia by mask is preferable if airway irritability does not develop. In longer procedures, the airway is best managed with an endotracheal tube. Intubating the trachea under moderately deep levels of anesthesia in conjunction with a muscle relaxant helps to avoid stimulating bronchial hyperactivity. The anesthesiologist occasionally will encounter copious and persistent tracheal secretions associated with intraoperative atelectasis (Fig 43–1). These respond to tracheal lavage and suctioning, postural drainage, and chest percussion (Fig 43–2).[6] Secretions should be collected in a sterile manner for culture and sensitivity, should subsequent antibiotic therapy be needed.

At the end of surgery the trachea is extubated when airway reflexes have returned and the child is awake. During transport and in the post-anesthesia recovery unit, supplemental oxygen should be administered and oxygen saturation monitored. Those caring for the child in the postoperative period must maintain close surveillance for postintubation croup, fever, atelectasis, pneumonia or signs of respiratory distress. The intravenous infusion should be continued until the child is taking oral fluids and it is apparent that respiratory complications do not threaten.

SUMMARY

A runny nose is not specific for an upper respiratory infection in a child and does not, when present alone, justify automatically canceling elective surgery in an otherwise healthy child. If other findings support the diagnosis of a URI, postponement should be strongly considered. However, in deciding whether or not to proceed, the anesthesiologist must consider the child's age, general health, and severity of symptoms as well as the surgery that is planned and whether tracheal intubation will be necessary. For infants less than a year old, when URI symptoms are marked, or when surgery is prolonged and tracheal intubation is required, postponement is the safest course. When surgery cannot be delayed, the parents must be informed of the potential for complications and the anesthesiologist must anticipate and be prepared to treat them.

REFERENCES

1. Tait AR, Knight PR: Intraoperative respiratory complications in patients with upper respiratory tract infections. *Can J Anaesth* 1987; 34:300–303.
2. Tait AR, Knight PR: The effects of general anesthesia on upper respiratory tract infections in children. *Anesthesiology* 1987; 67:930–935.
3. Picken JJ, Niewoehner DE, Chester EH: Prolonged effects of viral infections of the upper respiratory tract upon small airways. *Am J Med* 1972; 52:738–746.
4. DeSoto H, Patel RI, Soliman IE, et al: Changes in oxygen saturation following general anesthesia in children with upper respiratory infection signs and symptoms undergoing otolaryngological procedures. *Anesthesiology* 1988; 68:276–279.
5. Berry FA: The child with the runny nose: in Berry FA (ed): *Anesthetic Management of Difficult and Routine Pediatric Patients,* ed 2. New York, Churchill Livingstone 1990.
6. McGill WA, Coveler LA, Epstein BS: Subacute upper respiratory infection in small children. *Anesth Analg* 1979; 58:331–333.
7. Wood RA, Hoekelman RA: Value of chest x-ray as a screening test for elective surgery in children. *Pediatrics* 1981; 67:447–452.
8. Cohen MM, Cameron CB: Should you cancel the operation when a child has an upper respiratory tract infection? *Anesth Analg* 1991; 72:282–288.
9. Dueck R, Prutow R, Richman D: Effect of parainfluenza infection on gas exchange and FRC response to anesthesia in sheep. *Anesthesiology* 1991; 74:1044–1051.

10. Empey DW, Laitinen LA, Jacobs L, et al: Mechanisms of bronchial hyperreactivity in normal subjects after upper respiratory tract infection. *Am Rev Respir Dis* 1976; 113:131–139.
11. Collier AM, Pimmel RL, Hosselblad V, et al: Spirometric changes in normal children with upper respiratory infections. *Am Rev Respir Dis* 1978; 117:47–53.
12. Aquilina AT: Airway reactivity in subjects with viral upper respiratory infections. *Am Rev Respir Dis* 1980; 122:3–10.

44

Repair of Atrial Septal Defects

A 5-year-old, 15-kg, girl is scheduled for repair of an atrial septal defect (ASD). She is normally active for her age. Her parents are extremely apprehensive about the procedure and especially concerned about the child's postoperative pain. Hemoglobin, 13g/dL; hematocrit, 36%.

Recommendations by David A. Rosen, M.D., and Kathleen R. Rosen, M.D.

Defects in formation of the atrial septum make up one of the ten most common congenital heart lesions and account for 7% of all cases.[1] An ASD may be an isolated anomaly or part of a more complex lesion. The intra-atrial connection is located in the middle portion of the septum, secundum type, in 80% of cases. Defects of the lower part of the septum near the atrioventricular valves, primum type, are much less common. Twice as many females as males have ASDs. Atrial defects either arise sporadically in the population or cluster within families.[2]

NATURAL HISTORY

An ASD allows shunting of blood from the systemic circulation (left) to the pulmonary circulation (right). Although such children tend to be smaller than average, the magnitude of intra-atrial flow is usually hemodynamically insignificant, and the children are usually asymptomatic. Most ASDs are discovered when a routine physical examination reveals a murmur in the pulmonic region with a wide splitting of the second heart sound. Progressive pulmonary vascular changes resulting from increased pulmonary blood flow produce symptoms as the child gets older. During adolescence only a slight decrease in exercise tolerance has been described.[3] These changes do not usually become hemodynamically significant until the third decade of life, when congestive heart failure, occurring in 14% of cases, and dysrhythmias present in 20%, are manifested. The incidence of atrial arrhythmias is related to the degree of left-to-right shunting.[2] Pulmonary vascular disease has been noted to occur more rapidly in children who live at higher altitudes.[2]

Because intra-atrial pressures are normally low, ASD shunt flow is not turbulent and produces only minimal risk of subacute bacterial endocarditis (SBE). Antimicrobial prophylaxis against SBE is not recommended for the child with an uncomplicated ASD. Following ASD closure with prosthetic material, SBE prophylaxis is indicated for the first 6 months only. Unlike ventricular septal defects, ASDs generally do not close spontaneously.

PREOPERATIVE EVALUATION AND PREPARATION

The physical signs and symptoms associated with an ASD in a small child are frequently subtle. In the first decade, impaired physical growth may be the only sign observed. The child's current height and weight, both as absolute values and as related to percentile curves, provide important data. The alteration of pulmonary blood flow caused by even a small ASD predisposes the child to frequent and potentially serious upper and lower respiratory infections. A detailed pulmonary history and examination are essential.

Because congenital anomalies of the head and neck are frequently associated with congenital heart disease, careful evaluation of the airway is essential. Many patients presenting for ASD repair are between the ages of 5 and 10 years and are at risk for shedding of their deciduous teeth.

The preoperative diagnostic cardiac evaluation of the child with an ASD does not normally require cardiac catheterization. Chest x-ray findings are usually unremarkable. The atrial shunts are low-pressure shunts, and the superior and inferior venae cavae, representing a large capacitance bed, can absorb some of the shunt volume. If there is a large left-to-right shunt, pulmonary vascular markings are increased, and the heart takes on a triangular shape as a secondary effect of the enlarged pulmonary arteries. The electrocardiogram (ECG) usually demonstrates normal sinus rhythm with a slightly prolonged QRS complex and a rSr′ or rsR′ pattern.[4] Noninvasive two-dimensional color Doppler imaging has supplanted invasive procedures in the evaluation of specific intracardiac and extracardiac vascular anatomy for these patients.

Young children like this girl who present for ASD repair deserve special, gentle attention, preoperative education, and preparation. They are asymptomatic, generally healthy, and active and may not appreciate the need to fix this organ, which does not appear to be broken. Although they may not completely understand the seriousness, invasiveness, and risks of open heart surgery, they have a rudimentary appreciation of the significance of the heart for the human body. They also often reflect parental anxiety and stress. Terrorizing misconceptions about the perioperative course are not uncommon. Pain, discomfort, separation from family, and fear of death are all potential sources of stress.

The anesthesiologist has many resources for facilitating the child's passage from the active preoperative state to postoperative convalescence. There is no physiologic need for preoperative medication for children undergoing ASD repair, but it may ease separation, provide amnesia, and initiate analgesic control for the intraoperative and postoperative periods. Oral regimens may be just as effective as using needles, which frighten most small children.[5] Various combinations of opiates, benzodiazepines, phenothiazines, barbiturates, and other sedative drugs for preoperative medication have been described. If the preselected protocol has not achieved the desired effect, then premedication can be augmented in the holding area, before separation from the family, with midazolam and/or ketamine administered orally, intranasally, or parenterally.[6]

Pain control is vital to the proper management of children undergoing cardiovascular surgery, and effective pain management plans must be initiated preoperatively. It is important that the child have a realistic notion of what she will experience after the surgery. The anesthesiologist should explain to her honestly that despite efforts to minimize pain, there may still be some, but that effective treatment is readily available if requested. Positive examples and simple language are called for: "If you hurt, we will give you medicines to make the pain go away. These medicines can be put into plastic tubes so that you won't need a shot."

The preoperative period is the proper time to introduce a pain assessment tool that is appropriate for the child's age. For this normal 5-year-old child, we would use Beyer's "Oucher" scale for pain assessment .[7] It has a linear scale of 0 to 100 for children who are able to understand abstract relationships. The numerical system is complemented by a series of pictures of a young child in increasing degrees of distress. Patients are instructed to point to a picture of a child who feels as they do. This scale can be effective in children as young as 3 years of age.

ANESTHETIC MANAGEMENT

We have a simple motto for anesthesia in the child with congenital heart disease: anticipation is the key. Prepare for the unexpected. Even the child with an asymptomatic ASD has limited cardiac and pulmonary reserve when compared with the child without a cardiac malformation. Remember that children with ASDs are usually quite small for their age. Standard formulas used in the preselection of airway equipment may not be accurate. Smaller masks, laryngoscope blades, and endotracheal tubes may be required. Also, vascular access can be difficult in the patient with congenital heart disease. Having a large and varied supply of vascular catheters is wise. It is also important to have a few drugs such as atropine, succinylcholine, ketamine, and a nondepolarizing muscle relaxant ready for either intravenous or intramuscular administration. Drugs intended for intramuscular injection should be prepared in the most concentrated, undiluted, form available, and the syringes should be equipped with short (≤ 1 in.), small-bore (23 or 25 gauge) needles. Resuscitation equipment must be immediately available. A defibrillator capable of either synchronous or asynchronous operation should be ready for operation. The resuscitation drugs that should be prepared for all cardiac cases are 5% to 10% calcium chloride, epinephrine, phenylephrine, isoproterenol, sodium bicarbonate, and lidocaine. We recommend that anesthesia personnel unfamiliar with the pediatric dosages for these drugs calculate and post the doses for the specific patient before induction of anesthesia.

There is a risk of significant systemic or cerebral air embolism in the patient with an ASD despite the predominant left-to-right direction of shunt flow. All air must be removed from vascular infusion tubing, both central and peripheral. Air bubbles are attracted to sites of turbulent flow and may adhere to the walls of the tubing. The areas of greatest turbulence include stopcocks, tubing connections, latex side ports, and right-angle connectors. Air bubble filters are available, but they are not foolproof. Moreover, they must be placed distal to all potential injection sites and may slow infusion rates significantly. We recommend flushing of intravenous tubing during the initial anesthesia setup. The intravenous solution will warm slightly as it is exposed to the heat generated by lights and other electrical equipment and any dissolved air will tend to come out of solution. The intravenous apparatus should be reinspected just before the start of the procedure and purged again if necessary.

A traditional high-dose opiate "cardiac anesthetic" is not physiologically necessary in healthy children undergoing repair of an uncomplicated ASD. The child should be offered a choice of induction methods, but the anesthesiologist should be prepared to switch techniques if the induction is not proceeding as planned. A precordial stethoscope and pulse oximeter are adequate during induction. In many cases, inhalation induction with halothane in nitrous oxide and oxygen can be performed without arousing the child from the slumber provided by the preoperative medication. Intravenous thiopental or intravenous or intramuscular ketamine are suitable parenteral alternatives.

The interval between induction of anesthesia and the start of surgery is very busy. The remaining monitors are applied, and peripheral intravenous access is established. Two catheters of moderate to large diameter are desirable. Syringes should always be held upright and any air expressed before intravascular injection, to avoid the introduction of air. After endotracheal intubation, the indicated invasive procedures are performed. Placement of urinary, intra-arterial, and central venous catheters is essential.

The surgical approach to ASD may be by either a sternotomy or a thoracotomy. Although thoracotomy is often requested by female patients so that the scar can be hidden, the anesthesiologist should be aware that thoracotomy is much more painful. There is a risk of postoperative peripheral neurologic injury that is enhanced by long procedures and cooling during cardiopulmonary bypass (CPB). Proper patient positioning and appropriate padding are required.

Many techniques and anesthetic agents have been successfully utilized for ASD repair. Early postoperative extubation, either in the operating suite or upon arrival in the intensive care unit (ICU) should be anticipated. Any of the nondepolarizing neuromuscular blockers may be selected before CPB. Repeat dosage should maintain 1/4 twitches in the train-of-four. If additional blockade is required during or after CPB, we recommend atracurium because its metabolism will be inhibited during CPB with cooling and resume when the blood is returned to normal temperature.

Children given sufficient anesthesia will remain motionless and asleep during their procedure. If they do not have analgesia, the afferent sensory input of pain continues along the C fiber synapses in the spinal cord, and a C fiber pain reflex arc is established despite adequate anesthesia.[8] Prevention of this spinal hyperexcitability due to pain reflex requires much less medication than obliteration of the hyperexcitability reflex after it is present. We prefer to combine a potent inhalation agent, nitrous oxide, and an opiate, but discontinue the nitrous oxide prior to CPB. The opiate may be given intravenously or in the caudal peridural space.[9] There is no justification for withholding pain management because of the desire for extubation.

It is important to continue anesthesia during CPB. Repair of an ASD requires cooling to only 32°C, and this temperature alone does not provide anesthesia. Intravenous and/or inhalation agents may be used. CPB oxygenators interact with the anesthetic agents in a variable fashion. The membrane oxygenators manufactured by SciMed (Minneapolis) have the greatest potential for anesthetic uptake since they are made of silicon. Silicon components in any bypass circuit can bind significant amounts of lipophilic drugs. The capacity for fentanyl uptake by the SciMed membrane, for example, is 130 ng/cm^2 of membrane surface area.[10] Analgesia may be reliably produced by morphine because none of the currently made oxygenators have any affinity for morphine.

After successful weaning from CPB we prefer to maintain anesthesia with isoflurane and an opiate because of the minimal myocardial depression associated with these agents. At the end of surgery, residual neuromuscular blockade is reversed, and the child is extubated and taken to the ICU. An Ambu bag, oxygen tank, and airway and cardiac resuscitation equipment and drugs should accompany the patient during transport. We also monitor the ECG and direct arterial pressure en route.

POSTOPERATIVE PAIN MANAGEMENT

Traditionally, postoperative pain control was prescribed by the surgical team, usually infrequent narcotics as needed. A more active and aggressive approach by the anesthesiologist can bring about improvements in analgesia and postoperative recovery. The efficacy and safety of a continuous morphine infusion in children after cardiac surgery has been documented.[11] An infusion rate of 10 to 40 µg/hr will usually provide adequate analgesia without clinically significant respiratory depression. Supplemental incremental doses of morphine, 0.025 mg/kg, are administered when the pain score is 3/5 or more on the Oucher scale.

An alternative method, the use of epidural opiates, provides long-acting, good-quality pain relief with minimal side effects in children. The simplest approach to the pediatric epidural space is via the caudal canal. The caudal space in children is very easily entered and reduces the risks of potential dural puncture or compression caused by a hematoma. A single injection of morphine given caudally at the end of surgery can provide total pain control for a mean of 10 to 12 hours after cardiac surgery. The dose of preservative-free morphine is 0.075 mg/kg, diluted to 10 mL with preservative-free saline in children heavier than 12 kg.[12] The total volume is reduced to 5 mL if the dose of morphine is less than 1 mg. Our experience of 6 years with over 300 patients has confirmed the efficacy and safety of this procedure. Nausea and pruritus have occurred in 25% of patients. Metoclopramide, prochlorperazine, and nalbuphine have been used as antiemetics. Diphenhydramine and nalbuphine are effective in the treatment of pruritus. Urinary retention is difficult to assess because of the routine use of Foley catheters during cardiac surgery. Respiratory depression has occurred only twice, in patients who received an incorrect dose (0.1 mg/kg) as well as supplemental intravenous narcotics. Morphine is the opiate of choice when the drug is administered at a location distant from the actual site of pain. Lipophilic drugs do not diffuse as completely throughout the peridural space.

The period of maximal pain is the first 48 hours. The epidural method for postoperative analgesia can be extended through the use of a caudal epidural catheter. The catheter is placed in the caudal space as early as possible after the induction of anesthesia to minimize any possible bleeding problems during heparinization. The catheter is injected with preservative-free morphine as described above before the start of surgery. This dose is repeated every 10 hours during the first 48 hours. Alternatively, the catheter can be continuously infused. The initial bolus is reduced to 0.04 mg/kg, and a continuous infusion is maintained at 0.125 µg/kg/min for 48 hours. As with the continuous intravenous infusion of morphine, small 0.025-mg/kg boluses are given intravenously for breakthrough pain. If good pain control is established during the first 48 hours, a transition to oral analgesics is possible on the third postoperative day.

TRANSFUSION THERAPY

One final issue in this case is the administration of blood components. Bloodless cardiac surgery can now be offered to most children with adequate preoperative hemoglobin levels. The volume in the CPB circuit should be minimized so that the ratio of the patient's estimated blood volume to the volume in the pump will be less than 1.2:1. With this ratio, successful hemodilution can be achieved with avoidance of transfusion in 90% of children, regardless of size.[13] Patients may be hemodiluted on bypass to hematocrits as low as 15%. A brisk diuresis is initiated during CPB to quickly remove the excess priming fluid and restore the hematocrit as soon as possible. It is important to drain the CPB circuit completely and return all volume to the patient. Performing cardiac surgery on children without using blood components requires a team effort by anesthesiologists, surgeons, nurses, and perfusionists.

SUMMARY

In summary, the care of children during repair of an ASD must be meticulous. The selection of an anesthetic technique is flexible. These patients usually do not experience physiologic compromise during the procedure or early recovery phase. The anesthesiologist can have a major impact on the entire perioperative course through an aggressive prophylactic approach to pain management. Early, continuous pain control may decrease the total inpatient time to only 5 days. Both the patient and family will appreciate the anesthesiologist's effort to address two controversial issues: analgesia and avoidance of transfusion.

REFERENCES

1. Behrendt DM: Atrial septal defects, in Arciniegas I (ed): *Pediatric Cardiac Surgery*. St Louis, Mosby–Year Book, 1985, p 133.
2. Vick GW, Titus JL: Defects of the atrial septum, including the atrioventricular canal, in Garson A, Bricker JT, McNamara DG (eds): *The Science and Practice of Pediatric Cardiology*. Philadelphia, Lea & Febiger, 1990, pp 1023–1054.
3. Spire DW: *Understanding and Diagnosing Pediatric Heart Disease*. E Norwalk, Conn, Appleton & Lange, 1991.
4. Garson A Jr: *The Electrocardiogram in Infants and Children*. Philadelphia, Lea & Febiger, 1983.
5. Nicolson SC, Betts EK, Jobes DR, et al: Comparison of oral and intramuscular preanesthetic medication for pediatric inpatient surgery. *Anesthesiology* 1989; 71:8–10.
6. Wilton NCT, Leigh J, Rosen DA, et al: Preanesthetic sedation of preschool children using intranasal midazolam. *Anesthesiology* 1988; 69:972–975.
7. Beyer J, Aradine C: Content and validity of an instrument to measure young children's perceptions of the intensity of their pain. *J Pediatr Nurs* 1986; 1:386–395.
8. Wall PD: The prevention of postoperative pain. *Pain* 1988; 33:289–290.
9. Rosen KR, Rosen DA: Caudal epidural morphine for control of pain following open heart surgery in children. *Anesthesiology* 1989; 70:418–421.
10. Rosen DA, Rosen KR, Silvasi DL: In vitro variability in fentanyl absorption by different membrane oxygenators. *J Cardiothorac Anesth* 1990; 4:332–335.

11. Lynn AM, Opheim KE, Tyler DC: Morphine infusion after pediatric cardiac surgery. *Crit Care Med* 1984; 12:863–866.
12. Rosen KR, Rosen DA: Caudal epidural morphine for control of pain following open heart surgery in children. *Anesthesiology* 1989; 70:418–421.
13. Rosen DA, Rosen KR, Bove EL, et al: Hemodilution for heart surgery in children. *Anesthesiology* 1990; 73:A1242.

45

Multiple Trauma

A 6-year-old boy who was hit by a car is admitted to the emergency room. He is comatose but withdraws from painful stimuli. The left side of the chest and abdomen are contused, the mandible broken, and the left femur fractured. The emergency room physician requests that the child be intubated and sedated for computed tomography (CT) of the head, chest, and abdomen. Exploratory laparotomy and debridement of the femoral fracture are planned following the CT scan. The child has two 20-gauge peripheral intravenous catheters in place. Blood pressure, 65/45; pulse, 140; no laboratory data are available.

Recommendations by Peter J. Davis, M.D.

Patients with life-threatening injuries make up 10% to 15% of all hospitalized injured patients.[1] In children, accidents are the leading cause of death.[2] The initial survival of patients with severe trauma is related to control of the airway, support of the circulation, and restraint of increases in intracranial pressure (ICP).[3, 4] The Committee on Trauma of the American College of Surgeons recommends a two-part approach to trauma: a primary survey of the injuries with concomitant resuscitation and a secondary survey with definitive treatment.[5]

EVALUATION AND EARLY MANAGEMENT

During the primary survey and resuscitation, the patient's overall condition is immediately assessed, the airway established, adequate ventilation achieved, and the circulation stabilized. The role of the anesthesiologist in the care of the trauma patient is vital. The priorities in the early phase of trauma management are summarized by the mnemonic ABC—airway, breathing, and circulation. However, an adequate airway and sufficient oxygenation and ventilation must be accomplished without creating or exacerbating any neurologic injury, such as increased ICP or an unstable cervical spine. This particular patient presents with possible airway difficulties and breathing problems (pulmonary contusion, hemothorax, pneumothorax as evidenced by the external signs of trauma), circulatory instability, and an abnormal neurologic status.

Secretions, bleeding, a foreign body, or direct trauma can obstruct or partially obstruct the airway. Therefore, all trauma patients should have supplemental oxygen administered by face mask, tent, or nasal cannula until the extent of injury and respiratory compromise can be determined. Spinal cord injuries should be presumed in all trauma victims until adequate documentation of a normal cervical spine is obtained. Although the reported sensitivity of the lateral cervical spine radiograph is 0.8,[6] spinal cord injury may be present even in the absence of radiographic findings.[7] Thus, in-line immobilization of the neck with the head in a neutral position or application of a Philadelphia collar combined with sandbags and tape should be maintained for all trauma patients.

If the child is unconscious, is in a state of hypovolemic shock, has sustained major trauma to the head, face, neck, or chest, or has incurred a smoke inhalation injury or airway burn, then control of the airway with endotracheal intubation, cricothyrotomy, or tracheostomy is essential. Establishing an airway in a pediatric trauma patient involves four major considerations: aspiration, complicating neurologic injuries, compromised airway, and hemodynamic instability.

All trauma patients are at risk for aspiration of food, blood, or foreign bodies. Oral endotracheal intubation should be considered for most trauma patients. In those with stable vital signs, no signs or symptoms of increased ICP, a normal cervical spine, and a normal airway, a rapid-sequence intubation with preoxygenation and cricoid pressure can be performed. Care should be taken to avoid hyperextension or flexion of the neck. Thiopental, 4 mg/kg, or etomidate, 0.3 mg/kg, along with succinylcholine, 2 mg/kg, are appropriate in children less than 10 years of age, and atropine, 10 to 20 μg/kg, should be administered before induction to prevent the adverse cardiovascular effects of succinylcholine and laryngoscopy. Blind nasal intubation is strongly discouraged because of the child's large adenoids. Nasal intubation often creates a "groove adenoidectomy" and airway bleeding as well as adenoidal plugging and obstruction of the endotracheal tube. In addition, blind nasal intubation is seldom successful in children.

An understanding of factors affecting cerebral perfusion pressure (CPP), ICP, and cerebral blood flow (CBF) is important in the selection of anesthetic agents and techniques for establishing the airway. The CPP is the mean pressure of blood perfusing the brain and is defined as the mean arterial pressure minus the ICP. CPP and CBF are related by the compliance curve of the cranium. When compliance is high, small changes in blood flow have little effect on ICP, whereas when cranial compliance is low, small changes in blood flow can have dramatic effects on ICP.

Factors that affect CBF include the arterial partial pressures of oxygen and carbon dioxide, the mean arterial blood pressure, and anesthetic agents (Fig 45–1). Arterial carbon dioxide tension and CBF are directly related. Acute decreases in carbon dioxide result in marked cerebral vasoconstriction, a decrease in CBF, a decrease in ICP, and an increase in CPP. In the physiologic ranges, arterial oxygenation has little effect on CBF. However, at oxygen tensions less than 50 mm Hg, hypoxemia results in cerebral vasodilation, and at oxygen tensions greater than 300 mm Hg, hyperoxia is a vasoconstrictor. In normal adults, CBF is autoregulated over a mean blood pressure range of 50 to 150 mm Hg. At blood pressures less than 50 and greater than 150 mm Hg, there tends to be a linear relationship of CBF with pressure. In children, autoregulation of CBF also occurs, but at age-adjusted mean blood pressures. In trauma patients with increases in ICP, autoregulation is lost,

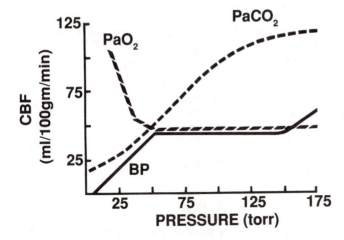

FIG 45–1.
Cerebral blood flow changes due to alterations in Pa_{CO_2} *(dashed line)*, Pa_{O_2} *(parallelogram dashes)*, and blood pressure *(solid line)*. When one variable is altered, the other two variables remain stable at normal values. (From Shapiro HM: *Anesthesiology* 1975; 43:445. Used by permission.)

and CBF changes passively with changes in blood pressure. Consequently, in patients with severe head injury who have lost autoregulation, increases in mean blood pressure either from noxious stimuli (such as laryngoscopy, surgery, suctioning of the endotracheal tube), inadequate anesthesia or from worsening cerebral edema increase the risk of cerebral ischemia.

Normally, CBF is closely linked to cerebral metabolic demand. Increases in metabolic demand promote increases in CBF, and conversely, decreases in metabolic demand decrease CBF. Anesthetic agents can significantly affect CBF and cerebral metabolism (Table 45–1). In general, all inhalation anesthetics uncouple CBF and metabolic demand. Inhalation anesthetics including nitrous oxide are cerebral vasodilators to various degrees and thus increase CBF and ICP. With the exception of ketamine, the intravenous anesthetics generally decrease ICP and CBF. Ketamine is a cerebrovasodilator and can increase CBF by 60%. Consequently, in patients with increased ICP, ketamine is contraindicated. In addition to anesthetic agents, the choice of muscle relaxants can also influence CBF. Nondepolarizing muscle relaxants have no effects on CBF, whereas succinylcholine increases both CBF and ICP.

Although all trauma patients are at risk for aspiration of gastric contents, patients with increased ICP and inadequate anesthesia during laryngoscopy are also at risk for recalcitrant ICP spikes and further neurologic impairment. If this child did not require intubation at the time of initial evaluation, anesthesia would be slowly induced with thiopental or etomidate and a nondepolarizing muscle relaxant administered. Gentle bag-and-mask ventilation with cricoid pressure would be maintained throughout the induction. A faster onset of action of neuromuscular blockade can be achieved by use of the priming principle or by administration of four to six times the 95% effective dose (ED_{95}) of the muscle relaxant at the time of induction. Because of the high doses of nondepolarizing muscle relaxants required with this approach, an agent with minimal cardiovascular side effects such as vecuronium would be preferable. After loss of the lash reflex, hyperventilation would be initiated and cricoid pressure maintained. Fentanyl, 2 to 4 µg/kg, and lidocaine, 2 mg/kg, are useful in ablating the stimulus of intubation.

If a nasogastric tube is not in place before intubation, the stomach and its contents should be decompressed by passage of an oral gastric tube. In patients with midface trauma or evidence of basilar skull or cribriform fractures, nasal gastric tubes are contraindicated. Once the airway is se-

TABLE 45–1.

Effects of Anesthetic Agents on Cerebral Circulation, Intracranial Pressure, and Cerebrospinal Fluid Dynamics*

Anesthetic Agent†	CBF‡	CMRO$_2$‡	Autoregulation	ICP‡
Intravenous				
Thiopental	↓ ↓	↓ ↓	Preserved	↓ ↓
Fentanyl (low dose)	—	—	Preserved	—
Etomidate	↓	↓	Preserved	↓
Lidocaine (nontoxic)	↓	↓	Preserved	↓
Droperidol	↓	—	Preserved	↓
Benzodiazepines	↓	↓	Preserved	↓
Ketamine	↑ ↑	—	Unknown	↑ ↑ §
Inhalation				
Nitrous oxide	↑ ¶	↑	Preserved	↑
Halothane	↑ ↑	↓	Abolished	↑ §
Enflurane	↑	↓	Abolished	↑ §
Isoflurane	↑	↓ ↓	Preserved, unless high dose	↑ §

*Adapted from Krane EJ, Domino KB: In Motoyama EK, Davis PJ (eds): *Smith's Anesthesia for Infants and Children,* ed 5. St Louis, Mosby–Year Book, 1990, p 558.
†All agents preserve responsiveness to carbon dioxide.
‡CBF = cerebral blood flow; CMRO$_2$ = cerebral metabolic rate for oxygen; ICP = intracranial pressure.
§The increase in ICP is dose related and blunted by hyperventilation.
¶The effect on CBF and ICP depends on the background anesthetic (volatile or barbiturate).

cured, all patients should be ventilated with 100% oxygen. The adequacy of oxygenation and ventilation should then be assessed by auscultation and analysis of arterial blood gases. The inspired oxygen concentration should be adjusted accordingly, and the arterial carbon dioxide levels titrated to between 25 and 30 mm Hg. Administration of other agents such as mannitol, furosemide, or calcium channel blockers as a part of the neurologic resuscitation is determined by the patient's underlying clinical condition.[8]

THE CHILD WITH A COMPROMISED AIRWAY

In a patient with a presumed abnormal airway who is hemodynamically stable and neurologically intact, a different approach to airway management is required. Spontaneous ventilation must be maintained during endotracheal intubation. Because the causes for an abnormal airway are numerous, the anesthesiologist must be well prepared for the unexpected. Several laryngoscope blades must be immediately available. The Bullard laryngoscope, a fiber-optic telescope configured with a mirror and a curved blade, may be useful in some patients because it does not require the tracheal, oral, and pharyngeal axes to be aligned. Fiber-optic techniques can also be used successfully, although these require more practice and expertise. Blind nasal intubation is strongly discouraged. In addition to the previously cited reasons, it can further compromise a patient by converting a partially dislocated larynx to a completely dislocated larynx. It must be remembered that any trauma patient with a compromised airway has a life-threatening injury. In patients with an obvious or presumed difficult airway complicated by shock or increased ICP or those in whom the anesthesiologist believes that the airway cannot be secured after the induction of anesthesia, tracheostomy or cricothyrotomy under local anesthesia is the safest way to establish the airway. Consequently, appropriately trained personnel must be immediately available when attempts to secure the airway are made.

RESTORATION OF INTRAVASCULAR VOLUME

After the airway has been established and adequate ventilation achieved, restoration of the circulation becomes the next priority. Hemorrhage and hypovolemic shock result in decreases in mean arterial pressure, regional perfusion, and oxygen and nutrient delivery and stimulate anaerobic metabolism. Tissue hypoxia and acidosis stimulate compensatory mechanisms that increase ventilation, heart rate, and contractility. Consequently, the early clinical signs of shock are tachycardia, decreased pulse pressure, delayed capillary refill, mottled skin, cold extremities, and an altered sensorium. Ninety-five percent of children over 1 year of age have a systolic blood pressure greater than 80 mm Hg. Nevertheless in early shock, arterial blood pressure can remain stable until 20% of the blood volume is lost (Fig 45–2). Thus, even with a normal blood pressure, a pediatric trauma patient may be in shock. A child in shock with flat neck veins is volume depleted. If the neck veins are distended, the differential diagnosis includes pneumothorax, pericardial tamponade, myocardial contusion, and air embolism. Treatment with a thoracostomy tube, pericardiocentesis, and prevention of air entrainment should be instituted immediately.

If the primary cause of shock is hypovolemia resulting from blood loss, then the initial treatment is fluid resuscitation. Intravenous access should be immediately attempted, and the largest possible venous catheter should be inserted. Cutdown on a saphenous or femoral vein should be performed if percutaneous peripheral venous cannulation is not easily achieved. Internal jugular and subclavian vein catheterizations are difficult to perform during the initial resuscitation and are discouraged because of the potential complications of pneumothorax and hemopneumothorax. Both of

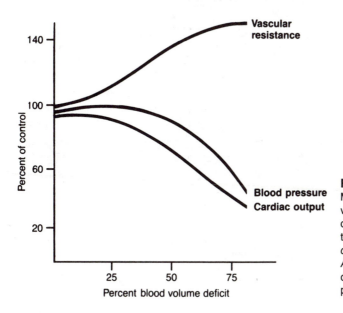

FIG 45–2.
Model of cardiovascular response to hypovolemia from hemorrhage. (From Chameides L, et al (eds): Recognition of respiratory failure and shock anticipations, in *Cardiopulmonary Arrest Textbook of Pediatric Advanced Life Support.* Chicago, American Heart Association, 1990, p. 5. Used by permission.)

these complications can further exacerbate any underlying pulmonary or hemodynamic instability. Therefore, these invasive, percutaneous approaches should be attempted only as a last resort and only by experienced personnel. Intraosseous infusion, a temporizing but lifesaving maneuver, can be initiated when intravenous access is difficult. In this technique a 13- to 16-gauge bone marrow needle is inserted percutaneously into the distal or proximal end of the tibia. Fluid infusion rates of 17 to 40 mL/min can be achieved. In addition to fluid administration, intraosseous infusions can also provide an alternative route for drug administration.[9, 10]

The initial fluid used in resuscitation should be crystalloid. A balanced salt solution, Ringer's lactate, is administered in a 20-mL/kg bolus over a period of 5 to 10 minutes. If there is not a rapid clinical response with a decrease in heart rate, an increase in blood pressure, and a decrease in capillary filling time and shock still remains, then a repeat 20-mL/kg fluid bolus is administered. If there is still no clinical response after the second fluid bolus, then type-specific blood or type O, Rh-negative blood is administered, 10 to 20 mL/kg. Additional volume resuscitation is guided by the clinical response as well as by laboratory values such as hemoglobin, hematocrit, and arterial blood gas tensions.

Failure to reverse the signs of shock indicates continuing hemorrhage. The use of military antishock trousers (MAST) in pediatric patients remains controversial. In some patients MAST can preserve central blood pressure and stabilize pelvic fractures, but their use can also create compartment syndromes and respiratory insufficiency. Continued shock despite aggressive fluid resuscitation is an indication for exploratory laparotomy. However, re-evaluation of the patient for other possible causes such as pneumothorax, pericardial tamponade, or spinal shock should also be undertaken.

DEFINITIVE CARE

After the primary survey is completed and resuscitation has stabilized the patient, the secondary survey and definitive care begin. It is during this time that diagnostic studies such as a CT scan or angiography are performed. Management during these diagnostic studies focuses on vigilant patient monitoring. Vital signs must be obtained frequently and recorded while diagnostic procedures are being conducted. In addition, if large volumes of fluid are required, repeat measurements of blood gas tensions and hematocrit are essential. Because trauma patients are frequently exposed to cool environmental temperatures in resuscitation areas and diagnostic procedure rooms, as well as cold fluid administration during the resuscitation, hypothermia frequently occurs. Thus, the anesthesiologist must be aware of the possibility of hypothermia and attempt to prevent or correct it should it occur. In addition to patient monitoring devices, anesthetic equipment and anesthetic agents necessary to administer general anesthesia must be available in the procedure room. Surgical team members should accompany the patient and be present in the room during the procedure in case an unforeseen emergency develops.

The anesthetic agents administered during diagnostic studies and any subsequent surgical procedures will be determined by the patient's overall condition. Postoperatively, he should be monitored in an intensive care unit.

REFERENCES

1. Gere M, (ed): *Resources for optimal care of the injured patient.* Chicago, American College of Surgeons, 1990, p. 15–18.
2. Nakayama DK, Davis PJ: Pediatric trauma, in Motoyama EK, Davis PJ, (eds): *Smith's Anesthesia for Infants and Children,* St. Louis, Mosby-Year Book, Inc., 1990.
3. Jaffe D, Wesson D: Emergency management of blunt trauma in children. *N Engl J Med* 1991; 324(21):1477–1482.
4. Trunkey D: Initial treatment of patients with extensive trauma. *N Engl J Med* 1991; 324(18):1259–1263.
5. Subcommittee of Advanced Trauma Life Support of the American College of Surgeons Committee on Trauma. *Advanced Trauma Life Support Student Manual,* American College of Surgeons, 1989, pp 267–268.
6. Ross SE, et al.: Clearing the cervical spine: Initial radiologic evaluation. *J Trauma* 1987; 27:1055.
7. Pang D, Wilberger JE: Spinal cord injury without radiographic abnormalities in childen. *J Neurosurg* 1982; 57:114.
8. Krane EJ, Domino KB: Anesthesia for neurosurgery, in Motoyama EK, Davis PJ, (eds): *Smith's Anesthesia for Infants and Children,* St. Louis, Mosby-Year Book, Inc., 1990.
9. Hodge D III, Delgado-Paredes C, Fleisher G: Intraosseous infusion flow rates in hypovolemic "pediatric" dogs. *Ann Emerg Med* 1987; 16:305.
10. Spivey WH: Intraosseous infusions. *J Pediatr* 1987; 111:639.

46

Posterior Fossa Craniotomy

A 6-year-old, 20-kg boy is scheduled for posterior fossa craniotomy. His presenting complaint was headaches. He is alert. Hemoglobin, 13.8 g/dL; hematocrit, 42%.

Recommendations by Sulpicio G. Soriano, M.D., M.S.Ed., and Mark A. Rockoff, M.D.

Brain tumors are the most common solid tumors occurring during childhood and rank second only to leukemia as the most common malignancy in children. Although most central nervous system (CNS) tumors in adults are supratentorial, the majority in children are located in the posterior fossa. Cerebellar astrocytomas and medulloblastomas are the most frequent lesions and account for almost half of all pediatric CNS tumors. Malignancies affecting the brain stem (astrocytoma and ganglioglioma) and fourth ventricle (ependymoma) occur less frequently.[1]

These space-occupying lesions often obstruct cerebrospinal fluid (CSF) flow and result in increased intracranial pressure (ICP). Brain stem structures vital to the control of respiration, heart rate, and blood pressure may be affected. Management of these physiologic variables during surgical resection often makes the intraoperative course challenging.

PREOPERATIVE EVALUATION

The initial signs and symptoms of a CNS tumor can be subtle. Headache, vomiting, irritability, and ultimately, lethargy may occur as a result of hydrocephalus. Infants may present with an inappropriate increase in head circumference. Localizing signs of brain stem and cerebellar pathology include cranial nerve palsies, ataxia, and nystagmus.

Recent advances in high-resolution computed tomography (CT) and magnetic resonance imaging (MRI) have aided the diagnosis and localization of CNS tumors.

The preoperative evaluation should include a careful review of the medical history. Respiratory, cardiac, and renal pathology can alter the anesthetic management of these patients. The presence of a cardiac defect may worsen the sequelae of venous air embolism and should be a consideration in positioning for surgery. Preoperative medications such as antibiotics and anticonvulsants should be continued intraoperatively. The patient's fluid status should be carefully reviewed. Inadequate hydration secondary to prolonged vomiting, poor appetite, and iatrogenic dehydration produced by fluid restriction or diuretics is not uncommon. Symptoms of diabetes insipidus such as unexpected bed wetting and nocturnal drinking should be sought. An accurate weight is necessary to guide drug administration and to aid in the assessment of blood loss and volume replacement. The baseline blood pressure, heart rate, respiratory rate, and temperature should be noted. The physical examination must also include a neurologic assessment. The child's mental status and ability to cooperate with anesthetic induction are paramount in deciding the type and amount of premedication necessary. Focal neurologic signs such as motor weakness, gag reflex, and pupillary responsiveness and equality should be assessed.

Significant blood loss may occur during a craniotomy. Therefore, laboratory data should include a hematocrit, platelet count, and determination of prothrombin and partial thromboplastin times. Blood should be typed and crossmatched, with one adult-sized unit generally being adequate. A determination of serum electrolytes, blood urea nitrogen, and osmolality can be helpful in assessing preoperative fluid status and anticipating problems with the administration of diuretics or osmotic agents. These laboratory tests are essential in patients with tumors near the pituitary gland. Diabetes insipidus may be subtle and result in significant problems with fluid and electrolyte homeostasis.

The preoperative management of a child with a CNS tumor usually includes steroid treatment such as dexamethasone, up to 1 mg/kg/day, to reduce brain swelling. Palliation of hydrocephalus by preoperative shunting of CSF provides more time to prepare the patient for a major tumor resection by decreasing the ICP prior to craniotomy. However, placement of a CSF shunt is not without complications in this setting. Among the potential complications are a delay in definitive treatment, dissemination of malignant cells through the shunt, infection or obstruction involving the shunt tubing, and transtentorial herniation occurring in a cephalad direction. Furthermore, many patients with a posterior fossa tumor do not require a shunt following tumor resection. Therefore, most neurosurgeons do not insert a CSF shunt prior to tumor resection, but can drain CSF acutely, if necessary, at the time of surgery.

ANESTHETIC MANAGEMENT

The major anesthetic considerations in a patient with a posterior fossa tumor are avoiding intracranial hypertension, monitoring the competence of brain stem function, and preventing and, if necessary, treating venous air embolism.

Premedication

The child's mental status and degree of disability will influence the need for and tolerance to premedication. Good rapport with the patient and parents will help immeasurably, although this may be difficult to develop when admission to the hospital occurs on the same day as surgery.

Obtunded patients should not receive any preoperative sedation. Those with nausea and vomiting are at increased risk for aspiration pneumonitis and require a rapid-sequence induction with cricoid pressure. It is usually easy to insert an intravenous catheter preoperatively in patients who should have an intravenous induction since they are frequently lethargic. However, most children undergoing a posterior fossa craniotomy will be alert and anxious and frequently benefit from preoperative sedation.

Premedication is best administered in a preoperative holding area adjacent to the operating room in the presence of the anesthesiologist. For this reason, rapid-acting agents are desirable. Midazolam, 0.5 to 0.75 mg/kg, may be given orally approximately 20 minutes prior to induction. Alternatively, methohexital, 20 to 30 mg/kg, can be administered rectally to small children (between about 9 months and 5 years of age) and induces sleep in less than 10 minutes. Methohexital should be avoided in children with psychomotor, temporal, or complex mixed seizure disorders because it can induce convulsions in these circumstances.[2] Thiopental, in similar doses, may be used instead. Parental presence during inhalation induction may be an alternative to traditional premedication. In older children, a small intravenous catheter can be inserted following injection of a local anesthetic. Sedatives such as midazolam can then be slowly titrated to relieve anxiety.

Induction of Anesthesia

As with premedication, the child's preoperative neurologic status will influence the type of induction selected. If the patient is alert, then almost any well-tolerated induction may be appropriate. If the patient has no intravenous access, anesthesia can be induced with halothane, nitrous oxide, and oxygen by mask. Airway obstruction and hypoventilation should be avoided since intracranial hypertension will be exacerbated by hypercarbia and hypoxia. Once sedation has occurred, an intravenous catheter can then be inserted.

If the patient has intravenous access, a variety of induction agents can be used. Thiopental is the traditional drug of choice. Dosage is dependent upon the child's mental status as well as the amount of premedication used. In unpremedicated children, induction doses generally range from 5 to 7 mg/kg. Although its use in children is not currently approved, propofol can be an effective alternative. Neuromuscular blockade can be accomplished with a nondepolarizing muscle relaxant. Pancuronium is the preferred relaxant since its prolonged duration of action is advantageous for neurosurgical procedures and its vagolytic effect is helpful in avoiding bradycardia in children. The child should be hyperventilated to lower ICP and anesthesia deepened with supplemental doses of fentanyl, 2 to 5 μg/kg, or thiopental, 1 to 2 mg/kg, to blunt the sympathetic responses to laryngoscopy and intubation.

If the patient is at increased risk for aspiration pneumonitis, a rapid-sequence induction is appropriate. Since rapid, complete muscle relaxation is necessary, succinylcholine is usually the muscle relaxant of choice. There is controversy regarding succinylcholine-induced intracranial hypertension.[3, 4] However, this issue is clinically insignificant if adequate anesthesia and muscle relaxation are provided prior to laryngoscopy and endotracheal intubation. Contraindications to the use of suc-cinylcholine are malignant hyperthermia susceptibility and recent denervation injuries that may re-sult in acute hyperkalemia. In these circumstances, a large dose of atracurium or vecuronium can produce ideal intubating conditions within 2 minutes.[5]

For a 6-year-old child, a 5.5-mm uncuffed endotracheal tube is usually appropriate. The tube should produce an air leak with positive airway pressures of 20 to 30 cm H_2O. A nasotracheal tube is less likely to be displaced and more easily secured, especially in patients in the prone position. Proper positioning of the endotracheal tube is essential because extremes of neck flexion or exten-sion can produce bronchial intubation or accidental extubation. The eyes should be lubricated with a sterile ophthalmic solution and taped closed. A gastric tube should be inserted to suction the stom-ach contents. It is useful to permit the tube to drain passively during the procedure to reduce bowel gas during prolonged procedures, especially when an uncuffed endotracheal tube is used.

Application of a skull holder is painful and will require supplemental anesthesia with thiopental or fentanyl. Local anesthesia with epinephrine injected into the scalp and periosteum can minimize scalp blood loss and provide supplemental analgesia.

Monitoring

Standard monitoring includes a precordial (and then esophageal) stethoscope, electrocardiogram (ECG), temperature probe, noninvasive blood pressure monitor, pulse oximeter, and end-tidal car-bon dioxide ($ETco_2$) analyzer. A peripheral nerve stimulator should be applied and checked after the induction of anesthesia but prior to the administration of muscle relaxants to ensure proper place-ment and function. An arterial catheter should be inserted for continuous blood pressure monitoring and sampling of blood gases, electrolytes, osmolality, glucose, and hematocrit. A 22-gauge catheter is adequate and can be placed in the radial, dorsalis pedis, or posterior tibial artery closest to the anesthesiologist. For patients in the sitting position, a central venous catheter can be helpful. Oth-erwise, a second peripheral intravenous catheter is usually adequate. Although external or internal jugular veins can be cannulated, impaired venous return from the operative site may result, espe-cially in small children. Cannulation of the brachial vein is a better route in older children, and the femoral vein can be easily catheterized in patients of all ages. A chest x-ray should be obtained to ensure proper placement of the catheter. The catheter tip should be positioned at the superior vena cava–right atrium junction. Catheters should not be permitted to remain in the heart because of an increased risk of myocardial perforation with prolonged use. A urinary catheter should be inserted into the bladder to assess urine output and permit complete drainage.

Transesophageal echocardiography is the most sensitive method of detecting vascular air en-trainment.[6] However, small transducers needed for children are not readily available. Currently, a precordial Doppler device is the preferred monitor for children. The sensor can be applied over the right sternal border at the level of the fourth intercostal space. The characteristic noise that occurs with intravascular air can be demonstrated by the rapid intravenous injection of agitated saline into a central or peripheral intravenous catheter. If the patient is prone, the Doppler probe can be placed between the spine and scapula. Another important monitor for detecting air emboli is capnography. A sudden decrease in $ETco_2$ without a decrease in blood pressure is supportive of venous air embo-lism (VAE) in a paralyzed patient whose ventilation is controlled. Changes in the ECG, arterial blood pressure, or the quality of heart tones heard with an esophageal stethoscope are late and ominous signs (Fig 46–1). As the height of the operative site increases above the level of the heart, the danger of air entrainment increases.

Positioning

Fortunately, most pediatric neurosurgeons position children prone for posterior fossa craniotomy. The sitting position is still occasionally utilized by some neurosurgeons, usually for children older than 3 years of age with midline lesions.

Prior to draping, it is important to pad all pressure points and be certain that the endotracheal tube and all intravascular catheters and tubing are secure and accessible. Extreme head flexion may occur with positioning. This can lead to bronchial intubation and occasionally will produce signs of brain stem compression. Careful auscultation of breath sounds is mandatory, and adequate clearance between the patient's chin and sternum should be ensured.

Maintenance of Anesthesia

The effects of various anesthetic agents on ICP have been reviewed extensively.[7] All volatile anesthetics are potent cerebral vasodilators and can increase ICP when used in high concentrations. Halothane produces a greater increase in cerebral blood flow (CBF) than does isoflurane. However, it is the best agent for inhalation induction in children. High concentrations of enflurane should be avoided because seizures may occur in the presence of hypocarbia. Isoflurane is the volatile agent of choice for maintenance of anesthesia. Fentanyl in combination with nitrous oxide and muscle relaxants provides a hemodynamically stable state of anesthesia. Fentanyl, 10 μg/kg prior to the incision and approximately 2 to 3 μg/kg/hr, blunts most sympathetic responses to surgery and leads to a calm and prompt emergence from anesthesia.

Since hypercarbia can exacerbate intracranial hypertension, ventilation should be controlled and $Paco_2$ maintained at approximately 30 mm Hg. Neuromuscular blockade should be ensured with a nondepolarizing muscle relaxant such as pancuronium. Patients receiving chronic anticonvulsant therapy may have increased muscle relaxant requirements.[8]

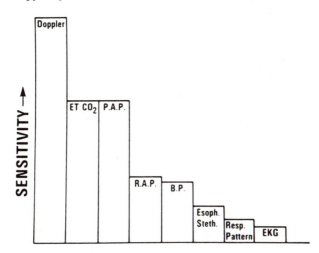

FIG 46–1.
Relative sensitivity of monitors for venous air embolism. *ET CO₂* = end-tidal carbon dioxide; *P.A.P.* = pulmonary artery pressure; *R.A.P.* = right atrial pressure; *EKG* = electrocardiogram. (From Ryan JF, et al (eds): *A Practice of Anesthesia for Infants and Children*, ed 1. Orlando, Fla, Grune & Stratton, 1986. Used by permission.)

Blood loss is difficult to assess during a craniotomy because of insidious bleeding from scalp edges, the use of copious amounts of irrigating solution, and the inability to collect lost blood or easily visualize the entire surgical field. Serial hematocrit values should be obtained to help determine blood loss. Transfusion is not necessary during most craniotomies in otherwise healthy children. A colloid solution such as 5% albumin can be administered if necessary. Since normal saline is slightly hypertonic to blood (osmolality of 308 mOsm), it may be a better fluid replacement than Ringer's lactate solution (osmolality of 272 mOsm). When intracranial hypertension is present, furosemide, 0.1 to 0.2 mg/kg, or mannitol, 0.25 to 1.0 g/kg, can be effective adjuvants to hyperventilation in reducing brain volume. A serum osmolality of 300 to 310 mOsm/kg is a reasonable goal. Hypokalemia and hypernatremia can develop after repeated doses of these agents.

COMPLICATIONS

Vital structures located in the posterior fossa (Fig 46–2) can be irritated or injured during the procedure. Respiratory control centers can be damaged during surgical dissection.[9] Stimulation of

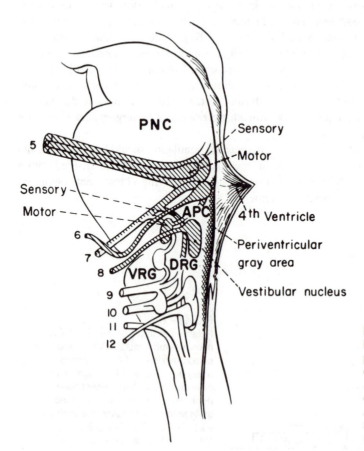

FIG 46–2.
Brain stem structures located in the posterior fossa. *PNC* = pneumotaxic center; *APC* = apneustic center; *VRG* = ventral respiratory group; *DRG* = dorsal respiratory group. (From Artru AA, Cucchiara RF, Messick JM: *Anesthesiology* 1980; 52:83. Used by permission.)

the nucleus of cranial nerve V produces hypertension and tachycardia, whereas vagal nucleus stimulation induces bradycardia. Injury to the vagal nucleus can also result in postoperative vocal cord paralysis. Continuous blood pressure and ECG monitoring are essential to detect encroachment on these vital structures. Table 46-1 lists the effects of manipulation of structures in the posterior fossa, although these motor responses will not be detectable in paralyzed patients.

One of the most significant complications associated with craniotomy is VAE. Raising the operative site above the heart reduces bleeding and brain swelling; however, it also increases the propensity for air entrainment into venous and bony sinuses. Small amounts of air can be filtered by the lungs, but rapid entry of a large volume of air can lead to right ventricular outflow tract obstruction and subsequent decreased cardiac output. In one study of children undergoing craniectomy for craniosynostosis, there was a 66% incidence of VAE detected by precordial echocardiography[10] even though the patients were all in the supine position. There were no deaths or untoward neurologic sequelae in the series. However, the relatively large head size of infants often places the operative site of a craniotomy above the heart, even when patients are supine or prone.

A potentially devastating consequence of VAE is paradoxical air embolism. In an autopsy study of 965 normal hearts, a probe-patent foramen ovale existed in 27% of the specimens.[11] When right atrial pressure exceeds left atrial pressure, a conduit for right-to-left atrial flow occurs. This is also possible in children with congenital heart defects. In addition, animal studies have shown that transpulmonary passage of air can occur.[12] Arterial air emboli can produce cerebral and coronary artery obstruction and lead to stroke and myocardial infarction.

TABLE 46-1.

Effects of Manipulation in the Area of the Brain Stem*

Brain Stem Area	Signs	Monitor†
CN† V	Motor-jaw jerk	EMG, visualization
	Sensory hypertension, bradycardia	Arterial pressure, ECG
CN VII	Facial twitch	EMG, visualization
CN X	Hypotension, bradycardia	Arterial pressure, ECG
CN XI	Shoulder jerk	EMG, visualization
Pons, medulla	Brain stem compression	BAER, SSEP
	Ectopic cardiac foci	ECG
	Hypertension/ hypotension	Arterial pressure
	Tachycardia/ bradycardia	ECG
	Gasp, irregular respirations	Stethoscope, ETco$_2$

*Adapted from Cucchiara RF, Michenfelder JD: *Clinical Neuroanesthesia.* New York, Churchill Livingstone Inc, 1990.
†CN = cranial nerve; EMG = electromyography; BAER = brain stem auditory evoked response; SSEP = somatosensory evoked potentials; ECG = electrocardiography; ETco$_2$ = end-tidal carbon dioxide.

If VAE occurs, treatment must be prompt and aggressive. The surgeon must be immediately notified so that the operative field can be covered with bone wax or filled with saline to prevent further entrainment of air. Since nitrous oxide can expand air bubbles, its use should be discontinued immediately. The head of the table should be lowered below the level of the heart. Hypotension must be treated aggressively with fluid administration and pressor support when necessary. Chest compressions may be required to maintain cardiac output. If the patient has a central venous catheter, an attempt should be made to aspirate air to aid the diagnosis of VAE and to reduce its volume whenever possible. However, the yield for aspirating air is low because most air goes into the right ventricular outflow tract and out the pulmonary circulation.

POSTOPERATIVE CARE

Reversal of neuromuscular blockade should be accomplished only after removal of the skull holder, application of the surgical dressing, and securing access to the airway. Small doses of fentanyl (1 µg/kg) may be given shortly before emergence to help prevent coughing. Unlike adults, most children do not develop hypertension after a craniotomy if adequate doses of of narcotics are administered. Gastric contents should again be aspirated. Neuromuscular function, cranial reflexes, and spontaneous respirations must be adequate prior to extubation of the trachea. Posterior fossa lesions and surgical manipulations can result in brain stem dysfunction. Postextubation vocal cord paralysis may present as stridor or airway obstruction.

Close observation in an intensive care unit (ICU) with staff capable of caring for children is crucial for the prevention and early detection of postoperative problems. Transient cranial nerve or brain stem dysfunction may result from surgical manipulation or postoperative bleeding. Obstructive hydrocephalus can also develop insidiously after posterior fossa craniotomy. Therefore, serial neurologic examinations should be performed.

Common postoperative problems include respiratory depression, fluid and electrolyte disorders, and arterial hypertension. Postoperative pain is minimal in this group of patients; therefore potent narcotics are generally not required. Children with persistent vomiting should be evaluated for evidence of intracranial pathology. An antiemetic such as droperidol can be used in small doses (10 µg/kg) to alleviate nausea. Most patients require only one night of observation in the ICU.

REFERENCES

1. Kadota RP, Allen JB, Hartman GA, et al: Brain tumors in children. *J Pediatr* 1989; 114:511–519.
2. Rockoff MA, Goudsouzian NG: Seizures induced by methohexital. *Anesthesiology* 1981; 54:333–335.
3. Cottrell JE, et al: Intracranial hemodynamic changes after succinylcholine administration in cats. *Anesth Analg* 1980; 62:1006–1009.
4. Lanier WL, Milde JH, Michenfelder JD: Cerebral stimulation following succinylcholine in dogs. *Anesthesiology* 1986; 64:551–559.
5. Lennon RL, Olson RA, Gronert GA: Atracurium or vecuronium for rapid-sequence endotracheal intubation. *Anesthesiology* 1986; 64:510–513.

6. Muzzi DA, Losasso TJ, Black S, et al: Comparison of a transesophageal and precordial ultrasonic Doppler sensor in the detection of venous air embolism. *Anesth Analg* 1990; 70:103–104.

7. Michenfelder JD: *Anesthesia and the Brain.* New York, Churchill Livingstone Inc, 1988.

8. Tempelhoff R, Modica PA, Jellish WS, et al: Resistance to atracurium-induced neuromuscular blockade in patients with intractable seizure disorders treated with anticonvulsants. *Anesth Analg* 1991; 71:665–669.

9. Artru AA, Cucchiara RF, Messick JM: Cardiorespiratory and cranial-nerve sequelae of surgical procedures involving the posterior fossa. *Anesthesiology* 1980; 52:83–86.

10. Harris M, et al: Venous embolism during craniotomy in supine infants. *Anesthesiology* 1987; 67:816–819.

11. Hagen PT, Scholz DG, Edwards WD: Incidence and size of patent foramen ovale during the first 10 decades of life: An autopsy study of 965 normal hearts. *Mayo Clin Proc* 1984; 59:17–20.

12. Vik A, Brubakk AO, Hennessy TR, et al: Venous air embolism in swine: Transport of gas bubbles through the pulmonary circulation. *J Appl Physiol* 1990; 69:237–244.

47

Epidermolysis Bullosa

A 6-year-old girl with epidermolysis bullosa is scheduled for surgical separation of acquired syndactyly of the hand. There are bullous areas on all extremities. The child is small for her age (18 kg) and very intelligent. Hemoglobin, 9.8 g/dL; hematocrit, 29%.

Recommendations by Alfonso E. Yonfa, M.D.

Epidermolysis bullosa (EB) includes a number of inherited conditions that can generally be distinguished by their clinical and genetic features. The anesthetic considerations are similar and significant.

TYPES OF EPIDERMOLYSIS BULLOSA

The disorder may be divided into two autosomal dominant forms and two autosomal recessive forms: the dominant simplex form, the dominant dystrophic or hypertrophic form, the recessive dystrophic form, and epidermolysis bullosa lethalis.

Dominant Simplex Form

In the dominant simplex form of EB, vesicles arise at sites of friction or trauma. The nails become dystrophic in about 20% of patients. The lesions heal with no severe scarring or pigmentation. This form of EB is usually noticed during the neonatal period or during infancy. After the patient is about 3 years of age, the bullae usually form only on the hands and feet. The oral mucosa of these patients can be affected, but is not usually severely involved.

Hypertrophic Form

The dominant dystrophic, or hypertrophic, form is characterized by flat, pink, scar-producing bullae on the ankles, knees, hands, elbows, and feet. Milia are common and the nails are usually thick and dystrophic. Bullae occur in the oral mucosa in 20% or fewer of the patients with this form of EB. Most authorities agree that the teeth of these patients do not exhibit enamel malformations.

Recessive Dystrophic Form

In the recessive dystrophic form, bullae form at sites of pressure or trauma. These bullae are usually seen at or shortly after birth; they collapse and leave bleeding surfaces. Secondary infection and fluid loss through the lesions seriously endanger the patient. Severe anemia and amyloidosis often occur and make the prognosis unfavorable.

Healing of bullae occurs with scarring, milia formation, and pigmentation changes (Fig 47–1). The nails may be grossly involved, dystrophic, or absent. Hyperhydrosis of the palms and soles sometimes occurs. The hair may be deficient. Eye changes include shrinkage of the conjuntiva, non-specific blepharitis, conjunctivitis, and keratitis with corneal opacity and vesicle formation. Bullae may occur in the larynx and pharynx and produce hoarseness and dysphagia. Esophageal stricture and obstruction may occur.

Severe deformity and contractures of the hands, feet, elbows, and knees is common (Fig 47–2). The oral mucosa is involved in over a third of patients. Scarring of the oral mucosa from previous bullae results in loss of buccal and lingual mobility or oral soft tissues. The oral mucosa often appears thick, gray, and smooth.

Several authors have reported that the teeth have defective enamel, are more susceptible to dental caries, and may be delayed in eruption and exfoliation. These findings and their frequency need further documentation. There appears to be no direct correlation between the severity of enamel changes in the teeth and the severity of the skin lesions in a given patient.

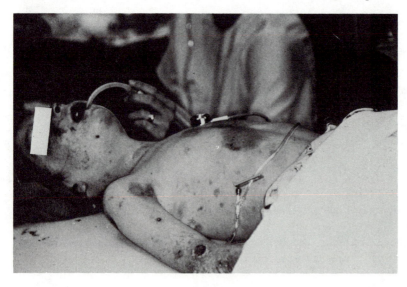

FIG 47–1.
Multiple cutaneous lesions in child with epidermolysis bullosa.

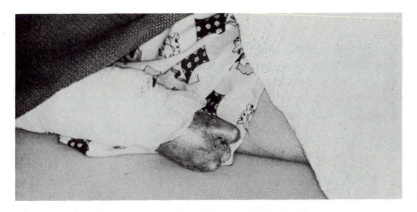

FIG 47–2.
Contracture formation and syndactyly in same child.

EB Lethalis

The final type, EB lethalis, is characterized by neonatal onset, death within the first three months, and absence of milia, pigmentary changes, or scarring. It is possible that this type is a severe form of recessive dystrophic EB. Hemorrhagic vesicles are noted in the base of the fingernails within the first few hours of life and nails are soon lost. This is followed by involvement of the trunk, extremities, umbilicus, face, and scalp. The palms and soles are not affected. Fragile hemorrhagic oral bullae are found in nearly all children, especially at the junction of the hard and soft palate.

PATHOPHYSIOLOGY

The etiology of the disease is unknown and there is no specific effective treatment. Some patients may be given steroids, but they are used infrequently. Phenytoin may be prescribed to reduce the activity of the collagenase that appears to be responsible for the blister formation. Therapy is supportive and directed at skin care and management of complications such as anemia, infection, and malnutrition.

These children frequently require anesthesia for surgical procedures. Dental restorations, esophagoscopy and dilatation, reconstructive procedures of the extremities, cystoscopy, and eye examinations are among the more common procedures.

PREOPERATIVE PREPARATION

When treatment requires general anesthesia, each person involved must be conscious of his or her role and of the general goals of the procedure. A team concept with frequent communication is essential. The team includes the parents, physicians, dentists, nurses, and other health care professionals who are to participate in the child's care.

To decrease the parents' anxiety, it is valuable for them to meet other families whose children with EB have undergone surgery. The family should come to the hospital for a preadmission visit. The parents and the patient can become acquainted with the hospital, the equipment, and the personnel of the operating and recovery room. To reduce the incidence of nosocomial infection, a one-day admission approach is preferred.

The operative consent signed at the preadmission evaluation should include consent for tracheostomy. Preoperative laboratory work consists of a urinalysis, complete blood count, and, when indicated, chest radiographs. Preoperative medication, may not be required. However, the use of midazolam by mouth, 0.5 mg/kg given with a sip of a soft drink and administered 10 to 30 minutes prior to induction of anesthesia, has proven to be useful in our experience.

ANESTHETIC MANAGEMENT

Most procedures are performed with general anesthesia. Local infiltration is contraindicated due to the risk of bullae formation and skin sloughing. Regional blocks are best avoided when the possible complications and risks are weighed against the benefits.

Monitoring should be adequate and kept to a reasonable minimum. No tape or adherent strips may be used in placing intravenous (IV) catheters, ECG leads, or oximeter probes. Properly padded and applied, a pneumatic tourniquet and blood pressure cuff can usually be used without producing bullae. The skin should be prepared by pouring appropriate solutions over the extremity. Conventional scrubbing is contraindicated.

There are several anesthetic considerations. Among them are malnutrition, electrolyte imbalance, anemia, secondary skin infection, amyloidosis, and porphyria. Once the patient has been thoroughly evaluated and every attempt made to restore a relatively normal physiologic status, elective surgical or dental procedures can be considered. The technical aspects of the anesthetic administration are very important. Each patient requires an individualized approach.

Intravenous and intramuscular ketamine[1-5] have been used as a sole anesthetic agent when muscle relaxation was not required. Glycopyrrolate is an excellent antisialagogue.[6] For most procedures, inhalation anesthesia and endotracheal intubation are employed.

The child is brought to the operating room in the hospital bed, which should be prepared with a sheepskin and foam padding. A parent may be allowed to accompany the child until anesthesia induction begins. This both decreases anxiety and gains the child's cooperation, thus avoiding the need for restraints during induction. After local preparation of the skin with sterile water or saline, an IV cannula is placed in the dorsum of the hand or wrist. Although barbiturates have been used without incident, some investigators have considered their use contraindicated because of the reported association with porphyria. However, this association has been questioned.[5, 9-11]

When general anesthesia with inhalation induction is decided upon, airway management represents a major challenge. Induction may be achieved by delivering high flow anesthetic gases with a mask held above the face,[7] and then gradually establishing mask and finger contact on the face, which has been lubricated with hydrocortisone cream. The use of oropharyngeal and nasopharyngeal airways and esophageal stethoscopes or temperature probes should be avoided. If endotracheal intubation is required, it must be gentle and atraumatic and performed only by a well-trained individual. A Macintosh laryngoscope blade is preferred to a straight blade to decrease the potential for supraglottic obstruction should epiglottic bullae form as a result of contact with the laryngoscope blade.

After the patient is well anesthetized, intubation can be accomplished with or without a muscle relaxant. I prefer to intubate the trachea without use of a muscle relaxant because it may be difficult to maintain pressure with the mask and adequately ventilate a paralyzed patient. No complications have been reported with succinylcholine despite the theoretical risk of hyperkalemia in patients with extensive tissue injury. If muscle paralysis is required, it is probably better to select a nondepolarizing agent. Lidocaine, 1.5 to 2 mg, should be given IV to reduce spasm or cough during intubation. An endotracheal tube is selected that is a half size smaller than usually appropriate for the child's age group. The length of the tube is precalculated to avoid carinal stimulation. These precautions are taken to avoid the potential requirement for emergency tracheostomy if upper airway obstruction should occur secondary to tracheal edema, hematoma, or bullae formation. Nasotracheal intubation is best avoided. The tube position should be verified, breath sounds ausculated, and the tube secured with umbilical tape passed around the neck and tied or pinned. No adhesive tape should contact the patient's skin.

Prior to extubation, fiberoptic endoscopy may be carried out to visualize the vocal cords and retropharynx for possible bullae formation. If the tissues are in satisfactory condition, another dose of lidocaine, 1.5 to 2 mg/kg, should be given IV and extubation performed while the child is deeply anesthetized to prevent laryngospasm. Gentle application of low continous positive-airway pressure can be maintained as the child gradually emerges from anesthesia. She should be transferred to the protected bed and transported to the recovery room. As soon as the child is awake, the parent may be allowed to participate in her postoperative care.

REFERENCES

1. Hamann RA, Cohen PJ: Anesthetic management of a patient with epidermolysis bullosa dystrophica. *Anesthesiology* 1971; 34:389–391.
2. Lee C, Nagel EL: Anesthetic management of a patient with recessive epidermolysis bullosa dystrophica. *Anesthesiology* 1975; 43:122–124.
3. LoVerme SR, Oropollo AT: Ketamine anesthesia in dermolytic bullous dermatolysis (epidermolysis bullosa). *Anesth Analg* 1977; 56:398–401.
4. Milne B, Rosales JK: Anesthesia for correction of esophageal stricture in a patient with recessive epidermolysis bullosa dystrophica: Case report. *Can Anaesth Soc J* 1980; 27:169–171.
5. Reddy AR, Wong DH: Epidermolysis bullosa: A review of anesthetic problems and case reports. *Can Anaesth Soc J* 1972; 19:536.
6. Idvall J: Ketamine monoanesthesia for major surgery in epidermolysis bullosa: Case report. *Acta Anaesthesiol Scand* 1987; 7:658–660.
7. Fisk GC, Kern IB: Anaesthesia for oesophagoscopy in a child with epidermolysis bullosa: Case report. *Anaesth Intensive Care* 1973; 1:297.
8. Kelly RE: Regional anesthesia in children with epidermolysis bullosa dystrophica (letter). *Anesthesiology* 1988; 68:469.
9. Tomlinson AA: Recessive dystrophic epidermolysis bullosa. *Anaesthesia* 1983; 38:485.
10. Kaplan R, Strauch B: Regional anesthesia in a child with epidermolysis bullosa. *Anesthesiology* 1987; 67:262.
11. Spargo PM, Smith GB: Epidermolysis bullosa and porphyria. *Anesth Analg* 1988; 67:297.

48

Fontan Procedure

A 6-year-old, 15-kg girl with a diagnosis of tricuspid atresia (Type Ib) is scheduled for a Fontan procedure. She previously had a Glenn shunt. Although she is able to attend school, she cannot participate in any extracurricular activities. Hemoglobin, 17 g/dL; hematocrit, 54%.

Recommendations by Frederick A. Burrows, M.D.

To correctly manage any patient with a congenital cardiac lesion, it is essential that the anesthesiologist be familiar with the child's pathophysiology and understand the implications of any palliative procedures she had previously. Preoperative consultation with the attending cardiologist and cardiovascular surgeon may be necessary before the anesthesiologist can completely appreciate the nuances of the defect and potential implications of the condition.

THE CARDIAC LESION

Tricuspid atresia (TA) is an uncommon form of congenital cardiac lesion that accounts for only 3% of all congenital heart disease.[1,2] Patients with TA have complete agenesis of the tricuspid valve with no direct communication between the right atrium and right ventricle. An interatrial defect, hypoplasia of the right ventricle, and a communication between the systemic and pulmonary circulation, usually a ventricular septal defect (VSD), are invariably present.[1-4] The etiology of TA is unknown.

TA is slightly more common in males (55%).[5] As in all patients with congenital heart lesions, it is important to look for other noncardiac anomalies. Extracardiac anomalies are present in 20% of patients with TA and most often involve the gastrointestinal or musculoskeletal systems.[6] TA has also been associated with the cat-eye syndrome,[7] Christmas disease,[8] Down syndrome, and asplenia.[6]

Intrauterine growth retardation is present in 4% and prematurity, conceptual age less than 36 weeks, in 6%.[6]

There are three main types of TA (Fig 48–1). The clinical picture in TA with diminished or normal pulmonary blood flow is one of cyanosis and its sequelae, whereas in those with excessive pulmonary blood flow, it is acyanosis and heart failure. The latter is a less common form of presentation that often goes unrecognized until the patient is a few months old. It is characteristic of infants with the D-transposition form of defect.

In patients, such as the one presented here, who have a type Ib defect (Fig 48–2,A), central cyanosis is the most frequent presenting sign and often occurs at birth or within the first month of life. The cyanosis results from the obligatory right-to-left shunt through the atrial septal defect. Its intensity is largely dependent on pulmonary blood flow. Cyanosis is most severe in infants with an intact ventricular septum or pulmonary stenosis and least severe in those with a large VSD and heart failure (Types Ic and IIc). Hypoxemia, when severe, is associated with acidemia and leads to hyperventilation caused by stimulation of arterial and cerebral chemoreceptors. Cyanosis may be minimal or absent in patients with transposition of the great arteries and significant pulmonary blood flow. In older patients, chronic hypoxemia results in secondary polycythemia and its consequences.[2, 9–11]

The treatment of patients with TA is surgical. Palliative surgery for all types of TA is designed to improve blood flow. When pulmonary blood flow is too low, palliation increases pulmonary blood flow and thereby encourages development of the pulmonary vascular bed and improves systemic oxygen saturation. When pulmonary blood flow is too high, palliation decreases pulmonary blood flow and the risk of developing pulmonary vascular occlusive disease, a consequence of high pulmonary blood flow and pressure.[12]

Type Ib TA is the most common.[13] Patients with this congenital heart lesion are cyanotic and have pulmonary stenosis, decreased pulmonary blood flow, and a small VSD. Palliative surgery is designed to increase pulmonary blood flow and systemic oxygen saturation and is indicated after they have sustained one or more documented hypoxic spells or have significant or progressive hypoxemia. Palliative surgery, rather than a definitive procedure, may be indicated initially in patients with one or more of the following: increased pulmonary vascular resistance, young age, small pulmonary arteries, atrioventricular valve incompetence, poor ventricular function, and myocardial hypertrophy. Palliative surgery for infants under 1 month of age usually involves a central aortopulmonary shunt with prosthetic material or a subclavian-to-pulmonary artery anastomosis, (a Blalock-Taussig shunt). For those between 1 month and 1 year of age, a Blalock-Taussig shunt is performed. After 1 year of age, a Blalock-Taussig shunt or an anastomosis of the right main pulmonary artery to the superior vena cava, a Glenn shunt,[12, 13] is the preferred procedure. The patient under consideration had a Glenn shunt.

The Glenn procedure, also referred to as cavopulmonary anastomosis or partial right heart bypass, is the most physiologic shunt. The procedure consists of end-to-side anastomosis of the superior vena cava to the right pulmonary artery with complete or partial ligation of the junction of the right atrium and the superior vena cava (Fig 48–2,B). Unlike systemic-to-pulmonary artery shunts, the Glenn shunt increases effective pulmonary blood flow at a low pressure while decreasing total pulmonary blood flow and ventricular volume load.[12]

The Glenn shunt has proved safe; the early mortality rate is only 1%. It is simple to perform, improves oxygen saturation, does not increase pulmonary artery pressure or cardiac work, and grows without distorting the pulmonary artery.[12]

Tricuspid Atresia with Normally Related Great Arteries

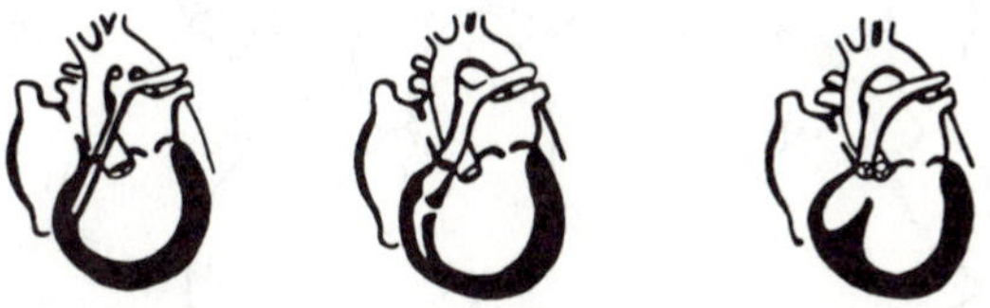

Morphological Type	I(a) Pulmonary atresia with intact ventricular septum	I(b) Pulmonary stenosis, small ventricular septal defect	I(c) Pulmonary stenosis, large ventricular septal defect
Pulmonary Blood Flow	decreased	decreased	normal or increased
Incidence	10%	50%	10%

Tricuspid Atresia with D Transposition of the Great Arteries

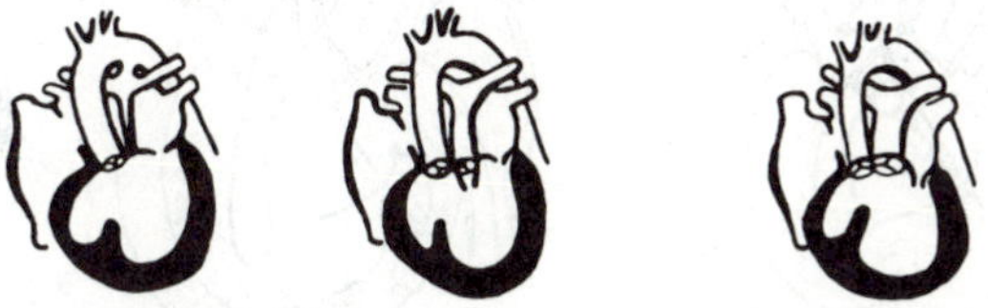

Morphological Type	II(a) Pulmonary atresia, ventricular septal defect	II(b) Pulmonary stenosis, ventricular septal defect	II(c) No pulmonary stenosis, ventricular septal defect
Pulmonary Blood Flow	decreased	normal or decreased	increased
Incidence	2%	8%	17%

Tricuspid Atresia with L Transposition of the Great Arteries

Morphological Type	III(a) Pulmonary / Subpulmonary stenosis	III(b) Subaortic stenosis
Pulmonary Blood Flow	decreased	increased
Incidence	rare	rare

FIG 48–1.
Incidence of morphologic types of tricuspid atresia with the effect of specific lesion on pulmonary blood flow. (Adapted from Vlad P: Tricuspid atresia, in Keith JD, Rowe RD, Vlad P (eds): *Heart Disease in Infancy and Childhood,* ed 3. New York, Macmillan Publishing Co Inc, 1978, pp 518–541.)

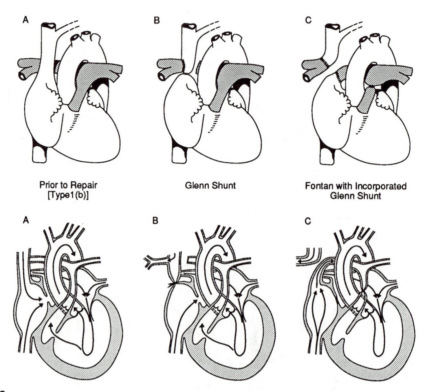

FIG 48–2.

Stages in the repair of type 1b tricuspid atresia: **A,** before repair; **B,** after establishment of a Glenn shunt; and **C,** after Fontan repair. The *arrows* represent the pattern of blood flow through the heart and lungs during each stage.

In general, the Glenn procedure is used only in children with irreparable malformations since taking it down during definitive repair, while feasible, adds to the risk of the repair.[14, 15] It is also an unsatisfactory operation for infants under 6 months of age because their pulmonary arteries are too small. Moreover, in the neonate, the pulmonary vascular resistance may also be elevated, and perfusion from a low-pressure systemic venous vessel may not be possible.[12]

A major disadvantage of the classic end-to-end Glenn shunt, such as the patient described here has undergone (Fig 48–2,B), is the vulnerability of the isolated left pulmonary artery. The residual blood flow into the artery, particularly with the addition of a subsequent shunt, may be sufficient to cause an increase in pulmonary vascular resistance. Alternatively, too little flow over a prolonged period may lead to inadequate growth of the left pulmonary artery. Both conditions can jeopardize a future Fontan operation, and both may be avoided with the use of a bidirectional Glenn shunt. This shunt is an end-to-side anastomosis of the superior vena cava to the ipsilateral pulmonary artery in which the pulmonary arteries remain in continuity[12, 16] (Fig 48–3).

As is evident from the patient presented here, the benefits of a Glenn shunt gradually diminish, usually 6 to 8 years after the anastomosis, at which time some additional procedure is necessary.[17] There are many interrelated reasons for this phenomenon. In some patients, gradual enlargement of collateral venous channels between the superior vena cava and the inferior vena cava occurs, thus

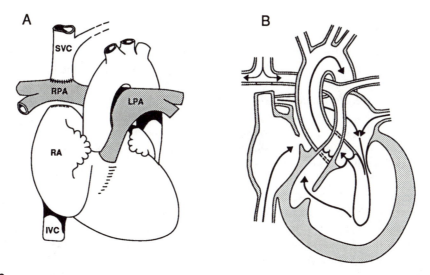

FIG 48–3.
A, schematic of a bidirectional cavopulmonary anastomosis (Glenn shunt) showing the end-to-side anastomosis of the superior vena cava *(SVC)* to the ipsilateral pulmonary artery. The junction of the SVC to the right atrium *(RA)* is oversewn. The pulmonary arteries are in continuity. *RPA* = right pulmonary artery; *LPA* = left pulmonary artery; *IVC* = inferior vena cava. **B,** the *arrows* represent the pattern of blood flow through the heart and lungs.

diminishing the flow through the anastomosis. More often, there is a reduction in blood flow through the contralateral lung either from actual narrowing of the channel (VSD, pulmonary stenosis or shunt) or simply from its failure to grow with the child. Decreased pulmonary blood flow leads to decreased oxygen saturation, polycythemia, increased viscosity, and in turn, diminished flow through the nonpulsatile Glenn shunt.[17]

THE FONTAN PROCEDURE

A Fontan operation has been chosen for the child as the next appropriate surgical step. The Fontan procedure directs vena cava blood to the lungs, while only oxygenated blood returns to the left heart.[18] A right atrial-to-main pulmonary artery direct anastomosis or conduit, with or without a valve, channels the systemic venous return directly into the lung. The atrial septal defect is closed and the main pulmonary artery ligated just above the pulmonary valve. The existing Glenn anastomosis does not have to be disturbed (see Fig 48–2,C). In patients with a systemic-to-pulmonary artery arterial shunt, this shunt must be closed to reduce pulmonary pressure and avoid excessive pulmonary flow.

Patient selection for a Fontan procedure is paramount: special attention must be given to anatomic variations, timing of the operation, pulmonary artery size and resistance, and technical considerations.[19, 20] Candidates are usually between the ages of 4 and 15 years. Patients with a mean preoperative pulmonary artery pressure greater than 15 to 20 mm Hg, pulmonary vascular resistance greater than 4 Wood units/m^2, an ejection fraction less than 0.45, or ventricular end-diastolic pressures greater than 15 mm Hg are poor candidates for Fontan procedures and should be considered for other palliation. With normal or low left atrial pressure, only a small rise in right atrial pressure is necessary to produce adequate pulmonary and systemic flow.

The benefits of a Fontan repair are improved systemic oxygenation and a reduction in the obligatory diastolic load borne by the ventricle that is required to fill systemic and pulmonary circuits. A given level of hypoxemia provides a stimulus to polycythemia that increases with age; thus the deleterious effects of increased blood viscosity become more evident in older children. The compensatory ventricular dilation that must occur in a parallel circuit places that ventricle in an unfavorable position on the Starling curve. Thus, a diastolic load is imposed that, over time, will lead to progressive ventricular dysfunction. Establishing a series circuit in these children will improve oxygenation and favorably alter ventricular geometry as a result of decreased blood volume demands. Glenn shunts, which are not mandatory in the majority of patients but may be advantageous in some, can be incorporated into the Fontan procedure.[21]

Two criteria that clearly influence operative and late results are preoperative pulmonary arteriolar resistance and left ventricular diastolic function. Various criteria exist for the determination of a child's suitability for a Fontan repair. The relatively strict selection criteria proposed by Choussat et al.[19] (Table 48–1) are associated with excellent results. However, acceptable results have been obtained in patients not satisfying one or more of these original criteria.[22] Repair before 4 years of age has been suggested since it may avoid the development of left ventricular dysfunction.[23] Patients older than 15 years of age have successfully undergone repair.[24] Preservation of normal sinus rhythm and contractile atria have not been uniformly mandatory for good results.[25, 26]

Before surgery, pulmonary wedge angiograms, if feasible, can provide important information about the ability of the pulmonary vasculature to accommodate a Fontan repair. A frozen pathologic section from a lung biopsy specimen taken intraoperatively can provide further immediate information about the suitability of the pulmonary vasculature should the patient be considered a borderline candidate.[27]

PREOPERATIVE CONSIDERATIONS

The problems presented by a cyanotic patient with TA relate to her adaptation to chronic hypoxemia, including polycythemia, increased blood volume and vasodilation, neovascularization, and alveolar hyperventilation with chronic respiratory alkalosis.[9] Polycythemia increases the hematocrit and viscosity of the blood and, subsequently, systemic and pulmonary vascular resistance. An increase in hematocrit increases the oxygen-carrying capacity of the blood, but when the hematocrit exceeds 60%, the increased viscosity decreases cardiac output and impairs oxygen delivery, thereby further stimulating red blood cell production. These patients are at increased risk of cerebral and renal thrombosis, particularly if they become dehydrated,[2, 10] and may present preoperatively with a history of thrombotic episodes, residual defects, or both. Patients whose hematocrits exceed 60% to 70% may benefit from preoperative erythropheresis. The anesthesiologist should undertake this procedure in consultation with cardiologists and surgeons. These patients require adequate preoperative hydration and intravenous fluid therapy should begin with the institution of preoperative fasting.

Such cyanotic patients may also have coagulopathies. These are due, in part, to decreased levels of platelets and fibrinogen,[11] which increases the risks of intraoperative and postoperative bleeding.

TABLE 48–1.

Selection Criteria for Fontan Repair*

Mean pulmonary artery pressure <20 mm Hg
Pulmonary vascular resistance <4 Wood units/m^2
Age 4 to 15 yr
Normal sinus rhythm
Left ventricular ejection fraction >0.60
Diameter of the pulmonary artery/aorta ≥0.75
Normal systemic venous drainage
Adequate right atrial volume
No mitral valve dysfunction
No hemodynamic impairment from prior shunts

*Adapted from Choussat A, Fontan F, Besse P, et al: Selection criteria for Fontan's procedure, in Anderson RH, Shinebourne EA (eds): *Pediatric Cardiology 1977*. Edinburgh, Churchill Livingstone, Inc, 1978; pp 559–566.

The need for sedative premedication must be individually assessed and discussed. Many children are mature enough and do not require premedication. Some prefer no or light sedation. Younger children may benefit greatly from preoperative sedation, which makes parental separation and induction of anesthesia less traumatic for the parent, child, and operating room staff.

When sedative premedication is used, our team prefers diazepam, pentobarbital, or midazolam administered orally. Where possible, the drug is administered by a parent. Frequently the child is asleep by the time of separation from the parent. Another potential advantage is the amnestic properties of the drug. These advantages may be important when a young patient requires further operative procedures.

ANESTHETIC MANAGEMENT

For induction of anesthesia, patients should be monitored by means of a noninvasive blood pressure device, an electrocardiograph, a precordial stethoscope, an axillary temperature probe, and pulse oximetry. Many different techniques can be used to safely anesthetize cyanotic children.[28, 29] For sicker and younger children, particularly neonates, high-dose narcotic anesthesia has been shown to safely and effectively blunt cardiovascular and stress responses to anesthesia and surgery.[30–33] Ketamine has also been shown to be safe and to have relatively little effect on hemodynamics in young children with congenital heart disease.[28, 29, 34] Inhalation agents, including nitrous oxide, reduce blood pressure and depress the myocardium to greater degrees than do ketamine[28] and narcotics.[29] Inhalation techniques are also useful in more vigorous children with less severe forms of the disease.[28, 29]

Anesthesia can be safely maintained with either a narcotic, inhalation, or a combined technique, the choice is dependent upon the pre-existing cardiovascular status of the patient. A narcotic technique has the theoretical advantage of producing less myocardial depression and greater cardiac stability in the presence of pre-existing myocardial dysfunction. This patient would receive fentanyl, 50 to 100 μg/kg, and a benzodiazepine such as diazepam, 0.4 mg/kg, have neuromuscular paralysis induced with pancuronium, and receive a supplemental inhalation agent, halothane or isoflurane, as required. We have found that this technique provides adequate anesthesia and analgesia and enables early postoperative extubation.

After the induction of anesthesia and establishment of a stable anesthetic state, the patient is intubated nasotracheally. Two large-bore peripheral intravenous catheters are inserted and arterial cannulation established. Central venous cannulation can be performed, but in the presence of a Glenn shunt, the pressure will reflect only the superior vena caval pressure rather than the right atrial pressure. The catheter can be useful in monitoring right pulmonary artery pressures after the Fontan repair and for the administration of drugs.

Additional monitoring includes rectal, esophageal, and nasopharyngeal temperature readings reflecting core, perfusion, and cerebral temperatures, respectively. Peripheral skin temperature readings indicate peripheral perfusion. The greater the gradient between the peripheral and the core temperatures, the poorer the peripheral perfusion. The usefulness of end-tidal carbon dioxide monitoring is limited in cyanotic patients because of the presence of and the lack of stability of the end-tidal–to–arterial carbon dioxide gradient.[35, 36]

POSTBYPASS MANAGEMENT

Before weaning the patient from cardiopulmonary bypass, transthoracic left and right atrial pressure monitoring catheters are placed to aid postoperative management. Once the patient is weaned from cardiopulmonary bypass, pulmonary perfusion is dependent upon the gradient from the right atrium and the superior vena cava to the left atrium.

The two most important features in the hemodynamics of children who have had a Fontan operation are the left atrial pressure, which reflects the diastolic properties of the ventricle and the function of the systemic atrioventricular valve, and the pulmonary vascular resistance.[37–40]

Pulmonary blood flow is phasic, with a substantial proportion occurring during diastole. Changes in diastolic compliance of the ventricle therefore affect the pulmonary blood flow. Decreases in ventricular diastolic compliance, as occur with altered ventricular geometry or diastolic dysfunction, reduce pulmonary blood flow and therefore preload in the ventricle and result in a decrease in cardiac output. Postoperatively, the volume output of the ventricle must meet only the demands of the systemic circuit, and thus end-diastolic volume is substantially reduced. As the end-diastolic volume decreases, an alteration in ventricular geometry takes place. In some children, the resulting small, hypertrophic ventricle exhibits diastolic dysfunction that was not present at a higher end-diastolic volume.[37–40]

These patients are extremely sensitive to and have a limited ability to compensate for changes in pulmonary vascular resistance. Before repair, the parallel-circuit physiology (see Fig 48–2, A and B) shunts blood away from the lungs when pulmonary vascular resistance increases, thus resulting in hypoxemia. After repair, series-circuit physiology (Fig 48–2,C) replaces the parallel-circuit physiology, and such shunting is not possible. An increase in pulmonary vascular resistance is manifested by a decrease in cardiac output caused by the limited return of blood to the systemic ventricle. This can be described by the following equation:

$$Q_p = (P_{pa} - P_{la})/R_p$$

where Q_p is the pulmonary blood flow, P_{pa} is pulmonary artery pressure, P_{la} is left atrial pressure, and R_p is pulmonary vascular resistance. Common postoperative causes of increased pulmonary vascular resistance include hypoxia, hypercarbia or acidosis, and the mechanical effects produced in the pulmonary artery bed by excessive positive airway pressure and positive end-expiratory pressure or extrinsic pulmonary compression from sources such as pneumothorax and hemothorax or pleural effusions.[37-40]

In the period after cardiopulmonary bypass, the cardiac output can be increased by altering the various variables in the equation. The pulmonary artery pressure (P_{pa}), which is represented by the right atrial or superior vena cava pressure, can be increased by volume loading, thereby increasing the $P_{pa}-P_{la}$ gradient. The left atrial pressure (P_{la}) can be lowered to increase the gradient by improving left ventricular function with inotropic agents such as dopamine or afterload-reducing agents such as sodium nitroprusside or amrinone.

Under ideal conditions, the postoperative right atrial pressure should be less than 20 mm Hg and the gradient between the right atrium and left atrium less than 5 mm Hg. A right atrial pressure greater than 20 mm Hg is associated with a poor prognosis because it implies systemic ventricular dysfunction, and this requires treatment with inotropic agents.[39] A right-to-left atrial pressure gradient greater than 5 mm Hg suggests obstruction of pulmonary blood flow from the right atrium to the left atrium.[37-40]

When the pulmonary artery pressure is less than the right atrial pressure, stenosis at the anastomosis between the right atrium and the pulmonary artery is likely and may be amenable to surgical revision. The obstruction can also be at the level of the pulmonary resistance vessels, in which case the pulmonary artery pressure should equal the right atrial pressure. Obstruction at the resistance vessels can be due to structural causes such as pulmonary vascular occlusive disease or inadequate development of the pulmonary vasculature. Such obstruction is fixed but may regress in the ensuing months to years. Obstruction at the resistance vessels can also be reactive. This reactivity may result in an initial high pulmonary vascular resistance (R_p) that will decrease in the first few days after surgery.

A ventilatory pattern that minimizes mean airway pressure is preferable to maximum pulmonary blood flow. Techniques such as short inspiratory-to-expiratory ratios and the adjustment of positive end-expiratory pressure to the minimal levels necessary to maintain functional residual capacity at normal levels facilitate a low R_p. Minute alveolar ventilation should be adjusted to maintain normocapnia or hypocapnia to further reduce R_p. Other factors that increase R_p and should be aggressively treated include hypoxia, acidemia, hypothermia, and pleural or peritoneal fluid accumulations. R_p may be further reduced by hemodilution or the use of pulmonary vasodilators such as nitroglycerin or sodium nitroprusside. Hemodynamically unstable patients may require continued paralysis and sedation to control fluctuations in R_p.[41] Early extubation is advantageous because it introduces negative intrathoracic pressure, thereby facilitating both venous return and decreasing R_p. One group has shown that early extubation is feasible in more than 50% of these patients.[42]

The importance of atrial contractions is controversial. It has been suggested that a normal sinus rhythm may assist pulmonary artery flow and help maintain a low left atrial pressure in patients who have high preoperative atrial pressures,[19, 43] but it has also been suggested that atrial contractions may actually impede pulmonary blood flow by creating turbulence in patients whose atrial pressures were low preoperatively.[25, 26]

The application of phasic external compression to the lower portion of the body with antishock air pants has been recommended because they relocate peripherally sequestered fluid to the central circulation.[44] This technique appears to augment venous return, decrease the requirement for a large fluid volume infusion, and decrease the incidence of fluid sequestration caused by inadequate right-sided hemodynamics. In our center, the pants have been useful only in very high-risk patients.

POSTOPERATIVE CONSIDERATIONS

Fluid retention with pleural and pericardial effusions is a common postoperative complication. The cause of this fluid retention is unclear but may be related both to the elevated systemic venous pressure and to the activation of inflammatory mediators during cardiopulmonary bypass. Pleural effusions require drainage until the effusion stops. Effusion usually ceases after only a few days but, in up to 30% of patients, may be prolonged. Pericardial effusion can usually be treated with intermittent pericardiocentesis. Persistent recurrence, which occurs in 10% of patients exhibiting pericardial effusion, is an indication for a pericardial window.[45]

Arrhythmias occur postoperatively in up to 50% of patients. Many are transient, do not cause hemodynamic instability, require no intervention, and resolve by the seventh postoperative day. However, significant arrhythmias, particularly supraventricular tachycardias, do occur. Control of the arrhythmias is not difficult to achieve, with the exception of rapidly accelerated junctional rhythms, which are frequently associated with a fatal outcome.[46] The incidence of arrhythmias increases from about 15% on the seventh postoperative day, to 25% after 5 years, and to 37% at 7.5 years after surgery.

Thrombotic complications can occur along the suture lines or other parts of the Fontan repair. Formation of a thrombus in the right atrium or pulmonary artery is a particularly dangerous late complication that is often fatal.[47, 48] These thrombi may be treated by surgical excision or with streptokinase.[48] Cerebral infarction has also been reported.[49] This event may be embolic, associated with arrhythmias, thrombotic, or associated with thrombocytosis or congestive heart failure. Oral anticogulant therapy may be required for several months postoperatively until the patient's hemodynamics have improved and such complications are unlikely.

A protein-losing enteropathy associated with chronic diarrhea and hypoalbuminemia, as well as generalized edema, has also been associated with this procedure.[50] The mechanism of this complication is probably related to higher-than-normal systemic venous pressure resulting in increased lymph production in the drainage area of the inferior vena cava and obstruction of lymph drainage because of high pressure in the superior vena cava and thoracic duct.

The operative mortality rate in good-risk patients is less than 5%.[20, 24] The risk of the operation increases with an increasing number of risk factors and may be as high as 20% to 30%.[23, 24, 51] Perioperative mortality is usually related to compromised pulmonary blood flow, residual shunts, or inadequate cardiac output.[52] Late mortality occurs in approximately 10% of survivors, usually in the first 5 years after the operation, and is most often related to residual obstruction or intracardiac shunts.[52]

Approximately 15% of patients require reoperation for residual intracardiac lesions after a Fontan operation, most commonly in the first year after surgery.[53–55] Reoperation may be required for obstructed atriopulmonary communication, a residual shunt, a dehisced patch, subaortic stenosis, or increasing insufficiency of an atrioventricular valve.

Patients who survive the operation generally do very well. Ninety-eight percent are in the New York Heart Association class I or II, and 97% attend school or work at regular jobs.[24, 56] Most require no medication.

REFERENCES

1. Rosenthal A, Dick M II: Tricuspid atresia, in Adams FH, Emmanouilides GC, Riemenschneider TA (eds): *Heart Disease in Infants, Children, and Adolescents,* ed 4. Baltimore, Williams & Wilkins, 1989, pp 348–361.
2. Nadas AS, Fyler DC: *Pediatric Cardiology,* ed 3. Philadelphia, WB Saunders Co, 1972, pp 565–568.
3. Rowe RD, Freedom RM, Mehrizi A, et al: *The Neonate with Congenital Heart Disease.* Philadelphia, WB Saunders Co, 1983, pp 1186–1203.
4. Gasul BM, Arcilla RA, Lev M: Tricuspid atresia, in Gasul BM, Arcilla RA, Lev M (eds): *Heart Disease in Children. Diagnosis and Treatment.* Philadelphia, JB Lippincott, 1966, pp 565–685.
5. Dick M, Fyler DC, Nadas AS: Tricuspid atresia: Clinical course in 101 patients. *Am J Cardiol* 1975; 36:327–337.
6. Fyler DC, Buckley LP, Hellenbrand WE, et al: Report of the New England regional infant cardiac program. *Pediatrics* 1980; 65(suppl):375–461.
7. Freedom RM, Gerald PS: Congenital cardiac disease and the "cat eye" syndrome. *Am J Dis Child* 1973; 126:16–18.
8. Lawson R, Rullman D, Brodeur M, et al: Tricuspid atresia with Christmas disease (hemophilia B). Report of a case. *J Thorac Cardiovasc Surg* 1975; 69:585–588.
9. Theodore J, Robin ED, Burke CM, et al: Impact of profound reduction of Pao$_2$ on O$_2$ transport and utilization in congenital heart disease. *Chest* 1985; 87:293–302.
10. Phornphutkul C, Rosenthal A, Nadas AS, et al: Cerebrovascular accidents in infants and children with cyanotic congenital heart disease. *Am J Cardiol* 1973; 32:329–334.
11. Kontras SB, Sirak HD, Newton WA Jr: Hematologic abnormalities in children with congenital heart disease. *JAMA* 1966; 195:611–615.
12. Trusler GA, Williams WG, Cohen AJ, et al: The cavopulmonary shunt. Evolution of a concept. *Circulation* 1990; 82(suppl 4):131–138.
13. Vlad P: Tricuspid atresia, in Keith JD, Rowe RD, Vlad P (eds): *Heart Disease in Infancy and Childhood,* ed 3. New York, Macmillan Publishing Co Inc, 1978, pp 518–541.
14. Pacifico AD, Kirklin JW: Take-down of cava-pulmonary artery anastomosis (Glenn) during repair of congenital cardiac malformations. Report of 5 cases. *J Thorac Cardiovasc Surg* 1975; 70:272–277.
15. Rohmer J, Quaegebeur JM, Brom AG: Takedown and reconstruction of cavopulmonary anastomosis. *Ann Thorac Surg* 1977; 23:129–134.
16. Bridges ND, Jonas RA, Mayer JE, et al: Bidirectional cavopulmonary anastomosis as an interim palliation for high-risk Fontan candidates. Early results. *Circulation* 1990; 82(Suppl 4):170–176.
17. Williams WG, Rubis L, Trusler GA, et al: Palliation of tricuspid atresia. Potts-Smith, Glenn, and Blalock-Taussig shunts. *Arch Surg* 1975; 110:1383–1386.
18. Fontan F, Baudet E: Surgical repair of tricuspid atresia. *Thorax* 1971; 26:240–248.
19. Choussat A, Fontan F, Besse P, et al: Selection criteria for Fontan's procedure, in Anderson RH, Shinebourne EA (eds): *Pediatric Cardiology 1977.* Edinburgh, Churchill Livingstone Inc, 1978, pp 559–566.
20. Fontan F, Deville C, Quaegebeur J, et al: Repair of tricuspid atresia in 100 patients. *J Thorac Cardiovasc Surg* 1983; 85:647–660.
21. Pennington DG, Nouri S, Ho J, et al: Glenn shunt: Long-term results and current role in congenital heart operations. *Ann Thorac Surg* 1981; 31:532–539.

22. Mair DD, Hagler DJ, Puga FJ, et al: Fontan operation in 176 patients with tricuspid atresia. Results and a proposed new index for patient selection. *Circulation* 1990; 82(Suppl 4):164–169.

23. Mayer JE Jr, Helgason H, Jonas RA, et al: Extending the limits for modified Fontan procedures. *J Thorac Cardiovasc Surg* 1986; 92:1021–1028.

24. Humes RA, Mair DD, Porter CJ, et al: Results of the modified Fontan operation in adults. *Am J Cardiol* 1988; 61:602–604.

25. Behrendt DM, Rosenthal A: Cardiovascular status after repair by Fontan procedure. *Ann Thorac Surg* 1980; 29:322–330.

26. de Leval MR, Kilner P, Gewillig M, et al: Total cavopulmonary connection: A logical alternative to atriopulmonary connection for complex Fontan operations. Experimental studies and early clinical experience. *J Thorac Cardiovasc Surg* 1988; 96:682–695.

27. Burrows FA, Rabinovitch M: The pulmonary circulation in children with congenital heart disease: Morphologic and morphometric considerations. *Can Anaesth Soc J* 1985; 32:364–373.

28. Greeley WJ, Bushman GA, Davis DP, et al: Comparative effects of halothane and ketamine on systemic arterial oxygen saturation in children with cyanotic heart disease. *Anesthesiology* 1986; 65:666–668.

29. Laishley RS, Burrows FA, Lerman J, et al: Effect of anesthetic induction regimens on oxygen saturation in cyanotic congenital heart disease. *Anesthesiology* 1986; 65:673–677.

30. Hickey PR, Hansen DD: Fentanyl- and sufentanil-oxygen-pancuronium anesthesia for cardiac surgery in infants. *Anesth Analg* 1984; 63:117–124.

31. Hickey PR, Hansen DD, Wessel DL, et al: Blunting of stress responses in the pulmonary circulation of infants by fentanyl. *Anesth Analg* 1985; 64:1137–1142.

32. Hickey PR, Hansen DD, Strafford M, et al: Pulmonary and systemic effects of nitrous oxide in infants with normal and elevated pulmonary vascular resistance. *Anesthesiology* 1986; 65:374–378.

33. Moore RA, Yang SS, McNicholas KW, et al: Hemodynamic and anesthetic effects of sufentanil as the sole anesthetic for pediatric cardiovascular surgery. *Anesthesiology* 1985; 62:725–731.

34. Morray JP, Lynn AM, Stamm SJ, et al: Hemodynamic effects of ketamine in children with congenital heart disease. *Anesth Analg* 1984; 63:895–899.

35. Burrows FA: Physiological dead space, venous admixture and the arterial to end-tidal carbon dioxide difference in infants and children undergoing cardiac surgery. *Anesthesiology* 1989; 70:219–225.

36. Lazzell VA, Burrows FA: Stability of the intraoperative arterial to end-tidal carbon dioxide partial pressure difference in children with congenital heart disease. *Can J Anaesth* 1991; 38: 859–865.

37. DiSessa TG, Child JS, Perloff JK, et al: Systemic venous and pulmonary arterial flow patterns after Fontan's procedure for tricuspid atresia or single ventricle. *Circulation* 1984; 70:898–902.

38. Ishikawa T, Neutze JM, Brandt PWT, et al: Hemodynamics following the Kreutzer procedure for tricuspid atresia in patients under two years of age. *J Thorac Cardiovasc Surg* 1984; 88:373–379.

39. Sanders SP, Wright GB, Keane JF, et al: Clinical and hemodynamic results of the Fontan operation for tricuspid atresia. *Am J Cardiol* 1982; 49:1733–1740.

40. Kirklin JW, Barratt-Boyes BG: Tricuspid atresia, in Kirklin JW, BG (eds): *Cardiac Surgery. Morphology, Diagnostic Criteria, Natural History, Techniques, Results, and Indications*. New York, John Wiley & Sons Inc, 1986, pp 857–888.

41. Burrows FA, Klinck JR, Rabinovitch M, et al: Pulmonary hypertension in children: Perioperative management. *Can Anaesth Soc J* 1986; 33:606–628.

42. Barash PG, Lescovich F, Katz JD, et al: Early extubation following pediatric cardiothoracic operation: A viable alternative. *Ann Thoracic Surg* 1980; 29:228–233.

43. Nakazawa M, Nakanishi T, Okuda H, et al: Dynamics of right heart flow in patients after Fontan procedure. *Circulation* 1984; 69:306–312.

44. Heck HA Jr, Doty DB: Assisted circulation by phasic external lower body compression. *Circulation* 1981; 64:118–122.

45. Britton LW, Mayer JE, Galinanes M, et al: Effusive complications of Fontan procedures (abstract). *Circulation* 1986; 74:49.

46. Kürer CC, Tanner CS, Norwood WI, et al: Perioperative arrhythmias after Fontan repair. *Circulation* 1990; 82(suppl 4):190–194.

47. Dobell ARC, Trusler GA, Smallhorn JF, et al: Atrial thrombi after Fontan operation. *Ann Thorac Surg* 1986; 42:664–667.

48. Dajee H, Deutsch LS, Benson LN, et al: Thrombolytic therapy for superior vena caval thrombosis following superior vena cava-pulmonary artery anastomosis. *Ann Thorac Surg* 1984; 38:637–639.

49. Mathews K, Bale JF Jr, Clark EB, et al: Cerebral infarction complicating Fontan surgery for cyanotic congenital heart disease. *Pediatr Cardiol* 1986; 7:161–166.

50. Hess J, Kruizinga K, Bijleveld CMA, et al: Protein-losing enteropathy after Fontan operation. *J Thorac Cardiovasc Surg* 1984; 88:606–609.

51. Mair DD, Rice MJ, Hagler DJ, et al: Outcome of the Fontan procedure in patients with tricuspid atresia. *Circulation* 1985; 72(suppl 2):88–92.

52. Sade RM: Tricuspid atresia, in Sabiston DC, Spencer FC (eds): *Gibbon's Surgery of the Chest*. Philadelphia, WB Saunders Co, 1981, pp 457–479.

53. Coles JG, Kielmanowizc S, Freedom RM, et al: Surgical experience with the modified Fontan procedure. *Circulation* 1987; 76(suppl 3):61–66.

54. Kirklin JK, Blackstone EH, Kirklin JW, et al: The Fontan operation. Ventricular hypertrophy, age, and date of operation as risk factors. *J Thorac Cardiovasc Surg* 1986; 92:1049–1064.

55. Laks H, Milliken JC, Perloff JK, et al: Experience with the Fontan procedure. *J Thorac Cardiovasc Surg* 1984; 88:939–951.

56. Humes RA, Porter CJ, Mair DD, et al: Intermediate follow-up and predicted survival after the modified Fontan procedure for tricuspid atresia and double-inlet ventricle. *Circulation* 1987; 76(suppl 3):67–71.

49

Masseter Spasm

A 6-year-old, 22-kg girl is anesthetized for an appendectomy. Anesthesia is induced with 75 mg thiopental. Atropine, 0.2 mg, and succinylcholine, 20 mg, are then administered. The anesthesiologist is unable to open the patient's mouth to perform laryngoscopy. Blood pressure, 90/60 mm Hg; pulse, 120; oxygen saturation, 98%.

Recommendations by Barbara W. Brandom, M.D.

It is presumed that the difficulty encountered in opening this patient's mouth is due to spasm of the masseter muscles. Therefore, the child must have demonstrated normal mouth opening prior to the administration of succinylcholine.

DIFFERENTIAL DIAGNOSIS OF MASSETER SPASM

Masseter spasm is an increase in tension of the masseter. The most strict definition is that this tension is so great that the jaw cannot be forced open. Therefore, the definition is subjective. By this definition the child described in this case did experience masseter spasm. Although masseter spasm occurs in pediatric patients most often after the administration of succinylcholine following induction of anesthesia with halothane, it may occur after the administration of barbiturates and other anesthetic agents.[1]

Once anesthetic drugs have been administered, there are several reasons why the mouth may resist opening by the anesthesiologist. Increased tension in the masseter may accompany "light" anesthesia. The dose of thiopental is less than 3.5 mg/kg. The child with normal circulatory function often requires a larger dose of thiopental to induce anesthesia than does the adult. A dose of 4 to 6 mg/kg may be expected to produce a loss of the lash reflex in an unpremedicated healthy child.[2, 3] Loss of the lash reflex is a sign of depression of reflex activity but occurs at a lighter plane of an-

337

esthesia than is required to facilitate intubation without neuromuscular blockade. If more potent anesthetics are not administered, intravenously or via the lungs, the child's reflexes will rapidly become more active. Thus, after the administration of 75 mg of thiopental, without premedication or administration of other general anesthetic agents, we may assume that the child was lightly anesthetized.

To facilitate intubation of the trachea in the lightly anesthetized child it is essential to administer enough neuromuscular blocking drug to induce complete paralysis of the masseter. If there is a difference between the response of the adductor pollicis and the masseter to a bolus of succinylcholine, the masseter is more sensitive, and blockade will occur more rapidly in the masseter.[4] Therefore, if after the administration of succinylcholine no movement of the thumb can be evoked, neuromuscular transmission in the masseter should be fully blocked.

If neuromuscular function is not tested after administration of succinylcholine, the anesthesiologist can only guess that the drug has produced neuromuscular blockade in the masseter. The dose of succinylcholine administered, 20 mg, is equivalent to 0.9 mg/kg in this child. This dose is at least twice the 95% effective dose (ED_{95}) of succinylcholine in the child during balanced anesthesia.[5] However, the ED_{95} is the estimated dose that will produce 95% blockade of evoked neuromuscular function in the average patient. It is customary to administer larger multiples of the ED_{95} of succinylcholine. For example, a dose of 1 mg/kg of succinylcholine in the adult is equivalent to more than three times the ED_{95}. Marked variability in the degree of neuromuscular blockade produced by a smaller dose of succinylcholine has been observed.[5, 6] One possible reason is variability in the function of pseudocholinesterase. As well as a genetic variation in pseudocholinesterase activity that results in a 30% more rapid degradation of substrate than usual, there are many acquired causes of increases in pseudocholinesterase activity.[7] Elevations in pseudocholinesterase function may be more common in the pediatric than in the adult population.[8] The authors of a recent study of succinylcholine, which included two pediatric patients who were markedly resistant to the effects of this drug, suggested that a dose of at least 2 mg/kg of succinylcholine should be administered to facilitate intubation during nitrous oxide-narcotic-sedative anesthesia in the pediatric patient.[5]

The timing of laryngoscopy in this case may have been less than optimal. The onset of blockade of neuromuscular function is expected to occur in the masseter before it occurs in the adductor pollicis.[9] Yet, at the same time that neuromuscular transmission is blocked, there is an increase in the tension of the masseter that acts to close the jaw.[9-13] If the anesthesiologist waited until there was no evoked movement of the thumb, laryngoscopy might have been attempted at the time when tension in the masseter was greatest.[10] Although the average child with normal pseudocholinesterase function would have no neuromuscular function in the masseter for several minutes after intravenous administration of this dose of succinylcholine, the increased tension of the masseter could preclude laryngoscopy. During anesthesia with potent inhalation agents the increase in resting tension that follows the administration of succinylcholine has been noted to range from undetectable to so strong that the mouth can not be opened (Fig 49-1).[11] The increased masseter tension can be exacerbated by increased epinephrine concentrations in the blood.[14] Thus the difficulty experienced in opening this child's mouth could be a normal response to succinylcholine. The scenario of "light" anesthesia in an "emergency" procedure may make a perceptible increase in jaw tension after the administration of succinylcholine more likely.

In summary, the differential diagnosis of the inability to open the mouth after the administration

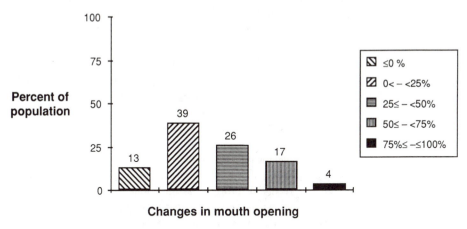

Mouth opening changes after succinylcholine

FIG 49–1.
Distribution of mouth opening in a sample population. (From Van Der Spek AFL, Fang WB, Ashton-Miller JA, et al: *Anesthesiology* 1988; 69:11–16. Used by permission.)

of succinylcholine includes anatomic abnormalities that make jaw opening difficult under any circumstances, inadequate anesthesia, inadequate paralysis, and increased tension secondary to the administration of succinylcholine.

POTENTIAL ASSOCIATION WITH MALIGNANT HYPERTHERMIA

It has been claimed that 50% of patients who experience masseter spasm are susceptible to malignant hyperthermia (MH) as indicated by in vitro caffeine-halothane contracture testing.[1] Certainly MH can be triggered by the administration of succinylcholine, and masseter spasm is an expected result of the administration of succinylcholine. However, the incidence of MH and masseter spasm in the general population of pediatric anesthetics differs by close to two orders of magnitude. Given the results of a recent review of over 42,000 anesthetics in which succinylcholine was administered to pediatric patients anesthetized with potent inhalation agents,[15] one might argue that masseter spasm is likely to be associated with enough damage to muscle to produce measurable myoglobin release and elevation of creatine phosphokinase levels in the blood postoperatively, but much less likely to be associated with the metabolic aberrations indicative of MH.

ANESTHETIC IMPLICATIONS

The most immediate implication of masseter spasm in this case is that an attempted rapid-sequence induction has failed. Cricoid pressure should be maintained. If a nasogastric tube is in place, it should be allowed to drain by gravity. Ventilation with 100% oxygen should be performed with low peak airway pressures. The anesthesiologist then faces the first decision of whether surgery should be continued or cancelled. In this case, there is an emergent need for surgery. The patient's vital signs and oxygen saturation are acceptable. Therefore, more anesthetic should be administered either intravenously or by inhalation. If paralysis is evident in the patient's hands or feet, it is certainly futile to administer more succinylcholine. The increase in jaw tension may last as long as paralysis induced by succinylcholine (Fig 49–2).[11] The anesthesiologist can wait for jaw rigidity to dissipate spontaneously. However, there have been cases where jaw rigidity persisted longer than the anticipated surgery (personal experience at Children's Hospital of Pittsburgh). An alternative is to administer a nondepolarizing neuromuscular blocking agent. My clinical opinion is that this is rapidly followed by improved jaw mobility, but I cannot separate my experience with atracurium-induced paralysis following masseter spasm from the possibility that the spontaneous resolution of the increased tension was also rapid.

After the airway is secured, the anesthesiologist should be concerned with documentation of vital signs, including temperature. It is likely that this patient, with the clinical signs of appendicitis, had a fever preoperatively. She also received atropine during induction of anesthesia. The usual measures utilized to maintain body heat in the pediatric patient should be avoided. She should remain outside the occlusive drapes in so far as possible. There should be a mattress under the patient that could be turned to cooling temperatures. It is up to the anesthesiologist to decide whether the degree of abnormality in vital signs warrants symptomatic treatment of fever or tachycardia. Respiratory parameters such as tidal volume, respiratory rate, fresh gas flow, and inspired and expired

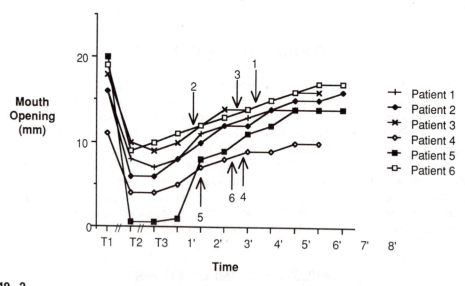

FIG 49–2.
Changes in mouth opening over time in six patients who received 1.5 mg/kg succinylcholine intravenously and who had mouth opening reduction of 50% or more at T2 or T3. T1 is the time at which baseline measurements were taken, T2 represents the loss of adductor pollicis twitch to ulnar nerve stimulation, and T3 is 45 seconds after T2 followed by intervals of 1 minute. *Arrows* indicate a return of the first visible twitch in each patient. (From Van Der Spek AFL, Fang WB, Ashton-Miller JA, et al: *Anesthesiology* 1988; 69:11–16. Used with permission.)

carbon dioxide concentrations must be documented. As anesthesia proceeds, there is usually a decrease in core temperature and a decline in expired carbon dioxide tension. If this does not occur and tachycardia unrelated to the surgical stimulus persists, a venous blood sample should be obtained to assess acid-base status. Since the anesthesiologist can proceed with these evaluations of physiologic status, the only reason not to proceed with emergency surgery would be that no dantrolene was available.

If there is significant respiratory or metabolic acidosis out of proportion to the degree of fever, the anesthesiologist should presume that the patient is developing MH and administer dantrolene while continuing with a "nontriggering" anesthetic. It is noteworthy that in the group of 57 pediatric patients who had anesthesia continued without the administration of dantrolene after isolated masseter spasm occurred,[15] a relatively mild mixed acidosis was documented with average values of P_{CO_2}, 50 mm Hg; pH 7.23; and base deficit, 6 mEq/L. Yet these patients had no adverse response to anesthesia other than myoglobin in their serum and/or urine. The decision to administer dantrolene has implications beyond the immediate prophylaxis against MH. The hypotonic effects of dantrolene can persist for hours. The medical record will label the patient who has received dantrolene for suspected MH, MH susceptible until proved otherwise.

Masseter spasm may be accompanied by evidence of injury to muscle without significant evidence of MH. Injury to muscle reflected by elevation of serum creatine phosphokinase levels is nonspecific. However, injury to muscle will be of clinical significance if sufficient myoglobin is released to threaten renal function. Myoglobin appears in the blood within minutes after the administration of succinylcholine. The presence of myoglobinuria can be assessed by dipstick of the urine for blood. A positive reaction with Hematest (orthotolidine) indicates the presence of myoglobin or hemoglobin. If the test findings are negative, there is no significant amount of myoglobin in the urine. If the results are positive, generous urine output should be ensured while further diagnostic tests are performed.

When masseter spasm complicates the induction of anesthesia for emergency surgery, more vigilance is required in the management of the anesthetic and the postoperative care of the patient. It is much more difficult to know what the implications of this anesthetic complication should be for the future anesthetic management of the patient and her family. It is necessary to document all relevant signs and physiologic and laboratory parameters in the medical record. If the label of MH susceptibility is applied, it may be difficult and costly for the family to remove it. However, it is often simple to adjust an anesthetic plan to avoid drugs most likely to induce an episode of MH.

REFERENCES

1. Larach MG, Rosenberg H, Larach DR, et al: Prediction of malignant hyperthermia susceptibility by clinical signs. *Anesthesiology* 1987; 66:547–550.
2. Coté CJ, Goudsouzian NG, Liu LMP, et al: The dose response of thiopental for the induction of general anesthesia in unpremedicated children. *Anesthesiology* 1981; 55:703–705.
3. Jonmarker C, Westrin P, Larsson S, et al: Thiopental requirements for induction of anesthesia in children. *Anesthesiology* 1987; 67:104–107.
4. Plumley MH, Bevan JC, Saddler JM, et al: Dose-related effects of succinylcholine on the adductor pollicis and masseter muscles in children. *Can J Anaesth* 1990; 37:15–20.

5. Meakin G, McKiernan EP, Morris P, et al: Dose-response curves for suxamethonium in neonates, infants and children. *Br J Anaesth* 1990; 62:655–658.

6. Liu LMP, DeCook TH, Goudsouzian NG, et al: Dose-response to intramuscular succinylcholine in children. *Anesthesiology* 1981; 55:599–602.

7. Whittaker M: Cholinesterase, in *Monographs in Human Genetics,* vol 11. New York, S Karger AG, 1986, pp 14, 73, 74.

8. Hutchinson AD, Widdowson EM: Cholinesterase activities in the serum of healthy British children. *Nature* 1954; 169:284–285.

9. Saddler JM, Bevan JC, Plumley MH, et al: Jaw muscle tension after succinylcholine in children undergoing strabismus surgery. *Can J Anaesth* 1990; 37:21–25.

10. Leary NP, Ellis FR: Masseteric muscle spasm as a normal response to suxamethonium. *Br J Anaesth* 1990; 64:488–492.

11. Van Der Spek AFL, Fang WB, Ashton-Miller JA, et al: Increased masticatory muscle stiffness during limb muscle flaccidity associated with succinylcholine administration. *Anesthesiology* 1988; 69:11–16.

12. Van Der Spek AFL, Fang WB, Ashton-Miller JA, et al: The effects of succinylcholine on mouth opening. *Anesthesiology* 1987; 67:459–465.

13. Van Der Spek AFL, Reynolds PI, Fang WB, et al: Changes in resistance to mouth opening induced by depolarizing and nondepolarizing neuromuscular relaxants. *Br J Anaesth* 1990; 64:21–27.

14. Pryn SJ, Van Der Spek AFL: Comparative pharmacology of succinylcholine on jaw, eye, and tibialis muscle. *Anesthesiology* 1990; 73:A859.

15. Littleford JA, Patel LR, Bose D, et al: Masseter muscle spasm in children: Implications of continuing the triggering anesthetic. *Anesth Analg* 1991; 72:151–160.

50

Near-Drowning

A previously healthy 6-year-old boy falls through the ice while skating with a friend. A period of about 30 minutes elapses before the ambulance team arrives and commences cardiopulmonary resuscitation (CPR). On arrival at the local hospital 10 minutes later he remains pulseless and apneic, and the electrocardiogram (ECG) shows a flat tracing. He is intubated and ventilated with 100% oxygen, and aggressive cardiac resuscitation is continued. Arterial blood gas pH, 7.08; rectal temperature, 24°C.

Recommendations by Peter N. Cox, M.B., Ch.B., F.F.A.R.C.S., F.R.C.P.(C)

With annual deaths amounting to over 2,000,[1] drowning ranks as the number two cause of accidental death in children in the United States. Often more devastating, however, are those who survive the initial insult only to die at a later stage or to be left with a severe neurologic deficit. It has been estimated that for every child who dies, eight survive and, of this number, one or two will survive in a persistent vegetative state. The impact economically, both in terms of years of productive life lost and the direct dollar cost to society is enormous, not to mention the emotional effect of a childhood death or impaired survival on the family.[2]

The thrust of research over the past 20 years has been aimed at improving the quality of the survivors by more widespread knowledge of resuscitation techniques and more effective in-hospital treatment regimens. Since neither has made a significant difference to outcome, more recent research has focused on attempting to find prognostic indicators to guide the emergency room physician's dilemma of whether to resuscitate or not and, if commenced, at what stage to abandon further attempts at resuscitation. An excellent, well-referenced review of near-drowning may be found in the work of Bohn.[3]

THE HISTORY

As in this case, most drowning victims would have CPR initiated at the scene of the accident. Because the degree of neurologic injury is directly related to the duration of hypoxemia, the emergency room physician should attempt to establish the period of submersion, important but often unreliable information. More important is ascertaining the presence or absence of vital signs at the scene of the accident and at what stage vital signs were first detected after initiation of CPR. Where the drowning occurred may be an important guide to water temperature and its effect on final outcome. Whether the drowning occurred in fresh or salt water, while of experimental and theoretical interest, has not been shown to be of clinical significance.[4] Both may damage the alveolar capillary basement membrane, inactivate surfactant, and lead to a picture of noncardiogenic pulmonary edema.

EMERGENCY ROOM MANAGEMENT

In the pulseless victim arriving in the emergency room full resuscitative measures should be taken, including immediate intubation and ventilation with 100% oxygen and the use of appropriate cardiac drugs and sodium bicarbonate. Since a metabolic acidosis is invariably present, sodium bicarbonate should be used empirically if blood gas results are not available. Intravenous fluid should be given in sufficient quantities to replace sequestered fluid and maintain adequate blood pressure. Inotropic drugs may be added once filling volumes are adequate. Overhydration may aggravate the existing brain injury and should therefore be avoided. Because large quantities of water may be swallowed prior to loss of consciousness, it is important that the stomach be emptied to decrease the risk of further fluid and electrolyte shifts and to prevent aspiration of gastric contents. In the presence of hypothermia the heart is unlikely to respond to resuscitative efforts and is also prone to arrhythmias. Active rewarming should therefore commence as early as possible in the resuscitation. A rapid and thorough clinical examination should be performed to exclude medical conditions that may have precipitated the drowning process. A minimal number of diagnostic studies is indicated and should include a chest x-ray and determination of arterial blood gases, hematocrit, electrolytes, blood urea nitrogen, and creatinine. These act both as a baseline and as a guide to resuscitation.

Selection of the method of rewarming is guided principally by the patient's clinical status and the measured rectal temperature. A low-temperature thermometer must be used. Passive surface warming, or limiting of further heat loss, is reserved for the mildly hypothermic patient with a temperature greater than 35°C. Active surface rewarming, or the addition of exogenous heat by water mattress or immersion in warm water, is indicated for more severe cases of hypothermia in which the temperature is 33 to 35°C and the circulation intact. Patients with inadequate circulation require rapid active core warming. Warmed intravenous fluids (40°C) and warmed humidified inspired gases (40 to 45°C) are the most effective and least invasive of these methods of rewarming. Lavage of body cavities, i.e., peritoneal, gastric, rectal, and pleural, with warm fluids is well described and very effective but rarely necessary. Although partial cardiopulmonary bypass has been used for rewarming, it is usually not a practical option. Previous controversy over the appropriate rate of rewarming and the associated risk of cardiac arrhythmias and after-drop, or further core cooling, has now largely been resolved. Numerous studies demonstrate that with appropriate and meticulous management of fluid shifts, rapid active rewarming of the severely hypothermic patient is both safe and effective.[5]

The questions of whether and when to discontinue resuscitation have no easy answers. A number of retrospective studies have attempted to correlate both clinical findings and measured physiologic variables with outcome. These variables include duration of submersion, rapidity and aggressiveness of resuscitation, Glasgow Coma Scale (GCS) scores on arrival, pH in the emergency room, and fixed dilated pupils. Of these, the only factor that appears to be positively correlated with a good outcome is the presence of vital signs in the emergency room.[4, 6–8] However, a core temperature of less than 33°C at presentation may be associated with a full recovery in an apparently lifeless child with a GCS score of only 3 or 4. Furthermore, the diagnosis of death may be difficult to distinguish from the clinical effects of hypothermia. Based on this information, we recommend that aggressive CPR be continued at least until the core temperature is 33°C in children who have sustained hypothermic submersion of less than 1 hour in duration. If appropriate resuscitation and rewarming cannot increase the core temperature after 60 minutes, we would desist. Likewise, if there is no spontaneous cardiac output at a temperature of 33°C and after a period of 60 minutes, further attempts at resuscitation should be abandoned.

Unfortunately, the outcome for children presenting in the emergency room with vital signs absent after warm-water drowning is dismal. While it is often possible to achieve sinus rhythm with sufficiently aggressive resuscitation in this group of patients, the poor potential for intact neurologic recovery should be considered. Current evidence would suggest that at best the outcome of this group is a persistent vegetative state and therefore to continue resuscitation beyond a reasonable period as described above is inappropriate.

INTENSIVE CARE MANAGEMENT

While all patients with a significant history of near-drowning should be admitted to a general ward for at least 24 hours of observation, any patient who has required CPR, has abnormal arterial blood gas values, or has abnormal chest x-ray findings should be admitted to an intensive care unit. The goal of therapy in the hospital is to minimize further organ damage due to the initial insult and possible complications arising from this. Since many of the therapeutic interventions required to support these patients carry their own inherent risk, physicians should be wary of not further aggravating the injury.

The extent of the neurologic injury is directly related to the duration of hypoxia. While it makes theoretical sense that prompt restoration of adequate oxygen supply, reduction of oxygen demand, and control of intracranial pressure should prevent further injury and allow cells with reversible damage to recover, this has not been borne out in practice. Aggressive cerebral protection protocols using induced hypothermia, barbiturate coma, and monitoring and control of intracranial pressure have not been shown to be superior to less aggressive management protocols.[9, 10] Intracranial pressure monitoring has, however, taught us that certain preventable factors, including hypercarbia, overhydration, hypertension, hypoxia, hyperthermia, and seizures, may increase intracranial pressure and cerebral oxygen requirements and therefore jeopardize viable neurologic tissue. Our current therapeutic regimen is therefore aimed at preventing these factors. Controlled hyperventilation to a $Paco_2$ of 25 to 30 mm Hg is combined with adequate oxygenation and fluid restriction to 30% of maintenance. Muscle relaxants are used to prevent rises in intracranial pressure secondary to abnormal movements, and body temperature is kept in the normal range. If the patient presents with or develops seizure activity, phenobarbital or phenytoin is added in appropriate doses. We continue this mode of treatment for 24 to 36 hours, at which point we discontinue the use of muscle relaxants, normalize the CO_2, and do a repeat neurologic assessment. Patients who show neurologic improvement are weaned further, whereas those showing no improvement or who have abnormal movement have a baseline electroencephalograph (EEG) and somatosensory evoked potentials performed and therapy continued for a further 24-hour period before reassessment and possible discontinuation of aggressive support.

The etiology of the lung injury in near-drowning is multifactorial, with hypoxemia being the major clinical consequence. Aspiration of fluid induces disruption of the capillary basement membrane and inactivation of pulmonary surfactant. Resultant pulmonary edema leads to decreased pulmonary compliance, increased intrapulmonary shunting, loss of lung volume, and a ventilation-perfusion mismatch that is manifested clinically as respiratory distress syndrome (RDS). This initial damage may be further aggravated by oxygen and ventilator therapy. Goals of treatment are therefore to maintain adequate oxygenation while minimizing the risks of oxygen toxicity and barotrauma. If the spontaneously breathing patient cannot maintain a Po_2 of 60 mm Hg with an Fio_2 less than 0.4, positive-pressure ventilatory support is indicated. Positive end-expiratory pressure (PEEP) is the mainstay of this support and is an effective means of recruiting alveoli and increasing the functional residual capacity (FRC). Mechanical ventilation may be required, and it is effectively achieved with conventional modes of ventilation.

It cannot be overemphasized that *oxygen in high concentrations, i.e., Fio_2 greater than 0.5, is toxic* and plays a major role in the development of RDS. Aggressive use of PEEP and acceptance of somewhat lower Po_2 values, in the range of 60 mm Hg, may minimize this risk.

Near-drowning victims are at increased risk of infection both from exogenous and endogenous sources. As well as aspiration of potentially contaminated water, the hypoxic insult may damage the integrity of the gut mucosa and allow translocation of bacteria normally confined to the gastrointestinal tract. It has also been demonstrated that hypothermia per se impairs host defense mechanisms and reduces the release of neutrophils from bone marrow.[9] It is not our policy to use prophylactic antibiotics routinely, but rather to institute them for specific indications. Careful monitoring for septic complications including daily cultures of blood, sputum, and urine should be performed.

OUTCOME

Many studies over the last 20 years have attempted to define predictors of poor prognosis. Numerous variables have been studied, often with conflicting results. However, in the normothermic, comatose near-drowned patient, the absence of vital signs and the presence of a severe acidosis in the emergency room is consistently associated with a poor outcome. Hypothermia may impart a degree of cerebral protection, and this group of patients should be rewarmed and stabilized prior to the definitive assessment of coma.

REFERENCES

1. Wintemute GJ: Childhood drowning and near-drowning in the United States. *Am J Dis Child* 1990; 144:663–669.
2. Guyer B, Ellers B: Childhood injuries in the United States: Mortality, morbidity and cost. *Am J Dis Child* 1990; 144:649–652.
3. Bohn DJ: Resuscitation after near-drowning and exposure, in Baskett PJF (ed): *Monographs in Anaesthesiology: Cardiopulmonary Resuscitation.* Amsterdam, Elsevier Science Publishers, 1989.
4. Modell JH, et al: Clinical course of 91 consecutive near drowning victims. *Chest* 1976; 70:231.
5. Edsall DW: Treatment of hypothermia. *JAMA* 1980; 244:1902.
6. Biggart MJ, Bohn DJ: Effect of hypothermia and cardiac arrest on outcome of near-drowning accidents in children. *J Pediatr* 1990; 117:179–183.
7. Jacobsen WK, et al: Correlation of spontaneous respiration and neurologic damage in near-drowning. *Crit Care Med* 1983; 11:487–489.
8. Kemp AM, Sibert JR: Outcome in children who nearly drown: A British Isles study. *Br Med J* 1991; 302:931–933.
9. Bohn DJ, et al: Influence of hypothermia, barbiturate therapy, and intracranial pressure monitoring on morbidity and mortality after near-drowning. *Crit Care Med* 1986; 14:529–534.
10. Nussbaum E, Maggi JC: Pentobarbital therapy does not improve neurologic outcome in nearly drowned, flaccid-comatose children. *Pediatrics* 1988; 81:630–634.

51

Laser Surgery for Laryngeal Papillomas

A 6-year-old, 20-kg girl is scheduled for laryngoscopy and probable excision of laryngeal papillomas. She is hoarse but in no respiratory distress. Hemoglobin, 13.5 g/dL; hematocrit, 37.5%.

Recommendations by T.C.K. Brown, M.D., F.A.N.Z.C.A., F.C.A. (UK)

Stridor is the result of abnormal airflow through the larynx. It can be due to postintubation stenosis, a functional disturbance of the larynx due to damage to nerves or muscles, extrinsic compression, swelling of the mucosa, infection, the presence of a foreign body, or a growth within the larynx such as a papilloma. A hoarse voice may be an accompanying symptom, particularly if the vocal cords are involved.

If there is significant obstruction associated with the lesion, the accessory muscles of respiration may be used. There may be a tracheal tug or indrawing of the lower portion of the thorax on inspiration. The breathing pattern may be modified to allow gas flow in and out past the obstruction. The general principle of pressure = flow × resistance is helpful in considering the clinical features. The obstruction will require a greater negative pressure in inspiration to maintain the same respiratory flow, or there will be slower flow if the same pressure is generated.

THE HISTORY AND PHYSICAL EXAMINATION

A preoperative history and examination are important. A papilloma is usually slow growing, so the symptoms develop gradually. Papillomas may grow on any part of the larynx and may be sessile or pedunculated. If the latter is between the vocal cords, aphonia may develop. It is important to assess the severity of obstruction because this may influence the choice of anesthesia. While indirect laryngoscopy can be helpful, it may be difficult for a 6-year-old to cooperate. It may be easier to demonstrate the lesion with fiber-optic laryngoscopy. Lateral and anteroposterior (AP) x-ray films of the neck may show the presence of a foreign body if it is radiopaque, or soft-tissue radiographs or a computed tomographic (CT) scan can demonstrate the location of a mass. It is uncommon to pursue the diagnosis to this extent since laryngoscopy will usually reveal the problem. A diagnostic laryngoscopy can be performed with the patient under anesthesia; if a papilloma is found, microlaryngeal laser surgery can then take place.

There is a choice whether or not to use premedication. In some centers parents attend induction of anesthesia. If the parent wants to attend and is assessed as being able to cope, premedication will not usually be needed. If the parents do not attend, some anesthesiologists administer premedication. The choice depends on local tradition and drug availability. An oral benzodiazepine can provide anxiolysis and amnesia. Some children, particularly those coming for repeat removal of papillomas, elect to have no premedication.

ANESTHETIC MANAGEMENT

There are several options for the anesthetic technique. These include inhalation induction and maintenance, intravenous induction with thiopental followed by inhalation anesthesia, and intravenous anesthesia with propofol infusion and fentanyl or alfentanil. Ventilation may be controlled and a muscle relaxant utilized. Whichever technique is used, once the level of anesthesia is deep enough to allow laryngoscopy, the vocal cords should be sprayed with 4% lidocaine, up to 4 mg/kg. Occasionally high plasma levels over 10 μg/mL have been recorded with this dose, although the mean peak level in children is usually below 6 μg/mL.[1]

Inhalation induction and maintenance with halothane is usually regarded as the safest approach, especially if a significant degree of obstruction is present. In such cases uptake is slow and induction prolonged. Care should be taken to ensure that the pupils are central before spraying the vocal cords with local anesthetic; otherwise laryngeal spasm may occur. The concentration of halothane should be increased as tolerated to 4% until laryngoscopy can be performed. It is desirable to have intravenous access and to administer atropine to prevent the bradycardia that occurs with deep halothane anesthesia and with laryngoscopy.

If the degree of obstruction is not serious, anesthesia may be induced with thiopental or another intravenous agent. A small dose of succinylcholine can be given to undertake preliminary diagnostic laryngoscopy. If it is decided to proceed to laser therapy, halothane can be introduced as the patient's ventilation is assisted while the relaxant wears off.

The problem with inhalation anesthesia for these procedures is atmospheric pollution. However, this can be significantly reduced by placing a suction device near the patient's mouth or at the laryngoscope exit during laser microsurgery.

Hepatitis following repeat halothane anesthesia in children is exceedingly rare,[2, 3] and it has not occurred in our patients having repeated laser surgery. One patient has had nearly 200 anesthetics for treatment of papillomas.

The intravenous technique with propofol and alfentanil or fentanyl obviates the atmospheric pollution and is a useful alternative. It has the advantage of slowing respiration, which makes directing the laser easier. A minor problem is that the dose of propofol varies widely between patients,[4] as does the dose of midazolam, which some anesthesiologists use as an alternative.

When muscle relaxants and intermittent positive-pressure breathing (IPPB) are used, intubation or jet ventilation is required. The small airway in this patient precludes the use of a special microsurgery tube. Any tube will obstruct the operator's view, and the laser will ignite most tubes, especially if high oxygen concentrations are present.[5] Tubes wrapped in foil or special nonflammable tubes can be used in older patients. Metal tubes are safe from ignition but, if not made nonreflective, can reflect laser beams so that other tissues can be damaged. Jet ventilation carries a higher risk of barotrauma, especially in children.

Fires have occurred during microlaryngeal laser surgery, with tubes igniting in the presence of high oxygen concentrations. Ideally an inhalation agent should be delivered in air with only enough oxygen added to maintain adequate oxygen saturation.

My choice of anesthesia is to use a halothane or thiopental induction, depending on the degree of obstruction. Atropine is administered intravenously, and deep halothane-in-air is supplemented with local anesthesia. I would maintain spontaneous ventilation without intubation. This provides optimal surgical exposure and avoids the fire hazard and the likelihood of postoperative laryngeal edema.

Monitoring should include at least precordial stethoscopy because heart sounds become softer as cardiac output decreases if anesthesia becomes too deep, as well as pulse oximetry. Careful clinical observation of the patient is essential. Other precautions should include protection of the upper teeth with a mouthguard and protection of the eyes with tape to prevent corneal abrasion by the drapes.

When the microlaryngoscope is inserted, the gases can be insufflated via a catheter placed into the light carrier or via a nasal catheter in the back of the pharynx out of view of the laser beam. As the procedure progresses, the halothane concentration can be reduced, although a higher-than-expected concentration is often needed because the surgeon's suction apparatus removes some of the anesthetic.

Occasionally a child presents with very severe obstruction, and a tracheostomy may be required. On rare occasions this must be performed as an emergency procedure. It should be done with a small endotracheal tube in place if one can be inserted. The microlaryngeal laser surgery can then be performed with the anesthetic administered via the tracheotomy. Some tracheostomy tubes are flammable if hit by a laser beam in the presence of a high oxygen concentration. Care must be taken to place a moist barrier between the lesion being lasered and the tracheotomy tube, and a high oxygen concentration must be avoided. Alternatively, a metal tracheotomy tube can be used.

These patients require careful postoperative observation. Supplemental oxygen should be administered. The chance of developing postoperative laryngeal edema is less with laser excision than with previously employed surgical methods. It will also be reduced by avoiding endotracheal intubation.

The natural history of the disease is for the papilloma to recur. In some patients, papillomas regress spontaneously after a year or two, but in others they persist for years and the children require repeated anesthetics. Antiviral agents have been tried with limited success.

It must also be remembered that the staff must be protected from eye damage by wearing protective glasses. Accidentally misdirected or reflected laser beams can be a source of injury to personnel as well as patients.

REFERENCES

1. Eyres RL, Bishop W, Oppenheim RC, et al: Plasma lignocaine concentration following topical laryngeal application. *Anaesth Intensive Care* 1983; 11:23.
2. Wark H: Postoperative jaundice in children. *Anaesthesia* 1983; 38:237.
3. Wark H, O'Halloran M, Overton J: Prospective study of liver function in children following multiple halothane anaesthetics. *Br J Anaesth* 1986; 58:1224.
4. Leslie K, Crankshaw DP: Potency of propofol for loss of consciousness after a single dose. *Br J Anaesth* 1990; 64:734.
5. Snow JC: Fire hazards of tubes with laser. *Anesth Analg* 1976; 55:146.

52

Lung Biopsy and AIDS

A 2-year-old boy with documented acquired immunodeficiency syndrome (AIDS) is scheduled for open lung biopsy to confirm the diagnosis of *Pneumocystis carinii* infection. Blood pressure, 85/45; pulse, 120; respirations, 35 and labored; temperature, 38.5° C. Hemoglobin, 7.5 g/dL; hematocrit, 22%; WBC count, 2,500; platelet count, $30,000 \times 10^9$/L.

Recommendations by Kim R. Weigers, M.D., Charles H. Lockhart, M.D.

First described in 1982, pediatric acquired immunodeficiency syndrome (AIDS) cases have continued to increase at an alarming rate. The Centers for Disease Control (CDC) documented approximately 3400 pediatric AIDS cases as of December, 1992.[1] More and more of these children will be admitted to hospitals and will require a variety of operative procedures, including central venous access placement, open lung biopsy, bronchoscopy, and various gastrointestinal (GI) procedures. It is imperative that anesthesiologists have a clear understanding of the disease process and clinical implications, before and during administration of an anesthetic.

AIDS

The causative agent of AIDS is the human immunodeficiency virus (HIV), a human T-lymphotropic retrovirus. As the virus duplicates and the disease process continues, T-lymphocytes are damaged or destroyed, leading to cell-mediated immunodeficiency. The development of a variety of opportunistic infections, including *Pneumocystis carinii*, cytomegalovirus, atypical mycobacterial infections, and herpes virus, as well as unusual malignancies (Kaposi's sarcoma being the most common) are hallmarks of the disease. Diagnosis of HIV infection is accomplished with enzyme-linked immunosorbent assay (ELISA) and Western blot tests, which detect antibody to HIV-1 virus.[2] It is important to remember that all infants born to HIV-positive mothers, while not actually having the disease, will have the HIV antibody for anywhere from 6 to 15 months, due to transplacental transmission of maternal IgG. Of these infants, approximately 30% to 40% will become infected and progress to producing their own antibody after 15 months. Since the source of antibody production is unknown for those children under 15 months, all pediatric patients under 15 months born to HIV-positive mothers should be considered infected and appropriate precautions taken. While over 80% of the children are infected secondary to transplacental exposure, other sources of transmission include transfusion and coagulation factor therapy, 13% and 5%, respectively.[3]

Clinically manifested infections with the AIDS virus are varied and often devastating. Unquestionably, the primary organ system affected in HIV-infected children are the lungs. Of the many opportunistic infections that occur, *Pneumocystis carinii* is the most prevalent and damaging.

Pneumocystis carinii PNEUMONIA

With few exceptions, *Pneumocystis carinii* pneumonia (PCP) only afflicts the immunocompromised or immunosuppressed patient. Early diagnosis is imperative because the mortality from respiratory failure of untreated PCP approximates 100%. Prognosis is related to severity of pulmonary impairment, as reflected by the degree of hypoxia at the time of diagnosis. Thus, an early aggressive approach to diagnosis and treatment is recommended.

Initial signs and symptoms of PCP are fever up to 40° C and nonproductive cough, followed by tachypnea, dyspnea, and coryza. Although cyanosis and severe respiratory distress occur later, early arterial blood gas analysis demonstrates abnormalities disproportionate to early clinical findings. Right-to-left intrapulmonary shunting of blood due to infiltration of alveoli by organisms and inflammatory exudate leads to arterial hypoxemia accompanied by respiratory alkalosis. A chest x-ray generally shows diffuse bilateral interstitial infiltrates. Early in the disease, the infiltrates are central in location and may not be thought clinically significant. However, a high index of suspicion, because of this patient's underlying disease, should lead to further aggressive efforts at diagnosis.

The diagnosis of PCP usually depends on microscopic identification of the organism in lung tissue. Serologic determinations for antiginemia have improved reliability but are not regarded as diagnostic. The organisms reside in the alveoli and are usually not found in the bronchial tree. Because of this, identification in sputum or bronchial washings is unreliable. Deep endobronchial brush biopsy and closed lung biopsy have been used; however, open lung biopsy has consistently proven the most reliable for recovery of the organism. Following diagnosis, trimethoprim-sulfamethoxazole (Bactrim) is the treatment of choice.

NONPULMONARY MANIFESTATIONS OF HIV INFECTION

Cardiac involvement is being recognized more frequently in HIV-infected children.[3] Manifestations include right and left ventricular dysfunction, pericardial effusion, dysrhythmias, pericarditis, and myocarditis. Echocardiograms are often abnormal. Interestingly, some children develop an exaggerated heart rate and blood pressure response to medication, possibly due to an autonomic neuropathy.

Many pediatric patients will develop CNS abnormalities with HIV infection.[3] These include a progressive encephalopathy and motor dysfunction characterized by spasticity, pseudobulbar signs, movement disorders and cerebellar signs, and loss of milestones and behavioral changes. Other serious neurologic complications associated with HIV infection are primary CNS lymphomas, stroke, and bacterial infections. Unlike adults, opportunistic infections of the CNS system are rare in the pediatric population.

Renal changes are significant in children with documented HIV infection. From 5% to 10% of patients will develop nephrotic syndrome with proteinuria, hypoalbuminemia, and edema. A small percentage subsequently progress to a full-blown picture of renal failure. Gastrointestinal alterations secondary to HIV infection often present with failure to thrive due to chronic diarrhea, as well as mucocutaneous candidiasis, which is reported to occur in up to 75% of patients. Hepatitis also occurs in these children.[3]

Hematologic manifestations are varied, sometimes culminating in depression of all cell lines. Anemia, thrombocytopenia, lymphopenia, and neutropenia are due to a variety of causes including malnutrition, chronic disease, drug therapy, and primary marrow failure. Drugs administered to HIV infected patients, such as zidovudine (AZT) and trimethoprim-sulfa methazole (Bactrim), may actually contribute to some of the hematologic alterations. Other nonspecific manifestations that may be present are lymphadenopathy, enlarged parotid glands, and craniofacial dysmorphic features making careful examination of the airway essential.

PREVENTION OF HIV INFECTION

Without a cure on the horizon and the high mortality rate associated with AIDS, two very important questions arise for anesthesiologists caring for these patients: (1) How do we protect ourselves? (2) How do we protect our patients? Universal precautions should be adhered to at all times while caring for all patients with potentially transmissible diseases. These include wearing gloves, fluid-resistant masks, face shields or protective eyewear, and gowns.[4, 5] The incidence of seroconversion from a needle puncture of an HIV-positive patient is approximately 1:200, mandating meticulous disposal of needles, scalpels, and other sharp instruments used in the operating room. Needles should never be recapped by hand and a puncture-resistant container must be available for proper disposal of all sharp instruments. Availability of emergency ventilation devices to prevent direct mouth-to-mouth contact with any infected patients is important. Even if protective gloves are worn, thorough handwashing by all health care workers is necessary to prevent further spread of the disease. Every health care institution should have a protocol detailing procedures to be followed when an employee sustains an accidental needle puncture when caring for a patient known or suspected to be HIV-positive.

Though blood and blood components represent the greatest risk for transmission of HIV, as well as hepatitis B and C, universal precautions should be followed for semen, vaginal secretions, human tissues, and other fluids, such as cerebrospinal, synovial, pleural, peritoneal, pericardial, and amniotic. In addition, any other fluid or bodily secretion, especially if contaminated with blood, must be handled in an appropriate fashion.

PREOPERATIVE EVALUATION

Preoperative assessment in this 2-year-old patient begins with a thorough history and physical examination. Auscultation of the chest is often misleading, with breath sounds being normal despite the patient being clinically dyspneic. Rales are not a common physical sign in the early stages of the disease. A chest x-ray is, of course, essential, to evaluate the extent of pulmonary involvement. Laboratory examination includes a CBC, serum electrolytes, BUN, urinalysis, creatinine level, and liver function studies. Arterial blood gases would be useful. Due to actual invasion of cardiac myocytes by the virus, a significant cardiomyopathy may be present and the echocardiogram may demonstrate ventricular dysfunction or chamber hypertrophy. An ECG would assist in diagnosing any dysrhythmia that might require further evaluation and treatment.

Careful examination of the airway is mandatory in these children. Generalized lymphadenopathy in the cervical and mandibular area, as well as parotid gland enlargement, may significantly distort upper airway anatomy or restrict temporomandibular joint movement, making laryngoscopy difficult. Use of the fiberoptic bronchoscope to facilitate intubation and control of the airway may be necessary.

When severe bone marrow suppression is present, significant anemia, thrombocytopenia, and leukopenia may exist. Although granulocyte transfusions are not generally recommended, transfusion with other blood components may be necessary preoperatively to correct anemia and thrombocytopenia. Transfusion with red blood cells (RBC) to correct anemia is encouraged to maximize oxygen-carrying capacity while minimizing the risk of volume overload and contamination with other potentially antigenemic or infectious factors carried in the buffy coat or plasma fractions. The hematocrit of donor RBC varies according to the method of concentration used in the blood bank. Simple gravity sedimentation, centrifugation, or differential centrifugation with cell washing may be utilized. The latter method usually provides a suspension of approximately 65% RBC in saline. Assuming a hematocrit of 65%, each 10 mL of RBC per kg of body weight infused should result in a 9% to 10% increase in the patient's hematocrit. This patient should receive a preoperative RBC transfusion of 15 mL/kg to increase his hematocrit to approximately 35%. Ideally, the blood would be given slowly, preferably in divided increments, 48 and 24 hours preoperatively. When time is critical, 10 mL/kg administered over two hours preoperatively is acceptable.

Platelet transfusion should be delayed until the immediate preoperative period. Guidelines vary for "safe" platelet count levels to assure adequate surgical hemostasis. This patient presents with $30,000 \times 10^9$/L, which would generally be the minimal acceptable level. Concentrations of $100,000 \times 10^9$/L are preferable. If not given preoperatively, platelet concentrates should be immediately available for use intraoperatively and postoperatively. Each unit of platelet concentrate has a volume of approximately 50 mL. Guidelines for administration are 1 unit of platelet concentrate for each square meter of body surface area, resulting in an increase in platelet count of approximately $10,000 \times 10^9$/L. One unit of concentrate per 10 kg of body weight should increase the count approximately $40,000 \times 10^9$/L.

Premedication should be administered judiciously because of preexisting pulmonary compromise and incipient respiratory failure. Midazolam, 0.5 mg/kg mixed in a flavored syrup, administered orally 30 to 40 minutes before surgery, is an effective anxiolytic without respiratory depression, at this dose and route of administration.

ANESTHETIC MANAGEMENT

Intraoperative considerations for this patient would include those normally employed in any child undergoing thoracotomy. Placement of an arterial catheter should be considered both for blood pressure monitoring and blood sampling during surgery and postoperatively when there is high risk of respiratory failure due to progressive lung disease and the superimposed thoracotomy incision.

Induction can be accomplished either by inhalation of volatile anesthetics or IV administration of anesthetic agents. An inhalation induction must be completed in an orderly fashion, with 0.5% increments of halothane being added every 6 to 10 breaths. Addition of nitrous oxide would be helpful in reducing halothane requirements and speeding induction, but must be considered in light of the pulmonary disease and need for supplemental oxygen. A slow induction should be anticipated because sensitive irritable airways will not tolerate sudden changes in halothane concentration. Patience is a virtue that will be rewarded by absence of cough, breath-holding, or laryngospasm. Following a successful induction, placement of an IV cannula should be completed under strict aseptic conditions as soon as possible.

An IV induction would be a favored alternative, especially for patients coming to the operating room with an IV in place. After application of all appropriate monitors, atropine, 0.01 mg/kg, should be administered to prevent bradycardia and subsequent hypotension during the operative procedure. For induction, either thiopental, 4 to 5 mg/kg, or propofol, 2 to 3 mg/kg, could be chosen, followed by a nondepolarizing muscle relaxant once control of the airway has been obtained. Titration of narcotics, such as fentanyl or morphine, would be of benefit in controlling the intraoperative stress response and managing postoperative pain.

Following intubation, controlled positive-pressure ventilation will be necessary due to the nature of the procedure. The dosage requirement for volatile agents, either halothane or isoflurane, may be attenuated by concomitant use of muscle relaxants and narcotics during the operative procedure. Any significant end-organ damage due to the disease process may have an effect on metabolism and the subsequent half-life of IV agents.

POSTOPERATIVE CARE

The decision concerning postoperative ventilation must be based on preoperative evaluation of the severity of the pulmonary disease, intraoperative blood gas and lung compliance assessments, and the degree of surgical intervention. Consideration should be given to intraoperative intercostal nerve block with bupivacaine to minimize immediate postoperative respiratory compromise due to chest wall splinting secondary to pain. In any case, it is likely that immediate extubation in the operating room will be difficult and perhaps inadvisable in most instances. However, the anesthetic plan outlined will not preclude early extubation in the recovery room. This may be further facilitated by the IV administration of an analgesic such as fentanyl, 1 to 2 μg/kg, as the operation approaches conclusion. Weaning from the ventilator should be accomplished as soon as possible. This may be feasible in the recovery room in one to two hours, or it may require several days of respiratory support concurrent with treatment of the primary disease. The ability to maintain spontaneous ventilation, adequate oxygenation, and an appropriate level of consciousness with protective airway reflexes present are the parameters to be assessed.

The adequacy of spontaneous ventilation is evidenced by maintenance of a normal Pa_{CO_2} with a reasonable respiratory rate. Weaning from ventilatory support may best be accomplished by decreasing the rate of intermittent mandatory ventilation (IMV) while observing for evidence of respiratory distress and measuring arterial blood gases. During IMV, the possibility of interstitial air leak or pneumothorax must be kept in mind. Poor lung compliance may result in high airway pressures during positive-pressure ventilation. Although the affected side will be partially protected by closed chest tube drainage, contralateral lung barotrauma can also occur. A chest roentgenogram and physical examination are necessary immediately prior to extubation. During the weaning process, arterial oxygenation should also be evaluated. The Pa_{O_2} should be in the normal range, with an F_{IO_2} of 0.4 or less.

The perioperative mortality for patients with *Pneumocystis carinii* pneumonia subjected to open lung biopsy has been reported to be as high as 2.5%. While progression of PCP is a major factor in mortality, expert anesthetic and postoperative respiratory management can substantially reduce the risk.

REFERENCES

1. Morbidity and Mortality Weekly Report 1992; 41:28–29.
2. Husson RN, Comeau AM, Hoff R: Diagnosis of human immunodeficiency virus infection in infants and children. *Pediatrics* 1990; 86:1–9.
3. Schwartz D, Schwartz T, Cooper E, et al: Anaesthesia and the child with HIV infection. *Can J Anaesth* 1991; 38:626–633.
4. Kunkel SE, Warner MA: Human T-cell lymphotropic virus type III (HTLV-III) infection: How it can affect you, your patients and your anesthesia practice. *Anesthesiology* 1987; 66:195–207.
5. Warner MA, Kunkel SE: Human immunodeficiency virus infection. *Anesthesiol Clin North Am* 1989; 7:795–810.

53

Open Eye Injury

A healthy 7-year-old, 30-kg boy sustained an open eye injury while playing. The accident occurred one-half hour after he ate lunch. The ophthalmologist thinks the eye is salvageable and surgery should be performed as soon as possible. The child is crying uncontrollably. Hemoglobin, 12 g/dL; hematocrit, 36%.

Recommendations by Lawrence S. Berman, M.D

Ophthalmic injuries are the most common cause of loss of vision in children. In many cases, vision can be saved by primary repair of the laceration. Because the alternative to primary repair is enucleation and the repair should be done as soon as possible to prevent infection and loss of ocular contents, maximum effort is made to operate without delay.[1] A detailed examination of the child's eye is frequently postponed until after the induction of anesthesia. The eye should be protected with a shield until the repair.

Injuries that penetrate the eye present two problems for the anesthesiologist: loss of the ocular contents and thus blindness in the eye, and regurgitation and aspiration of gastric contents with the induction of anesthesia.

With an open eye, the intraocular pressure (IOP) is essentially zero.[2] Any factor that increases, IOP in an intact eye may cause loss of the intraocular contents. IOP may be influenced by anesthetics, pressure from extraocular structures, stress, or choroidal volume.

EFFECTS OF ANESTHETIC AGENTS ON INTRAOCULAR PRESSURE

Halothane,[3] enflurane,[4] and isoflurane[5] in combination with nitrous oxide and oxygen have been shown to decrease or have no effect on IOP. Thiopental,[6] when given alone, has also been found to decrease IOP. Ketamine has varied effects on IOP.[7] In one study, ketamine, 8 mg/kg administered intramuscularly, decreased IOP. The authors suggested that the decrease was due to relaxation and cooperation by the patients during control measurements. In another study, IOP increased after intramuscular administration of ketamine, 5 mg/kg,[8] and peaked at 15 minutes in patients accustomed to the procedures of IOP measurement preoperatively and not premedicated. Since ketamine is also associated with nystagmus and blepharospasm, it may not be the ideal agent for induction in this case. Pressure from extraocular structures can also affect IOP. One previous study[7] suggests that a patient's struggling may increase IOP.

Succinylcholine without pretreatment with nondepolarizing muscle relaxants increases IOP.[9] This may be due either to muscle fasciculations caused by succinylcholine, which increase the pressure of the eye, to the cardiorespiratory stress of intubation, or to a direct effect of succinylcholine on the eye. The efficacy of attenuating the rise in IOP induced by succinylcholine by pretreatment with nondepolarizing muscle relaxants is controversial.[9] A 10-year experience in which a small dose of nondepolarizing muscle relaxant was administered prior to succinylcholine has been reported without a single instance of expulsion of global contents or aspiration of gastric contents.[10]

In one study, rapid-sequence induction of anesthesia using thiopental, 5 mg/kg, with either succinylcholine or atracurium caused no increase in IOP with either technique.[11] Induction was accomplished within 25 seconds, and the trachea was intubated at 60 seconds. IOP was raised from a baseline of 13.0 mm Hg by only 0.2 mm Hg at 1 minute. The IOP continued to increase 0.93 mm Hg at 2 minutes and then proceeded to fall. When atracurium was used for rapid-sequence induction, the patients were intubated at 2 minutes. IOP fell 4.7 mm Hg at 1 minute and 4.8 mm Hg at 2 minutes after induction. In general, nondepolarizing muscle relaxants alone do not raise IOP. Pancuronium[12] and fazadinium[13] do not raise IOP, and curare actually lowers it.[12]

Another group looked at rapid-sequence induction with either atracurium, 1.0 mg/kg, or vecuronium, 0.2 mg/kg.[14] While both groups of patients showed a fall in IOP, from 19 to 17 mm Hg following atracurium, and 23 to 17 mm Hg following vecuronium, the IOP began to increase after that and 1 minute after intubation rose to 24 mm Hg after atracurium and 27 mm Hg after vecuronium. The authors stressed that the anesthesiologist should minimize the cardiovascular stress of intubation as reflected by increases in blood pressure and heart rate. A follow-up study[15] in which sufentanil or fentanyl was administered in conjunction with thiopental for rapid-sequence inductions with the same muscle relaxants showed no rise in IOP. This lack of increase may have been due to blockade of an increase in blood pressure by the narcotics.

Within the physiologic range, changes in choroidal volume with changes in blood pressure usually have little effect on IOP.[2] However, changes in venous pressure may markedly affect IOP. An increased central venous pressure as the result of laughing, crying, or straining against an endotracheal tube may cause choroidal blood volume to increase immediately. A cough can produce an IOP of 40 mm Hg or more, which may be sufficient to cause the loss of ocular contents through a lacerated eye.

ASPIRATION OF GASTRIC CONTENTS

Aspiration of gastric contents poses a grave risk to the child with a full stomach and may account for up to 25% of anesthetic-related deaths.[16] Measures to decrease the risk of aspiration are to delay surgery until the stomach empties, perform an awake intubation, or use a rapid-sequence induction. Waiting for the stomach to empty may increase the risk of blindness in the injured eye. In addition, pain and anxiety may slow gastric emptying. Struggling and coughing during an awake intubation would increase IOP and risk loss of the ocular contents. Therefore, a rapid-sequence induction is the procedure of choice.

Attempts should be made to decrease the risks of aspiration. Premedicating the patient with 0.3M sodium citrate[17] to neutralize the gastric acid and the administration of H_2 receptor antagonists to modify gastric pH may be beneficial. Cimetidine, 7.5 mg/kg, is effective in decreasing the pH of gastric fluid if given 1 to 3 hours preoperatively.[18] While these drugs are of some assistance, they will not prevent aspiration. Although the gastric pH will be increased and the volume of fluid may be decreased, particles of partially digested food may also be present and can, in fact, cause more extensive lung damage.

RAPID-SEQUENCE INDUCTION

A rapid sequence induction consists of preoxygenation, induction of general anesthesia, administration of a muscle relaxant to facilitate endotracheal intubation, and rapid and accurate endotracheal intubation. Pressure should be applied to the cricoid before the induction of anesthesia and continued until the intubation is complete and the cuff of the endotracheal tube inflated if a cuffed tube is used, and the position of the tube verified by auscultation and/or capnography. Cricoid pressure may prevent regurgitation of gastric contents into the oropharynx despite an intraesophageal pressure of 100 cm H_2O.[19] Suction may be lifesaving in the event of emesis, and the suction apparatus must be set up and checked before induction.

Laryngoscopy and endotracheal intubation should be performed as soon as the patient is adequately relaxed. One indication of relaxation is the cessation of spontaneous ventilation. A nerve stimulator also assists in indicating the loss of muscle function. If possible, the patient should breathe 100% oxygen for 3 to 5 minutes before induction. He will then be adequately oxygenated, and no attempt should be made to assist ventilation prior to intubation. An alternative to breathing oxygen for several minutes is to have the patient breath 100% oxygen while taking four deep breaths.[20] This will provide denitrogenation equivalent to breathing 100% oxygen at rest. Mask ventilation is avoided because air may be forced into the stomach, thereby increasing intragastric pressure and the risk of vomiting and aspiration.

Although not the technique of choice, inhalation induction can be performed with halothane if an intravenous cannula cannot be inserted preoperatively.[21] As respiration becomes depressed, gentle assistance may be given if the airway is adequate and ventilation does not expand the stomach. As anesthesia deepens and the patient relaxes, gentle endotracheal intubation may be performed without the aid of a muscle relaxant. After the trachea has been intubated, the intravenous catheter is inserted and a muscle relaxant administered. Although risky, this technique may be necessary in a patient in whom vascular access has not been established and whose crying and struggling may lead to loss of the intraocular contents.

The correct size of endotracheal tube is important. Too large a tube is difficult to insert and might increase the risk of complications such as croup or subglottic stenosis. A loose-fitting tube may make ventilation difficult and may not protect the airway from aspiration of stomach contents. The addition of a cuff to an endotracheal tube improves the fit of the tube and helps prevent aspiration. Cuffed endotracheal tubes may be used in children over 6 to 7 years of age. A tube size 0.5 mm smaller than the calculated size should be used.[22] A high-volume, low-pressure cuff may decrease the risk of tracheal damage from the tube.

Heavy premedication should be avoided. Atropine, 0.015 to 0.02 mg/kg, should be administered to minimize the risk of bradycardia secondary to the oculocardiac reflex,[23] but it can be given intravenously during or shortly after induction of anesthesia.

PREFERRED ANESTHETIC TECHNIQUE

An intravenous route should be obtained preoperatively. The child is already crying uncontrollably, and little further increase in IOP may be anticipated when inserting the catheter. After noninvasive monitoring devices are applied, the child then breathes 100% oxygen for 3 to 5 minutes. Atropine, 0.02 mg/kg, should be given prior to induction and tachycardia noted. A small dose of a nondepolarizing muscle relaxant, such as vecuronium, 0.01 mg/kg, is also administered approximately 3 minutes prior to induction. Cricoid pressure should be applied and thiopental, 4 mg/kg, and succinylcholine, 1.5 to 2.0 mg/kg, administered rapidly. Upon cessation of spontaneous ventilation, usually 45 to 60 seconds, the child's trachea is intubated with a 5.5-mm cuffed endotracheal tube. The cuff should be inflated and the lungs ventilated. Upon assurance that both lungs are being ventilated and after identifying CO_2 by capnography or mass spectroscopy, cricoid pressure may be removed. An alternative to using succinylcholine would be the administration of vecuronium, 0.1-0.15 mg/kg, or atracurium, 0.5 mg/kg, for muscle relaxation prior to intubation.

Anesthesia can be maintained with any inhalation agent. A potential intraoperative complication is initiation of the oculocardiac reflex—bradycardia with pressure on the globe or tension on the eye muscles. Treatment includes atropine, 0.02 mg/kg intravenously, and temporary cessation of surgical manipulation.

Extubation under deep anesthesia may decrease coughing at that time but may also increase the risk of aspiration. Because most patients tend to cough later if they are extubated early,[2] the patient is best extubated only after adequate muscle strength and airway reflexes have been demonstrated.

REFERENCES

1. Paton D, Goldberg MF: *Management of Ocular Injuries*. Philadelphia, WB Saunders Co, 1976, pp 205–214.
2. Holloway KB: Control of the eye during general anesthesia for intraocular surgery. *Br J Anaesth* 1980; 52:671.
3. Al-Abrak MH, Samuel JR: Further observations on the effects of general anaesthesia on intraocular pressure in man: Halothane in nitrous oxide and oxygen. *Br J Anaesth* 1974; 46:756.
4. Runciman JD, Bowen-Wright RM, Welsch NH, et al: Intraocular pressure changes during halothane and enflurane anaesthesia. *Br J Anaesth* 1978; 50:371.
5. Ausinsch B, Graves SA, Munson ES, et al: Intraocular pressures in children during isoflurane and halothane anesthesia. *Anesthesiology* 1975; 42:167.
6. Joshi C, Bruce DL: Thiopental and succinylcholine: Action on intraocular pressure. *Anesth Analg* 1975; 54:471.

7. Ausinsch B, Rayburn RL, Munson ES, et al: Ketamine and intraocular pressure in children. *Anesth Analg* 1976; 55:773.

8. Yoshikawa K, Murai Y: The effect of ketamine on intraocular pressure in children. *Anesth Analg* 1971; 50:199.

9. Cook JH: The effect of suxamethonium on intraocular pressure. *Anaesthesia* 1981; 36:359.

10. Libonati MM, Leahy JJ, Ellison N: The use of succinylcholine in open eye surgery. *Anesthesiology* 1985; 62:637.

11. Edmondson L, Lindsay SL, Lanigan LP, et al: Intra-ocular pressure changes during rapid sequence induction of anaesthesia. *Anaesthesia* 1988; 43:1005.

12. Al-Abrak MH, Samuel JR: Effects of general anaesthesia on the intraocular pressure in man: Comparison of tubocurarine and pancuronium in nitrous oxide and oxygen. *Br J Ophthalmol* 1974; 58:806.

13. Couch JA, Eltringham RJ, Magauran DM: The effect of thiopentone and fazadinium on intraocular pressure. *Anaesthesia* 1979; 34:586.

14. Schneider MJ, Stirt JA, Finholt DA: Atracurium, vecuronium, and intraocular pressure in humans. *Anesth Analg* 1986; 65:877.

15. Stirt JA, Chiu GJ: Intraocular pressure during rapid sequence induction: Use of moderate-dose sufentanil or fentanyl and vecuronium or atracurium. *Anaesth Intensive Care* 1990; 18:390.

16. Salem MR, Wong AY, Collins VJ: The pediatric patient with a full stomach. *Anesthesiology* 1973; 39:435.

17. Cunningham AJ: Intraocular pressure-physiology and implications for anaesthetic management. *Can Anaesth Soc J* 1986; 33:195.

18. Goudsouzian N, Coté CJ, Liu LMP, et al: The dose-response effects of oral cimetidine on gastric pH and volume in children. *Anesthesiology* 1981; 55:533.

19. Salem MR, Wong AY, Fizzotti GF: Efficacy of cricoid pressure in preventing aspiration of gastric contents in paediatric patients. *Br J Anaesth* 1972; 44:401.

20. Gold MI, Duarte I, Muravchick S: Arterial oxygenation in conscious patients after 5 minutes and after 30 seconds of oxygen breathing. *Anesth Analg* 1981; 60:313.

21. McGoldrick KE: Pediatric anesthesia for ophthalmic surgery, in Bruce RA Jr, McGoldrick KE, Oppenheimer P (eds): *Anesthesia for Ophthalmology.* Birmingham, Ala, Aesculapius Publishing Co, 1982, p 75.

22. Motoyama EK, Davis PJ (eds): *Smith's Anesthesia for Infants and Children,* ed 5. St Louis, Mosby–Year Book, 1990, p 273.

23. Arthur DS, Dewar KMS: Anaesthesia for eye surgery in children. *Br J Anaesth* 1980; 52:681.

54

Craniopharyngioma

An 8-year-old, 40-kg girl with a recurrent craniopharyngioma is scheduled for craniotomy and tumor excision. She developed diabetes insipidus following her initial craniotomy 1 year ago. Current medications are desmopressin (DDAVP), levothyroxine, and prednisone. Hemoglobin, 12.2 g/dL; hematocrit, 36.5%.

Recommendations by Patricia Harper Petrozza, M.D.

Craniopharyngiomas are the most common suprasellar tumors in children. The appropriate management of this histologically benign lesion is a subject of much controversy in neurosurgical circles due to the high incidence of postoperative endocrine and psychosocial problems following attempts at complete surgical excision. Traditionally, the tumor is described as arising from embryonic cell rests of Rathke pouch, an incompletely involuted hypophyseal-pharyngeal duct. Although this embryologic origin has been challenged, groups of tumor cells can be found lying within the pituitary stalk and extending from the hypothalamus to the pituitary gland. The tumor thus insinuates itself into the substance of the hypothalamus.[1]

THE SURGICAL PROCEDURE

At the time of initial craniotomy the goal is complete excision of the tumor with the operating microscope. Often, however, the resection is limited because a definitive line between tumor and normal tissue is obscure and the tumor adheres to blood vessels and the hypothalamic stalk. For this reason, prior to the regular use of the microscope, recurrence rates were as high as 40%. Recent large series of surgical patients indicate that the recurrence rate is now approximately 10%.[2]

Surgery for a recurrent craniopharyngioma can be considered high risk. The neurosurgical literature indicates that despite microsurgical technique and modern hormone replacement, a mortality rate of 40% within 1 year is sustained by children who require a second or subsequent craniotomy for tumor recurrence.[3] Difficulty of surgical dissection at the second procedure is the primary factor in the poor outcome. The requirement for a ventriculoperitoneal or ventriculoatrial shunt perioperatively also increases the likelihood of a poor outcome. Hydrocephalus in this setting most likely reflects hypothalamic invasion by the tumor.

Some degree of endocrine impairment is to be expected in the majority of patients following the initial craniotomy for craniopharyngioma (Fig 54–1). In patients in whom radical total excision is attempted, postoperative diabetes insipidus is almost invariably present, while as many as 80% of the children may also experience deficiencies of growth hormone (GH) and thyroid-stimulating hormone (TSH). Seventy-five percent of the children will lack adrenocorticotropin (ACTH) to stimulate cortisol production.[4] Although replacement hormones are available for each of these conditions, endocrine crises primarily related to acute cortisol deficiency can be provoked by stimuli such as a minor respiratory illness and, if unrecognized, lead to untimely mortality.

Even in patients with apparently successful initial surgical resection, injury to the hypothalamic-pituitary complex causes many behavioral problems including short-term memory loss, emotional immaturity, and sexual immaturity.[5] Occasionally children will have uncontrolled anger or

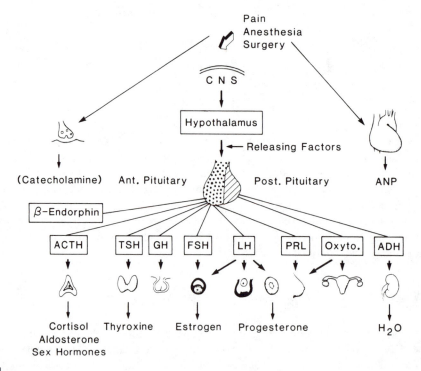

FIG 54–1.
Hypothalamic-pituitary axis and hormones. CNS = central nervous system; ACTH = adrenocorticotropic hormone; TSH = thyroid-stimulating hormone; GH = growth hormone; FSH = follicle-stimulating hormone; LH = leutinizing hormone; PRL = prolactin; Oxyto. = oxytocin; ADH = antidiuretic hormone; ANP = atrial natriuretic peptide. (From Roizen MJ: *Anesthesia for Patients With Endocrine Disease.* Philadelphia, WB Saunders Co, 1987. Used by permission.)

aggression and hyperphagia. The latter disturbance is apparently related to hyperinsulinism and damage to the ventromedial areas of the hypothalamus.[6]

CLINICAL PRESENTATION

Visual symptoms are the most common reason an initial medical examination is sought for children with craniopharyngiomas. In a recent series of 74 patients, 45 had visual field defects, while 24 had papilledema on initial presentation.[2] Headache is also a common symptom related to obstructive hydrocephalus. The intimate relationship of the pituitary stalk, optic chiasm, and cerebrospinal fluid (CSF) pathways can be readily appreciated (Fig 54–2). An interesting seesaw nystagmus in which one eye moves upward and rotates inward while the other eye moves downward and rotates outward is also seen in patients with craniopharyngioma and anatomically places the lesion near the diencephalon.

Both computed tomography (CT) and magnetic resonance imaging (MRI) scans are valuable in evaluating the patient preoperatively.[7] CT scans are particularly useful for the diagnosis of small tumors and allow the identification of cystic components within partially calcified tumors. The MRI scan helps the surgeon determine the relationship of the neoplasm to the surrounding structures and the direction of growth (Fig 54–3). Patients will often require cerebral angiography to define the relationship of the intracranial arteries and tumor. The blood supply most often arises from small branches of the anterior cerebral, anterior communicating, or posterior communicating arteries.

During the initial preoperative assessment, diagnostic tests reveal GH deficiency to be the most common endocrine abnormality. Careful questioning will also reveal the existence of diabetes insip-

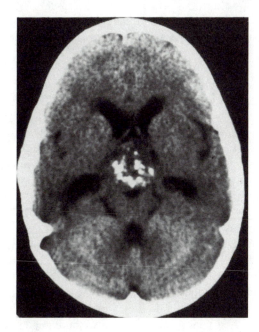

FIG 54–2.
CT scan of a 6-year-old child with a craniopharyngioma. Note the presence of tumor calcifications and hydrocephalus.

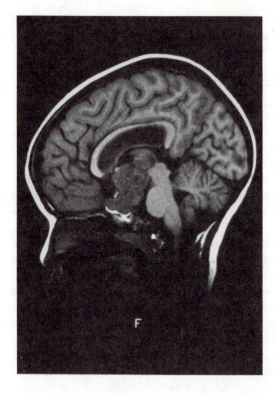

FIG 54–3.
MRI scan of a 4-year-old child with a craniopharyngioma. Note the extent of tumor and displacement of the hypothalamic-pituitary structures.

idus in approximately 20% of the patients before the initial craniotomy. A radioimmunologic assay (RIA) of plasma vasopressin is available if clinical signs of polyuria and hyperosmolality are inconclusive.

PREOPERATIVE EVALUATION

In the case of a patient who presents with a recurrent craniopharyngioma, the preoperative assessment must include a careful examination for signs of increased intracranial pressure and obstructive hydrocephalus. A recent history of nausea and vomiting should be sought and the presence of papilledema noted. Attempts at establishing rapport with a child who may exhibit difficult behavior are encouraged.

An endocrine profile and assessment is especially important because the children often have manifestations of panhypopituitarism. Diabetes insipidus is generally well controlled with desmopressin acetate (1-D-amino-8-D-arginine vasopressin [DDAVP]) administered intranasally. Clinically, if the patient does not complain of thirst or frequent nocturia and the serum sodium level as well as serum osmolality are normal, the syndrome is under good control. The dose of DDAVP is carefully titrated for each patient, with intranasal administration of 5 to 20 μg twice daily. Since DDAVP has a duration of 12 to 24 hours, aqueous vasopressin in a dose of 5 to 10 units administered subcutaneously or intramuscularly may be preferred perioperatively because the duration of action is 4 to 6 hours, which allows easier titration in the operating room setting where fluid retention is extremely detrimental.[8]

Adrenal insufficiency due to a lack of ACTH or corticotropin-releasing hormone (CRH) results from damage to the pituitary-hypothalamic axis. Clinical signs of inadequate cortisone replacement include fatigue, hypotension, diarrhea, vomiting, and dehydration. A small heart may also be seen on chest radiography. Standard prednisone therapy in children with adrenal cortical insufficiency is 5 to 6 mg/m^2/day administered orally in two to three divided doses. During times of stress or surgery, it is necessary to administer cortisol replacement at two to four times the normal level.[9]

Evidence for hypothyroidism should also be sought, including levels of thyroid hormone and a clinical assessment noting skin changes, bowel alterations, and bradycardia. Standard replacement therapy is levothyroxine, 100 μg/m^2 once daily. The half-life of levothyroxine approaches 1 week.

In addition to concerns about the intracranial pathology and the endocrine state of the child, the anesthesiologist should note the administration of phenytoin or other anticonvulsants, particularly if a bifrontal craniotomy approach is anticipated. The large surgical area and vascular structures involved necessitate blood component availability. It is also advisable to discuss with the surgeon the planned approach, most often a bifrontal craniotomy necessitating retraction on the frontal lobes, and whether or not a perioperative CSF shunt will be utilized.

ANESTHETIC MANAGEMENT

Ideally, an intravenous infusion with normal saline is begun in the preoperative holding area the morning of surgery. Carefully titrated doses of midazolam, 0.01 to 0.03 mg/kg, or fentanyl, 0.5 to 1.0 μg/kg, can be administered to ease separation anxiety for the patient and family. While the presence of emotional immaturity may be anticipated, the induction is best performed in the operating room following the placement of noninvasive monitors. Induction is accomplished with thiopental, 3 to 4 mg/kg, followed by vecuronium, 0.1 mg/kg. If the child has a recent history of vomiting, a rapid-sequence induction utilizing 0.3 mg/kg of vecuronium may be appropriate. During mask ventilation and while awaiting the onset of neuromuscular blockade, up to 5 μg/kg fentanyl is administered. After lidocaine, 1.5 mg/kg, is administered intravenously, intubation is accomplished by using a cuffed endotracheal tube with minimal balloon occlusion pressure. Following induction, an arterial catheter is placed as well as a central venous pressure (CVP) catheter, preferably through an antecubital vein. The CVP catheter allows assessment of intraoperative volume status and large intravenous access in the case of significant intraoperative hemorrhage. A Foley catheter is also inserted.

When the pinhead holder is placed, cardiovascular responses are blunted with the administration of 10 to 20 μg/kg alfentanil. As the operating table is turned for surgical positioning, the patency of all intravenous catheters and tubing is reassessed. The arterial transducer should be leveled at the foremen magnum, or external auditory meatus. Breath sounds are rechecked to be sure that the endotracheal tube has not slipped into a mainstem bronchus during surgical positioning. Efforts are made to keep the child warm with blankets, a heated water mattress, and fluid warming. At this juncture, a blood gas sample is evaluated with the aim of maintaining the Pa$_{CO_2}$ between 25 and 30 mm Hg. The electrolyte status and blood glucose are also assessed at this time.

Perioperative endocrine management includes the administration of hydrocortisone sodium succinate, 30 mg/m^2, shortly after the intravenous infusion is begun. Hydrocortisone sodium succinate, 10 mg/hr, is administered throughout the procedure. The patient's thyroxine dose is given on the morning of surgery despite the drug's relatively long half-life because the patient may be unable to eat for some time postoperatively. GH, if necessary, may also be administered in the preoperative period.

Diabetes insipidus is managed perioperatively by eliminating the morning dose of DDAVP and administering the short-acting form of vasopressin, aqueous pitressin in a dose of 0.05 to 0.1 unit/kg subcutaneously every 4 to 6 hours intraoperatively. Despite possible uneven absorption, this regimen addresses surgical concerns about water intoxication, and vasopressor side effects are uncommon in this setting. During the operation, urinary volume, specific gravity, and serum electrolytes are assessed hourly, and glucose are also determined. Normal saline is the maintenance fluid of choice.

Surgical incision is anticipated by increasing the level of fentanyl to approximately 10 µg/kg and adding small concentrations of isoflurane. Pancuronium would be utilized for intraoperative muscle relaxation. Because craniopharyngiomas often invade or are continuous with the third ventricle and a CSF leak can be anticipated through the diaphragm sella with surgical manipulation, nitrous oxide is best avoided so that air/nitrous oxide collections do not accumulate in areas where CSF has been displaced.

Intraoperative events of concern are the exacerbation of diabetes insipidus, hemorrhage related to manipulation of the large blood vessels of the anterior circle of Willis or the sphenoid sinus, and hypothalamic dysfunction manifested primarily as poor temperature regulation. Intraoperative diabetes insipidus would be characterized by prodigious amounts of urine, as much as 0.5 L/hr with a specific gravity less than 1.005 and a rising serum sodium concentration. As mentioned previously, intraoperative management with intramuscular and subcutaneous injections of vasopressin, 0.05 to 0.1 µg/kg, is effective temporary management of this condition.

An infusion of nitroglycerine or sodium nitroprusside should be available for use in the event of profuse hemorrhage. Mean arterial blood pressure may be lowered to aid in the control of surgical bleeding. Computerized electroencephalographic monitoring in this instance assists in the detection of ischemia and possible intraoperative damage to the carotid vessels.

POSTOPERATIVE MANAGEMENT

If the operative course has been relatively uneventful without major hemorrhage or brain swelling, planned extubation of the child is appropriate. Eliminating isoflurane while maintaining a stable blood pressure to decrease microsurgical bleeding may entail the use of labetalol, 0.1 to 1.0 mg/kg, or a nitroglycerine infusion. At the end of the procedure, muscle relaxant action is reversed, and the child is extubated when responsive. Careful postoperative management requires vigilance for diabetes insipidus, hypothalamic dysfunction, seizures, and possible subdural hematoma related to overzealous CSF drainage.

Thrombosis and spasm of the carotid arteries have been demonstrated following craniopharyngioma resection, and the brief appearance of the syndrome of inappropriate antidiuretic hormone secretion 2 to 3 days postoperatively has also been noted. Careful attention to the neurologic examination and fluid and electrolyte status is the hallmark of postoperative care for this child.

REFERENCES

1. Laws ER Jr: Craniopharyngiomas: Diagnosis and treatment, in Sekhar LN, Schramm VL Jr (eds): *Tumors of the Cranial Base: Diagnosis and Treatment*. New York, Futura Publishing Co Inc, 1987.
2. Baskin DS, Wilson CB: Surgical management of craniopharyngiomas: A review of 74 cases. *J Neurosurg* 1986; 65:22–27.
3. Yasargil MG, Curcic M, Kis M, et al: Total removal of craniopharyngiomas: Approaches and long-term results in 144 patients. *J Neurosurg* 1990; 73:3–11.
4. Lyen KR, Grant DB: Endocrine function, morbidity, and mortality after surgery for craniopharyngioma. *Arch Dis Child* 1982; 57:837–841.
5. Danoff BF, Cowchock FS, Kramer S: Childhood craniopharyngioma: Survival, local control, endocrine and neurologic function following radiotherapy. *Int J Radiat Oncol Biol Phys* 1983; 9:171–175.
6. Bucher H, Zapf J, Torresani T, et al: Insulin-like growth factors I and II, prolactin, and insulin in 19 growth hormone–deficient children with excessive, normal, or decreased longitudinal growth after operation for craniopharyngioma. *N Engl J Med* 1983; 309:1142–1146.
7. Pigeau I, Sigal R, Halimi P, et al: MRI features of craniopharyngiomas at 1.5 tesla: A series of 13 cases. *J Neuroradiol* 1988; 15:276–287.
8. Roizen MF: *Anesthesiology Clinics of North America: Anesthesia for Patients With Endocrine Disease*. Philadelphia, WB Saunders Co, 1987.
9. Wilson JD, Foster DW: *Williams Textbook of Endocrinology*. Philadelphia, WB Saunders Co, 1985.

55

Post-tonsillectomy Bleeding

An 8-year-old boy who had a tonsillectomy 5 days previously is brought to the emergency room by his parents who state that he has been spitting up bright red blood for about an hour and vomited "a lot" of blood clots and food on the way to the hospital. The otorhinolaryngologist sees brisk bleeding from the right tonsillar fossa and wants to take the child directly to the operating room. While the emergency room nurse notifies operating room, the surgeon notifies you and then inserts a 22-gauge intravenous cannula. Pulse, 125; respirations, 28; blood pressure, 110/70. No laboratory results are available.

Recommendations by Frederic A. Berry, M.D.

Postoperative bleeding is one of the most worrisome complications of tonsillectomy and adenoidectomy. Bleeding occurs at two major time periods: primary bleeding develops within the first 24 hours, and secondary bleeding occurs 2 or more days postoperatively. In a recent study, 7 of 2,011 patients experienced a primary tonsillar hemorrhage.[1] Six of the 7 bled within 3 1/2 hours after the operation, and 1 bled 7 hours later. Twenty-nine of the 2,011 patients had a secondary hemorrhage, with 2 of the 29 bleeding from the area of adenoid excision.

EVALUATION AND PREPARATION OF THE PATIENT

The anesthesiologist must begin to formulate a clinical picture of the child from the history and vital signs and be prepared to decide several issues immediately after the child arrives in the operating suite. The major issue is the timing of anesthesia and surgery. The answer will be determined by the volume status of the patient and the degree of ongoing hemorrhage. The question of volume status is difficult to answer from the history, but the initial assumption must be that the child may have had significant blood loss. The fact that he is spitting up bright red blood suggests an arterial source for the hemorrhage. The parents stated that he had vomited "a lot" of blood clots, but under these circumstances a moderate amount of blood goes a long way. The degree of volume depletion is not clear without further information.

The anesthesiologist should be preparing for the case as the child is being transported. This means setting up a large-bore suction and another intravenous catheter with a balanced salt solution not containing dextrose. A quick history and examination of the child when he arrives in the operating room will provide rapid information about the volume status. Time must be taken to explain to him who you are and what is happening. This explanation should be reinforced at every step of the procedure. If the child is sitting up and talking with the parents, this would indicate that the volume deficit is not severe. If he is lying down and has pale conjunctiva and an altered state of consciousness, it is evident that there has been considerable blood loss and rapid resuscitation is indicated.

If the history indicates that the child became dizzy when standing, this would be significant. The presence of orthostatic hypotension reflects a loss of at least 20% of the circulating blood volume and mandates aggressive fluid therapy. A 25-mL/kg bolus of balanced salt solution should be given as quickly as possible. This can be accomplished through the existing 22-gauge needle with a syringe and stopcock. On the other hand, depending on how well the intravenous catheter runs, it might be appropriate at this point to start another. If the child was able to walk into the emergency room and could stand without developing orthostatic hypotension, this would indicate that the degree of blood loss was not major and that surgery could proceed immediately while a 10- to 15-ml/kg bolus of balanced salt solution is being administered.

The physical examination may be useful in determining the patient's blood volume. The pulse of 125 and respiratory rate of 28 strongly suggest an outpouring of catecholamines in response to either volume depletion or from the excitement and/or terror of the situation. The blood pressure of 110/70 mm Hg is normal, but that does not necessarily mean that the blood volume is normal. It may only indicate that the compensatory mechanisms of the body have been activated to maintain the circulation. In the presence of the endogenous vasopressors angiotensin II, antidiuretic hormone (ADH) or vasopressin, epinephrine, and norepinephrine, the blood pressure may be normal and the pulse elevated but the circulating blood volume still compromised. Almost all anesthetic techniques interfere with the normal compensatory circulatory mechanisms and may lead to a hypotensive episode in a hypovolemic patient.

LABORATORY EVALUATION

There is enormous controversy about what is indicated for routine preoperative laboratory investigation of hemostasis in patients having tonsillectomy and adenoidectomy. Since bleeding is one of the most serious complications, the physician needs to evaluate this possibility preoperatively. There are two major schools of thought relative to this issue. One group believes that the patient's personal and family history is sufficient to determine whether a bleeding tendency is present. If there is, then laboratory studies are indicated to determine the nature of the problem.[2, 3] The second group believes that a routine hemostatic assessment including a prothombin time (PT), partial thromboplastin time (PTT), platelet count, and a bleeding time is necessary.[4] However, when a patient comes back with postadenotonsillectomy bleeding, the question of whether a bleeding diathesis is present certainly arises. If there is serious question whether a hemostatic defect is contributing to the bleeding, the above studies should be obtained. At times, nonspecific "oozing" can be caused by an unrecognized underlying hemostatic defect. The empirical administration of desmopressin (DDAVP) may help bring the bleeding under control.[5] DDAVP has been used to correct bleeding abnormalities associated with von Willebrand disease, disorders of platelet function, and mild hemophilia A. It should be remembered though that DDAVP, which is a synthetic vasopressin, may result in the retention of free water. Seizure activity due to the development of acute dilutional hyponatremia has been reported in children who received hypotonic intravenous fluids along with the DDAVP therapy. The administration of a balanced salt solution will avoid this problem.

The hematocrit may provide information about the amount of hemorrhage. The actual value should be considered in light of the background. The history suggests that bleeding began in the preceding several hours. A moderate amount of compensatory transcapillary refill would have occurred, along with activation of the renin-angiotensin-aldosterone system to stimulate the kidney to conserve sodium and water. A normal hematocrit of 35% to 38% would suggest that the tonsillectomy had been rather bloodless and the current bleeding was moderate, probably less than 5% to 10% of the blood volume. If the hematocrit is 30% to 35%, this would indicate that either the previous surgery was relatively bloody or the present bleeding is moderately severe. A hematocrit below 30% indicates significant blood loss of at least 15% to 20% of blood volume, either acutely or in addition to the previous loss.

VOLUME REPLETION

If the hematocrit is significantly below 30%, 10 to 15 mL/kg of blood should be administered through a blood warmer and repeated as indicated by vital signs and a second hematocrit. If the child's blood type is not available or there is any question about the degree of volume depletion, then O-negative blood should be requested and used immediately. In the interim, immediate volume resuscitation with a balanced salt solution without dextrose should be initiated. Dextrose is eliminated from all perioperative fluids because of the danger of enhancing any neurologic damage that may occur with an ischemic episode.[6, 7]

If the child's vital signs are stable, surgery can proceed. However, the author has never seen a child exsanguinate from a "bleeding tonsil" while aggressive fluid resuscitation was being undertaken to better prepare him for surgery. If severe volume depletion is suspected, adequate fluid resuscitation should be accomplished before proceeding. In the hypothetical situation of severe arterial bleeding from the tonsilar bed causing blood loss more rapid than could be replaced, it might be possible for the surgeon to put pressure on the area with a gauze pad on a clamp while resuscitation continued.

ANESTHETIC TECHNIQUE

Monitors should be applied as the child is being evaluated and fluid infused. In general, anesthetics decrease the body's ability to compensate for volume loss. The volatile anesthetics are both myocardial depressants and vasodilators. Narcotics are also vasodilators. Barbiturates interfere with the sympathetic nervous system and, in the face of a contracted blood volume with enhanced sympathetic activity, may cause severe hypotension. Positive-pressure ventilation decreases venous return, thereby reducing cardiac output. In short, most anesthetics will reduce blood pressure. In the face of normovolemia, the blood pressure reduction may be as much as 30% with volatile anesthetics. However, in the face of hypovolemia and volume contraction, the blood pressure might fall much lower with even minimal amounts of anesthetic. The anesthetics are a test of blood volume. If the patient is thought to be normovolemic and has normal induction of anesthesia and an excessive drop in blood pressure, then this would suggest that he was not fully volume repleted. On the other hand, if blood pressure follows the expected drop with the induction of anesthesia, this would indicate that the blood volume was normal.

The anesthesiologist may be faced with the extremely rare but exsanguinating hemorrhage that threatens the life of the child because of the inability to replace blood as fast as it is being lost. Appropriate anesthesia would be oxygenation during the administration of 1 to 2 mg/kg of ketamine followed immediately by 2 mg/kg of succinylcholine intravenously. Cricoid pressure should be applied. A large-bore suction, turned on and immediately available, is essential. The above-described technique is extremely hazardous and should only be undertaken in the face of life-threatening hemorrhage. This is a true "crash" intubation.

If the patient can be adequately volume repleted and his vital signs stabilized, the anesthetic problem will be that of a child with a full stomach and a bleeding tonsillar bed. The anesthesiologist must be prepared for a rapid-sequence induction and a difficult intubation because the bleeding may preclude a good view of the larynx and vocal cords. Preoxygenation can be accomplished with the patient in the sitting position or in the lateral position with the bleeding side down. A large-bore suction should be activated and made immediately available. If there is any question about the adequacy of the volume replacement, ketamine is the induction agent of choice in a dose of 1.5 to 2 mg/kg. Otherwise, thiopental, 4 mg/kg, can be used. Succinylcholine, 1.5 to 2 mg/kg, is the muscle relaxant of choice in order to rapidly gain control of the airway. The succinylcholine should be preceded by a nondepolarizing muscle relaxant such as curare or atracurium, 0.05 mg/kg, in order to reduce the muscle pain following succinylcholine administration. In addition, this will reduce the intragastric pressure and the danger of regurgitation. Cricoid pressure should be applied in the usual manner. The formula for the correct size of endotracheal tube is 16 plus age divided by 4. A cuffed endotracheal tube is preferable in this situation. The presence of a cuff reduces the size of the endotracheal tube. For this patient, I would use a 5-mm tube with a cuff. In addition, I would have a stylet in the endotracheal tube even though there was no apparent history of difficulty with intubation during the previous anesthetic.

The blood pressure after induction will often reflect the volume status. If the pressure is the same or increases, then a volatile agent and nitrous oxide can be used. This would indicate that volume repletion has been adequate. Careful titration of the blood pressure and anesthetic agent is indicated. If the child becomes hypotensive after induction, this indicates a fluid deficit, and he should receive another 10 to 15 mg/kg of blood or balanced salt solution. Securing the tonsillar bleeder can usually be accomplished fairly rapidly, so either atracurium or vecuronium is the muscle relaxant of choice. The maintenance anesthetic would be nitrous oxide with either halothane or isoflurane.

The author recalls a unique case in which a child was returned to the operating room on three occasions because of what the parents described as bright red bleeding. The child had a significant reduction in hematocrit with the first two bleeding episodes, and it was necessary to reanesthetize her to find and control the bleeding. The operative course in both of the previous procedures was benign and the bleeding site not impressive. The child was discharged from the hospital and bled again 2 days later. The third time around, the induction was carried out as described above. The hematocrit was in the high 20s, and the child was adequately volume repleted. After the induction of anesthesia and securing of the airway, again no bleeding could be determined. It was noted that after induction on all three occasions there was a normal drop in blood pressure of 20% to 30%. Therefore, 15 mg of ephedrine was given to this 35-kg patient. The heart rate and blood pressure increased to hypertensive levels, and the bleeding point became evident in the posterior aspect of the tonsilar bed and was ligated. There were no further bleeding problems.

EXTUBATION OF THE TRACHEA

The major postoperative consideration is extubation of the trachea in the presence of a full stomach. The dangers of aspiration in this particular case are of airway obstruction with particulate matter or blood clots. The blood would buffer the acid of the stomach. The passage of a large-bore orogastric tube during anesthesia to empty the stomach will decompress the volume of gastric fluid but does not guarantee that the stomach is empty. The oral route for the gastric tube is preferred in order to bypass the area of surgery. The stomach must still be considered full, even if there is no further return from the orogastric tube.

Awake extubation is the technique of choice to ensure that the child will be able to control his airway and reflexes. One of the problems with awake extubation is that the patient may react on the endotracheal tube but not be sufficiently alert to control his airway reflexes. Lidocaine, 1.5 mg/kg, should be given intravenously to depress the airway reflexes while the effects of the inhalation anesthetic are being dissipated. This dose may be repeated in 5 to 10 minutes, if necessary, and the child extubated when his eyes are open and he is responding to commands and pulling at the endotracheal tube.

SUMMARY

The major problems of the post-tonsillectomy patient are volume depletion with the need for resuscitation and a full stomach with a bleeding tonsillar bed. Understanding these problems will enable the anesthesiologist to tailor the resuscitation and anesthetic methods to meet these needs.

REFERENCES

1. Colclasure JB, Graham SS: Complications of outpatient and adenoidectomy: A review of 3,340 cases. *Ear Nose Throat J* 1990; 69:155–160.
2. Kaplan EB, Sheiner LB, Boeckmann AJ, et al: The usefulness of preoperative laboratory screening. *JAMA* 1985; 253:3576–3581.
3. Barber A, Green D, Gallozzo T, et al: The bleeding time as a preoperative screening test. *Am J Med* 1985; 78:761–764.

4. Bolger WE, Parsons DS, Potempa L: Preoperative hemostatic assessment of the adenotonsillectomy patient. *Otolaryngol Head Neck Surg* 1990; 103:396–405.

5. Smith TJ, Gill JC, Ambruso DR, et al: Hyponatremia and seizures in young children given DDAVP. *Am J Hematol* 1989; 31:199–202.

6. Drummond JC, Moore SS: The influence of dextrose administration on neurologic outcome after temporary spinal cord ischemia in the rabbit. *Anesthesiology* 1989; 70:64–70.

7. Nakakimura K, Fleischer JE, et al: Glucose administration before cardiac arrest worsens neurologic outcome in cats. *Anesthesiology* 1990; 72:1005–1011.

56

Splenectomy and Idiopathic Thrombocytopenic Purpura

An 8-year-old, 40-kg boy with idiopathic thrombocytopenia is scheduled for splenectomy. Despite therapy with prednisone and intravenous gamma globulin, he continues to have purpura and now presents with an intracranial hemorrhage resulting in mild hemiparesis. Hemoglobin, 11.2 g/dL; hematocrit, 33.5%; platelets, $40,000 \times 10^9$/L; prothrombin time (PT) and partial thromboplastin time (PTT), normal.

Recommendations by Richard B. Siegel, M.D., and
Robert P. Castleberry, M.D.

Idiopathic thrombocytopenic purpura (ITP) of childhood is a bleeding diathesis that results from a decrease in circulating platelets caused by increased peripheral destruction in the presence of normal marrow production and the absence of other underlying systemic disorders. ITP is a subclass of immune thrombocytopenia that is characterized by immunoglobulin-platelet interactions as the etiology of thrombocytopenia.

CLINICAL MANIFESTATIONS OF ITP

Clinically, patients are categorized as acute or chronic, depending on the duration of thrombocytopenia, less or more than 6 months, respectively.[1] These two groups typically demonstrate different clinical characteristics at diagnosis. The patient with acute ITP frequently presents between the ages of 2 and 6 years with the sudden onset of purpura, epistaxis, or bleeding from the gingiva. The platelet count is often less than $20,000 \times 10^9$/L. Males and females are equally affected. In contrast, individuals with chronic ITP are usually older at the time of diagnosis, experience a more insidious onset of symptoms, and have a milder course, with platelet counts commonly greater than $30,000 \times 10^9$/L. In the chronic group there is a 3:1 predominance of females to males.

The immunologic nature of ITP was suggested when it was demonstrated that plasma from affected patients induced thrombocytopenia when transfused into normal subjects.[2] The disorder was linked to immune mechanisms by identifying an IgG globulin that when adsorbed onto normal platelets, resulted in decreased in vivo platelet survival.[3] Other techniques have identified platelet antibodies in 50% to 90% of patients with ITP.[4] It has been suggested that the putative molecule is an antigen-antibody complex rather than an isolated immunoglobulin.[5] At any rate, it is clear that antibodies adherent to the platelet surface are responsible for the thrombocytopenia.

The causes of cross-reacting antibodies are most likely heterogeneous. Because approximately 75% of children with acute ITP have a history of an antecedent infection,[6, 7] the antibody is considered to be immune in origin. The primary source of antibody production seems to be the spleen,[8] although the bone marrow has also been implicated.[9]

The principles of managing the patient with acute vs. chronic ITP differ because of the previously described variations in the natural history of the entities. In either clinical category, platelet transfusions are generally unnecessary and ineffective.[10] Intercurrent life-threatening bleeding or surgical emergencies may be the only indications for such treatment.[1] When transfusions are necessary, consideration should be given to the use of directed and single-donor blood components.

Corticosteroids are frequently administered to the child with acute disease, particularly during the first weeks following diagnosis when the risk of serious hemorrhage is greatest. This form of treatment is particularly appropriate for children who at diagnosis have platelet counts of $10,000 \times 10^9$/L, active bleeding from any site, or a history of head injury or any violent trauma. The efficacy of steroids in preventing life-threatening hemorrhage remains unproved, however, because the data presently available are based on uncontrolled studies. Nevertheless, significant elevation of the platelet count in response to steroid therapy clearly occurs in children with ITP[10] and has been attributed to both immunosuppression[11] and diminished retention of affected platelets by the reticuloendothelial system.[3] The drug most commonly used is prednisone at a dosage of 2 mg/kg/day. Although the duration of therapy must be individualized according to response, an initial 2-week course with slow tapering of the dose is commonplace. Until recovery occurs, continuation of steroids on a long-term basis to prevent symptoms may be required in some patients. Interestingly, there is some evidence that prolonged steroid treatment may delay recovery of acute ITP.[7]

Therapy with intravenous gamma globulin may be considered, especially in children who have not responded to steroids. The doses of intravenous gamma globulin range from 0.5 to 2 g/kg/day for 2 to 5 days. The mechanism of action is still unclear.

The typical clinical course of acute ITP, that is, spontaneous and permanent remission within 6 months, usually obviates other immunosuppressive agents or splenectomy. Life-threatening hemorrhage, especially intracranial bleeding, is an indication for emergency splenectomy. Our experience and that of others indicates that such episodes are rare in spite of low platelet counts and that the tendency to hemorrhage in these children is less than in children with thrombocytopenia due to inadequate platelet production.[8, 9]

In chronic cases, the decision in favor of surgery is influenced not only by a patient's dependency upon steroids or intravenous gamma globulin but also by life-style issues. Splenectomy becomes the treatment of choice when a child aged 5 years or more continues to have intermittent exacerbations of purpura or to have unacceptable limitations of activities. Chances of spontaneous recovery are particularly low in this group of patients. The 70% remission rate observed following splenectomy[10] reflects the removal of the principal site not only of platelet destruction but also of antibody production. However, splenectomy has been associated with a 1% incidence of fatal postsplenectomy sepsis, which may be higher in children under the age of 5 years.[11] Therefore, postponing surgery until the child is older than age 5 is advisable. The degree to which this complication is attenuated by the administration of pneumococcal vaccine, Hib (*H. influenzae* type b) vaccine, and postsplenectomy prophylactic penicillin remains to be determined in controlled trials. Appropriate surgical management of the patient with chronic ITP who has previously received steroids will be outlined subsequently.

In the unlikely event that splenectomy should fail in the chronic patient, various immunosuppressive drugs, including vincristine, have been recommended.[12] Because this is an uncommon occurrence in pediatric patients, the role of these agents in childhood ITP has not been clearly defined.

ANESTHETIC MANAGEMENT

With reference to the above case, several preoperative studies should be performed prior to providing anesthesia for the surgical procedure. A careful history will provide much useful information regarding associated conditions and alert the anesthesiologist to potential anesthetic problems.

Minimally, a PT, PTT, and platelet count should be obtained within 4 hours of surgery. Bleeding time is not essential because these patients are known to have a low platelet count. A chest x-ray is important in order to have a baseline should postoperative pneumonia occur. Any further studies should be based on the patient's history, signs and symptoms, and the physical examination.

The patient's mental status and strength following the hemiparesis that resulted from the previous intracranial hemorrhage must be fully documented. The degree of increase in intracranial pressure should be assessed. While an intracranial bleed is unlikely to result in hypovolemia in this age group, the examination should be directed toward discovering whether concurrent bleeding in other areas has created this additional problem.

Preoperative medication would depend on the child's mental status prior to surgery. Consultation with the patient's hematologic team will give insight into specific needs. As our method of preoperative preparation, we prefer to outline the planned course of anesthesia to the patient and family rather than depend on sedation. Patients presenting for emergency surgery are not sedated.

Because of the associated bleeding problems, intramuscular premedication should be avoided. If sedation is used, we prefer to administer oral benzodiazepines the night before and the morning of surgery. Emergency patients are given metoclopramide, 0.2 mg/kg, and ranitidine, 0.75 mg/kg intravenously. An intravenous infusion is usually started prior to the patient's arrival in surgery. Intravenous premedication can also be administered in the anesthesia staging area, if necessary. An anticholinergic would be administered intravenously.

This patient, who has a history of steroid therapy, would be prepared with steroids prior to surgery. The average cortisol production rate is 12 ± 2 mg/m^2/day. With adrenocorticotropic hormone (ACTH) stimulation, this can increase 10 to 15 times. Therefore, a dose of 225 mg/m^2 day is used in patients subjected to stressful situations. It is preferable, if at all possible, to maintain a continuous infusion of steroids based on this dose over a 24-hour period by utilizing a suitable intravenous pump.[13] In order to avoid bleeding associated with intramuscular injections, we prefer not to give intramuscular steroids. An alternative method would be the oral administration of steroids the morning of surgery with the preoperative benzodiazepine. Should the need arise, it is important that steroids for intravenous injection be available in the operating room.

Prior to induction of anesthesia, adequate blood components, specifically platelets and red blood cells (RBCs) and/or fresh whole blood must be available. The patient's blood volume is estimated to be between 3,000 and 3,250 mL. At least 2 units of fresh whole blood or RBCs should be readily available. The need for platelet administration will depend on the patient's status immediately prior to induction. We prefer to maintain the platelet count above 30,000/μL and transfuse the patient accordingly. If a patient requires platelets, they are best given upon arrival in the operating room or during surgery since their effective half-life is brief.

One unit of platelets per square meter will raise the platelet count by 10,000 to 15,000 $\times$ 10^9/L. The height and weight of the patient will allow a calculation of the appropriate dose to elevate the platelet count to tolerable levels prior to and during surgery.[14]

The patient should be brought to the operating room and placed on the operating table in a supine position. Blood pressure, temperature, electrocardiogram, heart tones, end-tidal CO_2 pulse oximetry, and respiration should be monitored. Continuous electronic measurement of blood pressure by oscillometric technique is helpful; however, care must be exercised not to perform these measurements too frequently, such as every minute, because significant bleeding can occur from the tourniquet-like action of the blood pressure cuff. Invasive hemodynamic monitors are used depending upon the patient's condition.

Following adequate preoxygenation, anesthesia should be induced with a benzodiazepine, short-acting narcotics, and/or barbiturates. Intravenous lidocaine is useful in patients with increased intracranial pressure. The use of succinylcholine following intracranial hemorrhage and hemiparesis must be considered because elevation of potassium levels has been reported in this patient population. We prefer to avoid succinylcholine and use pancuronium or another nondepolarizing agent to facilitate intubation. An oral endotracheal tube should be placed under direct laryngoscopy. Extreme care must be exercised during laryngoscopy to avoid trauma to the gingiva, oral mucosa, and tongue because of the decreased platelet count. After ascertaining proper tube position, the tube should be secured. Maintenance of anesthesia can be accomplished with an inhalation agent and/or intermittent narcotics.

Care must be taken during positioning of the patient because ecchymosis and bleeding can result from undue pressure. When monitoring the patient's temperature, we prefer to use a skin probe to prevent bleeding that might be induced by a stiff rectal or tympanic probe. An esophageal stethoscope–temperature probe combination can be used and inserted under direct vision to avoid trauma to the oropharynx.

Fluid management would consist of replacing calculated fluid deficits according to time without intake (NPO) plus a maintenance rate of 5 mL/kg/hr, or 200 mL/hr in this patient. The fluid deficit should be replaced at a rate of 50% during the first hour, 25% during the second hour, and 25% during the third hour which would probably be in the recovery room.

Introduction of a nasogastric tube must be accomplished with extreme care because severe epistaxis and nasal bleeding can occur. We prefer to use an orogastric tube under direct vision and insert it after the splenectomy has been accomplished.

Should hypotension occur and not respond to appropriate fluid and anesthetic management, the use of large doses of intravenous steroids should be considered. Five to 15 mg/kg of hydrocortisone should be administered rapidly. Other appropriate supportive drugs can be added as required to treat the hypotension. The patient should be examined for signs of recurrent intracranial hemorrhage.

On termination of the procedure, the patient should be transported to the recovery room or intensive care unit where monitoring is continued. He should be observed closely for infection. An overall mortality of 2.4% from overwhelming sepsis has been reported.[15] The authors reported serious infections in 6% of the patients reviewed, with an overall mortality of 3.3% following splenectomy. Severe gastrointestinal hemorrhage, massive epistaxis, and massive hematuria have been reported during the intraoperative and immediate postoperative periods.[16]

REFERENCES

1. McMillan CW: Platelet and vascular disorders, in Miller DR, Pearson HA, Baehner RL, et al (eds): *Blood Diseases of Infancy and Childhood.* St Louis, Mosby–Year Book, 1978, pp 707–717.
2. Harrington WJ, Minnich V, Hollingsworth JW, et al: Demonstration of a thrombocytopenic factor in the blood of patients with thrombocytopenic purpura. *J Lab Clin Med* 1951; 38:1.
3. Shulman NR, Marder VJ, Weinrach RS: Similarities between known antiplatelet antibodies and the factor responsible for thrombocytopenia in idiopathic purpura: Physiologic, serologic, and isotopic studies. *Ann N Y Acad Sci* 1965; 124:499.
4. Movassaghi N, Moorhead J, Leikin S: Antiplatelet antibodies in childhood idiopathic thrombocytopenic purpura. *Am J Dis Child* 1979; 133:257.
5. Lightsey AL: Thrombocytopenia in children. *Pediatr Clin North Am* 1980; 27:293.
6. Clemen DH, Diamond LK: Purpura in infants and children. *Am J Dis Child* 1953; 85:259.
7. Lusher JM, Zuelzer WW: Idiopathic thrombocytopenic purpura in childhood. *J Pediatr* 1966; 68:971.
8. Bussel JB: Autoimmune thrombocytopenic purpura. *Hematol Oncol Clin North Am* 1990; 4:181.
9. Harber LA, Slichter SJ: The bleeding time as a screening test for evaluation of platelet function. *N Engl J Med* 1972; 287:155–159.
10. Simons SM, Main CA, Yaish HM, et al: Idiopathic thrombocytopenic purpura in children. *J Pediatr* 1975; 87:16.
11. Singer DB: Postsplenectomy sepsis. *Perspect Pediatr Pathol* 1973; 1:285.
12. Lusher JM, Iyer R: Idiopathic thrombocytopenic purpura in children. *Semin Thromb Hemost* 1977; 3:175.
13. Fass B: Glucocorticoid therapy for nonendocrine disorders: Withdrawal and "coverage." *Pediatr Clin North Am* 1979; 26:251–256.
14. Richards JDM, Thompson DS: Assessment of thrombocytopenic patients for splenectomy. *J Clin Pathol* 1979; 32:1248–1252.
15. Ein SH, Shandling B, Simpson JS, et al: The morbidity and mortality of splenectomy in childhood. *Ann Surg* 1977; 185:307–310.
16. Zerella JT, Martin LW, Lampkin BC: Emergency splenectomy for idiopathic thrombocytopenic purpura in children. *J Pediatr Surg* 1978; 13:243–246.

57

Coarctation of the Aorta

An 8-year-old, 41-kg boy is admitted for correction of coarctation of the aorta. The diagnosis was initially made during a routine precamp physical. Blood pressure in the arms is 140/90 and 160/95; pulses in the lower extremities are weak. Hemoglobin, 13 g/dL; hematocrit, 40%.

Recommendations by James W. Bland, Jr., M.D., and Thomas J. Mancuso, M.D.

Coarctation is a congenital constriction of the aorta that varies from partial to complete and may involve a long or short segment. Obstruction may be located anywhere beyond the aortic valve but most commonly occurs at the junction of the ductus arteriosus and the aortic arch, just distal to the origin of the left subclavian artery.[1]

COARCTATION OF THE AORTA

A useful classification of the different forms of coarctation is based on the location of the ductus in relation to the coarcted segment of the aorta.[2] Preductal or infantile-type coarctations involve a longer segment of aortic wall, are more frequently heralded by the onset of congestive heart failure in early infancy, and are often associated with other congenital cardiac defects such as a patent ductus arteriosus, ventricular septal defects, hypoplastic left heart variants, and transposition of the great arteries. Postductal or adult-type coarctations rarely present in early infancy as congestive heart failure and are less often associated with other hemodynamically significant cardiac defects, although a bicuspid aortic valve is not unusual. It should be noted that the designation infantile or adult type is not absolutely accurate because some infants do demonstrate the narrow or discrete segment type of coarctation while some older children may have the long-segment form.

More often than not, the coarctation produces almost total obliteration of the aortic lumen. Survival depends upon the development of a network of collateral arteries that connect the brachiocephalic vessels with the descending thoracic aorta. The major collateral pathways involve the arteries around the shoulder girdle and those within the muscles of the chest wall, particularly the intercostal and internal mammary systems. The extensive anastomoses of these vessels account for the rib notching seen on chest x-ray film and the not infrequent physical finding of multiple bruits and thrills over the infrascapular areas of the back.

Some form of congenital heart disease occurs in approximately 1 of every 123 live births (0.8%) in North America.[3] Coarctation of the aorta is not a rare defect and accounts for 5% to 8% of all patients with congenital heart disease.[4] It was first described in the late 18th century, but it was not until 1945 that successful surgical correction was reported.[5] The overall incidence of coarctation is higher in males, approximately 2:1,[4] but the male:female ratio of cases diagnosed in infancy is about equal.[4, 6] Isolated coarctation in females may be associated with Turner syndrome.

Associated cardiac anomalies should always be suspected in patients with coarctation. Patency of the ductus arteriosus has been reported in 64%, ventricular septal defects in 32%, transposition of the great arteries in 10%, and atrial septal defects in 6.5%.[2] Isolated coarctation occurs in only 18% of patients presenting with signs and symptoms during the first year of life. Other associated cardiac defects include aortic stenosis and/or insufficiency and mitral valve disease. Cerebral aneurysms are not uncommon. The presence of a bicuspid aortic valve is probably more prevalent than previously recognized, as high as 85% in some series.[7, 8] Noncardiac anomalies are not rare in patients with coarctation and include hypospadias, clubfoot, ocular defects, and Turner syndrome.[1, 9]

PREOPERATIVE EVALUATION

Information pertinent to the conduct of anesthesia should be recorded by the anesthesiologist in the patient's hospital record. This information includes significant history, medications, physical findings, laboratory data, chest radiography report, graphics results, cardiac catheterization and angiography data, preoperative orders and premedication, anesthetic management plan, and immediate postoperative management plan. When questions arise as to the specific type of repair planned or when observations such as fever, superficial skin infections, or abnormal laboratory data suggest that surgery may be deferred, the surgeon should be informed.

The preoperative medication plan, the induction procedure, and the postoperative management plan, including pain therapy, should be explained in appropriate detail to the child and his family. Preoperative teaching by the cardiac nurse clinician and the nurse expected to care for the child in the intensive care unit is often most helpful to both patient and family.

The older child with coarctation of the aorta is usually asymptomatic, the diagnosis usually being made when weak or absent pulses in the lower extremities are noted along with hypertension in the arms and lower blood pressure in the legs. A gradient of 20 mm Hg or greater between the arms and legs indicates significant obstruction. The history is often unremarkable. Uncommonly, the child complains of leg cramps upon vigorous exertion. Children with uncomplicated coarctation should have normal exercise tolerance and demonstrate normal growth and development. As with any patient undergoing anesthesia, current or recent medications should be noted by the anesthesiologist and the decision made whether to continue or to stop them in the perioperative period.

Besides weak or absent pulses in the lower extremities and a measurable difference in blood pressure between the arms and legs, there may be a short systolic murmur, generally heard best along the left upper sternal border, that is transmitted to the back and may actually be heard best over the spine between the scapulae. A systolic ejection murmur over the right upper sternal border transmitted to the suprasternal area and into the carotid arteries plus an ejection click heard at the apex suggests the presence of a bicuspid aortic valve. However, a bicuspid aortic valve does not always produce a murmur. A diastolic murmur over the base of the heart indicates aortic valve insufficiency. In patients with extensive collaterals, there will be thrills and murmurs, systolic or continuous, over the course of the intercostal arteries and the midback.

The physical examination by the anesthesiologist should, of course, include a determination of adequate opening of the mouth and neck mobility, the presence of loose or missing teeth, enlarged tonsils, or the presence of an upper respiratory infection. Any abnormal lung sounds should be investigated further. The right radial artery should be checked by an Allen test to ascertain integrity of the palmar arch.

In isolated coarctation of the aorta, frank cardiomegaly, as evidenced by an increased cardiothoracic ratio, is unlikely. However, other radiologic changes may be noted. The presence of adequate collateral blood flow around the coarcted segment is indicated by notching of the ribs posteriorly, usually the fourth to the eighth. Rib notching is nearly always bilateral.[10] If the coarctation is located distal to the left subclavian artery, bilateral notching occurs; if the constriction is proximal to the left subclavian or if its orifice is involved in the coarctation, rib notching will be seen only on the right side. An aberrant right subclavian artery that arises as the last of the brachiocephalic vessels from the aortic arch is found in 1% of coarctations.[11] Left-sided rib notching is seen when the aberrant right subclavian artery originates distal to the coarcted segment. The implication of the latter anomaly relates to placement of the blood pressure cuff and arterial monitoring catheter, as will be discussed subsequently. Rib notching is found in 75% of adult patients with coarctation, but its incidence in children varies.[10] It should be kept in mind that coarctation is not the only cause of rib notching since it is also seen in other disease entities. Defects resulting in decreased pulmonary blood flow, such as tetralogy of Fallot and pulmonary atresia, may produce rib notching as a consequence of collateral flow to the ischemic lungs. It may also occur following a Blalock-Taussig or other systemic-to-pulmonary artery shunt.[12] On the lateral chest radiograph, retrosternal scalloping by enlarged collaterals may be present.

After successful repair of coarctation in children, rib notching regresses rapidly and usually disappears within 6 to 12 months.[13] Persistence or the recurrence of notching 2 years or more postoperatively suggests recoarctation.[14]

Other radiologic findings include the "figure 3 sign," or "double aortic knob," as seen at the left lateral border of the aorta in the frontal view (Fig 57–1). This is caused by traction of the ligamentum arteriosus just proximal to the constricted segment, a tortuous left subclavian artery, and poststenotic dilation distal to the coarctation. The barium-filled esophagus may also show indentation by dilatation of the aorta proximal and distal to the coarctation, the "E" sign. The ascending aorta appears prominent in some patients, although this is not a constant finding.[15] On the lateral chest radiograph, there may be a prominent indentation of the barium-filled esophagus that is caused by poststenotic dilatation beyond the coarctation and the already mentioned retrosternal scalloping caused by collaterals.

Electrocardiographic (ECG) findings in isolated coarctation may well be normal, but there is

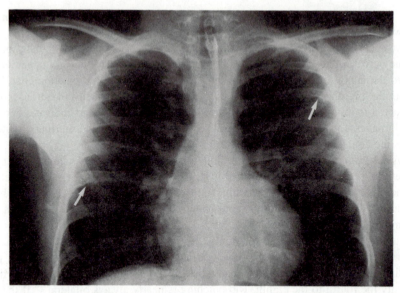

FIG 57–1.
A posteroanterior (PA) chest film shows mild cardiomegaly with left ventricular prominence. The barium-filled esophagus demonstrates the "E" sign, while the mediastinum shows the "3" sign. *Arrows* indicate rib notching. (Courtesy of Dr. Turner I. Ball, Jr., Radiology Department, Henrietta Egleston Hospital for Children, Atlanta.)

sometimes evidence of moderate left ventricular hypertrophy manifested as increased voltage in the left precordial leads[2, 4] (Fig 57–2). Exercise ECG may unmask ST segment and T wave changes and suggest ischemia, but normal recordings during exercise in patients with isolated coarctation are not unusual.[4]

It has been said that the clinical diagnosis of coarctation is easier to make than the echocardiographic diagnosis.[4] The role of M-mode echocardiography in coarctation is sometimes helpful in recognition of a bicuspid aortic valve as well as in estimation of left ventricular wall thickness and the shortening fraction. Two-dimensional echocardiography may also provide evidence of left ventricular measurements reflecting increased afterload, but imaging of the region of the coarctation is technically difficult. The major justification of the time and effort required to obtain meaningful echocardiographic studies in patients with coarctation is to provide additional confirmation that the coarctation is indeed in the usual location and may eliminate the necessity for catheterization and provide the surgeon with confidence in planning the usual incision for the operative approach.

The role of magnetic resonance imaging in evaluating patients before and after repair of coarctation remains to be elucidated (Figs 57–3 and 57–4). Some reports suggest that it is a useful method for detection and localization of the area of narrowing and poststenotic dilatation.[4, 16, 17] Its ultimate clinical value may be in the follow-up of patients with repaired coarctation, either surgically or after balloon angioplasty, to identify aneurysm formation, aneurysmal enlargement, or distortion of the aorta.[18]

Cardiac catheterization and angiocardiography are performed to rule out associated defects, determine the adequacy and site of the major collateral channels around the coarctation, and define the anatomic type and location of the coarctation. Catheterization is particularly useful when there is an

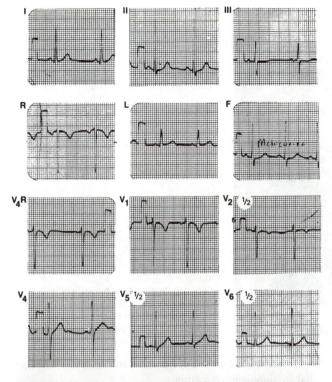

FIG 57–2.
The standard ECG shows a normal sinus rhythm with large R waves in the left precordial leads that are compatible with left ventricular hypertrophy. (Courtesy of Dr. Elizabeth Nugent, Cardiology Section, Henrietta Egleston Hospital for Children, Atlanta.)

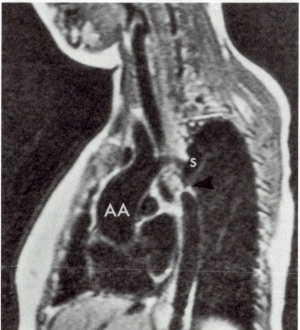

FIG 57–3.
Sagittal MRI showing an area of coarctation indicated by an *arrow*. Dilation of the ascending aorta *(AA)* and proximal subclavian artery *(S)* and hypoplasia of the transverse arch are evident. (Courtesy of Shelli Bank, M.D., Department of Radiology, Egleston Children's Hospital, Atlanta.)

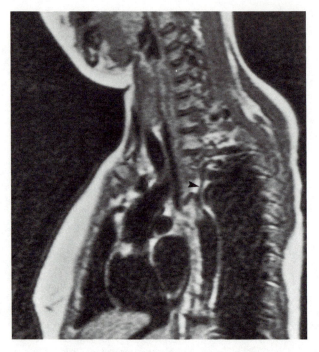

FIG 57–4.
Large collateral vessel in a patient with co-
arctation *(arrow)*. (Courtesy of Shelli Bank,
M.D., Department of Radiology, Egleston
Children's Hospital, Atlanta.)

absence of rib notching, it is difficult to image the site of narrowing on echocardiography, and significant associated defects cannot be excluded by noninvasive methods.

The anesthesiologist should note the pressure gradient across the narrowed segment and the
range of blood pressures recorded proximal to the coarctation during the catheterization procedure,
as well as those recorded elsewhere in the patient's record. This will help determine an acceptable
range of blood pressure during the surgical repair. Any abnormality in the origin of the brachiocephalic vessels should be appreciated so that the proper site for monitoring blood pressure during surgery can be selected. Arterial pressure tracings above the coarctation typically show elevation of
systolic, diastolic, and mean pressures with widening of the pulse pressure. Pressure tracings below
the area of narrowing are usually damped with low systolic and narrow pulse pressures. Calculated
cardiac output in isolated coarctation should be normal, and calculated peripheral resistance proximal to the lesion will usually be moderately elevated.

PREOPERATIVE ORDERS AND PREMEDICATION

The recent trend away from prolonged fasting prior to surgical procedures is a welcomed advance to most pediatric anesthesiologists. It now appears, based on several current reports, that it is
safe for many otherwise healthy pediatric patients to be allowed clear liquids up to 2 hours prior to
induction of anesthesia.[19–22] Our present regimen is to order clear liquids as desired after midnight
on the day of surgery and to offer up to 180 mL 2 hours prior to the scheduled procedure.

The use of sedatives, tranquilizers, narcotics, and anticholinergic drugs prior to induction of anesthesia in the pediatric patient remains largely a matter of personal choice. Premedication is not necessary for all children. Sedatives, narcotics, and even some tranquilizers may produce an alarmingly dysphoric reaction in some children that makes separation from parents and induction of anesthesia more difficult. Many children will accept an intravenous induction, with thiopental administered via a skillfully introduced small-bore needle, rather than experience a painful intramuscular injection. The child's previous hospital experiences often influence the selection of premedicant and induction drugs. Some older children will request "the needle" rather than "the mask." Discussion with the older child will make the choice easier and more acceptable to both patient and parents if a calm, sympathetic, and reassuring approach is used during the preoperative visit.

Traditionally, children over 1 year of age who are having major thoracic surgery have been given substantial preoperative sedation, usually an orally administered sedative or tranquilizer and an injection of a narcotic-anticholinergic combination.[23-25] It is now common practice in our institution, as well as in many other pediatric centers, to use oral premedication almost exclusively.[26-28] The guidelines for oral premedication are summarized in Table 57-1.[29]

ANESTHETIC MANAGEMENT

Either intravenous induction using thiopental, 3 to 4 mg/kg, or propofol, 2 to 3 mg/kg,[30] or an inhalation induction with oxygen–nitrous oxide and halothane should be safe and effective in the patient with uncomplicated coarctation. Ketamine is not considered an appropriate induction agent because of its sympathomimetic properties, which may increase the blood pressure, pulse rate, and cardiac output as well as systemic and pulmonary vascular resistances.[31, 32] If an inhalation induc-

---

TABLE 57-1.

Oral Premedication Guidelines*

1. The pharmacy prepares a mixture of **meperidine** and **atropine** in a palatable syrup
   A. For patients older than 12 months:
      0.4 mL contains 3 mg meperidine and 0.02 mg atropine (1 mL contains 7.5 mg meperidine and 0.05 mg atropine)
      Dosage: 0.4 mL/kg body weight (maximum volume, 14 mL)
   B. For patients younger than 12 months:
      Atropine alone may be used and is taken from the multiple-dose vial and given orally
      Dosage: 0.02 mg/kg body weight (0.04 mg/mL)
2. Pentobarbital (Nembutal) may be useful as an added oral medication and administered in a dosage of 1 to 4 mg/kg

*An alternative to meperidine-atropine-pentobarbital oral premedication is midazolam, 0.2 to 0.5 mg/kg, with a maximum dose of 15 mg. The drug is withdrawn from the multiple-dose vial with a syringe by the nursing staff, mixed with a palatable syrup, and given orally 30 to 45 minutes prior to surgery.

tion is chosen, we usually begin by allowing the gas mixture to blow gently over the patient's face for several minutes by using the cupped hand instead of a mask. Once the child has become drowsy, the mask is placed on his face. Vital signs are monitored with a precordial stethoscope, blood pressure cuff applied to the right arm, pulse oximeter, and ECG. After the child is unconscious, two large intravenous catheters are inserted; tracheal intubation is accomplished after administration of a nondepolarizing muscle relaxant, either vecuronium, 0.1 mg/kg, or atracurium, 0.4 mg/kg.

Invasive monitors are inserted after the child is unconscious. Direct arterial blood pressure is monitored by using a 22-gauge cannula inserted into the right radial artery unless the right subclavian arises aberrantly. In that case, the right or left temporal artery may be used. Mean distal aortic pressure (DAP) is also usually monitored from a femoral artery site during the surgical procedure since inadequate distal aortic blood flow during aortic cross-clamping is one of two proposed causes of spinal cord ischemia during coarctation repair. The other is interruption of a critical segmental supply to the anterior spinal artery and cord.[33] Although a minimum DAP required to ensure adequate cord perfusion is unknown, 45 to 50 mm Hg has been recommended. Monitoring DAP probably contributes significantly to optimum intraoperative management of coarctation repair.[33] A low DAP may be improved by repositioning of aortic cross-clamps in some patients. Hypotensive agents, if required, may also be used more intelligently when both proximal and distal aortic pressures are known.

Central venous pressure is usually measured via a catheter placed in the right internal jugular vein. Urine output is monitored, and temperature is measured with rectal and nasopharyngeal or esophageal thermistor probes. A nerve stimulator is employed to monitor the level of neuromuscular blockade. Inspired oxygen is constantly measured by using an in-line oxygen analyzer, and end-tidal gas and vapor are monitored by using the mass spectrometer and capnograph. Ventilation is controlled during the operation, and the monitoring of end-tidal carbon dioxide is an important aid in assessing the adequacy of alveolar ventilation.

After induction, anesthesia is maintained by using a combination of a nondepolarizing muscle relaxant, oxygen–nitrous oxide, and halothane or isoflurane. Supplemental intravenous narcotics may also be administered: morphine, 0.1 to 0.15 mg/kg, or fentanyl, 1 to 3 μg/kg.

THE SURGICAL PROCEDURE

Definitive repair of isolated coarctation implies complete surgical relief of the obstruction and is usually undertaken between the ages of 4 and 6 years since by that time the aorta has achieved more than 50% of its growth potential and the wall is still elastic enough for primary anastomosis.[34, 35] Repair at an earlier age may be necessary if there is significant hypertension or congestive heart failure due to the coarctation.

There are several different surgical choices for repair of isolated coarctation, including resection with end-to-end anastomosis, a prosthetic interposition graft, patch aortoplasty, subclavian flap aortoplasty, and complete prosthetic bypass graft. All have some advantages as well as disadvantages.[34, 36–39]

The standard operation for localized coarctation is resection and end-to-end anastomosis with exposure and mobilization of the narrowed segment through a left thoracotomy. During opening of the chest and mobilization or the aorta, bleeding from collateral vessels may be extensive. Adequate blood must be ordered preoperatively and be immediately available in the operating room. Before the chest incision is made, if large collaterals are known to be present, blood should be hanging and in-line, with necessary equipment for rapid infusion immediately at hand. Adequate collateral vessels around the coarctation are important in minimizing or preventing neurologic and renal complications. The measurement of DAP by using a catheter in a femoral artery is extremely helpful in assessing distal flow during cross-clamping. A significant rise (>180 mm Hg) in proximal aortic pressure with a fall in DAP (<45 to 50 mm Hg) during test cross-clamping suggests inadequate collateral circulation. A test cross-clamping should always be performed before any "bridges are burned" during the repair to determine how high the proximal pressure will rise and how low the distal pressure will fall. Nitroprusside and propranolol should always be available for use during repair of uncomplicated coarctation, but our recent experience indicates that hypotensive agents are rarely if ever necessary. Moderate systemic hypothermia was advocated in the past to minimize the risk of spinal cord ischemia,[40] as was the use of various forms of left heart bypass.[41] These methods are not often employed today.

Once the repair has been accomplished, the anesthesiologist should be informed and preparations made for removing the cross-clamps. Blood should be available for rapid transfusion if unexpected excessive bleeding occurs. If vasodilators were used, they should be decreased or discontinued. The distal cross-clamp should be gradually removed first over a period of 2 or 3 minutes. Hemostasis should be carefully checked as the distal clamp is completely released. If significant bleeding is encountered, the distal clamp can be reapplied and the bleeding controlled. After the distal clamp is completely released, the proximal one is removed over a 3- or 4-minute period with the same hemostatic precautions. The blood pressure almost invariably falls with removal of the cross-clamps, but usually not alarmingly so if there has been adequate volume replacement during the course of the procedure.

POSTOPERATIVE CARE

Postrepair "rebound" hypertension may occur in the immediate postoperative period. If not managed properly, it may result in the postcoarctation syndrome which is characterized by abdominal pain, ileus, mesenteric arteritis, and bowel infarction. If unrecognized and untreated, this condition can be fatal. Two types of hypertensive responses in postoperative patients have been described.[42] In some patients, the elevation of blood pressure occurred early, 12 to 24 hours postrepair. In those in whom the elevation was delayed 2 to 3 days, it tended to last longer. The postcoarctation syndrome is more likely to be seen in patients with a delayed onset of hypertension. Characteristic of the delayed response are diastolic hypertension, with or without systolic elevation, and a good response to antihypertensive agents such as reserpine. We have not seen the syndrome in patients whose diastolic blood pressure was maintained within the normal range for age by using vasodilators and/or β-blocking agents and in whom decompression of the gastrointestinal tract was ensured by withholding early feedings and providing continuous nasogastric tube drainage for several days postoperatively. Other investigators[43] have reported resolution of hypertension and abdominal pain after the administration of antihypertensive agents.

The exact etiology of the two types of blood pressure responses in patients after coarctation repair is not clearly defined. It is suggested that the hypertension is caused by stimulation of sympathetic nerve fibers in the aortic isthmus that results in release of norepinephrine and causes juxtaglomerular cells to release renin, both resulting in elevation of systemic blood pressure. An additional effect in increased renin production may be the shunting of blood away from mesenteric arteries, thereby resulting in bowel ischemia and producing the abdominal symptoms.

We and others[44-46] feel that aggressive treatment of early postoperative hypertension decreases the likelihood that the postcoarctectomy syndrome will develop. Before undertaking treatment of hypertension following coarctation repair it is essential that other causes be excluded. These include residual coarctation after an imperfect repair, hypoxemia, hypercarbia, pain, and agitation. Many pharmacologic agents have been used to treat postoperative hypertension, including sodium nitroprusside, propranolol, captopril, reserpine, and hydralazine. Sodium nitroprusside is usually the first agent used, although there is the theoretical problem that it affects primarily vascular smooth muscle rather than attenuating the reflex response of norepinephrine release and increased plasma renin.[45] Recently, the successful use of esmolol, a short-acting β-blocker similar to propranolol has been reported as an adjunct to sodium nitroprusside when a second agent was required.[46, 47] Esmolol has a very short half-life of distribution (2 minutes) and elimination (9 minutes) and can be administered by continuous infusion. These agents are gradually weaned over several days postoperatively. During the weaning, oral antihypertensive agents such as propranolol and/or captopril are usually administered.

In an uncomplicated coarctation repair that has proceeded without significant intraoperative problems, we prefer early extubation in the operating room or the intensive care unit to avoid the stimulating effect of the endotracheal tube in an awakening child.

POSTOPERATIVE ANALGESIA

There are several options available for postoperative treatment of pain. The importance of adequate pain relief in children after thoracotomy has been reviewed.[48] Opioid analgesics are the mainstay of pain relief, and morphine remains the standard by which all other opioids are measured. In addition to intramuscular and intermittent and continuous intravenous infusion, both epidural and intrathecal morphine are utilized to treat postoperative pain in children who have undergone open heart surgery.[49-51] We have also used patient controlled analgesia (PCA) successfully in children as young as 4 years.

There are conflicting data regarding the efficacy and safety of continuous intrapleural administration of bupivacaine to children who have undergone thoracotomy.[52-54] We have employed it on some occasions but not enough to recommend its use. Our success has been better when using intercostal nerve blocks[55-57] performed by either the surgeon or an anesthesiologist. Before closure, the surgeon injects as far posteriorly as possible at the incision level and one or two segments above and below. Alternatively, the anesthesiologist can use a transcutaneous approach at the conclusion of the operation.

REFERENCES

1. Gersony WM: Coarctation of the aorta, in Adams FH, Emmanouilides GC, Riemenschneider TA (eds): *Moss' Heart Disease in Infants, Children and Adolescents,* ed 4. Baltimore, Williams & Wilkins, 1989, p 243.

2. Keith JD: Coarctation of the aorta, in Keith JD, Rowe RD, Vlad P (eds): *Heart Disease in Infancy and Childhood,* ed 3. New York, Macmillan Publishing Co Inc, 1978.

3. Mitchell SC, Korones SB, Bernendes HW: Congenital heart disease in 56,109 births. *Circulation* 1971; 43:323.

4. Garson AG, Bricker JT: Coarctation of the aorta and interrupted aortic arch, in Garson A, Bricker JT, McNamara DG (eds): *The Science and Practice of Pediatric Cardiology,* vol 2. Philadelphia, Lea & Febiger, 1990.

5. Crafoord C, Nylin G: Congenital coarctation of the aorta and its surgical treatment. *J Thorac Cardiovasc Surg* 1945; 14:347.

6. Brinsfield DE, Plauth WH: Clinical recognition and medical management of congenital heart disease, in Hurst JW, Logue RB, Schlant RC, et al (eds): *The Heart,* ed 4. New York, McGraw-Hill International Book Co, 1978.

7. Edwards JE: Coarctation of the aorta, in Gould SE (ed): *Pathology of the Heart,* ed 2. Springfield Ill, Charles C Thomas Publishers, 1960.

8. Tawes RL, Berr CL, Aberdeen E: Congenital bicuspid aortic valves associated with coarctation of the aorta in children. *Br Heart J* 1969; 31:127.

9. Campbell M, Polani PE: The etiology of coarctation of the aorta. *Lancet* 1961; 1:463.

10. Boone ML, Swenson BE, Felson B: Rib notching: Its many causes. *AJR* 1964; 91:1075.

11. Brynolf I, Crafoord C, Mannheimer E: Coarctation of the aorta proximal to both subclavian arteries: Case report of a six year old girl. *J Thorac Cardiovasc Surg* 1958; 35:123.

12. Campbell M: Unilateral rib notching from collateral circulation after division of the subclavian artery. *Br Heart J* 1958; 20:253.

13. Gooding CA, Glickman MB, Suydam MJ: Fate of rib notching after correction of aortic coarctation. *AJR* 1969; 106:21.

14. Hartman AF, Goldring D, Strauss AW, et al: Coarctation of the aorta, in Moss AJ, Adams FH, Emmanouilides GC (eds): *Heart Disease in Infants, Children, and Adolescents,* ed 2. Baltimore, Williams & Wilkins, 1977.

15. Sloan RD, Cooley RN: Coarctation of the aorta: The roentgenologic aspects of 125 surgically confirmed cases. *Radiology* 1953; 61:701.

16. Vick WG, Rokey R, Johnston DL: Nuclear magnetic resonance and positron emission tomography—Clinical aspects, in Garson A, Bricker JT, McNamara DG (eds): *The Science and Practice of Pediatric Cardiology.* Philadelphia, Lea & Febiger, 1990, p 855.

17. Boxer RA, LaCorte MA, Singh S, et al: Nuclear magnetic resonance imaging in evaluation and followup of children treated for coarctation of the aorta. *J Am Coll Cardiol* 1986; 7:1095.

18. Morrow WR, Vick GW III, Nihill MR, et al: Balloon dilation of unoperated coarctation of the aorta: Short and intermediate-term results. *J Am Coll Cardiol* 1988; 11:133.

19. Schreiner MS, Triebwasser A, Keon TP: Ingestion of liquids compared with preoperative fasting in pediatric outpatients. *Anesthesiology* 1990; 72:593.

20. Splinter WM, Stewart JA, Muir JG: The effect of preoperative apple juice on gastric contents, thirst, and hunger in children. *Can J Anaesth* 1989; 36:55.

21. Maltby JR, Koehli N, Ewen A, et al: Gastric fluid volume, pH, and emptying, in elective inpatients: Influences of narcotic-atropine premedication, oral fluid, and ranitidine. *Can J Anaesth* 1988; 35:562.

22. Meakin G, Dingwal AE, Addison GM: Effects of preoperative feedings on gastric pH and volume in children. *Br J Anaesth* 1987; 59:678.

23. Hansen DD: Anesthesia, in Sade RM, Cosgrove DM, Castaneda AR (eds): *Infant and Child Care in Heart Surgery.* St. Louis, Mosby–Year Book, 1977.

24. Bland JW, Williams WH: Anesthesia for treatment of congenital heart defects, in Kaplan JA (ed): *Cardiac Anesthesia.* Orlando, Fla, Grune & Stratton, 1979.

25. Koch F: Perioperative management of the pediatric cardiac patient, in Lake C (ed): *Pediatric Cardiac Anesthesia.* E Norwalk, Conn, Appleton & Lange, 1988.

26. Walters J, Christianson L, Betts EK, et al: Oral vs intramuscular premedication for pediatric inpatients. *Anesthesiology* 1983; 59:A454.

27. Brzustowicz RM, Denkin AN, Betts EK, et al: Efficacy of oral premedication for pediatric outpatient surgery. *Anesthesiology* 1984; 60:475.

28. Nicolson SC, Betts EK, Jobes DR, et al: Comparison of oral and intramuscular preanesthetic medication for pediatric inpatient surgery. *Anesthesiology* 1989; 71:8.

29. Bland JW, Brosius KK, Mancuso TJ, et al: Anesthesia for pediatric and neonatal thoracic surgery, in Kaplan JA (ed): *Thoracic Anesthesia,* ed 2. New York, Churchill Livingstone Inc, 1991, p 497.

30. Hannallah RS, Baker SB, Casey W, et al: Propofol: Effective dose and induction characteristics in unpremedicated children. *Anesthesiology* 1991; 74:217.

31. Tweed WA, Minuck M, Mymin D: Circulatory responses to ketamine anesthesia. *Anesthesiology* 1972; 37:613.

32. Reich DL, Silvay G: Ketamine: An update on the first twenty-five years of clinical experience. *Can J Anaesth* 1989; 36:186–197.

33. Watterson KG, Dhasmana JP, O'Higgins JW, et al: Distal aortic pressure during coarctation operation. *Ann Thorac Surg* 1990; 49:987.

34. Moulton AL: Coarctation of the aorta, in Arciniegas E (ed): *Pediatric Cardiac Surgery.* St Louis, Mosby–Year Book, 1985.

35. Moss AJ, Adams FH, O'Loughlin BH, et al: The growth of the normal aorta and of the anastomotic site in infants following surgical resection of coarctation of the aorta. *Circulation* 1959; 19:338.

36. Schuster SF, Gross RE: Surgery for coarctation of the aorta: A review of 500 cases. *J Thorac Cardiovasc Surg* 1962; 41:54.

37. Pennington DG, Liberthson R, Jacobs M, et al: Critical review of experience with surgical repair of coarctation of the aorta. *J Thorac Cardiovasc Surg* 1979; 77:217.

38. Hallman GL, Cooley DA: *Surgical Treatment of Congenital Heart Disease,* ed 2. Philadelphia, Lea & Febiger, 1975.

39. Kirklin JW, Pacifico AD: Surgical treatment of congenital heart disease, in Hurst JW, Logue RB, Schlant RC, et al (eds): *The Heart,* ed 4. New York, McGraw-Hill International Book Co, 1978.

40. Pontius RG, Brockman HL, Hardy EG, et al: The use of hypothermia in the prevention of paraplegia following temporary aortic occulsion: Experimental observations. *Surgery* 1954; 36:33.

41. Lusoto R, Kyllonen KEJ, Merikallio E: Surgical treatment of coarctation of the aorta with minimal collateral circulation. *Scand J Thorac Cardiovasc Surg* 1980; 14:217.

42. Sealy WC, Harris JS, Young WG, et al: Paradoxical hypertension following resection of coarctation of the aorta. *Surgery* 1957; 42:135.

43. Ho ECK, Moss AJ: The syndrome of "mesenteric arteritis" following surgical repair of aortic coarctation. *Pediatrics* 1972; 49:40.

44. Fox S, Pierce WS, Waldhausen JA: Pathogenesis of paradoxical hypertension after coarctation repair. *Ann Thorac Surg* 1980; 29:135.

45. Taylor SP: Aortic valve and aortic arch anomalies, in Lake CL (ed): *Pediatric Cardiac Anesthesia.* E Norwalk, Conn, Appleton & Lange, 1988, p 333.

46. Vincent RN, Click LA, Williams HM, et al: Esmolol as an adjunct in the treatment of systemic hypertension after operative repair of coarctation of the aorta. *Am J Cardiol* 1990; 65:941.

47. Smerling A, Gersony WM: Esmolol for severe hypertension following repair of aortic coarctation. *Crit Care Med* 1990; 18:1288.

48. Tyler DC: Respiratory effects of pain in a child after thoracotomy. *Anesthesiology* 1989; 70:873.

49. Berde CB, Sethna NF, Holzman RS, et al: Pharmacokinetics of methadone in children and adolescents in the perioperative period. *Anesthesiology* 1987; 67:A579.

50. Berde CB, Holzman RS, Sethna MB, et al: A comparison of methadone and morphine for post-operative analgesia in children and adolescents (abstract). *Anesthesiology* 1988; 69:768.

51. Rosen KR, Rosen DA: Caudal epidural morphine for control of pain following open heart surgery in children. *Anesthesiology* 1989; 70:418.

52. McIlvaine WB, Know RF, Fennessey PV, et al: Continuous infusion of bupivacaine via intrapleural catheter for analgesia after thoracotomy in children. *Anesthesiology* 1988; 69:264.

53. Rosenberg PH, Scheinin BMA, Lepantalo MJA, et al: Continuous intrapleural infusion of bupivacaine for analgesia after thoracotomy. *Anesthesiology* 1987; 67:811.

54. Stevens DS, Edwards WT: Management of pain after thoracic surgery, in Kaplan JA (ed): *Thoracic Anesthesia,* ed 2. New York, Churchill Livingstone Inc, 1991, p 570.

55. Rothstein P, Arthur CR, Feldman HS, et al: Bupivacaine for intercostal nerve blocks in children: Blood concentrations and pharmacokinetics. *Anesth Analg* 1986; 65:625.

56. Rice LJ, Hannallah RS: Local and regional anesthesia, in Motoyama ED, Davis PJ (eds): *Smith's Anesthesia for Infants and Children,* ed 5. St Louis, Mosby–Year Book, 1990.

57. Arthur DS, McNichol LR: Local anaesthetic techniques in paediatric surgery. *Br J Anaesth* 1986; 58:760.

58

Scoliosis and Ehlers-Danlos Syndrome

An 8-year-old girl with Ehlers-Danlos syndrome and kyphoscoliosis is scheduled for anterior spine fusion with Zielke instrumentation. She is small for her age (18 kg) and has severe kyphoscoliosis (Figs 58–1 and 58–2). Hemoglobin, 11.2 g/dL; hematocrit, 34%.

Recommendations by Geoffrey A. Lane, M.B., F.F.A.R.C.S.

The Ehlers-Danlos syndrome (EDS) refers to a group of connective tissue disorders caused by defects in collagen biosynthesis. The principal features include joint hypermobility, hyperelasticity of the skin, a tendency to bruising and bleeding, and poor wound healing causing characteristic broad "cigarette paper" scars. Death can occur from spontaneous arterial rupture or gastrointestinal perforation.

TYPES OF EHLERS-DANLOS SYNDROME

There is a wide range of severity of EDS. Patients with mild forms seldom require medical attention and may undergo surgery and pregnancy without problems. Extreme hyperextensibility may enable the patient to assume the remarkable postures of contortionists; the virtuosity of the violinist Nicolo Paganini has been attributed in part to features of EDS. Patients with severe forms may have severe disabilities, and surgery is fraught with complications and may be lethal.[1]

The classification of EDS into subgroups with characteristic patterns of inheritance, biochemical defects, and clinical manifestations of the disease, is useful in evaluating the surgical patient.[2] Ten different types are currently recognized,[3] and perioperative problems are especially likely in patients with EDS types I, IV, and VI. Type I (gravis) is distinguished by severe manifestations of

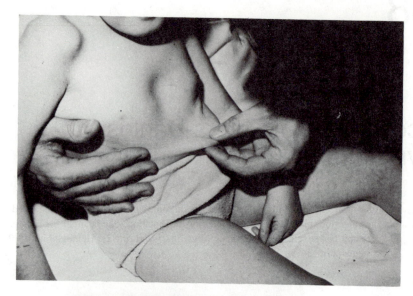

FIG 58−1.
Hyperelasticity of skin in a child with Ehlers-Danlos syndrome.

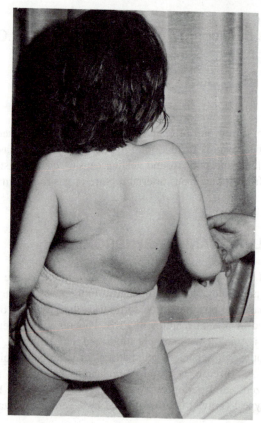

FIG 58−2.
Posterior view of the same child as in Figure 58−1 with marked kyphoscoliosis.

all of the clinical features, including skin hyperelasticity, bruising, and joint hypermobility. Surgery is complicated by poor wound healing and tissues that are extremely friable. Type IV (ecchymotic) is marked by a tendency for rupture of major blood vessels, severe bruising, and intestinal perforation. In these patients, surgery may be complicated by uncontrollable hemorrhage and should be avoided whenever possible. Fortunately, musculoskeletal disorders are uncommon. Type VI is noted for ocular manifestations, including fragility of the cornea and sclera, and kyphoscoliosis.

Less severe forms of EDS include type II (mitis), type III (benign hypermobile), type VIII (periodontal disease), and type X. Inheritance in most forms (including types I through IV and type VIII) is autosomal dominant but may be X-linked recessive (type V and IX) or autosomal recessive (types VI, VII and X).

While the most striking features of this patient may be the manifestations of EDS, kyphoscoliosis itself can cause significant cardiopulmonary problems that may be exacerbated by the surgical approach. The object of surgical correction is to apply suitable corrective forces on the spine to counter the developing curvature and to maintain the position by instrumentation or body casts until permanent fusion occurs through ossification.

The challenge in this case is to develop a management plan that recognizes the potential problems from EDS, together with the logistic problems of managing anesthesia for spine fusion and electrophysiologic monitoring of spinal cord function.

PREOPERATIVE EVALUATION AND PREPARATION

The first priority is to establish the type of EDS by appropriate consultation so that the patient's parents may receive sufficient counseling to participate effectively in the decision to operate. The decision to proceed with surgery must balance the hazards from the specific type of EDS against the risks of progression of both the kyphoscoliosis and the EDS. For this young patient with significant kyphoscoliosis, surgery will only become more difficult as time goes by. Surgery is likely the better option unless type IV EDS is diagnosed; in that case, the risk of arterial bleeding might be considered unacceptable.

Surgical correction of severe kyphoscoliosis usually requires both anterior and posterior spine fusion. Although there are advantages to completing both approaches during a single anesthetic in selected patients, the fragility of the tissues in patients with EDS suggests that the posterior fusion should be staged, ideally 10 to 14 days later.

The bleeding diathesis associated with EDS is usually caused by the connective tissue disorder affecting the walls of the blood vessels and is seldom amenable to treatment other than transfusion. However, coagulation defects do occur and merit investigation and correction to reduce the need for transfusion. Because patients with EDS may require major transfusions for minor surgical procedures, preoperative consultation with the transfusion service is necessary to ensure adequate supplies of blood components. Consideration should be given to intraoperative salvage and autotransfusion of shed blood. Preoperative collection of blood from this patient is unlikely to be useful in view of the volume of blood required and the problems with vascular access.

Cardiovascular features of EDS include mitral valve prolapse, which may require antibiotic prophylaxis because of the risks of bacterial endocarditis, and conduction defects. Various congenital cardiac anomalies have been associated with EDS, but they are uncommon. Echocardiography should indicate any potential problems.

Pulmonary function may be impaired by the kyphoscoliosis and complications of the EDS, including spontaneous pneumothorax. The evaluation should be based on the child's exercise tolerance, previous history of pulmonary complications, clinical examination, and pulmonary function test results. The patient should be in optimum condition for surgery. She may require preoperative physiotherapy and vigorous treatment of intercurrent chest infection.

Intraoperative risks include damage to the skin, eyes, and joints from improper positioning. Special attention should be directed to evaluating postural problems. With the cooperation of the patient and parents, a rehearsal of the likely intraoperative position may guide the subsequent arrangement of the patient's limbs, as well as application of protective devices and restraints.

The child with severe EDS may justly be apprehensive when contemplating major surgery. Minimizing anxiety by preoperative education and premedication is even more important than usual because a lack of cooperation during induction can cause tissue damage. Play therapy and tours of the hospital can be helpful, and the parents should be included since their anxieties are communicated to the child. We would consider having the parents present during induction and would include a visit to the induction room in the tour. Preoperative evaluations and consultations should be arranged on an outpatient basis, with admission on the day of surgery to minimize separation anxiety.

Premedication should be chosen according to the needs of the child and should probably be generous. The oral route is preferable to intramuscular injections, which may cause significant hematomas in patients with EDS.[1] Cherry-flavored oral midazolam, 0.75 mg/kg, provides excellent sedation in 15 to 25 minutes.

OPERATIVE MANAGEMENT

The major anesthetic considerations are provision of adequate vascular access and blood replacement; avoidance of positional injuries to the skin, eyes, and joints; and postoperative pulmonary care. The choice of individual anesthetic agents is determined by the need to avoid loss of the somatosensory evoked potentials (SSEPs) used to monitor spinal cord function. Hypertension should be avoided because of the risks of excessive bleeding and spontaneous arterial rupture.

During induction, the chief concerns will be intravascular access and intubation without tissue trauma. Intravenous induction with thiopental is the method of choice if a suitable vein can be identified. A halothane induction is often more acceptable to the child but should be avoided here because it causes long-lasting depression of SSEPs. A cautious inhalation induction with isoflurane may be necessary if vascular access is difficult, and it will be facilitated by adequate premedication. Percutaneous venous cannulation is often extremely difficult and may require a cutdown in patients with EDS. Central venous catheters are often recommended for spine fusions, but they should not be used for patients with EDS because there is a significant risk of perforation and hematoma formation in the neck or mediastinum. Two large peripheral catheters are essential since major blood loss may occur.

Intubation should be performed with care following the administration of a muscle relaxant to avoid the risks of trauma to the airway. Damage to the teeth can cause significant bleeding from the gums. The endotracheal tube should be secured carefully, preferably with waterproof adhesive tape to resist dislodgement by oral secretions. For any patient undergoing thoracotomy, it is especially important for the distal end of the tube to be midway between the carina and larynx to avoid the extubation or endobronchial intubation that may occur with changes in position.

MONITORING

Although arterial catheterization is advisable for patients having spine fusions, the risk of tears in the arterial wall in those with EDS is significant. Unfortunately, patients with the severe forms of EDS who would benefit most from an arterial catheter are also those at greatest risk for arterial damage. Arterial pressure can be monitored indirectly with a noninvasive automated monitor or with a Doppler transducer, and capnography will guide ventilation. The bladder should be catheterized and urine output monitored.

There is a risk that correction of the kyphoscoliosis may injure the cord; recovery of cord function has occurred when the distraction forces were relaxed immediately following loss of SSEPs. Spinal cord function is monitored during surgery by evoked responses to peripheral stimulation. The low voltage of the responses from scalp electrodes requires averaging of several hundred stimuli by a computer to separate responses from background noise. Most anesthetics depress SSEPs, but narcotics can be used, and 0.25% isoflurane may be acceptable.

POSITIONING

When the patient is turned to the lateral position, the limbs should be positioned carefully to avoid joint dislocation or hyperextension. They should be secured with care and the skin protected by properly positioned restraints and foam pads or sheepskin.

The eyes are especially prone to injury and should be protected with sterile ointment and the lids closed with adhesive tape. A foam "donut" placed under the face avoids pressure on the globe if a wedge is excised from the section under the orbit. Surgical drapes should be kept off the face by an "ether screen."

ANESTHETIC TECHNIQUE

Considerations in the choice of anesthetic technique include the following:

1. High F_{IO_2} to compensate for the collapsed lung tissue caused by retraction
2. Normotension or mild hypotension to avoid spontaneous arterial rupture and excessive bleeding
3. Low airway pressures to reduce the risks of pneumothorax, especially in the dependent lung

A high-dose narcotic infusion with nitrous oxide and 0.25% isoflurane is the preferred anesthetic and has the advantage of providing early postoperative analgesia. Muscle relaxation should be maintained with a nondepolarizing agent such as vecuronium or curare. The latter agent will also provide modest hypotension. Neuromuscular blockade should be monitored with a peripheral nerve stimulator.

Blood loss may be extensive and is likely to exceed the initial blood volume. The amount of blood and fluid replaced should be guided by estimates of blood loss, clinical observations, serial hematocrit determinations, and urine output. In addition to adequate supplies of blood, preparations for transfusion include the availability of blood warmers and pressure infusion devices for rapid transfusion. Component therapy with platelets and fresh frozen plasma may be indicated to prevent coagulopathy if massive bleeding does occur. Calcium administration may be required to prevent hypocalcemia and should be guided by ionized calcium concentrations.

POSTOPERATIVE CARE

The patient should be transferred to the intensive care unit postoperatively and ventilation assisted until pulmonary function is satisfactory, hemorrhage is controlled, and vital signs are stable. Intravenous narcotics should be used for pain relief.

REFERENCES

1. Dolan P, Sisko F, Riley E: Anesthetic considerations for Ehlers-Danlos syndrome. *Anesthesiology* 1980; 52:266–269.
2. McKusick VA: *Heritable Disorders of Connective Tissue,* ed 4. St Louis, Mosby–Year Book, 1972.
3. Byers PH: Disorders of collagen biosynthesis and structure, in Scriver CR, et al (eds): *The Metabolic Basis of Inherited Disease,* ed 6. New York, McGraw-Hill International Book Co, 1989.

59

Renal Transplantation

An 8-year old, 20-kg boy is scheduled for renal transplantation. He has been on hemodialysis for 11 months. Hemoglobin, 6.2 g/dL; hematocrit, 19%; Na, 142 mEq/L; K, 5.8 mEq/L; temperature, 37°C; pulse, 90; respirations, 22; blood pressure, 142/82 mm Hg.

Recommendations by Babu V. Koka, M.D.

Children undergoing renal transplantation pose many challenges to the anesthesiologist because end stage renal disease (ESRD) adversely affects almost all vital organ systems. In addition, ESRD alters the effects of various drugs used in anesthetic practice. Careful preoperative evaluation and preparation of the patient, as well as a knowledge of altered drug responses, are essential in planning and managing anesthesia.

END STAGE RENAL DISEASE

The incidence of ESRD in children under 16 years of age is two to three per million population. Common causes of renal failure in this group are congenital malformations of the kidney and urinary tract, glomerular disorders, and hereditary renal disease. Vascular disease and cortical or papillary necrosis are rare in children as compared with the adult population.

The onset of renal insufficiency is insidious, with subtle changes in the serum composition, renal function tests, and nutritional status. Early detection and treatment of underlying disease will prevent major complications in the initial stage. Management consists of dietary therapy and control of infection, hypertension, cardiac failure, and edema. Evolution of major complications such as malnutrition, significant growth arrest, osteodystrophy, severe fluid and electrolyte imbalances, or cardiovascular disturbances dictates a more aggressive therapeutic approach. Hemodialysis is initiated when the glomerular filtration rate (GFR) falls below 5 mL/1.73 m^2, serum creatinine is greater than 10 mg/dL, and blood urea nitrogen (BUN) is approximately 100 mg/dL.

RENAL TRANSPLANTATION

Dialysis or renal transplantation are the only two options for patients with ESRD. Long-term dialysis is associated with growth deficiencies, irreversible central nervous system (CNS) injury, and problems with vascular access. In contrast, renal transplantation improves the quality of life dramatically[1] and adequate growth and development are possible.[2, 3] Kidney transplantation is much more cost-effective than dialysis over an extended time period. Renal transplantation is the treatment of choice for most children with ESRD and should be presented to the parents as the initial therapeutic choice. Early or "preemptive" renal transplantation can be performed antecedent to fulfillment of the criteria for initiation of dialysis in children suffering from disease states where renal failure would inevitably ensue. Such procedures are very successful and are associated with few complications. However, the timing of kidney transplantation can be controversial in children who are not yet uremic. There may be some benefit in delaying the transplant until after the commencement of dialysis. In small infants, delay is often necessary because it is difficult to find an appropriate donor.

Uremia is associated with suppression of the immune response. It has been suggested that graft survival might be increased if endogenous immunosuppression is induced. However, with the advent of current immunosuppressive agents and surgical techniques, early renal transplantation in children has been shown to be safe and effective in terms of patient and graft survival.[4, 5]

There is great disparity between need and the number of organs available for transplantation despite efforts to increase organ procurement by public awareness campaigns. In the United States alone, there are over 18,000 patients awaiting renal transplantation. In 1990, The National Organ Procurement and Transplantation Network (UNOS) reported that 9,560 renal transplants were performed in the United States: 7,787 from cadaveric donors and 1,773 from living donors.

The outcome of renal transplantation depends upon the donor source, the transplant center, and the type of immunosuppressive therapy employed. At the Children's Hospital in Boston, the overall actuarial survival rate is 91% at 1 year, 83% at 10 years, and 81% at 15 years.[6] In general, kidneys taken from living related donors seem to fare better than those from cadaveric donors. Graft retention is better, and mortality is lower. This difference is particularly evident in children where the 1-year graft survival rate for kidneys from living related donors is 88% and that from cadavers is 71%. Children less than 16 years of age and elderly patients over 60 have a lower graft survival rate (73%) as compared with the rate (79%) for patients aged 16 to 60 years following cadaveric transplantation. The sex of the recipient is not a significant factor in transplant outcome. However, the age and the sex of the donor seem to have some influence on graft survival. Kidneys taken from very young or very old donors seem to do poorly.[7] In young children, the 1-year graft survival rate of cadaver kidneys from donors less than 4 years of age is 50%, whereas it is 87% with kidneys from donors older than 4 years.[8] In the short term, the 1-year graft survival rates are the same for kidneys from male or female donors. However, long-term survival rates for patients who received kidneys from male donors seem to be better than when the donor is female. Other factors that influence the outcome of renal transplantation are opportunistic infections,[9] noncompliance with immunosuppressive protocols,[10] pretransplant transfusions, HLA-DR mismatch, donor race, and the cause of donor death.

In pediatric patients, matching the size of the donor organ with the recipient's proportions is critical. There are several problems when a small infant receives a large kidney from an adult donor. A substantial portion of the cardiac output will be diverted to the transplanted kidney since it possesses comparably large capacitance and low resistance. The relatively small caliber of the recipient's vessels may cause problems with vascular anastomosis. Closure of the abdomen is difficult when a large donor kidney is placed into a small abdominal cavity. Most of the surgical difficulties can be resolved by placing the kidney intra-abdominally. Cardiac output and renal perfusion must be maintained by aggressive volume expansion and appropriate drug therapy during the surgical procedure and in the immediate postoperative period.

PREOPERATIVE CONSIDERATIONS

Most children have undergone several surgical interventions prior to renal transplantation. Vascular access procedures are required for hemodialysis and nephrectomies are performed for severe hypertension, chronic infection, or malignancy. Some patients will require subtotal parathyroidectomy for secondary hyperparathyroidism.

The patient's fluid and electrolyte status must be carefully evaluated. An accumulation of fluid results in peripheral edema, congestive heart failure, and hypertension. In hypertensive patients, the blood pressure is exquisitely sensitive to changes in blood volume. An increase in blood volume may precipitate a hypertensive crisis. Conversely, a normal or low blood pressure in a previously uncontrolled hypertensive patient may signal hypovolemia. The status of hydration should be ascertained by a careful review of the history and physical examination, an accurate measurement of fluid intake and output, and determinations of weight before and after dialysis, serial electrolytes, hematocrit, and blood pressure.

Hyperkalemia is frequent in the late stages of uremia and is due to decreased excretion of potassium. Infection, acidosis, hemolysis, and increased tissue catabolism can further increase the serum potassium level. Serum potassium values must be interpreted cautiously in small children. Potassium levels may be falsely elevated due to hemolysis at the time blood is drawn. With spurious hyperkalemia the electrocardiogram is normal, in contrast to the profound changes in the electrocardiogram associated with actual elevation of the potassium level. As serum potassium levels increase, the electrocardiogram progressively shows peaked T waves, a widening QRS complex, decreased P waves, a prolonged PR interval, atrial standstill, and finally, ventricular asystole.

This patient has a serum potassium of 5.8 mEq/L, which could be hazardous because further increases of potassium may be induced by surgical trauma, acidosis, transfusions, hypoxemia, hypothermia, and infection. Aggressive efforts should be made to reduce the serum potassium level to 5.5 mEq/L in the immediate preoperative period. Methods of decreasing serum potassium levels are based on the urgency of surgery and the severity of the cardiac effects of hyperkalemia. Hemodialysis is the most effective method for reducing the serum potassium level in patients with ESRD. Ion exchange therapy with sodium polystyrene sulfonate (Kayexalate), 1 g/kg orally or as a retention enema, will reduce the serum potassium level by 1 mEq/L within 2 to 4 hours. Glucose, 1 to 2 g/kg, with insulin, 1 unit/4 g glucose, administered intravenously will rapidly lower the serum potassium by driving potassium into the liver. Calcium gluconate, 30 to 60 mg/kg, or calcium chloride, 10 to 20 mg/kg administered intravenously, will oppose the effects of hyperkalemia on the myocardium. Sodium bicarbonate, 1 to 2 mEq/kg administered intravenously, will promote intracellular transfer of potassium due to the increase in pH. The last two therapeutic interventions have a rapid onset and are quite effective; however the effect is transient.

Hypokalemia can also occur in patients with ESRD and may be due to a variety of causes such as diuretic therapy, poor dietary intake, specific renal tubular defects, or hyperaldosteronism secondary to volume depletion. Mild hyponatremia commonly results from hemodilution but does not usually require treatment. Hypocalcemia is frequent because of decreased absorption of calcium from the gastrointestinal tract due to reduced synthesis of 1,25-dihydroxycholecalciferol and to the decreased effectiveness of parathyroid hormone on the bone. However, tetany is rare and hypocalcemia by itself is not an indication for intravenous calcium supplementation. Hyperphosphatemia is common due to decreased excretion of phosphate. It is treated with aluminum hydroxide–containing antacids, which bind phosphate in the gastrointestinal tract. Serum magnesium levels may be elevated in patients ingesting normal amounts of magnesium. Measurement of serum calcium, magnesium, and phosphate levels in the preoperative period is recommended because all of the ions influence neuromuscular transmission and the action of neuromuscular blocking agents.

Mild metabolic acidosis is common in ESRD and usually persists despite dialysis. Partial correction of acidosis with sodium bicarbonate will give symptomatic relief from hyperpnea and altered sensorium.

Most of the above-mentioned fluid and electrolyte imbalances can be corrected by dialysis; therefore, the patient should be hemodialyzed prior to renal transplantation if already on a dialysis regimen. A fall in the predialysis BUN level from 60 to 90 mg/dL to a postdialysis value of 15 to 30 mg/dL can be expected with adequate dialysis.

A normochromic normocytic anemia due to decreased erythropoiesis, low erythropoietin production, shorter red cell life span, bleeding, and decreased utilization of iron is common in patients with ESRD. Fluid retention exaggerates the anemia. Hematocrit values of 15% to 20% and hemoglobin concentrations of 5 to 7 g/dL are frequent. This degree of anemia is well tolerated because of an increased cardiac output, shift of the oxygen-hemoglobin dissociation curve, and increases in 2,3-DPG levels. Hypoxemia is especially dangerous in patients with severe anemia. When the hemoglobin contents is low, oxygen-carrying capacity is reduced. In addition, patients with very low hemoglobin levels will not develop cyanosis, and the familiar visible warning of hypoxemia will not be displayed.

While the exact mechanisms are still unknown, transfusion exerts beneficial effects on allograft survival in patients as well as animal models. A recent report suggests that transfusion in which there is a common HLA haplotype or shared HLA-B and HLA-DR antigens induces tolerance to donor antigens.[11]

With the advent of more effective immunosuppressive agents, the clinical importance of transfusion prior to organ transplantation has declined.[12] Potential adverse effects of transfusion are inhibition of erythropoietin production, transmission of viral diseases, and transfer of HLA antigen by white blood cells. The blood volume remains normal or above normal in the presence of anemia and low red cell mass. Therefore, hypervolemia, which can precipitate a hypertensive crisis, should be conscientiously averted by frequent monitoring of blood pressure during transfusion.

Coagulation defects and prolonged bleeding times are common in patients with ESRD. These result from decreased platelet adhesiveness due to activation of platelet factor 3. The defects can be corrected by hemodialysis or platelet transfusion, and blood loss during the transplant procedure should not be excessive.

The incidence of hepatitis among children receiving hemodialysis is reported to be 10%, primarily due to repeated transfusion. Anesthesia personnel should be aware of the risk of transmission of hepatitis and possibly other viral infections and use appropriate precautions.

Hypertension and edema are more common in children with ESRD than in adults. High blood pressure is often the result of sodium and water excess and can be controlled by salt restriction, diuretics, and dialysis. Inappropriate administration of saline or blood may lead to severe hypertension and congestive heart failure. Many patients take antihypertensive medications such as hydralazine, propranolol, and diazoxide, as well as diuretics such as hydrochlorthiazide and furosemide. The duration, efficacy, and side effects of these drugs should be carefully evaluated preoperatively. It is essential that antihypertensive medication be administered until the time of surgery because an acute hypertensive crisis may develop if treatment is abruptly discontinued. In hypertensive emergencies, hydralazine, 0.1 to 0.5 mg/kg, or diazoxide, 2 mg/kg, can be administered intravenously.

Cardiac failure is managed by lowering the blood pressure, fluid restriction, the administration of diuretics, and the judicious use of digoxin. Because digoxin is not excreted by the kidney and is dialyzable, it should be used with caution. Digitalis toxicity may be masked by elevated serum potassium levels and can be aggravated by hypokalemia.

Patients who are taking steroids should receive normal maintenance doses preoperatively. The dose is increased during the procedure to cover increased demands due to stress as well as for an immunosuppressive effect. With the advent of cyclosporine, it is possible to avoid steroids in patients undergoing renal transplantation.

Children with ESRD are of small stature because growth and sexual maturation are delayed. Psychological and emotional development is often erroneously underestimated by unacquainted medical personnel due to the patient's diminutive outward appearance. These children, who in actuality are older than they look, often feel indignant about this miscalculation. The children may have profound psychological disturbances, and consideration should be given to these issues during the preoperative visit. Many patients view dialysis as a traumatic experience and kidney transplantation as a panacea. Adolescents usually have greater emotional difficulty than do younger children. The preoperative visit is best time to provide an honest description of procedures and the expected perioperative events. Preoperative sedation with midazolam is often extremely effective.

INTRAOPERATIVE MANAGEMENT

Initially, the patient should be monitored with a precordial stethoscope, pulse oximeter, blood pressure cuff, and electrocardiogram. Following the induction of anesthesia, a Silastic central venous catheter should be placed in the superior vena cava under strict sterile conditions to monitor central venous pressure in the perioperative period and for administration of antibiotics and immunosuppressive agents during the period of hospitalization. An arterial catheter is essential in a small child receiving a large adult kidney. After placement of a Foley catheter, the bladder should be filled with 100 to 200 mL of antibiotic solution. Immunosuppressive agents and antibiotics should be administered during this period.

During induction and positioning of the patient, care should be taken to avoid injury to brittle bones and teeth. Hemodialysis access sites should be shielded by ample padding to minimize pressure and prevent thrombosis with consequent loss of vascular access.

Most patients undergo rapid-sequence induction with cricoid pressure followed by endotracheal intubation. Gastric hypersecretion is frequent in patients with uremia. Gastrin levels are elevated because gastrin is normally degraded by the kidney. The risk of aspiration is increased in patients undergoing emergency renal transplantation or those with nausea and vomiting. In such situations a rapid sequence induction is imperative. Decreased hepatic synthesis and increased plasma volume reduce plasma pseudocholinesterase levels to 45% of normal. However, the prolonged action of succinylcholine has very little clinical significance. The administration of succinylcholine is best avoided when the serum potassium level is greater than 5.5 mEq/L. There are isolated reports of life-threatening hyperkalemia following succinylcholine administration in patients with ESRD. However, well-documented studies have demonstrated that the risk of hyperkalemia is no greater than in patients without renal disease.

Anesthesia should be induced with caution because patients who are volume depleted may experience significant hypotension due to myocardial depression and decreased systemic vascular resistance caused by the induction agents. Initiation of positive-pressure ventilation may further reduce venous return to the heart. Rapid volume expansion with a 5% albumin solution will usually correct the problem. Uremic patients are said to be sensitive to barbiturates because of an altered blood-brain barrier, decreased plasma protein binding, and abnormal cerebral metabolism. Consequently, the onset of anesthesia may be rapid. A lower dose of thiopental is usually adequate because less of the drug is bound to protein. Induction with inhalation agents is similarly rapid due to hyperventilation induced by metabolic acidosis. In patients receiving antihypertensive therapy, halothane can cause arrhythmias or produce hypotension.

Halothane can be used for induction in small children when an intravenous induction is not feasible. The use of halothane in the presence of liver disease is controversial. Isoflurane has the advantage of more rapid uptake and elimination, and it causes less myocardial depression. However, it is not suitable as an induction agent due to irritant effects on the airway. For maintenance of anesthesia, isoflurane is the agent of choice, either alone or with low-dose narcotics and a nondepolarizing muscle relaxant. Nitrous oxide can be administered to reduce the requirement for potent inhalation agents. However, disadvantages are bowel distension and a higher incidence of nausea and vomiting.

Elimination of muscle relaxants is delayed in patients with ESRD.[13] Therefore, monitoring of neuromuscular blockade with a blockade monitor is crucial. The responses to train-of-four and single-twitch stimulation should be observed frequently. Pancuronium can cause prolonged blockade when administered in high doses or in repeated doses. Vecuronium, which seems to have little hemodynamic impact and less cumulative effect,[14] has been used successfully in patients undergoing renal transplantation. Elimination of atracurium is not dependent upon renal or hepatic function because it is degraded by ester hydrolysis and spontaneous Hoffmann elimination. Atracurium seems to be an exemplary neuromuscular blocking agent for patients with hepatic or renal failure because of its elimination characteristics. It is important to recall that elimination of muscle relaxants and agents used to reverse neuromuscular blockade is retarded to the same extent. Therefore, there should be no problem with adequate and lasting reversal of neuromuscular blockade. If prolonged muscle paralysis should occur, the anesthesiologist should rule out excessive dosage of muscle relaxants and anesthetic agents, acidosis, hypocalcemia, and hypermagnesemia.

INTRAOPERATIVE COMPLICATIONS

Hypotension and arrhythmias may occur with unclamping of the aorta and vena cava and reperfusion of the kidney. The etiology is multifactorial. The ischemic lower half of the body or the newly transplanted kidney can release substances with vasodilatory properties, potassium, and lactic acid. Using an adult kidney in a small child in effect adds a large vascular bed capable of sequestering 25% to 40% of the patient's total blood volume. Finally, blood loss occurs if the vascular anastomoses leak. These effects can be minimized by early adequate volume expansion.

Maintenance fluid replacement is usually a 2.5% dextrose in 0.45% sodium chloride solution. Third-space fluid loss should be replaced with normal saline or a 5% albumin solution. Blood loss is replaced with red blood cells. Ringer's lactate should usually be avoided because it contains potassium. Small children receiving adult kidneys should receive fluid therapy sufficient to maintain a systolic blood pressure of 130 to 140 mm Hg and a central venous pressure of 15 to 18 cm Hg. Transplanted adult kidneys seem to function better if they are perfused at mean arterial pressures similar to adult values. Sodium bicarbonate and calcium may also be administered when the clamps are released. If hypotension persists in spite of volume expansion, a vasopressor such as dopamine or dobutamine can be used. Furosemide, 1 mg/kg, and mannitol, 0.5 g/kg, are administered if there is no urine output.

Kidneys from living donors become firm, turn red, and begin to function very quickly. Kidneys from cadaveric donors often take a little longer, and there may be a period of oliguria or anuria if the preservation time was prolonged. When the urine output is not satisfactory, every effort should be made to treat hypotension and hypovolemia. Other intraoperative problems include hypothermia, bleeding, and increased intra-abdominal pressure from placement of a large organ in a small abdominal cavity, which produces decreased venous return and inhibits diaphragmatic excursions.

POSTOPERATIVE CARE

The heart rate, arterial blood pressure, and central venous pressure should be continuously monitored and fluid and electrolyte status carefully regulated. Potassium, bicarbonate, calcium, phosphorus, and magnesium levels should be measured at 2- to 4-hour intervals. Urine output should be replaced with 2.5% dextrose in 0.45% sodium chloride. Blood glucose should be monitored closely because hyperglycemia can result from such replacement, especially when large volumes are required.

SUMMARY

Great strides have been made in solving most of the technical difficulties regarding surgery and anesthesia for renal transplantation in the past decade. Better systems of donor organ procurement[15, 16] and more equitable distribution of the organs are needed. Advances in immunosuppressive therapy should lead to enhanced graft survival. Experimental new fields such as acquired tolerance development[17] and cross-species transplantation are on the horizon.

REFERENCES

1. Morel P, Almond PS, Matas AJ, et al: Long-term quality of life after kidney transplantation in childhood. *Transplantation* 1991; 52:47–53.
2. Fennell RS, et al: Growth in children following kidney transplantation. *Pediatr Nephrol* 1990; 4:335–339.
3. Aschendroff C, Offner G, Winkler I, et al: Adult height achieved in children after kidney transplantation. *Am J Dis Child* 1990; 144:1138–1141.
4. Nevins TE, Danielson G: Prior dialysis does not affect the outcome of pediatric renal transplantation. *Pediatr Nephrol* 1991; 5:211–214.
5. Fitzwater DS, Brouhard BH, Garred D, et al: The outcome of renal transplantation in children without prolonged pre-transplant dialysis. *Clin Pediat* 1991; 30:148–152.
6. Kim MS, Jabs K, Harmon WE: Long-term patient survival in a pediatric renal transplantation program. *Transplantation* 1990; 51:413–416.
7. Koka P, Cecka JM: Sex and age effects in renal transplantation. *Clin Transplant* 1990; 10:437–446.
8. So SKS, et al: The use of cadaver kidneys for transplantation in young children. *Transplantation* 1990; 50:979–983.
9. Harmon WE: Opportunistic infections in children following renal transplantation. *Pediatr Nephrol* 1991; 5:118–125.
10. Ettenger RB, Rosenthol JT, Marik JC, et al: Improved cadaveric renal transplant outcome in children. *Pediatr Nephrol* 1991; 5:137–142.
11. van Twuyver E, et al: Pre-transplantation blood transfusion revisited. *N Engl J Med* 1991; 17:1210–1213.
12. Potter DE, Portale AA, Melzer JS, et al: Are blood transfusions beneficial in the cyclosporine era? *Pediatr Nephrol* 1991; 5:168–172.
13. Gramstad L: Atracurium, vecuronium and pancuronium in end-stage renal failure. Dose response properties and interactions with azathioprine. *Br J Anaesth* 1987; 59:995–1003.
14. Starsnic MA, Goldberg ME, Ritter DE, et al: Does vecuronium accumulate in the renal transplant patient? *Can J Anaesth* 1989; 36:35–39.
15. Najarian JS, Matas AJ: The present and future of kidney transplantation. *Transplant Proc* 1991; 23:2075–2082.
16. Veatch RM: The shortage of organs for transplantation. *N Engl J Med* 1991; 325:1243–1249.
17. Sachs DH: Specific transplantation tolerance. *N Engl J Med* 1991; 325:1240–1241.

60

Muscle Biopsy for Possible Malignant Hyperthermia

An 8-year-old boy is referred for muscle biopsy for the diagnosis of suspected malignant hyperthermia (MH). He was anesthetized at another hospital 6 weeks before for tonsillectomy. Following an inhalation induction with halothane-nitrous oxide-oxygen, he received 0.25 mg atropine and 50 mg succinylcholine. The anesthesiologist was unable to open the child's mouth to perform laryngoscopy. Another 50 mg succinylcholine was administered, but intubation was still impossible, and the anesthesiologist discontinued use of the anesthetic. On arrival in the recovery room the child's pulse was 150; rectal temperature, 37.5°C, and oxygen saturation, 96%. No blood gas results were obtained. The creatine phosphokinase (CPK) level 1 week later was 200 IU.

Recommendations by Henry Rosenberg, M.D.

Although MH was first described in 1960,[1] it was not until approximately 15 years later that the relationship between masseter spasm and MH was recognized. The interpretation of masseter spasm after succinylcholine administration, its relationship to MH susceptibility, and its differentiation from the normal increase in muscle tone that can be seen in children who receive succinylcholine persist as an important clinical and laboratory problem until this day. Most anesthesiologists, especially those interested in the management of patients with MH, feel that masseter muscle rigidity after succinylcholine administration is a warning sign for MH and that the response to that sign should include either discontinuation of the anesthetic or conversion to a nontriggering anesthetic technique. Given that approximately 1 in 200 children who receive an inhalation induction followed by succinylcholine will develop masseter muscle rigidity,[2, 3] this problem is a not infrequent indication for diagnostic muscle biopsy for evaluation of MH susceptibility.

MUSCLE BIOPSY TESTING PROCEDURES

Muscle biopsy for the diagnosis of MH was first described in the early 1970s. Since that time, the diagnostic procedure and techniques have been refined and standardized both in North America and Europe.[4] At present, there are approximately 23 muscle biopsy diagnostic centers for MH in North America. Although other diagnostic tests have been recommended or suggested, only the contracture test involving exposure of muscle biopsy specimens to caffeine or halothane has withstood the test of time. In this test, approximately 1.5 g of muscle tissue is excised from the vastus lateralis muscle, and bundles weighing 60 to 200 mg are mounted in a muscle bath at 37°C. After a period of equilibration, muscle tissue is exposed either to 3% halothane for a period of 4 minutes or to incremental doses of caffeine. The halothane contracture response is recorded, as is the contracture response to caffeine (Fig 60–1). Based on these contracture values, the diagnosis of MH is confirmed or ruled out.

Since 1987, representatives of the biopsy centers in North America have met on a regular basis to standardize the testing protocol in an attempt to define the sensitivity and specificity of this test. Initial studies in North America centered on defining the rate of false-positive results by using muscle biopsy specimens from patients not thought to be MH susceptible and undergoing peripheral orthopedic procedures, that is, control samples. From these studies it was determined that the most specific diagnostic tests for MH were the contracture response to 3% halothane, the contracture response to 2 mM caffeine, and the percentage of maximum increase in contracture response at 2mM caffeine.[5]

It was also determined that variations in interpretation of the results emanated from differences in individual biopsy centers. Therefore, each biopsy center must determine its own control and its own threshold values for determining MH susceptibility.

Most recently, by utilizing a contracture response of 0.6 g to 3% halothane and a 0.3-g contracture to 2m M caffeine as defining MH susceptibility, it has been possible to define the sensitivity and specificity of the contracture test. When data are used from those not anticipated to be MH susceptible as defined above and results from those who likely experienced an unequivocal episode of MH, the sensitivity of contracture testing is 100%, and the specificity is over 80%. These are excellent findings for a diagnostic test. In partial confirmation of these findings, two studies have shown that the likelihood of false-negative diagnosis by the caffeine-halothane contracture test is 0%.[6]

Muscle biopsy centers in Europe, the United States, and other parts of the world generally agree that contracture responses to halothane and caffeine are the most accurate way to diagnose MH susceptibility. The causes of false-positive responses need to be more clearly defined.

One drawback to the muscle biopsy contracture test is that fresh muscle specimens must be tested. Therefore, the biopsy samples must be obtained within 4 to 6 hours of testing. The biopsy may be performed either on an outpatient basis or with a 1-day hospital stay. The vastus lateralis muscle has, by tradition, been chosen for testing. It is unknown whether other muscles such as the rectus abdominis or gracilis muscles behave in a similar fashion to the vastus muscle.

Prior to performing a muscle biopsy, most centers require a detailed history and physical examination as well as a family history related to anesthesia experiences. A CPK level is often determined on the day of surgery or as part of the preadmission testing procedure. Some centers will seek a neurologic evaluation since a small percentage of patients will have a concomitant muscle

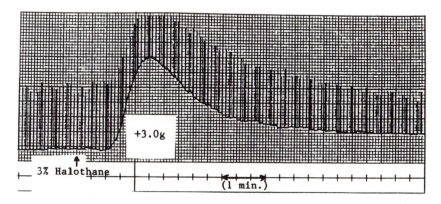

Abnormal Halothane Contracture

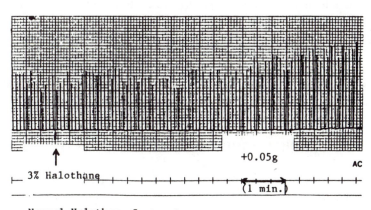

Normal Halothane Contracture

FIG 60–1.

An example of a contracture response to 3% halothane in a muscle specimen from an MH-susceptible patient *(top)* and a nonsusceptible patient *(bottom)*. On exposure to 3% halothane the MH muscle exhibits a 3-g contracture. (From Barash PG, Cullen BF, Stoelting RK (eds): *Clinical Anesthesia.* Philadelphia, JB Lippincott, 1989. Used by permission.)

disorder. The minimum age for muscle biopsy varies between centers, with a minimum weight of 20 kg accepted by our center. Others require the patient to be over 8 years of age.

ANESTHETIC MANAGEMENT FOR MUSCLE BIOPSY

Preparation of the anesthesia machine has been simplified in recent years following the demonstration that the machine can be purged of residual concentrations of inhalation agents by changing anesthesia tubing and flowing 10 L/min of oxygen for 10 minutes, if the fresh gas hose is changed. Twenty minutes is required if the fresh gas hose is not changed.[7] Vaporizers should be disconnected or drained prior to anesthesia. Preoperative administration of dantrolene is not recommended since there is some evidence that dantrolene may alter the contracture response to halothane. Similarly, calcium channel blockers and β-blockers may influence the contracture responses. Since the muscle biopsy is a superficial procedure involving one extremity, the procedure is imminently suitable to regional anesthesia techniques. Our preferences have been for femoral and lateral femoral cutaneous nerve blocks. More recently, we have been successful in using the block described by Dalens et al., termed the *fascia iliaca block*.[8] Spinal and epidural anesthesia may also be used.

For children who are uncooperative, generally below the age of 6 years, general anesthesia is induced intravenously with a rapidly acting agent and maintained with nitrous oxide and oxygen. Ketamine, propofol, narcotics, and barbiturates are appropriate intravenous induction agents. A narcotic and muscle relaxant such as atracurium or vecuronium are administered. Of course, the potent halogenated hydrocarbon anesthetics as well as ether, cyclopropane, and succinylcholine are triggering agents for MH and are avoided.

In our facility, the biopsy sample is obtained through an incision of approximately 2.5 in. in length. At the same time that the tissue is obtained for contracture testing, specimens are also obtained for histology and histochemistry.

The patient is observed in the recovery room in the usual fashion and discharged from the hospital in the evening if there are no complications. Older patients or those who may be experiencing more discomfort may be admitted overnight. The patient is able to ambulate on the evening of surgery and returns to full activity in approximately 10 days. The period of acute disability following muscle biopsy is usually 2 to 3 days, and the incidence of morbidity is extremely low.

INDICATIONS FOR MUSCLE BIOPSY

Masseter muscle rigidity is one of the most common indications for muscle biopsy. As in this patient, it is not unusual for the masseter muscle response to last for a brief period of time and for the patient to have a benign postoperative course. Elevation of the CPK concentration is expected on the evening of surgery, and peak levels occur within 24 hours. We have previously demonstrated that patients with CPK elevations above 20,000 IU have an extremely high likelihood of developing MH.[9] In such situations, we ensure that the CPK level has returned toward normal and recommend muscle biopsy since the patient may harbor an underlying myopathy.

The second most common reason for muscle biopsy is a family history of MH. Other reasons for biopsy include unexplained and unexpected postoperative myoglobinuria and intraoperative tachycardia, hypertension, and fever. Heat stroke, neuroleptic malignant syndrome, and unexplained elevation of CPK levels are other uncommon reasons for diagnostic biopsy.

WHY HAVE THE MUSCLE BIOPSY PERFORMED?

Some have questioned the value of muscle biopsy since after a suspicious episode such as the one described here, patients should be cautioned regarding susceptibility to MH and precautions would likely be taken should they need surgery or anesthesia in the future. Therefore, if the patient advises his anesthesiologist that he may be MH susceptible and appropriate precautions taken, the risk of MH is virtually nonexistent. However, not all practitioners are willing and able to care for MH-susceptible patients. Dentists, in particular, often object to caring for patients with MH susceptibility. Some smaller hospital facilities, rather than risk an MH episode, refer patients to another facility. This may cause inconvenience for the patient and his family. In addition, admission to the military and access to insurance coverage may be restricted. Finally and most importantly, another reason for muscle biopsy is the inherited nature of the syndrome. It is important to determine, with accuracy, whether other members of the family might be at risk of developing MH. Therefore, excluding the diagnosis of MH will eliminate inconvenience and anxiety in many individuals other than just the patient with the suspected history of MH.

Patients in whom the diagnosis of MH susceptibility is established from the contracture test are advised to wear a Medic-Alert bracelet and receive information from the Malignant Hyperthermia Association of the United States. They are also advised to caution other family members as to the likelihood or possibility of MH susceptibility, and they in turn should have muscle biopsy testing. An elevated CPK level in a close relative increases the likelihood of MH susceptibility dramatically. However, this increased CPK is not diagnostic of MH susceptibility, and certainly a normal CPK value does not indicate nonsusceptibility.

In the face of negative biopsy findings after an episode of masseter muscle rigidity, our current practice is to advise the patient that he is not at risk for MH. Since masseter rigidity induced by succinylcholine administration has never been recorded to be an inherited problem, other members of the family need not undergo muscle biopsy testing.

In conclusion, diagnostic muscle biopsy testing with the caffeine-halothane contracture test is currently the only accepted diagnostic test for MH. Unfortunately, the test involves freshly biopsied tissue. The sensitivity and specificity of the test is quite acceptable. When a muscle biopsy test is performed, it is important to evaluate the patient clinically and pathologically for other myopathic disorders. Fortunately, the test involves minimal risk to the patient and only a brief period of discomfort and disability. The results of testing have major health implications for the patient and his family.

REFERENCES

1. Denborough MA, Lovell RRH: Anaesthetic deaths in a family. *Lancet* 1960; 2:45.
2. Schwartz L, Rockoff MA, Koka BV: Masseter spasm with anesthesia: Incidence and implications. *Anesthesiology* 1984; 61:772.
3. Littleford JA, Patel LR, Bose D, et al: Masseter muscle spasm in children: Implications of continuing the triggering anesthetic. *Anesth Analg* 1991; 72:151–160.
4. Larach MG for the North American MH Group: Standardization of the caffeine halothane muscle contracture test. North American Malignant Hyperthermia Group. *Anesth Analg* 1989; 69:511–515.
5. Larach MG, Landis JR, Bunn JS, et al: Prediction of malignant hyperthermia susceptibility in low-risk subjects. *Anesthesiology* 1992; 76:16–27.
6. Allen GC, Rosenberg H, Fletcher JE: Safety of general anesthesia in patients previously tested negative for malignant hyperthermia. *Anesthesiology* 1990; 72:619–622.
7. Beebe JJ, Sessler DI: Preparation of anesthesia machines for patients susceptible to malignant hyperthermia. *Anesthesiology* 1985; 62:651.

8. Dalens B, Vanneuville G, Tanguy A: Comparison of the fascia iliaca compartment block with the 3 in 1 block in children. *Anesth Analg* 1989; 69:705–713.
9. Fletcher JE, Rosenberg H: In vitro interaction between halothane and succinylcholine in human skeletal muscle: Implications for malignant hyperthermia and masseter muscle rigidity. *Anesthesiology* 1985; 62:190.

61

Fractured Humerus

A 9-year-old boy who fell out of a treehouse 1 hour after eating dinner sustained a supracondylar fracture of the humerus. Immediate closed, possibly open, reduction is required because of an absence of the radial pulse. The parents ask whether a local anesthetic can be used because their older child vomited and aspirated during induction of anesthesia for an emergency procedure. No laboratory data are available.

Recommendations by Linda Jo Rice, M.D., and John T. Britton, M.D.

A supracondylar fracture is the most common elbow fracture in children. All degrees of displacement occur, and entrapment of the radial nerve can occur with reduction. Absence of the radial pulse, coolness, poor color, and pain on passive extension of the fingers indicates vascular compromise and requires emergent reduction of the fracture. If ischemia of the hand fails to resolve following reduction of the fracture, exploration of the antecubital fossa is mandatory.[1]

This child presents several problems. He has a full stomach, with a concomitant increased risk of vomiting and aspiration. In addition, there are no preoperative laboratory data. Finally, the surgery is a true emergency because the absence of a radial pulse indicates compromise of the brachial vessels; thus immediate reduction of the fracture is required to preserve vascular integrity to the hand.

THE FULL STOMACH

The increased risk of vomiting and aspiration is the major difference between an elective procedure and the same surgery performed on an emergent basis. The effect of trauma on gastric motility and emptying has been investigated in children.[2] The interval between the last oral intake and injury is important in determining the volume of gastric contents, and the sensation of hunger is not indicative of an empty stomach. Some patients have high gastric volumes after 8 hours of starvation. Therefore, it is recommended that all children who have general anesthesia following trauma have their airways protected with an endotracheal tube. A rapid-sequence induction is usually most appropriate.

If the time interval to surgery permits, preparation of the pediatric patient by the administration of antacids, H_2 blockers, and metoclopramide might be considered.[3, 4] These drugs have the same effects on gastric pH and gastric volume in pediatric patients as in adults. However, they are not commonly used in pediatric anesthesia practice. In this patient, there is insufficient time for them to exert maximum effects.

PREOPERATIVE LABORATORY EVALUATION

Recently, many traditional anesthetic practices have come into question, including routine preoperative laboratory determinations in asymptomatic pediatric patients. All studies appear to indicate that clinically significant anemia is very rare in otherwise healthy, well-nourished, active surgical patients.[5, 6] This is particularly true if the child is over 1 year of age. Mild anemia is not usually considered a contraindication to surgery because acceptable levels of hemoglobin appear to be on a downward trend as a result of the recognition of the risks of red blood cell transfusion.

This child sustained an injury that is unlikely to have a large amount of hidden blood loss. By history, he is otherwise healthy and is certainly active enough to break an arm! Therefore, it is not necessary to delay surgery until the hemoglobin level can be determined since the results are unlikely to alter anesthetic management. If statutory requirements make such a determination mandatory, a small amount of blood can be obtained when the intravenous catheter is inserted.

REGIONAL OR GENERAL ANESTHESIA?

This decision rests in large part on the maturity of the child and his and his parents' wishes. It is also dependent on the time required for surgery and the necessity to evaluate motor function following the surgical procedure. A regional anesthetic, even with a low concentration of local anesthetic, may make motor evaluation difficult. There is no reason, however, to avoid regional anesthesia for fear of undetected cast tightness causing impairment of the circulation because circulation checks are as effective as the presence of pain in detecting such a problem. Surgical procedures lasting up to 9 hours have been performed in sedated children under regional blockade. Keeping a child still and in the supine position for more than 2 hours becomes increasingly difficult unless large amounts of sedation are employed. This is undesirable in a patient with a full stomach.

REGIONAL ANESTHESIA

If the orthopedic surgeon has no objection to a regional block, the child and parents are psychologically appropriate for regional blockade as the sole anesthetic technique, and the anesthesiologist is skilled in regional anesthetic techniques, this is a reasonable choice. Appropriate sedation may be employed in a child, just as in an adult in similar circumstances. Children, however, benefit even more from a parent's presence during painful procedures than they might from pharmacologic intervention. Therefore, the parents are permitted to stay during placement of the intravenous catheter and the block. A great deal of verbal support and distraction is required during the procedure. Comic books or video tapes can be useful, as well as conversation regarding subjects of mutual interest.

The approaches to the brachial plexus block in children are the same as in the adult. One series of 200 children 5 years of age or less who were undergoing upper-extremity surgery involved axillary blocks only.[7] Twenty-seven of the children required no sedation, while the others received ketamine in varying doses. One microvascular procedure required 9 hours and was performed entirely with axillary blockade and sedation. Several children received blocks on multiple occasions, and they were well accepted by both patients and parents.[7] A lower incidence of nausea and vomiting has been reported when brachial plexus blockade and moderate sedation were employed for elective upper-extremity surgery than when general anesthesia was administered.[8] The success rate with regional blockade of the upper extremity is also high, 39 of 40 in one series.[9]

The brachial plexus is formed by nerves arising from C5–T1, passing through the intervertebral foramina, coursing laterally through the sulci of the transverse processes, and passing caudally between the anterior and middle scalene muscles of the neck. The fasciae of these muscles form an enclosed compartment. The nerve roots then subdivide to form the component parts of the plexus, which is eventually enclosed in a fascial sheath that includes the axillary artery. As in adults, the musculocutaneous nerve comes off high in the axilla. The ulnar nerve is posterior to the axillary artery, while the radial nerve is posterior and lateral and the median nerve is anterior.

The axillary approach to the brachial plexus would be chosen in this patient because it is easy to perform and does not require that paresthesias be elicited in this awake child. In addition, it almost always blocks the entire brachial plexus, in contrast to adults, where the radial and musculocutaneous nerves may be missed with this approach. Naturally, one should consult major textbooks before performing a block for the first time and should probably be facile with brachial plexus blockade in adults before utilizing this technique in children.

With the patient in the supine position the affected arm is gently abducted 90 degrees at the shoulder and flexed 90 degrees at the elbow. Prior to positioning the arm, an intravenous catheter is placed in the contralateral arm, and if necessary, small doses of midazolam are titrated, 0.05 mg/kg, for anxiolysis and cooperation. It is important to limit sedation so that the child can protect his airway if he vomits.

The parents should be placed on the side opposite the arm to be blocked so that they can provide comfort and aid in distraction. Using the left hand, the anesthesiologist palpates the arterial pulsation as high in the axilla as is practical. A skin wheal is raised with pH-adjusted local anesthetic to decrease the sting usually accompanying intradermal injections; pH adjustment does not decrease the onset time of the block. One milliliter of sodium bicarbonate is added to 9 mL of local anesthetic unless the local anesthetic is bupivacaine, in which case 0.1 mL of sodium bicarbonate is added to 9.9 mL of bupivacaine.

A 1-in. 23-gauge needle is inserted slowly at an angle of 45 degrees to the skin along an axis parallel to the artery. As the needle enters the fascia surrounding the neurovascular bundle of the axilla, a "pop" can be felt. If the needle is allowed to stand alone at that time, the transmitted pulsation of the artery will move it in a rhythmic fashion.[10] The needle is then carefully secured with the left hand, which is stabilized against the patient's arm. The syringe and intravenous extension tubing are carefully attached without moving the needle, and the initial aspiration is performed. The local anesthetic solution is injected with careful aspiration after each few milliliters are injected. The plexus is very superficial in a child, and care must be taken to not move the needle at all during the connection and injection. Following completion of the injection, the arm is carefully and slowly brought down to the side, with continuous pressure exerted below the site of injection to prevent distal spread of the solution.

The transarterial approach may also be employed. Here the artery is palpated with the left hand, and the needle is advanced through the artery while the anesthesiologist gently aspirates the syringe attached to the intravenous tubing. Once blood is aspirated, the needle is advanced until it passes through the artery, a distance of only a few millimeters. The tip of the needle should now be inside the sheath but outside the vessel. The local anesthetic is then injected into the sheath, with aspiration every few milliliters to ensure that the needle tip has not re-entered the vessel. Eliciting paresthesias or the use of a nerve stimulator is not useful in this situation because both are painful and even the most stoic child will flinch at the unexpected sensation.

Other approaches to the brachial plexus include the interscalene and parascalene approaches, both of which may be useful in the appropriate patient.[11, 12] Intravenous regional techniques are not useful for this procedure since the surgeon will want to palpate for a return of the radial pulse following reduction of the fracture.

Various dosage regimens have been proposed for regional blocks in children. A dose of 0.75 mL/kg of the local anesthetic of choice should provide good brachial plexus blockade.[13] The concentration must be sufficient to provide a motor block to facilitate reduction of the fracture. Lidocaine, 1.5%, lidocaine, 0.5% with 20 mg/10 mL of tetracaine crystals, or bupivacaine, 0.375%, all work equally well, although the "setup time" will differ.[10] It is important to calculate the total dose to ensure that toxic limits are not exceeded. The maximum dose of lidocaine with epinephrine is 7 mg/kg; for bupivacaine it is 3 mg/kg.

The average "setup" time for the block will be about 10 minutes. Once movement of the fractured arm is no longer painful, the patient can be taken to the operating room and the surgical site gently prepared. The block should be completely set after 20 minutes, with good analgesia and muscle relaxation evident. Again, a perfect block may not be sufficient in a child, who will require continued distraction and psychological support.

A tourniquet will not be required for closed reduction. However, if it is necessary to proceed with open reduction, a "ring block" high in the axilla is required to block the intercostobrachial and medial brachial cutaneous nerves so that the child will tolerate the tourniquet. Adjustment of the pH of the local anesthetic is necessary to avoid "stinging" sensations during the injection.

GENERAL ANESTHESIA

Should general anesthesia be indicated, this child with a full stomach will require rapid-sequence induction. For induction, thiamylal, 6 mg/kg, curare, 3 mg, atropine, 0.2 mg/kg, and succinylcholine, 2 mg/kg, would be appropriate. Following intubation, endotracheal tube placement is confirmed by both ET_{CO_2} and auscultation of the chest. Additional muscle relaxant and either a potent inhalation agent or intravenous narcotics are administered, keeping in mind that this surgical procedure might last as little as ½ hour or as long as 4 hours. Awake extubation would be planned in view of the full stomach. Antiemetic drugs may be of some value.

Alternatively, a combined technique of light general endotracheal anesthesia and brachial plexus blockade would be an excellent choice. At this point, a nerve stimulator might be employed after general anesthesia is induced.

SUMMARY

This child has a fractured arm with vascular compromise and a full stomach. Because he is healthy, we would not require preoperative laboratory evaluation since that would not alter anesthetic management. If the child, parents, and surgeons agree, a brachial plexus block with light sedation would be the anesthetic of choice. If any one of these three factors were not appropriate, a general anesthetic employing a rapid-sequence induction would be required. Anesthetic maintenance might still include a block and would certainly include measures for adequate postoperative pain management.

REFERENCES

1. Clement DA: Assessment of a treatment plan for managing acute vascular complications associated with supracondylar fractures of the humerus in children. *J Pediatr Orthop* 1990; 10:97.
2. Bricker SRW, McLuckie A, Nightingale DA: Gastric aspirates after trauma in children. *Anaesthesia* 1989; 44:721.
3. Coté CG, Goudsouzian NG, Liu LMP, et al: Assessment of risk factors related to the acid aspiration syndrome in pediatric patients—gastric pH and residual volume. *Anesthesiology* 1982; 56:70.
4. Lerman J, Christenson JK, Farrow-Gillispie AC: Effects of metoclopramide and ranitidine on gastric fluid pH and volume in children. *Anesthesiology* 1988; 69:A748.
5. O'Connor ME, Drasner K: Preoperative laboratory testing of children undergoing elective surgery. *Anesth Analg* 1990; 70:176.
6. Roy WL, Lerman J, McIntyre BG: Is preoperative haemoglobin testing justified in children undergoing minor elective surgery? *Can J Anaesth* 1991; 38:700.
7. Leak WD, Winchell SW: Regional anesthesia in pediatric patients: Review of clinical experience. *Reg Anesth* 1982; 7:64.
8. Wedel DJ, Krohn JS, Hall JA: Brachial plexus anesthesia in pediatric patients. *Mayo Clin Proc* 1991; 66:583.
9. King RS, Urquhart B, Urquhart B, et al: Factors influencing the success of brachial plexus block. *Reg Anesth* 1991; 15:63.
10. Winnie AW: *Plexus Anesthesia,* vol 1, in *Perivascular Techniques of Brachial Plexus Block.* Philadelphia, WB Saunders Co, 1990.
11. McNeely JK, Hoffman GM, Eckert JE: Postoperative pain relief in children from the parascalene injection technique. *Reg Anesth* 1991; 16:20.
12. Clayton ML, Turner DA: Upper arm block anesthesia in children with fractures. *JAMA* 1959; 169:99.
13. Eather KF: Regional anesthesia for infants and children. *Int Anesthesiol Clin* 1975; 13:19.

62

Bronchoscopy and Bronchography

A 9-year-old, 25-kg boy with repeated right middle lobe pneumonia is scheduled for bronchoscopy and bronchography. Old records are not available because he was previously hospitalized in another state. Hemoglobin, 9.8 g/dL; hematocrit, 29%.

Recommendations by Etsuro K. Motoyama, M.D.

Chronic obstruction of a bronchus may cause recurrent pneumonia and atelectasis confined to one or more lobes of the lung and can lead to localized bronchiectasis. The occurrence of these conditions in the right middle lobe, the most commonly affected site, is termed the *right middle lobe syndrome*. Bronchiectasis is a bronchial dilatation resulting from irreversible bronchial wall destruction that may require resection for successful treatment. Plain radiographic examination of the chest is usually nonspecific, and bronchography has been used to confirm the diagnosis.

Recently, the use of high-resolution, narrow-section computed tomography (CT) using 1.5- to 3.0-mm slices (instead of the conventional 10-mm slice) has become more common. Bronchiectasis can be diagnosed as effectively with the CT scan as with bronchography.[1-3] Consequently, bronchography is less commonly performed, although it is still used when the diagnosis is in question.

In most institutions, bronchography is performed in the radiology department, which is usually far from the main anesthetizing area and has inadequate facilities for administering anesthesia. Thus it is essential to make sure ahead of time that all necessary equipment is available and in good working order. A checklist for bronchography should include full cylinders of oxygen and nitrous oxide attached to the anesthesia machine (even though these gases may be piped into the fluoroscopy room), a functioning suction apparatus, electrocardiograph (ECG), pulse oximeter, capnograph, automatic blood pressure apparatus, other monitoring devices such as a nerve stimulator and temperature probe, and a flashlight with new batteries. In our institution, the necessary equipment and supplies, including an anesthesia machine, ECG and other monitors, and a well-stocked supply cart, are taken from the main anesthesia workroom in the operating suite to the radiology department, even though basic monitoring devices are available in the fluoroscopy room, to ensure that all equipment is in working order.

ANESTHETIC MANAGEMENT

Adequate sedation is desirable for bronchoscopy and bronchography in children because the strange surroundings and the hard, cold examining table in the fluoroscopy room are likely to cause apprehension, if not panic. Sedation also facilitates inhalation induction of anesthesia. For preanesthetic sedation, midazolam is most commonly administered, either intranasally, 0.2 mg/kg,[4] or orally, 0.5 mg/kg, with satisfactory results.

Anesthesia may be induced by mask with nitrous oxide and oxygen, followed by halothane. An intravenous infusion is established as soon as the patient becomes obtunded, and a vagolytic dose of atropine, 0.02 mg/kg, is given intravenously. Vital signs are monitored with a precordial stethoscope, pulse oximeter, ECG, capnograph, and blood pressure cuff. An automatic blood pressure measuring device with a digital readout is essential in the darkened fluoroscopy room. A heated humidifier should be incorporated into the anesthesia circuit to maintain body temperature and to humidify the upper airways. The nitrous oxide is then turned off, and the patient is paralyzed with an intubating dose of an intermediate-acting muscle relaxant such as atracurium, 0.5 mg/kg, or vecuronium, 0.1 mg/kg, while halothane, 1.5% to 2.0%, with oxygen is maintained. Dexamethasone, 0.4 mg/kg, is administered intravenously to minimize mucosal swelling.

BRONCHOSCOPY

Bronchoscopy is performed by using a ventilating bronchoscope with a sidearm (Fig 62–1) to which the anesthesia circuit is attached. Spontaneous breathing with any potent inhalation anesthetic provides inadequate gas exchange because of central respiratory depression and the added airway resistance of the bronchoscope and accessories. Thus, spontaneous breathing is of limited value except when it is specifically required for examination of vocal cord motion or for the diagnosis of conditions such as laryngotracheomalacia.

Adequate gas exchange can be maintained only with manual ventilation, provided that the proximal end of the bronchoscope is closed with a telescope or a glass obturator cap (Fig 62–1). Insertion of a Storz-Hopkins–type telescope into a bronchoscope[5] further impedes airflow through the bronchoscopy system and compromises gas exchange, even when ventilation is assisted or controlled through the side arm of the ventilating bronchoscope.[6–8] Ventilation may become difficult or inadequate. This may also occur when the bronchoscope is advanced beyond the carina into a mainstem or a lobar bronchus. Under such circumstances, the tip of the bronchoscope must be periodically pulled back into the midtrachea, or the telescope must be removed to allow unobstructed ventilation and restoration of proper gas exchange before bronchoscopic examination is resumed. For example, 30- to 60-second periods of hyperventilation and bronchoscopy are alternated to ensure sufficient gas exchange while the adequacy of oxygen saturation is continuously monitored by pulse oximetry. This technique requires good rapport and complete understanding between the anesthesiologist and the bronchoscopist.

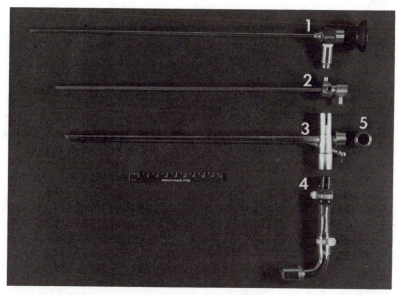

FIG 62–1.
Storz-Hopkins pediatric bronchoscopy assembly: *1,* Hopkins fiber-optic telescope; *2,* antifog sheath for the tele-scope; *3,* Storz ventilating bronchoscope, which accommodates both the telescope and sheath; *4,* adapter for the anesthesia circuit; *5,* glass obturator cap.

BRONCHOGRAPHY

For bronchography, an oral endotracheal tube is inserted immediately after the bronchoscope is removed. The endotracheal tube is securely taped and connected to an appropriate partial rebreathing circuit (Mapleson D or F) or a circle system via a right-angle connector with an open-end port covered with a perforated silicone rubber diaphragm. Halothane-oxygen anesthesia is maintained, and the patient's ventilation is controlled manually.

Until the mid-1980s a radiopaque catheter was inserted through the rubber diaphragm and advanced through the endotracheal tube into the appropriate bronchus under fluoroscopy. With this technique, placement of the catheter was guided by fluoroscopy without interrupting alveolar ventilation.

More recently, a small-caliber, flexible fiber-optic bronchoscope with a suction port has been available. This is inserted by the pediatric bronchologist into the endotracheal tube through the right-angle connector and rubber diaphragm and is advanced to the lobar or segmental bronchus to be examined (Fig 62–2). Dye is then injected through the suction port of the flexible bronchoscope. The smallest flexible bronchoscope available for this purpose has a 3.4-mm outside diameter (OD), which passes easily through a 5.0-mm-OD endotracheal tube without impairing controlled ventilation.

Bronchography can be performed through a rigid bronchoscope placed in the trachea. However, this technique is not recommended because it poses the unnecessary risk of inadequate ventilation and possible trauma to the airways as the child is turned back and forth in a darkened room with radiopaque material in the tracheobronchial lumen.

After bronchography is completed, an attempt should be made to aspirate the dye under fluoroscopy or through the flexible bronchoscope without traumatizing the tracheobronchial mucosa. The endotracheal tube is kept in place until the muscle paralysis is adequately reversed, the cough

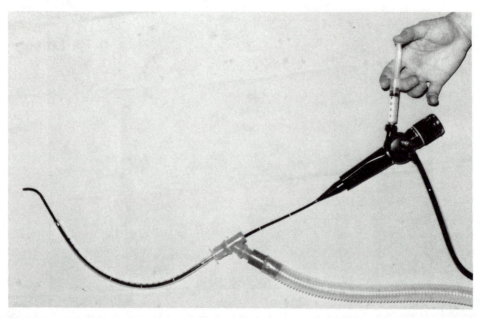

FIG 62–2.
Technique for bronchography. An ultrathin, flexible fiber-optic bronchoscope is introduced via the rubber diaghragm of a right-angle adapter and endotracheal tube into the desired bronchus while controlled ventilation continues uninterrupted. (From Motoyama EK: Anesthesia for ear, nose, and throat surgery, in Motoyama EK, Davis PJ (eds): *Smith's Anesthesia for Infants and Children,* ed 5. St Louis, Mosby–Year Book, 1990. Used by permission.)

reflex fully recovered, and spontaneous breathing resumed. Intravenous injection of lidocaine, 1.0 mg/kg, is useful because it reduces coughing and laryngospasm at the time of extubation. Inhalation of racemic epinephrine, 5 mL of a 0.5% solution in normal saline, is recommended if there is any sign of laryngeal irritation or stridor.

REFERENCES

1. Granier P, Maurice F, Musset D, et al: Bronchiectasis by thin-section CT. *Radiology* 1986; 161:95–99.
2. Silverman PM, Godwin D: CT/bronchographic correlations in bronchiectasis. *J Comput Assist Tomogr* 1987; 11:52–56.
3. Grenier P, Lenoir S, Brauner M: Computed tomographic assessment of bronchiectasis. *Semin Ultrasound CT MR* 1990; 11:430–441.
4. Wilton NCT, Leigh J, Rosen DR, et al: Preanesthetic sedation of preschool children using intranasal midazolam. *Anesthesiology* 1988; 69:972–975.
5. Saekely E, Farkas E: *Pediatric Bronchology.* Baltimore, University Park Press, 1978, pp 30–64.
6. Rah KH, Salzber AM, Boyan CP, et al: Respiratory acidosis with the small Storz-Hopkins bronchoscope: Occurrence and management. *Ann Thorac Surg* 1978; 27:197–202.
7. Widlund B, Walczak S, Motoyama EK: Flow-pressure characteristics of pediatric Storz-Hopkins bronchoscopes (abstract). *Anesthesiology* 1982; 57:417.
8. Motoyama EK: Anesthesia for ear, nose and throat surgery, in Motoyama EK, Davis PJ (eds): *Smith's Anesthesia for Infants and Children,* ed 5. St Louis, Mosby–Year Book, 1990, pp 649–674.

63

Osteogenesis Imperfecta

A 10-year-old, 20-kg boy with osteogenesis imperfecta (OI) is scheduled for multiple osteotomies and intramedullary rodding of the tibia. Both legs are deformed from multiple fractures (Fig 63–1), and he has kyphoscoliosis. Hemoglobin, 11.8 g/dL; hematocrit, 35%; temperature, 37.5°C pulse, 100.

Recommendations by Steven C. Hall, M.D.

OI is a rare, hereditary disease of bone that occurs in about 1 in 30,000 live births. It was originally classified on the basis of presentation at birth or early infancy as osteogenesis imperfecta congenita or as osteogenesis imperfecta tarda when patients presented later in childhood. The current classification includes four major classes based on the clinical profile.[1] Because the common underlying defect appears to be a quantitative and/or qualitative defect of collagen formation, there is a burgeoning literature trying to correlate the four clinical classes and specific genetic defects.[2]

CLINICAL MANIFESTATIONS

Type I, the most common type, presents with bone fragility, hearing loss, blue sclera, and autosomal dominant inheritance. Type II presents with severe, life-threatening fractures, is possibly autosomal recessive, and is usually associated with fetal or early neonatal demise. Type III also presents with severe skeletal deformities, autosomal recessive inheritance, and poor prognosis, although not as severe as type II. Type IV presents with bone fragility of variable severity, rare hearing loss, and autosomal dominant inheritance. Although these subtypes are broad guidelines to symptomatology, there is wide individual variation in clinical presentation, even within families.

The principal characteristic of OI is osteoporotic bones that fracture easily, sometimes with trivial trauma. The fractures classically are transverse and subperiosteal, often without much displacement. Because weight bearing, by itself, can cause the fractures, the long bones often show evi-

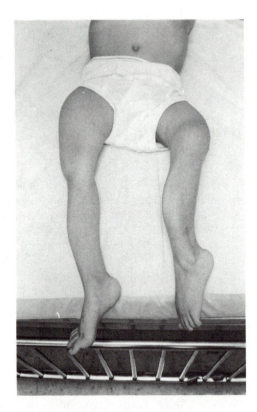

FIG 63–1.
Osteogenesis imperfecta in a 10-year-old boy.

dence of repeated fractures and consequent bowing. Kyphoscoliosis is common and may be severe enough to inhibit ventilation enough to cause cor pulmonale. Rib fractures can also contribute to restrictive chest wall defects. Because of the long-bone and spine abnormalities, these patients have a shortened stature. Fractures of the skull and face are also distinctive, with mandibular fractures being common and facial bone fractures rare. The skull is often a mosaic of bone islands, with frontal bossing and an overhanging occiput. This "helmet head" deformity functionally acts to flex the neck at rest.

Other aspects of connective tissue are also involved in OI. There can be considerable laxity of the joints, thin skin, and fragility of the tendons. Umbilical and inguinal hernias are relatively common in these patients. Of particular interest during airway maneuvers is the teeth. Teeth in patients with OI tend to be discolored, misshapen, and very brittle, fracturing easily with minor trauma. These patients can also have cardiac lesions such as atrial or ventricular septal defects, mitral insufficiency, and aortic insufficiency. There have also been reports of a higher incidence of cleft palate, hydrocephalus, and premature arteriosclerosis. Another area of interest to anesthesiologists is the potential for bleeding disorders. In some patients with OI, there is platelet dysfunction secondary to decreased release of platelet factor 3. Although the platelet count is normal, platelet adhesiveness is diminished.

Hyperthermia in children with OI has raised concern about malignant hyperthermia syndrome (MHS) in these patients. It appears that some patients with OI have hyperthermia and hyperhidrosis during general anesthesia that is not the same as MHS.[3] The signs disappear with discontinuation of the anesthetic and surface cooling. Both abnormal central nervous system control of temperature and abnormal cellular metabolism have been suggested. Some investigators have found elevated serum thyroxine levels, increased oxygen consumption, and elevated temperatures in these patients and have postulated that there is a generalized metabolic disturbance in some children with OI.[4] Confusing the issue is a paper reporting several patients with severe metabolic acidosis on induction, although not the classic picture of MHS.[5] Patients with both OI and MHS, or a clinical event that could be interpreted as such, have also been reported.[6] This has led to controversy about the potential for MHS in patients with OI. Although some authors feel that there is real risk of MHS in patients with OI, others feel that the evidence is not adequate to support this and that the occurrence of both OI and MHS in the same patient is coincidental.[7, 8] There is not a large body of evidence supporting a strong relationship between OI and MHS, although this may change with future studies.

Orthopedic management has become aggressive.[1] In the past, simple splinting was the primary treatment for fractures. Currently, a balanced approach of casting, bracing, physical therapy, and surgery is used for treatment of fractures, straightening of limbs, and strengthening of muscle mass to prevent fractures. These patients now come to the operating room for a variety of both elective and urgent procedures to stabilize long bones. There has been great interest in a variety of hormonal and pharmacologic modalities to strengthen bone and minimize fractures. Agents have included fluoride, vitamin D, calcitonin, and various gonadal hormones. However, there has yet to appear a pharmacologic agent that successfully improves these patients and their defects.

ANESTHETIC MANAGEMENT

A careful history is oriented toward the patient's skeletal system and past fractures. The amount of trauma necessary to cause a fracture is useful information when handling the child since there is wide individual variation. Also, a history of vertebral fractures will encourage obtaining preoperative cervical films to evaluate stability and the presence of deformities. A history of ventilatory problems or recurrent pneumonia may be an indication of significant rib cage and spine deformities. Exercise tolerance in the older child may give useful information about the progression of the child's disability and cardiopulmonary reserve.

Physical examination is also oriented to the skeletal system. Special attention is placed on examination of the head and neck. It is important to note the normal, comfortable position of the head at rest, the ability to open the mouth, any instability of the mandible, and the flexibility and range of motion of the cervical spine. During the chest examination, it is important to detect any evidence of pulmonary or cardiac disease. Previously undiagnosed murmurs should be evaluated before elective surgery. If there are signs of ventilatory impairment from kyphoscoliosis, rib fractures, or other thoracic cage deformities, pulmonary function testing is indicated.

Laboratory testing is largely determined by the history and physical examination. As mentioned, pulmonary function testing is indicated if there is a history of recurrent respiratory difficulties or the physical examination reveals severe bony abnormalities. Chest radiography is performed if there is a question of an acute pulmonic process vs. chronic changes. If there is a history of easy bruisability or bleeding, obtaining a bleeding time and coagulation profile is indicated.

There is no specific indication or contraindication for premedicants in these patients outside of the normal precautions for chronically ill children. Older literature suggests avoidance of atropine because of a tendency to decrease heat dissipation, but this has never been clearly demonstrated. Children with OI are usually not retarded and are quite appropriate in their reactions and fears. Older children are aware of their deformities and the various reactions these provoke in people. A calm, understanding approach to these children is necessary to reassure them and help them through the perioperative period. If sedation is indicated, it should be given.

Extreme care must be taken in positioning the patient. In particularly severe cases, movements as benign as changing a diaper have resulted in femoral fractures. Therefore, great care must be taken in moving and positioning the patient and all pressure points generously padded. In some cases, the patient's kyphoscoliosis or hydrocephalus may result in abnormal postures requiring support on the operating table in the form of blankets or towels. Tourniquets for facilitating vascular access or preventing blood loss must be applied carefully, if at all. There is a single case report of central retinal artery occlusion in a prone patient with the confounding variable of deliberate hypotension.[9] It is recommended that care be taken to avoid external pressure on the eyes if the patient is in the prone position.

These children are monitored in the same fashion as other children for anesthesia and surgery. Careful padding under the blood pressure cuff and anywhere else there is pressure on the patient's body will decrease the risk of fractures or abrasion of the thin skin. Although some have suggested eschewing the use of a blood pressure cuff to avoid the possibility of fracture, there is little evidence that this is necessary.

There are no specific contraindications to anesthetic agents, with one possible exception.[3] It is usually recommended that succinylcholine be avoided, if possible, to eliminate the risk of fasciculation-induced fractures. Although there have not been a large number of reported incidents demonstrating the danger of succinylcholine, it is reasonable to substitute a nondepolarizing relaxant, if clinically applicable.

There are multiple reasonable methods of anesthetic management for this particular patient. If there were questions about his airway, inhalation induction with halothane and nitrous oxide-oxygen would allow evaluation of the patency of the airway during spontaneous ventilation. Ketamine has been used in patients with OI to provide general anesthesia for minor procedures without airway manipulation. If the airway is not in question, intravenous induction with thiopental followed by a nondepolarizing muscle relaxant is a reasonable induction technique. Various combinations of nitrous oxide-oxygen, volatile agents, and narcotics have been used successfully for maintenance of anesthesia in these patients, with little to recommend one technique over the other. Probably the most important factor is the technique that produces the least upset in the child while ensuring controlled induction. Intravenous, inhalation, rectal, or intramuscular inductions are all possibilities. Regional anesthesia can be used in these patients, but the presence of vertebral fractures, a bleeding tendency, or long-bone fractures with minimal trauma such as turning to place the block increase the risk of these techniques.

Airway management can be one of the most challenging aspects of anesthetic care. Pressure by the face mask can cause mandibular or facial fractures, while teeth are easily broken during laryngoscopy. Extension of the head does convey some risk for cervical spine fracture.[1]

These patients often have increased frontal-occipital diameters, short necks, and barrel chests that make placement of a laryngoscope difficult. Fiber-optic laryngoscopy is a reasonable alternative to standard laryngoscopy.

Probably the most disturbing intraoperative complication that is unique to patients with OI is the appearance of hyperthermia, tachycardia, and tachypnea from increased metabolism, as discussed previously. This reaction is associated with normocarbia and easily controlled with surface cooling. If there is no response to cooling measures, an arterial blood gas measurement can be obtained to rule out the mixed metabolic/respiratory acidosis of MHS.

Ventilation-perfusion abnormalities are not uncommon in these children. Kyphoscoliosis, thoracic cage deformities, and recurrent infections contribute to varying degrees of abnormality. Humidified gases, tracheobronchial toilet, and positive end-expiratory pressure are useful in minimizing the abnormalities.

Children with OI usually have the normal range of responses to anesthetic and analgesic medications. However, they often have relatively weak respiratory muscles, kyphoscoliosis, and thoracic cage abnormalities, which decrease the margin of safety for ventilation. Because of this, extubation is prudent only when the patient is fully awake. Postoperative analgesia can be provided in a variety of ways, but the titration of small doses of narcotic is especially efficacious in providing pain relief with minimal depression.

REFERENCES

1. Gertner JM, Root L: Osteogenesis imperfecta. *Orthop Clin North Am* 1990; 21:151–162.
2. Edwards MJ, Graham JM: Studies of type 1 collagen in osteogenesis imperfecta. *J Pediatr* 1990; 117:67–72.
3. Libman RH: Anesthetic considerations for the patient with osteogenesis imperfecta. *Clin Orthop* 1981; 159:123–125.
4. Cropp GJA, Myers DN: Physiological evidence of hypermetabolism in osteogenesis imperfecta. *Pediatrics* 1972; 49:375–391.
5. Sadat-Ali M, Sankaran-Kutty M, Adu-Gyamfi Y: Metabolic acidosis in osteogenesis imperfecta. *Eur J Pediatr* 1986; 145:324–325.
6. Rampton AJ, Kelly DA, Shanahan EC, et al: Occurrence of malignant hyperpyrexia in a patient with osteogenesis imperfecta. *Br J Anaesth* 1984; 56:1443–1446.
7. Ryan CA, Al-Ghamdi AS, Gayle M, et al: Osteogenesis imperfecta and hyperthermia. *Anesth Analg* 1989; 68:811–814.
8. Brownell AKW: Malignant hyperthermia: Relationship to other diseases. *Br J Anaesth* 1988; 60:303–308.
9. Bradish CF, Flowers M: Central retinal artery occlusion in association with osteogenesis imperfecta. *Spine* 1987; 12:193.

64

Tonsillectomy and Fear of Injections

A 10-year-old, 35-kg girl is scheduled for tonsillectomy. She is terrified of "shots" but also of pain following surgery. Hemoglobin, 13 g/dL; hematocrit, 35%.

Recommendation by T.C.K. Brown, M.D., F.A.N.Z.C.A., F.C.A. (U.K.)

This 10-year-old probably has chronic or recurrent tonsillitis since it is relatively uncommon nowadays to perform this operation in a patient of this age. Her fear of injections probably stems from an unpleasant experience earlier in life. Immunizations are often the origin of the fear of needles. Intramuscular injections are more painful than are intravenous ones since pain is caused by splitting of muscle fibers.

PREOPERATIVE PREPARATION

The preoperative visit is particularly important, and the child, not the parents, should be the center of attention. She may be withdrawn, or put up a brave front, or admit that she "doesn't want any injections." The anesthesiologist should try to elucidate the cause of her fear. Is it related to a previous anesthetic experience or to unrelated injections? Did someone fail in attempts at venipuncture? Has she had a number of intramuscular injections? If the patient cannot explain the cause of her fear, perhaps the parents can. The possibility that the parents have used the threat of taking her to the doctor for an injection if she does not behave should be considered.

It is important to gain the child's confidence by reassuring her that you will care for her and minimize any discomfort. The anesthesiologist can discuss the alternative of an inhalation induction. If available, eutectic mixture of local anesthesia (EMLA) cream can be applied to the skin at the injection site. Even if an inhalation induction is selected by the patient, EMLA should be applied because of the possibility of rejection of the mask at the last moment. The child should be told that she will be asleep during the operation, that she will be awakened at the end, and that she will be given pain medication prior to her awakening.

The next decision relates to premedication. Most effective are intramuscular combinations of opioids and scopolamine; however, this requires a painful injection and triples the incidence of post-operative vomiting.[1]

A number of orally administered drugs have been used with varying success. In this age group, clinical studies have shown that diazepam and midazolam are not significantly better than a placebo.[2] Some children would benefit from sedation; however, it may be inadequate or ineffective and remove some of their inhibitions, possibly making them more difficult to manage than an unpremedicated child. Scopolamine and some benzodiazepines may produce amnesia even if the child is apprehensive at induction. Other drugs may produce a sleeping child who is very apprehensive if awakened. In addition, postoperative drowsiness slows recovery so that discharge from the recovery room or from a day surgical unit is delayed. Nasal midazolam[3] and sufentanil[4] as well as oral fentanyl have been used with success.

My choice of premedication for this patient would be oral diazepam, 0.3 mg/kg, with acetaminophen, 20 mg/kg, for analgesia 90 minutes preoperatively. I would also apply EMLA cream over a reasonably accessible vein on the back of the hand.

Children of this age should be able to cope, thus making the presence of the parents during induction unnecessary. A firm but caring approach of the anesthesiologist should be all that is required. The main group to benefit from parental presence are preschool children and the handicapped.

INDUCTION OF ANESTHESIA

If an inhalation induction was agreed upon, self-administration with a little assistance is indicated. Halothane is best; the concentration can be increased as tolerated to 4% to hasten induction. If the patient objects violently at this point and refuses an inhalation induction, a quick venipuncture with a 23- or 25-gauge needle followed by intravenous induction is kinder for the very frightened child. It is here that EMLA cream would be particularly valuable. A dose of thiopental of 6 to 7 mg/kg may be required since children require a larger dose[5] and the sympathetic response associated with apprehension causes increased cardiac output. With more rapid redistribution, more of the thiopental goes to the vessel-poor tissues such as the muscle.

Once anesthesia has been induced, a nondepolarizing relaxant such as atracurium may be administered. The dose must be appropriate since the 95% effective dose (ED_{95}) is somewhat higher for patients in this age group.[6] Morphine, 0.1 to 0.2 mg/kg, can now be given intravenously. The patient is ventilated with 70% nitrous oxide and oxygen and, when adequately paralyzed, is intubated with a 6.5 RAE tube.

If the patient is prepubertal, an uncuffed tube should be used. The correct size of tube is one that allows a minimal leak when positive pressure is applied. When there is an excessive leak, a size larger is indicated. The tube should be changed after the laryngoscope blade is in place and the larynx is in view so that there is minimal delay between breaths. If the tube is too big, laryngeal edema and stridor may develop postoperatively.

The use of an opioid, nitrous oxide, oxygen, and a nondepolarizing muscle relaxant allows rapid awakening. Residual neuromuscular blockade is reversed with atropine, 0.02 mg/kg, and neostigmine, 0.05 mg/kg. If an opioid is administered with an adequate concentration of nitrous oxide, awareness should not be a problem after thiopental induction. However, if this is a concern, a low concentration of inhalation agent can be added. The lower the concentration used, the more rapidly the patient recovers consciousness, and the less likely is laryngeal spasm on extubation.

An intravenous infusion is not essential for most tonsillectomies provided that blood loss is less than 5% of the patient's blood volume, the environmental temperature is not too high, and the period without fluid intake is not over 8 hours. The recent trend to allow clear fluid and juice intake up 2 to 3 hours before surgery[7] avoids the prolonged periods of fluid deprivation previously regarded as necessary.

POSTOPERATIVE ANALGESIA

Analgesia lasting well into the postoperative period can be obtained with the use of a local anaesthetic. It can be injected by the surgeon before the surgery and, if correctly placed, can help open the peritonsillar plane and make dissection easier. Alternatively, the anesthesiologist can spray local anesthetic over the raw tonsil fossa after the tonsils have been removed and the bleeding controlled. If the tip of a 21-gauge needle is bent at a right angle, it is possible to spray laterally into the upper and lower poles of the tonsil fossa. The equipment needed is thus simple, readily available, and cheap. One-half to 1 mL of 0.5% bupivacaine is sprayed on each tonsillar fossa. Bupivacaine has the advantage of a longer action than lidocaine and, with a maximum dose of 10 mg in 2 mL, toxicity is most unlikely.

Any excess local anaesthetic is removed by suction to prevent it from spilling into the pharynx. A concentration of 0.5% is used since the duration of action is longer with higher concentrations of topical local anaesthetic.[8] No complications have occurred in over 15 years that I have been using this technique. If properly applied to the tonsillar fossa, the local anesthetic provides postoperative comfort and allows early swallowing. Pain and the inability to swallow and drink postoperatively contribute to much of the misery that often follows tonsillectomy.

For additional postoperative analgesia, additional doses of morphine can be given intravenously if the needle or cannula remains in the vein. If a cannula with an injection port is placed in a forearm vein during anesthesia, it is comfortable and nonintrusive and can be used for an infusion if necessary. Alternatively, an oral or rectal analgesic such as acetaminophen, 20 mg/kg, can be given every 4 to 6 hours as required.

A postoperative follow-up visit can determine whether the approach taken was successful. It also provides positive encouragement in case future anesthetics are necessary and is an opportunity to find out whether there were any problems that can be avoided on future occasions.

REFERENCES

1. Rowley MR, Brown TCK: Postoperative vomiting in children. *Anaesth Intensive Care* 1982; 10:309.
2. Anderson BJ, Exarchos H, Lee K, et al: Oral premedication in children. A comparison of chloral hydrate, diazepam, alprazolam and placebo for day surgery. *Anaesth Intensive Care* 1990; 18:185–193.

438   T.C.K. Brown

3. Wilton NCT, Leigh J, Rosen DR, et al: Preanaesthetic sedation of preschool children using nasal midazolam. *Anesthesiology* 1989; 69:972–975.

4. Henderson JM, Brodsky DA, Fisher DM, et al: Preinduction of anesthesia in paediatric patients with nasally administered sufentanil. *Anesthesiology* 1987; 68:671–675.

5. Jonmarker C, Westrin P, Larsson S, et al: Thiopentone requirements for induction of anaesthesia in children. *Anesthesiology* 1987; 67:104–107.

6. Meretoja OA: Neuromuscular blocking agents in paediatric patients: Influence of age on the response. *Anaesth Intensive Care* 1990; 18:440–448.

7. Splinter WM, Stewart JA, Muir JA: The effect of preoperative apple juice on gastric contents, thirst and hunger in children. *Can J Anaesth* 1989; 36:55–58.

8. Robinson EP, Rex MAE, Brown TCK: A comparison of different concentrations of lignocaine hydrochloride used for topical anaesthesia of the larynx in the cat. *Anaesth Intensive Care* 1985; 13:137–144.

65

Appendectomy and Prader-Willi Syndrome

A 10-year-old boy with Prader-Willi syndrome (PWS) is scheduled for an appendectomy. He is mildly retarded, uncooperative, and obese (60 kg). He complains of pain when his abdomen is palpated and has been vomiting for 12 hours. Hemoglobin, 11.1 g/dL; hematocrit, 33.2%; white blood cell count, 22,000 × $10^3/\mu L$; serum glucose, 175 mg/dL; ketones, negative. Blood gases on room air: Pao_2, 58; $Paco_2$, 48; pH, 7.30; BE, −2.

Recommendations by Letty M.P. Liu, M.D.

The PWS is a multisystem disorder that was first described in 1956 by Prader, Labhart, and Willi.[1] This syndrome is seen in approximately 1:15,000 patients.[2] The exact prevalence is unknown because the diagnosis is based primarily on recognition of the clinical features. Major manifestations of PWS are linked to brain and autonomic nervous system abnormalities. They include infantile hypotonia; hypogonadism; obesity; psychomotor retardation; dysmorphic facial features such as strabismus, narrow bifrontal diameter, down-turned mouth, micrognathia, and almond-shaped palpebral fissures; short stature; short hands and feet; mental deficiency; and behavioral problems.[3, 4] Mild diabetes, premature coronary artery disease, scoliosis, hip dislocation, seizures, poor dentition, and abnormal regulation of body temperature are other conditions that may be present.[4-6] Although the presence or absence of anomalies and the severity of expression vary among patients with PWS, delayed development, hypotonia, and feeding problems are consistently seen during the first year of life.[7] Approximately half the patients with PWS have a deletion in chromosome 15.[4] If there is an abnormality in chromosome 15, the diagnosis can be confirmed in infancy.[8] In others, the diagnosis depends upon the development of additional manifestations of the syndrome. Early diagnosis allows measures to be instituted to control the child's weight and behavior before these factors become a significant problem. In addition, early diagnosis may enable medical personnel to assist the family in coping psychologically with an abnormal child.

PREANESTHETIC EVALUATION

The major factors that affect the anesthetic management of patients with PWS include hypotonia, abnormal carbohydrate and fat metabolism, mental and psychomotor retardation, behavioral problems, dysmorphic facies, cardiac abnormalities, and hyperthermia associated with anesthesia (Table 65–1).[9, 10] Hypotonia is a striking characteristic of infants with PWS. These babies frequently appear flaccid. They have a weak cough and cry and absent or poor reflexes. They feed poorly and tend to repeatedly aspirate feedings. Airway secretions are generally not a problem because saliva production is generally decreased.[4] Histologic and histochemical studies show no evidence of muscle disease, and electromyographic and neural conduction velocity findings are normal in most cases.[11, 12] With maturation, muscle tone improves, but patients still remain hypotonic.

The abnormalities in energy metabolism of patients with PWS may affect their anesthetic management. Because many of these patients have abnormal glucose tolerance test findings, they may be misdiagnosed as diabetics. Like the diabetic, patients with PWS can develop hypoglycemia if deprived of glucose for a prolonged period. Patients with PWS tend to use substrate for lipogenesis rather than to satisfy energy needs, even during fasting.[13] They have an increase in adipose tissue

TABLE 65–1.

Anesthetic Considerations in Prader-Willi Syndrome

Disorder	Problems
Hypotonia	Weak cough, repeated aspiration, failure to thrive
Obesity	Central distribution of fat, hypoventilation, ventilation-perfusion inequality, sleep apnea, hypertension
Mental and psychomotor retardation	Behavioral problems, language problems, learning disabilities
Dysmorphic facies	Micrognathia, poor anesthetic mask fit, difficult endotracheal intubation
Diabetes	Hyperglycemia, hypoglycemia
Cardiac anomalies	Arrhythmias, ischemia
Thermoregulatory disturbance	Hyperthermia, hypothermia
Poor dentition	Dental caries, dental malocclusion

lipoprotein lipase, which is the rate-limiting step in triglyceride uptake and storage by fat cells. Patients with PWS are distinguished from diabetics and patients who are simply obese by such characteristics as hypotonia, decreased reflexes, mental retardation, and dental caries,[14] features not usually associated with diabetics or the obese.

Children with PWS develop hyperphagia and generally start gaining weight rapidly between 1 and 4 years of age. The low energy expenditure is not due to a difference in energy utilization at the cellular level, but to their smaller fat-free mass.[15] If the oral intake is not controlled, obesity may become a serious problem. Fat is characteristically distributed centrally, i.e., around the abdomen, buttocks, and thighs. Grossly obese patients frequently hypoventilate, develop atelectasis, and have ventilation-perfusion inequalities. Ventilation may be further compromised in the patient with an acute abdomen as he attempts to minimize pain by splinting the abdomen. As in any obese patient, supine positioning may cause or intensify respiratory acidosis. Unless hypoxia and respiratory acidosis are severe, increasing the inspired oxygen concentration and assisting ventilation may be all that is necessary to return blood gases to normal values. Starting an intravenous infusion, establishing a good mask fit, maintaining a patent airway, and performing an atraumatic endotracheal intubation are additional challenges that may confront the anesthesiologist who cares for patients with PWS.

Behavioral problems such as temper tantrums, stubbornness, and impulsiveness are frequently seen in older children with PWS. These characteristics may present obstacles for the anesthesiologist. Obtaining the cooperation of these children may be difficult, and establishing rapport may be impossible. Preanesthetic medication may be necessary for these retarded children so that anesthesia can be induced atraumatically.

Common symptoms of patients with appendicitis include abdominal pain, fever, and vomiting. Depending on the length of illness and the severity of symptoms, dehydration and acid-base imbalance may or may not be present. In the severely ill patient with peritoneal irritation and protracted vomiting, blood volume may be markedly decreased. Serum electrolytes and pH may be abnormal and serum protein levels low. If possible, these abnormalities should be corrected before the child is brought to the operating room.

ANESTHETIC MANAGEMENT

A variety of drugs and anesthetic techniques can be used to anesthetize a patient with PWS and appendicitis. Understanding the patient's anomalies and surgical problem is crucial for optimal anesthetic management.

After obtaining the patient's medical history and performing a physical examination, attention should be directed to correcting biochemical abnormalities. Like this child, patients with PWS frequently have problems with ventilation. Those who are morbidly obese may not be able to lie flat because abdominal pressure from obesity may limit diaphragmatic excursion and thus cause them to be "short of breath." These patients may feel better if they are allowed to lie in a slight head-up position. Supplemental oxygen administered either through a nasal cannula or by face mask may help correct abnormalities in oxygenation.

The aim of premedication is to sedate the child without obtunding airway reflexes or further compromising ventilation or circulation. In this patient, the advantages of sedation must be balanced against the risk of obtunding a patient who probably has a "full stomach." If the child has an intravenous cannula in place, premedication can be administered by this route. Incremental doses are given until the desired degree of sedation is obtained. If the patient does not have an intravenous catheter in place, premedication may be administered orally, nasally, rectally, or intramuscularly. Oral premedication may not be effective since absorption is unpredictable in patients who are vomiting and in those with ileus. To avoid stressing patients with an injection, the intramuscular route should probably be reserved for children who cannot be sedated by other routes.

Premedicant drugs include barbiturates, hypnotics, and opioids. Tranquilizers such as midazolam will calm most patients, whereas barbiturates alone may intensify pain because of their antianalgesic properties. Adding a narcotic to the premedication regimen may decrease pain and provide additional sedation; however, narcotics should be used judiciously. This is especially true in patients with respiratory problems since indiscriminant administration of these drugs can easily lead to ventilatory failure. Intramuscular ketamine may be useful in patients with PWS, especially in those who have poor venous access and object to an inhalation induction. Ketamine may provide just enough sedation to allow an intravenous cannula to be inserted without compromising the patient's airway. Intramuscular ketamine may also be the best option for an extremely rambunctious uncooperative child.

General anesthesia is usually the anesthetic technique of choice for a patient with PWS. Obese patients may present technical difficulties because of their size when regional anesthesia is attempted. In addition, retarded patients with behavioral problems are frequently difficult to control when awake.

Since patients with appendicitis are prone to vomiting, they should be treated as having a "full stomach," and measures must be taken to protect the airway from possible aspiration of gastric contents. However, the patient's airway must be carefully evaluated prior to inducing anesthesia. Facial anomalies should be assessed to determine the ease of ventilation by face mask in the event that this may be necessary. If difficulty with intubation is anticipated, a rapid induction sequence may not be reasonable. Alternative methods of airway management should be considered. Awake oral or blind nasal intubation with sedation is an alternative. Another possibility is awake fiber-optic intubation. The optimal approach depends upon the skill and familiarity of the anesthesiologist with each technique.

If a rapid-sequence induction is planned, a short-acting barbiturate such as thiopental or newer agents such as propofol can be used to induce anesthesia. Aspiration during induction can be minimized by applying cricoid pressure, the Sellick maneuver,[16] while awaiting the onset of muscle relaxation.

Anesthesia can be maintained with a halogenated agent or with a balanced anesthetic technique. Although it is possible that children with PWS may be more sensitive to muscle relaxants, this has not been reported or studied. Any of the neuromuscular blocking agents can be used to achieve relaxation.

During anesthesia, attempts should be made to optimize the patient's ventilatory status. Assisted or controlled ventilation is indicated. Additional measures to improve ventilation include the use of positive end-expiratory pressure (PEEP) and large tidal volumes to keep alveoli patent. High airway pressure may be necessary to reopen atelectatic areas. Arterial blood gases should be determined and ventilation adjusted accordingly.

Because patients with PWS may have cardiac abnormalities such as coronary artery disease and conduction defects, there may be a narrow margin of safety should cardiac depression occur. Therefore, the anesthesiologist must avoid situations that could lead to a cascade of misfortunes that may potentially be irreversible.

Anesthetic care should include the monitoring of heart rate, heart and breath sounds, oxygen saturation, end-tidal carbon dioxide, the electrocardiogram, and temperature. In addition, neuromuscular function should be monitored in all patients who receive a muscle relaxant. The blood sugar content should be followed if the procedure is prolonged. Intravenous glucose is administered as needed. When repeated arterial blood samples must be drawn, placement of an arterial catheter is indicated.

POSTOPERATIVE CARE

At the end of the surgical procedure, any residual neuromuscular depression should be reversed and ventilatory function assessed. Since the risk of vomiting postoperatively is high in patients with appendicitis, especially this obese child, it is best for the patient to remain intubated until his airway reflexes return to baseline. Before he is extubated, he should be able to protect his airway. Airway reflexes do not usually return to their preanesthetic status until the patient is awake. If airway reflexes remain depressed even after the patient is awake or if ventilation is inadequate, the endotracheal tube should remain in place. Some patients may require mechanical ventilation for several hours after surgery.

In summary, the principal areas of concern to anesthesiologists caring for children with PWS are hypotonia, obesity, facial and airway anomalies, behavioral problems, and cardiorespiratory dysfunction. Anesthetic management should be individualized for each patient. In addition, the anesthesiologist must be knowledgeable about potential complications and be realistic about his or her own skills.

REFERENCES

1. Prader A, Labhart A, Willi H: Ein syndrome von adipositas, kleinwuchs, kryptorchismus und oligophrenie nach myatonieartigem zustand im neugeboranenalter. *Schweiz Med Wochenschr* 1956; 86:1260–1261.
2. Second Annual Prader-Willi syndrome scientific conference. *Am J Med Genet* 1987; 28:779–924.
3. Aughton DJ, Cassidy SH: Physical features of Prader-Willi syndrome in neonates. *Am J Dis Child* 1990; 144:1251–1254.
4. Cassidy SB, Ledbetter DH: Prader Willi syndrome. *Neurol Clin* 1989; 7:37–54.
5. Mackenzie JW: Anaesthesia and the Prader-Willi syndrome. *J R Soc Med* 1991; 84:239.
6. Page SR, Nussey SS, Haywood GA, et al: Premature coronary artery disease and the Prader-Willi syndrome. *Postgrad Med J* 1990; 66:232–234.
7. Clarren SK, Smith DW: Prader-Willi syndrome: Variable severity and recurrence risk. *Am J Dis Child* 1977; 131:789–800.
8. Ledbetter DH, Riccardi VM, Airhart SD, et al: Deletions of chromosome 15 as a cause of Prader-Willi syndrome. *N Engl J Med* 1981; 304:325–329.

9. Yamashita M, Koishi K, Yamaya R, et al: Anaesthetic considerations in the Prader-Willi syndrome: Report of four cases. *Can Anaesth Soc J* 1983; 30:179–184.

10. Milliken RA, Weintraub DM: Cardiac abnormalities during anesthesia in a child with Prader-Willi syndrome. *Anesthesiology* 1975; 43:590–592.

11. Gamstorp I: Metabolic neuropathies and myopathies in infancy and childhood. *Acta Neurol Scand Suppl* 1970; 46:117.

12. Dubowitz V: A syndrome of benign congenital hypotonia, gross obesity, delayed intellectual development, retarded bone age, and unusual facies. *Proc R Soc Med* 1967; 60:1006.

13. Johnsen S, Crawford JD, Haessler HA: Fasting hyperlipogenesis: An inborn error of energy metabolism in Prader-Willi syndrome. *Pediatr Res* 1967; 1:291–292.

14. Palmer SK, Atlee JL III: Anesthetic management of the Prader-Willi syndrome. *Anesthesiology* 1976; 44:161–163.

15. Schoeller DA, Levitsky LL, Bandini LG, et al: Energy expenditure and body composition in Prader-Willi syndrome. *Metabolism* 1988; 37:115–120.

16. Sellick BA: Cricoid pressure to control regurgitation of stomach contents during induction of anesthesia. *Lancet* 1961; 2:404–406.

66

Cholecystectomy and Sickle Cell Anemia

A 10-year-old, 25-kg boy with sickle cell anemia is scheduled for elective cholecystectomy. He has been admitted several times in the past with sickle cell crises. Hemoglobin, 6.5 g/dL; hematocrit, 19.5%; Hb S, 79%; reticulocyte count, 14%.

Recommendations by Susan Prince Watson, M.D.

Sickle cell anemia is an autosomal recessive disorder affecting 0.15% of black children in the United States. The cellular defect is the substitution of valine for glutamic acid at the sixth residue of the β-globin chain of hemoglobin. Deoxygenation of the red blood cells leads to intracellular Hb S polymer formation, deformation of erythrocytes, and obstruction of microvascular blood flow.[1] While this process is reversible with reoxygenation, irreversible membrane damage eventually occurs and leads to permanently sickled cells that are removed from the circulation by hemolysis and sequestration.[2, 3]

PREOPERATIVE EVALUATION

During the preoperative visit, the anesthesiologist should assess the extent of organ system involvement. Planning the perioperative management with the hematologist may be helpful.

Cerebrovascular accidents occur in about 6% of patients and have a very high recurrence rate. Chronic transfusion to reduce the Hb S level appears to be effective in reducing the risk of recurrence.

A decrease in pulmonary function occurs in association with a restrictive defect. Significant irreversible changes are uncommon in childhood, although acute respiratory infections are common.

Cardiovascular effects of sickle cell disease are primarily the result of chronic anemia. However, ST depression in response to exercise has been seen in children as young as 10 years.

Renal dysfunction occurs early in life, primarily from pathology in the renal medulla. Hyposthenuria, enuresis, nocturia, hematuria, and pyelonephritis occur in younger patients. End-stage renal disease may be seen in older patients.

Major damage to other organs is often evident in adulthood. Liver and biliary tract disease are the result of cholelithiasis, hepatic infarction, and transfusion-related hepatitis. Skeletal pathology, in particular, aseptic necrosis of the femoral head, is due to repeated infarctions. Retinopathy may lead to blindness.[3]

PREOPERATIVE PREPARATION

Sickle cell patients usually have a hemoglobin level of 6 to 9 g/dL, with 80% to 90% Hb S. Raising the hemoglobin and reducing the Hb S level are believed to decrease the perioperative complication rate.[4, 5] One group recommends partial exchange transfusion prior to cholecystectomy to a hematocrit of 30% to 36% and a Hb S level 30% or less.[6] A multicenter randomized study, the "Pre-op Transfusion Study in Sickle Cell Disease," is currently underway to assess the efficacy of these therapeutic maneuvers on perioperative morbidity and mortality. The optimal Hb S and hemoglobin levels to minimize perioperative complications remain to be defined.

Avoiding dehydration is essential to minimize the risk of sickling. Intravenous fluids should be administered at one and a half times maintenance during the fasting period.[7]

Premedication should be individualized. Adolescents with sickle cell anemia may have exaggerated depression and anxiety. Tolerance to narcotics may occur if painful crises have been frequent. Optimal premedication provides satisfactory sedation without hypoxia, hypercarbia, or hypotension.

INTRAOPERATIVE CARE

Anesthetic care for patients with sickle cell disease includes ensuring normal oxygenation and ventilation, attention to blood pressure and blood volume, and maintenance of body temperature. No particular anesthetic agent has proved superior to others in comparative studies.

The patient should be positioned on the operating table with a warming mattress in place. Noninvasive monitors should be placed prior to induction of anesthesia. The child is preoxygenated, and an induction agent chosen to minimize cardiovascular side effects is administered. A nondepolarizing muscle relaxant (pancuronium, atracurium, vecuronium, or pipecuronium) is selected, depending on the expected length of the procedure. Anesthetic maintenance with an inhalation agent allows flexibility in the administration of oxygen during the procedure. Hyperventilation should be avoided since hypocarbia will produce undesirable cerebral vasoconstriction. End-tidal CO_2 monitoring is recommended.

At the conclusion of the operation, the action of the muscle relaxant should be reversed and the patient extubated awake and alert prior to transfer to the recovery room. Oxygen administration and pulse oximetry should be continued during transport to minimize the risk of hypoxemia.

POSTOPERATIVE CARE

Oxygen should be administered in the recovery room to compensate for increased oxygen consumption during recovery. Maintenance of normal circulation, ventilation, and oxygenation continue to be important.

Pulmonary problems appear to be the greatest cause of postoperative morbidity. Careful consideration should be given to narcotic administration to provide satisfactory analgesia without excessive respiratory depression. The use of patient-controlled analgesia, epidural analgesics, and/or local anesthetics may be helpful.

With attention to all the details of perioperative care, complications in sickle cell patients can be minimized.

REFERENCES

1. Rogers GP: Recent approaches to the treatment of sickle cell anemia. *JAMA* 1991; 256:2097–2101.
2. Davis JR, Vichinsky EP, Lubin BH: Current treatment of sickle cell disease. *Curr Probl Pediatr* 1980; 10:1–64.
3. Smith JA: The natural history of sickle cell disease. *Ann N Y Acad Sci* 1991; 565:104–108.
4. Burrington JD, Smith MD: Elective and emergency surgery in children with sickle cell disease. *Surg Clin North Am* 1976; 56:55—71.
5. Janik J, Seeler RA: Perioperative management of children with sickle hemoglobinopathy. *J Pediatr Surg* 1980; 15:117–120.
6. Esseltine DW, Baxter MRN, Bevan JC: Sickle cell states and the anaesthetist. *Can J Anaesth* 1988; 35:385–403
7. Luban NLC, Epstein BS, Watson SP: Sickle cell disease and anesthesia, in Gallagher TD (ed): *Advances in Anesthesia,* vol 1. St Louis, Mosby–Year Book, 1984.

67

Myelomeningocele and Orthopedic Surgery

A 10-year old girl with a myelomeningocele is scheduled for a tendon transfer and osteotomy of the hip. She has a functioning ventriculoperitoneal shunt. Her mother states that she required a blood transfusion when a similar procedure was performed 1 year ago. Hemoglobin, 11.2 g/dL; hematocrit, 35%.

Recommendations by Lucille A. Mostello, M.D.

The typical child with a repaired myelomeningocele is a frequent visitor to the operating room. Most have a voluminous medical history and a complicated physical examination.

MYELOMENINGOCELE

Myelomeningocele, a saclike protrusion of spinal fluid, meninges, and neural elements through the vertebral arches, predominantly in the lumbosacral area, is part of a spectrum of embryologic abnormalities generically classified as spinal dysraphism and commonly referred to as spina bifida. The number of children born with this condition is declining, less than 1 per 1,000 births. The frequency of additional cardiorespiratory anomalies is not increased, but there is an association with some elements of the VATER syndrome (vertebral defects, imperforate anus, tracheoesophageal fistula, and radial and renal dysplasia) and cleft lip/palate.

To prevent infection, most American neurosurgeons today repair the back lesion in the neonatal period. Progressive hydrocephalus is present in 70% to 80% of patients, and cerebrospinal fluid (CSF) shunting, usually to the peritoneum, is performed during the first year of life. Seizures occur in about 20% of shunted patients but in nearly half who have had shunt infections.

Nearly all patients have the associated Chiari II deformity consisting of various degrees of downward displacement of the brain stem and cerebellum below the foramen magnum. Decompression surgery is advocated in the fewer than 15% of patients who become symptomatic with significant stridor, cranial nerve dysfunction, apnea, hypoventilation, and/or dysphagia. The majority of deaths in infancy are related to untreatable hindbrain dysfunction, which in severe cases may be attributed to the absence of cranial nuclei, as part of a picture of brain stem dysgenesis, or neuronal infarction secondary to the elongated and angulated arterial tree. Additionally, there are reports of abnormal ventilatory patterns during sleep in 72% of *asymptomatic* infants with myelomeningocele.[1] Adolescents with the Chiari malformation may have abnormal ventilatory responses to hypercapnia; some patients also exhibit depressed hypoxic ventilatory responses as well.[2]

Most children with a repaired myelomeningocele have normal intelligence, but about 25% have an IQ below 80. The child with spina bifida tends to maintain a level of reading and spelling skills while falling behind in mathematical calculation and visual-spatial skills.[3]

Almost all children will have some component of neurogenic bladder dysfunction and frequent urinary tract infections. Clean intermittent catheterization on a regular basis and pharmacologic management have markedly reduced the requirement for urinary tract diversions and the incidence of renal failure, once the most common cause of death after infancy.

A periodic monitoring program in the setting of a comprehensive, coordinated, multidiscipline follow-up clinic is used as a basis of assessment in these complicated patients.[4] For example, while the majority of patients with spina bifida have a tethered cord present on imaging, surgery is only warranted when deterioration of the neurologic status is detected as changes in muscle power, scoliosis, spasticity, pain, or urinary function. The abnormalities of nervous innervation at the spinal cord lesion lead to severe deformities of joints and muscles, lack of mobility, and orthopedic interventions,[5] as in this case where a dislocated hip is treated to improve ambulation. Because areas without sensation are particularly vulnerable to injury, the patient with spina bifida may develop skin breakdown or decubiti.

PROBLEM OF ALLERGY TO LATEX

Since 1989 there has been a steady increase in reports of anaphylaxis to latex. Health care workers, occupationally exposed individuals, as well as patients with either spina bifida or congenital genitourinary deformities appear to be at risk[6-8] for unknown reasons. The onset of sensitivity may be insidious, but in many cases the first manifestation is anaphylactic shock. Despite this limitation, a detailed history of allergic responses to rubber products is the mainstay of diagnosis. Skin tests and the radioallergosorbent test (RAST) for latex-specific immunoglobulin E (IgE) can confirm the sensitivity, but the predictive value of a positive test result with a negative history is unknown.[8]

A poll of children's hospitals by the Centers for Disease Control indicated that more than 75 patients with either myelomeningocele or congenital genitourinary dysplasias had suspected anaphylactic reactions to latex products in 1990.[9] A survey by the New England Myelodysplasia Association demonstrated that the percentage of children who had allergic reactions as manifested by rash, urticaria at the contact site, watery eyes, wheezing, or respiratory arrest, to rubber catheters, balloons, or gloves was 18% to 28% in five area clinics in a sample of 187 families.[10] Our prospective study showed that children with spina bifida are more likely than control surgical patients to have IgE specific to latex antigens (34% vs. 11%).[11]

In the past, preservatives and stabilizer chemicals that are added to the sap (latex) of the rubber tree in the manufacturing process accounted for reactions to rubber products that were manifested as contact dermatitis and referred to as type IV or cell-mediated hypersensitivity. In 1979, anecdotal reports of urticaria also began to appear; thus, type I hypersensitivity reactions to rubber products were suspected and then confirmed when IgE specific for latex peptides of various molecular weights was found.[12] IgE sensitizes the surfaces of mast cells and basophils; when antigen bridges two IgE molecules, there is a release of stored histamine and newly synthesized arachidonic acid metabolites. Progression of this reaction to anaphylaxis is unpredictable but dependent on such factors as the route of administration and the amount of antigen.[13] The known mediators function as vasoactive, bronchoconstrictive, and chemotactic agents with a range of reactions from pruritus and urticaria to shock and death.

Our current management follows an algorithm format (Fig 67–1). If any clinical history of allergic responses to rubber products, unexplained urticaria, or unusual allergy-like responses during surgery is known, we use premedication (Table 67–1) and avoid latex products as much as possible. A similar protocol has reduced the incidence of reactions,[14] but no drug regimen can be protective in all cases. We believe that a positive RAST test result can be a good predictor of potential latex allergy in a high-risk group. Since a standardized skin test for latex allergy is not yet available, we use the RAST, the results of which may not be available preoperatively. For these patients with unknown test status, we avoid latex products intraoperatively, but we do not premedicate. Those with negative histories *and* negative RAST test results are usually treated in a conventional manner,

SPINA BIFIDA AND LATEX ALLERGY

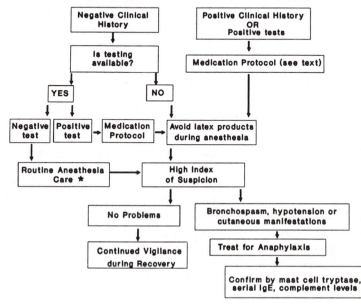

FIG 67–1.
Algorithm for the management of patients with spina bifida. The *asterisk* indicates that surgeons are advised to use nonlatex gloves if the peritoneum is handled.

TABLE 67–1.

Medication Protocol

A. *Ideal regimen prior to anesthesia:*

Diphenhydramine:	1 mg/kg po or IV q6h at 13, 7, and 1 hr preoperatively
Prednisone:	1 mg/kg po q6h at 13, 7, and 1 hr preoperatively or substitute hydrocortisone, 4 mg/kg IV for any dose
Ranitidine:	2 mg/kg po or 1 mg/kg IV q12h at 13 and 1 hr preoperatively

B. *Modified regimen:* Only one dose of each drug is administered intravenously 1 hr prior to anesthesia

C. *Postoperatively,* the regimen continues for 12 hr

D. *No regimen guarantees protection!*

but we advise the surgeons to use nonlatex gloves if significant peritoneal contact is anticipated. We always maintain a high degree of vigilance for allergic phenomena in *all* patients with spina bifida.

PREOPERATIVE EVALUATION

Special attention is given to evaluating the functioning of the ventriculoperitoneal shunt. The most common symptoms of shunt failure, vomiting, lethargy, headache, irritability, and anorexia, can be confused with viral illness. Moreover, there are no clinical signs in a quarter of patients with shunt failure.[15] The question of antibiotic prophylaxis for patients with CSF shunts remains a controversial one, but neurosurgeons are less likely to recommend antibiotics for orthopedic procedures when the shunt is directed to the peritoneum rather than to the atrium.

The level of mobility, particularly ambulation, will help determine the level of cardiovascular fitness. The degree of pulmonary compromise, mainly restrictive impairment, is related to the amount of scoliosis. It is very important to examine these children without back braces and when they are not supported in specially designed wheelchairs. A casual inspection often underestimates the severity of the spinal deformities.

An isolated laboratory finding of bacteriuria is expected if the patient undergoes clean intermittent catheterizations. The diagnosis of a urinary tract infection requires confirmatory signs such as fever, leukocytosis, or white cells in the urine.

For most osteotomies, a preoperative blood sample is typed and then reserved for crossmatch if necessary. If transfusion is likely, as in this case, and the child is cooperative, autologous blood can be deposited preoperatively. Many pediatric centers collect and process partial units, less than 500 mL, drawn from patients weighing less than 50 kg. As an alternative, a family member may donate the blood to be used. Both options require advance planning.

Repeated hospitalizations and operations often leave emotional scars. The child may have specific preferences for anesthesia, worries about postoperative pain and vomiting, or other concerns that need to be addressed in the presence of parental support.

CAN CONDUCTION ANESTHESIA BE ADMINISTERED?

Most anesthesiologists would choose general anesthesia for children. Epidural anesthesia is technically difficult due to alterations in landmarks. In addition, the spread of local anesthetic in a space filled with adhesions is unpredictable. In contrast, spinal anesthesia has been successfully employed.[16] The potential for neural damage is a primary consideration if needle entry is at the level of a functioning spinal cord. Regional techniques are more safely accomplished in an awake or mildly sedated patient who can respond to paresthesias. Because minor sequelae might cloud the evaluation of tethered cord syndromes, major regional techniques are best reserved for the neurologically stable, well-motivated, mature patient.

GENERAL ANESTHETIC TECHNIQUE

High levels of anxiety must be addressed by the use of premedication or an environment where parents can be present at induction. An intravenous catheter placed in an anesthetic limb is well tolerated but frequently not feasible due to scars from previous surgery. Following oral premedication with midazolam, 0.75 mg/kg, vascular access or inhalation induction would be less upsetting. Rectal methohexital has been used successfully but should be administered cautiously since there have been several unexplainable instances of very rapid induction and apnea in patients with spina bifida.[17]

Tetraplegia has occurred with hyperflexion during positioning for posterior decompressions of the Chiari II lesions.[18] Neurologic damage due to hyperflexion or hyperextension of the neck in patients with Chiari type I lesions has also been reported.[19, 20] Nonetheless, despite the frequent presence of a Chiari II malformation, intubation maneuvers have not been implicated as a cause of morbidity in patients with spina bifida. More common is the difficulty in positioning patients with severe kyphosis for intubation. After intubation, careful attention to positioning must continue with padding of bony prominences and supporting contracted limbs to minimize skin ischemia and breakdown.

Succinylcholine has been shown not to alter plasma potassium levels in children with spina bifida when administered following a thiopental induction.[21] The authors speculated that congenital denervation retards the maturation process of muscle, including the cholinergic muscle receptor sites. Similarly, autonomic hyperreflexia, of concern in spinal cord–injured patients with lesions at T10 and above, is not seen in patients with spina bifida.

A Foley catheter of silicone rubber is the only special monitor that is strongly suggested. In addition to following the amount of urinary output and by inference, cardiac output, it is helpful to drain a small, noncompliant, neurogenic bladder to reduce ureteral reflux. In addition, if a transfusion is administered, the characteristics of the urine can be observed.

No special restrictions on anesthetic agents are necessary. Nondepolarizing neuromuscular blocking agents are helpful because almost half of these patients have some form of spasticity in the upper or lower limbs.

Transfusion is seriously considered when the intraoperative hemoglobin level falls below 8 g/dL. Severe hemodilution, although tolerated by the cardiovascular system, may not be ideal for the neurologically impaired.

As regards the problem of latex allergy, a high degree of suspicion should be maintained if hypotension, increased airway pressure, or cutaneous changes occur. A well-planned protocol for the rapid treatment of anaphylaxis, with emphasis on epinephrine administration and fluid resuscitation, has been established[22] and is constantly being updated and refined.[13] Because latex allergy may only account for approximately 10% of allergic responses during anesthesia,[23] it is still prudent to draw appropriate blood specimens and thoroughly investigate each incident.[24]

POSTOPERATIVE CARE

The extent of postoperative pain in a patient who has partial lumbar sensation is unpredictable. For a child over 8 years of age who can understand preoperative instructions, we offer patient-controlled analgesia with morphine. Whatever pain control measures are chosen, they should minimize obtundation of consciousness, which might delay the evaluation of shunt malfunction.

Deep-vein thrombosis has been reported in patients with spina bifida postoperatively. The combination of weak extremities, spica casting, hypercoagulation in the postsurgical state, and urinary tract infection sets the stage for thrombosis, particularly in the iliac veins.[25]

REFERENCES

1. Ward SL, Jacobs RA, Gates EP, et al: Abnormal ventilatory patterns during sleep in infants with myelomeningocele. *J Pediatr* 1986; 109:631–634.
2. Swaminathan S, Paton JY, Ward SL, et al: Abnormal control of ventilation in adolescents with myelodysplasia. *J Pediatr* 1989; 115:898–903.
3. Wills KE, Holmbeck GN, Dillon K, et al: Intelligence and achievement in children with myelomeningocele. *J Pediatr Psychol* 1990; 15:161–176.
4. Liptak GS, Bloss JW, Briskin H, et al: The management of children with spinal dysraphism. *J Child Neurol* 1988; 3:3–20.
5. Mazur JM, Menelaus MB: Neurologic status of spina bifida patients and the orthopedic surgeon. *Clin Orthop* 1991; 264:54–64.
6. Gold M, Swartz JS, Braude BM, et al: Intraoperative anaphylaxis: An association with latex sensitivity. *J Allergy Clin Immunol* 1991; 87:662–666.
7. Slater JE: Rubber anaphylaxis. *N Engl J Med* 1989; 320:1127–1130.
8. Sussman GL, Tarlo S, Dolovich J: The spectrum of IgE-mediated responses to latex. *JAMA* 1991; 265:2844–2847.
9. Centers for Disease Control: Anaphylactic reactions during general anesthesia among pediatric patients— United States, January 1990–January 1991. *MMWR* 1991; 40:437.
10. Meeropol E, Kelleher R, Bell S, et al: Allergic reactions to rubber in patients with myelodysplasia. *N Engl J Med* 1990; 323:1072.

11. Slater JE, Mostello LA, Shaer C: Rubber-specific IgE in children with spina bifida. *J Urol* 1991; 146:578–579.

12. Morales C, Basomba A, Carriera J, et al: Anaphylaxis produced by rubber glove contact. *Clin Exp Allergy* 1989; 19:425–430.

13. Bochner BS, Lichtenstein LM: Anaphylaxis. *N Engl J Med* 1991; 324:1785–1790.

14. Nguyen DH, Burns MW, Shapiro GG, et al: Intraoperative cardiovascular collapse secondary to latex allergy. *J Urol* 1991; 146:571–574.

15. Kirkpatrick M, Engleman H, Minns RA: Symptoms and signs of progressive hydrocephalus. *Arch Dis Child* 1989; 64:124–128.

16. Broome IJ: Spinal anaesthesia for caesarean section in a patient with spina bifida cystica. *Anaesth Intensive Care* 1989; 17:377–379.

17. Yemen TA, Pullerits J, Stillman R, et al: Rectal methohexital causing apnea in two patients with meningomyeloceles. *Anesthesiology* 1991; 74:1139–1141.

18. Di Rocco C, Rende M: Chiari malformations, in Raimondi AJ, Choux M, Di Rocco C (eds): *The Pediatric Spine II*. New York, Springer-Verlag NY Inc, 1989, p 86.

19. Dong ML: Arnold-Chiari malformation type I appearing after tonsillectomy. *Anesthesiology* 1987; 67:120–122.

20. Vlcek BW, Ito B: Acute paraparesis secondary to Arnold-Chiari type I malformation and neck hyperflexion. *Ann Neurol* 1987; 21:100–101.

21. Dierdorf SF, McNiece WL, Rao CC, et al: Failure of succinylcholine to alter plasma potassium in children with myelomeningocoele. *Anesthesiology* 1986; 64:272–273.

22. Levy JH: Allergic reactions during anesthesia. *J Clin Anesth* 1988; 1:39–46.

23. Leynadier F, Pecquet C, Dry J: Anaphylaxis to latex during surgery. *Anaesthesia* 1989; 44:547–550.

24. Weiss ME, Adkinson NF, Hirshman CA: Evaluation of allergic drug reactions in the perioperative period. *Anesthesiology* 1989; 71:483–485.

25. Bernstein ML, Esseltine D, Azouz EM, et al: Deep venous thrombosis complicating myelomeningocele: Report of three cases. *Pediatrics* 1989; 84:856–859.

68

Supraclavicular Node Biopsy and Mediastinal Mass

A 10-year-old, 38-kg boy is scheduled for supraclavicular node biopsy. He also has a large mediastinal mass. The presumed diagnosis is non-Hodgkin's lymphoma. Biopsy is necessary prior to initiation of therapy. The child is sitting upright and breathing 40 times per minute. Hemoglobin, 9.5 g/dL; hematocrit, 28.5%.

Recommendations by Lynne R. Ferrari, M.D.

ETIOLOGY

In the pediatric population, the mediastinum is the primary site of involvement in 16% to 36% of non-Hodgkin's lymphoma and 54% to 81% of Hodgkin's lymphoma.[1] Although lymphomas constitute the largest group of masses that arise in the anterior mediastinum in children, other masses that may present in this location include teratomas, cystic hygromas, thymomas, hemangiomas, sarcomas, desmoid tumors, pericardial cysts, and diaphragmatic hernias of the Morgagni type (Table 68–1).

To understand the pathophysiology of the anterior mediastinum, it is important to be familiar with the anatomy. The mediastinum is defined as the extrapleural space in the thorax that is bounded anteriorly by the sternum, posteriorly by the thoracic vertebrae, superiorly by the thoracic inlet, and inferiorly by the diaphragm. Structures contained within the mediastinum that may undergo compression from an enlarging mass are the trachea and the mainstem bronchi, superior vena cava, aortic arch, main pulmonary artery, and a portion of the heart itself.[2]

TABLE 68–1.

Masses Located in the Anterior Mediastinum

Lymphoma
Sarcoma
Thymoma
Teratoma
Hemangioma
Cystic hygroma
Desmoid tumor
Pericardial cyst
Diaphragmatic hernia

PREOPERATIVE CONSIDERATIONS

Patients with anterior mediastinal masses may present with varied signs and symptoms referable to both the cardiovascular and respiratory systems (Table 68–2). The symptoms are directly related to the location and size of the mass, as well as the degree of compression of surrounding structures.[3] The most commonly observed respiratory symptom is cough, especially in the supine position, which results from anterior compression of the trachea by a mass located in the anterior mediastinum. Infants less than 2 years of age are more likely to experience wheezing as a sign of tracheal compression, whereas children older than 2 years of age usually present with malaise, cough, fever, and a neck mass. Other respiratory findings in patients of all ages include tachypnea, dyspnea, stridor, retractions, decreased breath sounds, and cyanosis on crying, all of which should alert the anesthesiologist to some degree of airway compromise that may worsen when positive intrathoracic pressure is generated.

Cardiovascular symptoms result from compression of the aortic and pulmonary vessels, as well as the right atrium and right ventricle. This can lead to both hypotension secondary to inadequate cardiac filling and restricted pulmonary blood flow resulting in poor oxygenation despite adequate ventilation. Findings referable to the cardiovascular system include fatigue, headache, hypotension

TABLE 68–2.

Symptoms of an Anterior Mediastinal Mass

Cough
Stridor
Wheezing
Retractions
Tachypnea
Cyanosis
Dyspnea
Malaise
Decreased breath sounds
Superior vena cava syndrome
New onset of cardiac murmur

or pallor in the supine position, a feeling of light-headedness, superior vena cava syndrome (facial edema, cyanosis, jugular venous distension), and the appearance of a new murmur, especially in the area of the pulmonary valve. It is essential that the anesthesiologist search for these signs and symptoms when interviewing and examining patients with mediastinal masses in an attempt to ascertain the degree of respiratory and cardiovascular compromise present. Patients with minimal symptoms can have catastrophic intraoperative events if subtle indicators are overlooked.

When the diagnosis of malignancy is suspected, an initial step is bone marrow aspiration under local anesthesia. This may provide the diagnosis but can be inconclusive, necessitating examination of tissue samples from the mass itself or adjacent lymph nodes. Although infiltration of a local anesthetic may be attempted for superficial tissue sampling in the older patient, general anesthesia is generally required in the younger child. The depth of sedation required to render the small child amenable to tissue biopsy during infiltration of local anesthesia is such that spontaneous ventilation may be depressed. It is therefore preferable to administer general anesthesia and secure the airway with an endotracheal tube.

In the absence of a tissue diagnosis it is difficult to justify empirical treatment with radiation therapy. Several cases of failure to make a tissue diagnosis after radiation therapy have been reported. Many childhood tumors, including lymphomas, are extremely radiosensitive and shrink markedly following a single treatment, thus reducing the likelihood of perioperative complications. However, the determination of an accurate diagnosis of tumor cell type is essential prior to initiation of chemotherapy and determination of the optimal treatment regimen. Even when preoperative radiation is limited to the central mantle of a mediastinal mass, there may be enough scatter of the radiation beam to compromise the accuracy of diagnosis in tissues taken from peripheral samples. The risk of this approach is that the patient may receive a suboptimal chemotherapy/radiation treatment regimen.[4]

In addition to the history and physical examination of the patient, laboratory and noninvasive radiologic testing should be completed prior to the induction of anesthesia and surgery. A complete blood count should be obtained to evaluate oxygen-carrying capacity and to detect evidence of bone marrow infiltration by the tumor (increased white blood cell count), which may lead to a decrease in platelet production. Intraoperative platelet transfusion should be considered to ensure surgical hemostasis and prevent hematoma formation, which may compress an already compromised airway in a patient with thrombocytopenia. Posteroanterior- and lateral-view chest radiographs taken in the erect position will allow the extent of the mass to be appreciated, and the superior and inferior margins of the mass to be noted. In the event of total tracheal occlusion on induction of anesthesia, insertion of a rigid bronchoscope or endotracheal tube beyond the mass to re-establish patency of the airway may be the only effective measure if the inferior limit of the mass is located above the carina.[5] A computed tomographic (CT) scan of the chest is valuable in determining the size of the tumor, evaluating compression and distortion of adjacent structures, and measuring tracheal cross-sectional area. Subclinical airway compression, however, can only be identified by CT scan in 50% of pediatric patients (Fig 68–1,A and B).

In children, small decreases in the cross-sectional area of the trachea will result in large increases in airway resistance, thus explaining early obstructive symptomatology in this patient group. Although the chest radiographs and CT scan are informative, they are static measurements and do not predict alterations in anatomy and physiology that can occur in the anesthetized state.[6] The patient with respiratory compromise can compensate for this in the awake state by generating a nega-

POSTERIOR

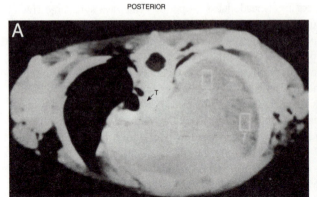

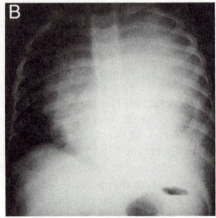

ANTERIOR

FIG 68–1.
A, chest radiograph of a 10-year-old male with non-Hodgkin lymphoma. **B,** CT scan of the chest in the same patient. Note the displacement of the trachea *(T)* to the right.

tive intrathoracic pressure during spontaneous respiration. In this state the diaphragm descends, the trachea is elongated, and the thorax expands, thereby decreasing compression of the airway by the tumor mass. Absence of airway compression on CT scans or chest radiographs in the awake, spontaneously breathing patient does not guarantee a patent airway after anesthetic induction. The flow-volume loop, when measured in both the supine and upright positions, is a dynamic examination at varying lung volumes and is the most sensitive predictor of changes that may occur under anesthesia. Maximal inspiratory and expiratory flow-volume curves can illustrate the degree of functional impairment present in individual patients as well as distinguish fixed from variable intrathoracic obstructions (Fig. 68–2). Transthoracic echocardiography is a noninvasive means by which the relation of the tumor to the heart and great vessels can be determined. Information generated from echocardiographic examinations regarding alterations in myocardial contractility as well as compression and distortion of adjacent structures may be helpful in identifying and correcting intraoperative events associated with changes in the patient's position.[7–9]

PREOPERATIVE PREPARATION

Solid food and milk products should be restricted for 12 hours prior to induction of anesthesia. Ingestion of clear fluids is permitted on an age-appropriate basis, with the shortest time period being 2 to 3 hours preoperatively. Although the routine practice of pediatric anesthesia discourages preoperative administration of an antisialagogue, one should be administered prior to anesthetic induction of the patient with an anterior mediastinal mass. Sedative premedication should not be administered since decreases in consciousness and inability to maintain maximal spontaneous respiration may result in worsening of airway obstruction. Intravenous access should be secured prior to the induction of anesthesia. If compression of the great vessels or the superior vena cava syndrome is suspected,

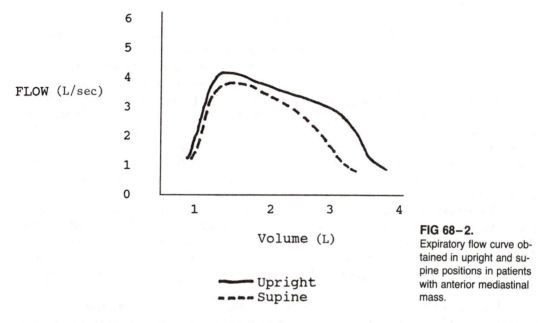

FIG 68–2.
Expiratory flow curve obtained in upright and supine positions in patients with anterior mediastinal mass.

the preferred site for insertion of an intravenous cannula is the lower extremity to allow adequate delivery of intravenous drugs in the event of total superior vena cava occlusion.[10] In the younger patient where an attempt to separate the child from the parents results in crying and struggling that may worsen pre-existing airway obstruction and cause hypoxemia, a small dose of intravenous ketamine, 0.5 to 1.0 mg/kg, may be administered with the caveat that spontaneous respirations must be maintained.

ANESTHETIC MANAGEMENT

Tracheal or bronchial obstruction can arise unexpectedly at any time during anesthesia and surgery, including induction, intubation, positioning, and extubation. Prior to inducing anesthesia, a functioning rigid bronchoscope and personnel who are experienced in its use should be present in the operating room. In the event of total tracheal compression by an anterior mediastinal mass, an attempt to regain control of the airway may be made by stenting the trachea via insertion of the rigid bronchoscope to a depth sufficient to bypass the obstruction.

On arrival in the operating room, standard monitoring devices are applied. If variations in blood pressure and oxygenation are present with minor changes in positioning, an arterial catheter should be inserted to observe beat-to-beat variability of blood pressure and obtain arterial blood for analysis.

Anesthesia is best induced with the child in the semi-Fowler or full sitting position since the supine position leads to decreased expansion of the rib cage and cephalad displacement of the diaphragm. Patients who are asymptomatic while awake may exhibit airway obstruction during anesthetic induction in the supine position, which is explained by a reduction in the dimensions of the thorax that limits the available space for the trachea relative to the tumor. In addition, inhalation anesthetic agents decrease chest wall muscle tone, which in turn decreases tracheal distending pressure, thus allowing collapse of the trachea to occur. The increase in central blood volume that accompanies the supine position can also lead to increased tumor volume and size, thus contributing to the potential for airway obstruction. The patient should spontaneously breathe increasing concentrations of halothane in oxygen via face mask until the anesthetic depth is sufficient to obtund pharyngeal reflexes. If it is possible to assist or control ventilation with positive pressure, the patient may be paralyzed and the trachea intubated. If positive-pressure ventilation is ineffective or controlled respiration results in airway obstruction, tracheal intubation should be performed without the aid of muscle relaxation. After auscultation and verification of proper endotracheal tube position, the patient may be lowered into the supine position. The adequacy of ventilation and blood pressure should be checked at frequent intervals until the optimum surgical position has been achieved. If transthoracic or transesophageal echocardiography is available in the operating room, the proximity of the mass to other vital structures may be observed during patient positioning (Fig. 68–3). If at any time a decrease in blood pressure occurs and causes an inability to oxygenate despite adequate ventilation or if an inability to provide adequate ventilation is encountered, the patient should be returned to the upright or lateral position. This will generally relieve airway obstruction caused by the tumor mass.

Anesthesia should be maintained with an inhalation agent in oxygen. If ventilation and oxygenation are acceptable, nitrous oxide may be introduced in an incremental fashion. If increased airway obstruction is encountered during attempted assisted or controlled ventilation, the patient should be allowed to breathe spontaneously throughout the surgical procedure. Fixed intravenous agents such as sedatives or narcotics that may delay emergence from anesthesia or depress spontaneous ventilation after surgery should be avoided. Intravenous fluid replacement should consist of isotonic solution in a sufficient volume to replace fasting deficits and hourly maintenance requirements throughout the surgical procedure. Intravascular volume should be preserved to ensure adequate cardiac filling and maintenance of acceptable cardiac output.

Extubation of the trachea at the conclusion of surgery and anesthesia carries the potential for

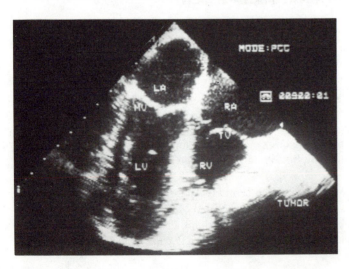

FIG 68–3.
Transthoracic ecdocardiograph of a patient with an anterior mediastinal mass. Note the proximity of the mass to the right-heart structures.

airway obstruction and must be approached with caution. The transition from general anesthesia to the awake state without an artificial airway can be as hazardous as the induction/intubation period. Pain, anxiety, and coughing during emergence can increase intrathoracic pressure and worsen pre-existing obstruction distal to the endotracheal tube. Tachypnea may increase turbulence in previously narrowed upper airways, thus limiting effective air exchange. Spontaneous ventilation should be present prior to any attempt at extubation of the trachea. The patient should be able to generate a negative intrathoracic pressure sufficient to maintain ventilation. If adequate blood pressure and oxygenation, as determined by pulse oximetry, cannot be easily maintained, extubation of the trachea should be delayed. If airway compromise is encountered at this time, however, and tissue has been obtained for diagnosis, it is now appropriate to institute antitumor therapy to diminish the size of the mass before tracheal extubation is attempted. The patient should be transferred to an intensive care unit for assisted ventilation and appropriate monitoring. Patients may be evaluated by means of clinical criteria and sequential chest radiographs. Often a single dose of radiation therapy and/or chemotherapy will shrink the mass sufficiently to allow safe tracheal extubation.

CONCLUSION

A combination of adequate preoperative patient evaluation, awareness of the anesthetic implications of anterior mediastinal masses, and a clear understanding of appropriate anesthetic management are essential. A previously well thought out plan of the conduct of general anesthesia, alternative management plans in the event of a complication, and a thorough understanding of the physiologic principles of this disorder will allow safe administration of anesthesia to this group of patients.

REFERENCES

1. Neuman GG, Weingarten AE, Abramowitz RM, et al: The anesthetic management of the patient with an anterior mediastinal mass. *Anesthesiology* 1984; 60:144–147.
2. Pullerits J, Holzman RH: Anaesthesia for patients with mediastinal masses. *Can J Anaesth* 1989; 36:681–688.
3. Azizkhan RG, Dudgeon DL, Buck JR, et al: Life-threatening airway obstruction as a complication to the management of mediastinal masses in children. *J Pediatr Surg* 1985; 20:816–822.
4. Ferrari LR, Bedford RF: General anesthesia prior to treatment of anterior mediastinal masses in pediatric cancer patients. *Anesthesiology* 1990; 72:991–995.
5. Mackie AM, Watson CB: Anaesthesia and mediastinal masses. *Anaesthesia* 1984; 39:899–903.
6. Halpern S, Chatten J, Meadows AT, et al: Anterior mediastinal masses: Anesthesia hazards and other problems. *Clin Lab Observ* 1983; 102:407–410.
7. Ferrari LR, Bedford RF: Anterior mediastinal mass in a pregnant patient: Anesthetic management and considerations. *J Clin Anesth* 1989; 1:460–463.
8. Marshall ME, Trump DL: Acquired pulmonic stenosis caused by mediastinal tumors. *Cancer* 1982; 49:1496–1499.
9. Keon TP: Death on induction of anesthesia for cervical node biopsy. *Anesthesiology* 1981; 55:471–472.
10. Janin Y, Wise BL, Schneider K, et al: Superior vena cava syndrome in childhood and adolescence: A review of the literature and report of three cases. *J Pediatr Surg* 1982; 17:290–295.

69

Colectomy and Postoperative Pain

An 11-year-old, 42-kg girl is scheduled for coloprotectomy for familial polyposis. Both she and her parents are worried about postoperative pain and ask whether there is any option other than intramuscular injections. Hemoglobin, 11 g/dL; hematocrit, 33%.

Recommendations by Norbert J. Weidner, M.D.

Familial adenomatous polyposis is an inherited autosomal dominant, non–sex-linked disease involving adenomatous polypoid proliferation of the colon and rectum. Inevitably all affected patients will develop malignant degeneration within the colon or rectum by the age of 50 years.[1] The severity of the disease and the probability of carcinoma vary among families.

The disease typically manifests symptoms near puberty. These symptoms include diarrhea, bleeding per rectum, abdominal pain, and anemia. Early in childhood the disease is asymptomatic, and the patient may undergo evaluation as a consequence of recognition of the disease in other family members.

Malignancy rarely occurs before late adolescence. Carcinoma has a reported incidence of less than 6% in the prepubescent population. However, as many as 60% of adults who come to surgery for familial polyposis will have carcinoma of the colon or rectum.[2]

Colectomy is reserved for any child who is symptomatic or for an asymptomatic child who has reached 10 to 15 years of age. Colectomy is indicated in early adolescence with ileostomy or endorectal pull-through as possible options for ileal terminus.

PREANESTHETIC EVALUATION

Preanesthetic evaluation should focus on recognizing the possible presence of anemia and assessing the patient's and her family's underlying level of anxiety. Accurate and supportive information regarding the procedure and postoperative experience will reduce the patient's anxiety. A short-acting benzodiazepine prior to the procedure may supplement the preoperative visit in those whom additional axiolysis is required.

The risks and benefits of the various techniques available for postoperative analgesia should be confidently and accurately outlined for the patient and her family in order to formulate a rational, acceptable plan for postoperative analgesia.

A technique of choice would be the placement of an epidural catheter intraoperatively for intraoperative and postoperative administration of local anesthetic and narcotic. The benefits of this approach vs. systemically administered narcotics are improved pulmonary function,[3, 4] improved oxygen saturation during sleep,[5] and earlier return of bowel function after abdominal surgery.[6]

INTRAOPERATIVE MANAGEMENT

Intraoperative management begins with the placement of noninvasive monitors. Induction of anesthesia can be accomplished either with a potent inhalation agent in combination with 70% nitrous oxide and 30% oxygen, or an intravenous induction may be chosen. Many older children dislike the experience of breathing the anesthetic and prefer an intravenous induction. Once the airway is secured, a nasogastric tube is inserted and the child turned to the lateral decubitus position in preparation for placement of an epidural catheter.

EPIDURAL ANALGESIA

Unlike adults, the epidural space is more superficial in children and correlates with patient age.[7] An 18-gauge Touhy needle and a 20-gauge catheter are easily managed in this age group. In a child weighing less than 20 kg, a 19-gauge short Touhy needle in conjunction with a 21-gauge catheter is preferred. A saline-filled glass syringe or specifically prepared loss-of-resistance plastic syringe is attached to the needle once the needle has punctured the skin. Continuous pressure on the syringe is advisable rather than needle advancement and intermittent pressure because of the short distance traversed and the lack of stiffness of the ligamentum flavum in children. A saline-filled syringe is chosen rather than an air-filled syringe to limit the potential for air embolism, particularly in smaller children. Patchy analgesia may result as a consequence of air bubbles preventing satisfactory contact between nerve rootlets and the local anesthetic solution.[8]

Catheter position is the main determinant of needle placement. A midline approach is chosen for interspaces below T10, while a paramedian approach is preferred for thoracic placement. The catheter is advanced a few centimeters into the epidural space. Although an epidural catheter may be advanced from the caudal space to the thoracic region in newborns, attempts to do so in older children are less successful.

After aspirating the catheter to ensure the absence of blood or cerebral spinal fluid, a test dose of local anesthetic, 0.1 mL/kg of 1% lidocaine with 1:200,000 epinephrine, is injected. Intravenous atropine may be administered prior to the epidural injection to enhance the response to an inadvertent intravascular injection. Significant false-negative responses can occur.[9] Following the test dose, local anesthetic administration into the epidural space should be performed in an incremental fashion.

The ability to monitor subarachnoid placement or intravascular injection is compromised because the epidural block is performed while the child is anesthetized. Spontaneous respirations serve as a marker for the development of a total spinal during initial drug administration. Once the catheter lies within the epidural space, it is secured by utilizing a clear adhesive dressing that allows visualization of the catheter during the subsequent postoperative period. A dose of 0.50 to 0.75 mL/kg of 0.25% bupivacaine plus epinephrine, 1:200,000, will block the selected dermatomes. The intraoperative period is managed with a light general anesthetic and controlled ventilation.

Reinjection of local anesthetic will be required approximately 90 to 120 minutes following the initial dose. There are two approaches to the timing of top-up injections. They can be given on the basis of pharmacokinetic properties and the duration of action of bupivacaine, or they may be given in response to physiologic evidence of inadequate analgesia. Repeat doses of approximately half the initial dose at 90-minute intervals will provide adequate analgesia and appropriate plasma concentrations of drug.[10]

POSTOPERATIVE MANAGEMENT

The choices for postoperative epidural analgesia are intermittent injection or continuous drug administration. Intermittent bolus administration of analgesia, usually preservative-free morphine, is a simple technique and requires no special equipment.[11, 12] However, a physician or trained nurse must be available to inject the catheter. With intermittent catheter injection, the epidural system is open periodically with the attendant risk of infection. Human dosing errors and variations in the quality of analgesia may occur with bolus dosing. In addition, the intermittent bolus technique does not favor the use of local anesthetic-narcotic mixtures. Continuous infusion of analgesia avoids variations in the quality of analgesia and allows the use of local anesthetic-narcotic combinations. By combining dilute solutions of a local anesthetic and narcotic, less total drug is utilized with theoretically fewer side effects. The need for infusion pumps and the technical problems inherent with their use may be viewed as a disadvantage.

The choice of narcotic depends on the operative site and catheter location. Lipophilic narcotics require that the catheter be placed near the dermatomes corresponding to the surgical site, whereas less lipid-soluble drugs offer greater flexibility with catheter placement while increasing the risk of opioid-related side effects such as respiratory depression. When the catheter is placed at the appropriate dermatome, less drug will be required to maintain adequate analgesia.

This patient is best managed by placement of the catheter in the epidural space corresponding to the middle of the incision with maintenance of a postoperative infusion of bupivacaine, 0.1%, and preservative-free morphine, 0.004%, at an infusion rate between 0.25 and 0.3 mL/kg/hr. Adjustments in the infusion rate should be made according to individual patient response. The bupivacaine dose should not exceed 0.5 mg/kg/hr. A morphine dose of 10 μg/kg/hr is usually adequate. The infusion can be continued for 3 to 5 days postoperatively or until the patient has regained use of the enteral route to provide analgesia.

Postoperative monitoring for epidural techniques continues to be controversial. At our hospital, we would monitor the patient on the ward. However, a coordinated system of management involving twice-daily physician visits in conjunction with a nursing staff trained in the care and monitoring of patients receiving epidural drugs is crucial to the safe and effective operation of this technique. Vital signs and motor blockade are monitored every 4 hours, while the respiratory rate and sedation are monitored hourly by the nursing staff. Respiratory depression or a depressed level of consciousness leads to physician assessment and intervention. It is crucial, with the use of epidural analgesia, that there be a support system within the hospital capable of providing immediate ventilatory support.[13, 14] Apnea monitors are utilized in children less than 6 months of age, and oximetry is provided for every patient receiving epidural opioids.

Side effects of epidurally administered narcotics can be anticipated. Urinary retention would be anticipated in this patient and should be managed with continuous urinary drainage. Pruritis can be managed with an antihistamine or low-dose naloxone as well as by changing or lowering the dose of epidural narcotic. Nausea and vomiting have not been a major problem with epidural administration, but if traditional antiemetics are ineffective, low-dose naloxone is recommended. Sedation and respiratory depression following epidural narcotics are of serious concern, and monitoring for respiratory depression outside the intensive care unit is essential.

Complications of local anesthetic administration are less frequent. Hypotension, unusual in children less than 8 years of age, may be managed by intravenous fluid administration. In spite of the use of dilute local anesthetic concentrations, some degree of motor blockade may occur. Care should be taken to ensure safety during ambulation and to protect the lower extremities from pressure injury during bed rest. Systemic toxicity to local anesthetics is uncommon with the continuous technique, and intermittent boluses of local anesthetics are not recommended.

OTHER ANALGESIC TECHNIQUES

An alternative technique would involve the administration of systemic narcotics both intraoperatively and postoperatively. Opioids remain the mainstay of clinical pain relief, and morphine continues to be the standard for opioid administration. New synthetic opioids may be more potent, but there is little evidence that they provide a wider margin of safety.

Agonist-antagonist drugs, although producing less respiratory depression, are less potent analgesics and demonstrate a ceiling effect above which further analgesia is not obtained.[15] The partial agonist buprenorphine has been examined in children[16] and found to be an effective analgesic with a slightly longer duration of action than morphine. Delayed respiratory depression with repeated intravenous administration of buprenorphine and a slightly higher frequency of nausea and vomiting do not favor its use over morphine.

Intermittent, on-demand, intramuscular analgesia, long the standard for postoperative analgesia, is appropriately being replaced by newer modes of opioid administration. Pharmacokinetic and pharmacodynamic principles point to the wide interpatient variation in narcotic analgesic needs. There exists as much as a fourfold difference in analgesic requirements for patients with the same postoperative stimulus.[17] In spite of wide interindividual variation in analgesic needs, there is a consistent intrapatient steady-state plasma concentration of opioid that defines a minimal effective analgesic concentration (MEAC).[18] The MEAC is not necessarily constant[19] and may, for example, be increased by movement, physiotherapy, ambulation, and coughing or decreased by distraction or other behavioral techniques.

Attempts to achieve an MEAC by intermittent intravenous opioid dosing are limited by the elimination half-life of the drug, which necessitates frequent administration, as well as by the time, interest, and bias of the medical staff attending the patient. Morphine must often be administered every 2 hours. Bolus intravenous dosing of narcotics is complicated by wide fluctuations in plasma opioid concentrations, which can give rise to toxicity, as well as periods of inadequate analgesia.

Attempts to overcome these limitations by constant opioid infusions have met with success.[20-22] However, frequent adjustment of the infusion rate to meet individual pharmacodynamics may result in increased side effects, overdosage, and respiratory depression. Patient-controlled analgesia (PCA), a system designed to accommodate a wide range of analgesic requirements, can be used to provide analgesia in children as young as 6 years of age[23] as well as adults.[24]

A suitable prescription for initiation of PCA with morphine involves establishing a level of analgesia by "loading" the patient with morphine, 0.05 mg/kg administered intravenously every 10 minutes, until the patient is comfortable. Subsequent morphine would be administered in a dose of 0.02 mg/kg with a lock-out interval of 10 minutes and a 4-hour limit of 0.25 mg/kg. In a study of 82 children receiving postoperative PCA morphine for analgesia, Berde utilized a basal continuous rate of 15 μg/kg/hr, which represented 30% to 50% of the average body requirements for children receiving a continuous infusion of morphine for postoperative or cancer pain. In contrast to adult studies,[25, 26] Berde's use of PCA plus a basal infusion did not increase the incidence of opioid-related side effects and provided a greater level of patient satisfaction.[27] The need for a continuous infusion is greatly diminished 48 hours after surgery.

Ketorolac tromethamine, a parenteral nonsteroidal anti-inflammatory drug, may serve as an adjunct to the systemic administration of narcotics. Ketorolac markedly diminishes the postoperative opioid requirement while lacking any intrinsic cardiorespiratory effects.[28, 29] Currently ketorolac is only available for intramuscular use, but future direction points toward intravenous use.[30]

Although PCA and epidural techniques may be beneficial,[31, 32] their implementation can be associated with significant side effects. Physicians and nursing staff involved in managing these techniques must vigilantly observe the patient for side effects as well as inadequate analgesia. A well-organized approach for managing these problems as well as a continuous educational program for those involved in administering these techniques are crucial for their safe operation. The absence of such a well-organized system precludes implementation of these techniques.

REFERENCES

1. Mayo CW, DeWeerd JH, Jackman RJ, et al: Diffuse familial polyposis of the colon. *Surg Gynecol Obstet* 1951; 93:87.
2. Williams RD, Fish JC: Multiple polyposis, polyp progression and carcinoma of the colon. *Am J Surg* 1966; 112:846.
3. Benhamou D, Samii K, Noviant Y: Effect of analgesia on respiratory muscle function after upper abdominal surgery. *Acta Anesthesiol Scand* 1983; 27:22.
4. Torda TA, Pybus DA: Extradural administration of morphine and bupivacaine. *Br J Anaesth* 1984; 56:141.
5. Catley DM, Thornton C, Jordan C, et al: Pronounced episodic oxygen desaturation in the postoperative period: Its association with ventilatory pattern and analgesic regimen. *Anesthesiology* 1985; 63:20.

6. Scheinin B, Asantila R, Orko R: The effect of bupivacaine and morphine on pain and bowel function after colonic surgery. *Acta Anaesthesiol Scand* 1987; 31:161.

7. Kosakay S, Kawajuchi R: Distance from skin to epidural space in children. *Jpn J Anesthesiol* 1974; 23:874.

8. Dalens B, Bazin JE, Haberer JP, et al: Epidural bubbles as a cause of incomplete analgesia during epidural anesthesia. *Anesth Analg* 1987; 66:679.

9. Desparmet J, Mateo J, Ecoffey C, et al: Efficacy of epidural test dose in children anesthetized with halothane. *Anesthesiology* 1990; 72:249.

10. Murat I, Montay G, Delleur MM, et al: Bupivacaine pharmacokinetics during epidural anesthesia in children. *Eur J Anesth* 1988; 5:113.

11. Ready LB, Oden R, Chadwick HS, et al: Development of an anesthesiology based postoperative pain management service. *Anesthesiology* 1988; 68:100.

12. Tyler D, Krane E: Postoperative pain management in children. *Anesthesiol Clin North Am* 1989; 7:155–170.

13. Ready LB, Edwards WT: Postoperative care following intrathecal or epidural opioids. II (letter). *Anesthesiology* 1989; 72:213.

14. Krane EJ: Delayed respiratory depression in a child after caudal epidural morphine. *Anesth Analg* 1988; 67:75.

15. Lloyd-Thomas AR: Pain management in pediatric patients. *Br J Anaesth* 1990; 64:85.

16. Maunuksela EL, Korpela R, Olkkola KT: Double blind multiple dose comparison of buprenorphine and morphine in postoperative pain in children. *Br J Anaesth* 1988; 60:48.

17. Austin KL, Stapleton JV, Mather LE: Relationship between blood meperidine concentration and analgesia response. *Anesthesiology* 1980; 53:460.

18. Dahlstrom B, Tamsen A, Paalzan L, et al: Patient-controlled analgesic therapy, Part IV: Pharmacokinetics and analgesic plasma concentrations of morphine. *Clin Pharmacokinet* 1982; 7:266.

19. Gourlay GK, Kowalski SR, Plummer JL, et al: Fentanyl blood concentration–analgesic response relationship in the treatment of postoperative pain. *Anesth Analg* 1988; 67:329.

20. Beasley SW, Tibballs J: Efficacy and safety of continuous morphine infusion for postoperative analgesia in the pediatric surgical ward. *Aust N Z J Surg* 1987; 57:233.

21. Bray RJ: postoperative analgesia provided by a morphine infusion in children. *Anaesthesia* 1983; 38:1075.

22. Lynn AM, Opheimke KE, Tyler DC: Morphine infusion after pediatric cardiac surgery. *Crit Care Med* 1984; 12:863.

23. Gaukroger PB, Tomkins DP, van der Walt JH: Patient-controlled analgesia in children. *Anaesth Intensive Care* 1989; 17:264.

24. White PF: Use of patient-controlled analgesia for management of acute pain. *JAMA* 1988; 259:243.

25. Owen H, Kluger MT, Plummer JL: Variables of patient-controlled analgesia. II. Concurrent infusion. *Anaesthesia* 1989; 44:11.

26. Sinatra R, Chung KS, Silverman DG, et al: An evaluation of morphine and oxymorphone administered via patient-controlled analgesia (PCA) or PCA plus basal infusion in postcesarean-delivery patients. *Anesthesiology* 1989; 71:502.

27. Berde C, et al: Patient-controlled analgesia in children and adolescents: A randomized prospective comparison with intramuscular administration of morphine for postoperative analgesia. *J Pediatr* 1991; 118:460.

28. Brandon Bravo LJC, et al: Comparative investigation into the effects on respiratory function of ketorolac and morphine. Presented at the International Symposium on Applied Physiology in Cardiorespiratory Emergencies, 1987, Rotterdam, The Netherlands.

29. Gillies GW, Kenny GN, Bullingham RE, et al: The morphine sparing effects of ketorolac tromethamine.

A study of a new, parenteral non-steroidal anti-inflammatory agent after abdominal surgery. *Anaesthesia* 1987; 42:727.

30. Olkkola KT, Maunuksela EL: The pharmacokinetics of postoperative intravenous ketorolac tromethamine in children. *Br J Clin Pharmacol* 1991; 31:182.

31. Wasylale T, Abbott F, Michael JM, et al: Reduction of postoperative morbidity following patient-controlled morphine. *Can J Anaesth* 1990; 37:726.

32. Yeager M, Glass DD, Neff R, et al: Epidural anesthesia and analgesia in high risk surgical patients. *Anesthesiology* 1987; 66:729.

70

Autologous Bone Marrow Harvesting

An 11-year-old, 38-kg girl with acute lymphoblastic leukemia (ALL) is scheduled for autologous bone marrow harvesting. She is currently in her second remission following chemotherapy. No suitable allogeneic bone marrow donor could be found. Hemoglobin, 11.5 g/dL; hematocrit, 34.5%. She is very apprehensive.

Recommendations by Susan G. Strauss, M.D., and Anne M. Lynn, M.D.

The childhood acute leukemias represent approximately 35% of all childhood malignancies. ALL accounts for about 80% of the acute leukemias in children and occurs most commonly between the ages of 1 and 10 years, with a peak incidence at 4 years.

ACUTE LYMPHOBLASTIC LEUKEMIA

A disease characterized by a predominance of immature lymphoid precursors, ALL is subclassified on the basis of cell morphology, surface phenotype, and karyotype of the malignant cells, as well as by the clinical presentation.[1] It is the most successfully treated leukemia. Treatment varies depending on the specific classification of the disease and the age of the patient. The likelihood of response and cure diminish with increasing age, although the age at which survival diminishes is ill-defined. The general strategy in attempting curative treatment of leukemia is to maximize the doses of cytotoxic agents to the limit of normal tissue tolerance. Therapy is generally divided into three phases: remission induction, central nervous system (CNS) prophylaxis, and treatment in remission. Complete remission is the absence of clinical signs and symptoms of disease and the presence of normal blood counts and a normocellular bone marrow with 5% or fewer blasts.

As a rule, the treatment of ALL uses combination chemotherapy for induction. The most effective combination has been vincristine and prednisone, which may induce complete remission in greater than 90% of pediatric patients with ALL. An additional agent(s) may be added, depending on the type of ALL and the risk group. When complete remission has been achieved, viable leukemic cells may still remain sequestered in virtually any organ, especially the brain, liver, and kidney. Therefore, the treatment strategy maintains cytoreductive therapy during complete remission. The CNS is the most common site of clinically apparent extramedullary leukemia. Because the incidence of CNS relapse increases with progressively longer periods of complete remission, therapy includes treatment of the CNS early in complete remission with intrathecal drugs such as methotrexate (MTX) or cytosine arabinoside (ARA-C), with or without cranial irradiation. Following cessation of therapy, the relapse rate ranges from 15% to 25%. Most relapses occur within the first year after treatment. Until recently, both hematologic and bone marrow relapse while under chemotherapy had a grim prognosis. Reinduction in this group of patients may require a three- or four-drug regimen, as well as high-dose intrathecal chemotherapy and craniospinal irradiation. Chemotherapy rarely produces long-term responses in patients who are in their second or subsequent remission. Bone marrow transplantation (BMT) has changed the outlook for these particular patients who are reinduced into complete remission.

BONE MARROW TRANSPLANTATION

BMT is playing an increasingly important role in the treatment of various hematologic malignancies. The use of marrow grafting in patients with leukemia permits the administration of drugs or radiation that are lethal to the host's hematopoietic system. Marrow transplantation from a major histocompatibility complex (MHC)-matched family member is the treatment of choice in ALL when a relapse has occurred during therapy.

ALL refractory to chemotherapy has been cured with both syngeneic (identical twin) and allogeneic BMT.[2] Despite very encouraging results when BMT is used to treat this disease, two major problems ensue: post-BMT relapse and life-threatening graft vs.host disease (GVHD). In attempts to overcome the problems of GVHD or in the absence of a suitable donor, autologous marrow transplantation (AMT) has offered hope of successfully treating leukemia where a second remission has been achieved.[3] The concept behind AMT includes removing the patient's own marrow during remission and storing it by using cryopreservation. The persistent leukemia is treated with ablative chemotherapy and occasionally radiation, and the patient is then rescued with infusion of her tumor-free marrow. If the stored marrow is contaminated with leukemic cells, the tumor cells may be eliminated by physical, immunologic, or other methods. AMT using marrow purged of leukemic cells by appropriate methods has been reported to be effective in patients with ALL in second or third remission.

THE TECHNIQUE OF BONE MARROW TRANSPLANTATION

Although there are no strict guidelines and standards for the techniques of marrow transplantation, most transplant physicians utilize similar methods for procuring and infusing the bone marrow.

The marrow aspirations take place in the sterile environment of the operating room. General anesthesia is utilized most often; however, regional techniques such as spinal, epidural, or caudal anesthesia have been used in adults. The donor is placed in the prone position, slightly flexed at the waist. Bone marrow is aspirated from the posterior iliac crests. It is not uncommon to also aspirate from the anterior iliac crests while the child is in the supine position if additional marrow is needed.[4] Some institutions give the patient 1,500 IU of heparin per square meter intravenously immediately preharvest. Single aspirates of 3 to 5 mL are collected repeatedly from multiple aspiration sites in children older than 5 years and approximately 2- to 3-ml aspirates in the children less than 5 years of age. The mean marrow harvest is 15 to 20 mL/kg. The marrow is then purged of leukemic cells if necessary, mixed with an anticoagulant, and cryopreserved. Intensive antitumor therapy is given once the patient has recovered from the anesthetic. If chemotherapy is given, very high doses of drugs that are quickly eliminated are administered. The marrow is returned via a central line following the elimination or inactivation of the drugs or, if radiotherapy is used, following cessation of treatment.

ANESTHETIC CONSIDERATIONS

There are several anesthetic considerations for patients who are in their second or subsequent leukemia remission. Treatment with various chemotherapeutic agents and radiation therapy may cause specific toxicities and sequelae that have an impact on preparation, intraoperative management, and postoperative patient care.[5] The anesthesiologist needs to know the side effects and interactions of the various chemotherapeutic agents because there is the potential for increased morbidity in patients who have received these drugs and undergo anesthesia for surgery (Table 70–1).

Doxorubicin (Adriamycin) and daunorubicin, highly toxic anthracycline antibiotics, may cause a severe dose-related and unpredictable cardiomyopathy. Acute myocardial injury from anthracycline administration can cause a sudden decrease in myocardial contractility. The myocardial damage can be mild, and possibly reversible, if contractile abnormalities are detected early and therapy with the drug is immediately discontinued. Severe injury may produce progressive, irreversible damage and death. Patients with anthracycline-induced cardiac dysfunction may develop congestive heart failure and have limited cardiac reserve. They tolerate neither intravascular volume shifts nor myocardial depressants well. Development of clinically apparent cardiomyopathy at doses less than 400 mg/m^2 is uncommon.[6] Perioperative cardiovascular complications are usually manifested as hypotension that cannot be explained by loss of circulating volume, surgical manipulation, or excessive concentrations of known myocardial depressants such as volatile anesthetic agents. Patient history, physical examination, and electrocardiography (ECG), combined with echocardiographic studies to evaluate the contractile state of the myocardium, have been used in an attempt to identify those patients at risk for perioperative cardiovascular complications. It has been found that the most reliable predictor of cardiovascular complications is a history of congestive heart failure.

Vincristine, a plant alkaloid, may cause neurotoxicity as evidenced by paresthesias, loss of deep tendon reflexes, ataxia, foot drop, and muscle wasting. The presence of a neuropathy may influence the anesthetic technique chosen, that is, general or regional anesthesia. In addition, preoperative documentation of any neuropathy is important should progressive changes or a new neuropathy occur postoperatively.

The use of high-dose steroids may cause suppression of the pituitary-adrenal axis. In conditions

TABLE 70–1.

Chemotherapeutic Agents Used in the Treatment of Acute Lymphoblastic Leukemia

Agent	End-Organ Toxicity	Physiologic Manifestations	Anesthetic Implications
Corticosteroid, e.g., prednisone	Pituitary-adrenal axis suppression Iatrogenic Cushing's syndrome	Hypertension, fluid retention, diabetes mellitus, obesity, inadequate endogenous glucocorticoid release during stress	Blood pressure monitoring, glucose monitoring, steroid coverage perioperatively
Vincristine	Neurotoxicity, myelosuppression	Foot drop, ataxia, paresthesias, constipation, IADH*, anemia/neutropenia/thrombocytopenia	Possibly avoid regional techniques, stool softeners if opiates given, strict attention to positioning and padding, check CBC*, platelet count
L-Asparaginase	Pancreatic/liver toxicity	Pancreatitis, diabetes mellitus, transaminase elevation, anaphylactic response	Glucose monitoring, possibly avoid halothane
Anthracycline antibiotics, e.g., doxarubicin (Adriamycin) daunorubicin	Cardiomyopathy, myelosuppression	Congestive heart failure, anemia/neutropenia/thrombocytopenia	Limited response to fluid loads, sensitivity to cardiac depressants, e.g., high-dose volatile agents, check CBC, platelet count
Methotrexate	Myelosuppression, liver toxicity, renal toxicity, gastrointestinal ulceration	Transaminase elevation, elevated BUN* and creatinine, stomatitis/esophagitis/enteritis	Possibly avoid halothane, avoid pancuronium/curare
6-Mercaptopurine	(See methotrexate entries above)		
ARA-C	Myelosuppression, cerebellar toxicity	Anemia/neutropenia/thrombocytopenia, ataxia	Check CBC, platelet count

*IADH = inappropriate antidiuretic hormone; CBC = complete blood count; BUN = blood urea nitrogen.

of excess glucocorticoids, the adrenal glands atrophy and cannot respond to stressful situations such as surgery by secreting more steroid. Clinically, very few patients who have suppressed adrenal function have cardiovascular problems such as labile blood pressure if they do not receive supplemental steroids perioperatively. However, there is little risk in administering supplemental glucocorticoids, and therefore, it is generally recommended.

Adequate venous access is another important consideration in this patient population. Inasmuch as up to one third of the child's circulating blood volume may be aspirated during a bone marrow harvest, rapid blood volume changes may occur. The medullary bone cavity from which the marrow is aspirated is a rich vascular network that is intimately connected to the peripheral circulation. The distribution of fluid and drugs injected via the intraosseous route is quite similar to that after intravenous injection.[7, 8] Conversely, aspiration of a large portion of an individual's marrow will be directly reflected as a loss of the circulating blood volume. Adequate venous access is necessary for rapid administration of fluids and/or blood in order to maintain hemodynamic stability.

In the early 1970s, the development of a Silastic right atrial catheter by Broviac and its subsequent modification by Hickman offered continuous circulatory access.[9] It is currently common practice to insert an indwelling central venous catheter soon after the diagnosis of leukemia in anticipation of the need for easy and frequent circulatory access for chemotherapy, antibiotics, blood components, and alimentation. Although most patients have central venous access, infection or malfunction may prevent its use or may have necessitated its removal.

Renal dysfunction from "tumor lysis syndrome" is a well-known complication of therapy. Leukemic cell lysis releases massive amounts of intracellular nucleic acids. Intrahepatic catabolism of the nucleic acids results in elevated serum levels and elevated urinary excretion of uric acid, which may precipitate in renal tubules and cause renal impairment. Adequate hydration and alkalinization of the urine with bicarbonate together with the administration of allopurinol prior to chemotherapy help to avert this complication. Should renal impairment ensue, it is usually short-lived; however, the presence of residual renal dysfunction should be ascertained before administering an anesthetic.

PREOPERATIVE EVALUATION AND PREMEDICATION

The preanesthetic visit will include a thorough medical evaluation and is also an opportunity to establish rapport and accomplish preoperative teaching. Evaluation of this child preoperatively should include a review of her chemotherapy protocol. The cumulative dose of Adriamycin or daunorobicin should be determined and an echocardiogram performed if her dose is ≥ 400 mg/m^2 or if a history and clinical symptoms of congestive heart failure are present. Corticosteroid therapy should be documented. Perioperative coverage is recommended if it has been 6 months or less since any steroid was taken.

The use of radiation therapy and the areas irradiated as well as the presence of CNS involvement should be noted. Evidence of any major reactions such as anaphylaxis to L-asparaginase or dystonic reactions from centrally acting antiemetics such as phenothiazines or metoclopramide should be sought. In addition, any major complications of therapy such as the occurrence of acute renal failure from tumor lysis syndrome and possible residual renal function compromise should be ascertained. Any hospitalizations not for chemotherapy such as pneumonia or sepsis, current medications, drug allergies, and past anesthetic experiences are evaluated.

Physical examination should be directed toward testing for neuropathy such as foot drop, weakness, or hypoesthesia and for cardiomyopathy. While hepatosplenomegaly may be seen initially with leukemia, at the time of harvesting bone marrow, the leukemia should be in remission and organomegaly not present. If craniospinal irradiation was part of the treatment protocol, evaluation should include assessment of temporomandibular and cervical spine mobility. Radiation fibrosis can cause progressive changes leading to limited mouth opening and difficulty with intubation if these areas were part of the radiation field.

Laboratory evaluation must include a platelet count and a white blood cell differential to assess myelosuppression from chemotherapy. Because marrow harvesting removes 25% to 35% of the effective blood volume, blood is typed and crossed-matched for the procedure. Cytomegalovirus

(CMV)-negative blood should be ordered. It has been shown that patients who are CMV-negative have a significantly lower rate of CMV infection when transfused with CMV-negative blood components. It is also necessary to irradiate all blood components prior to transfusion. Irradiation inactivates lymphocytes that could possibly contaminate the marrow inoculum being collected. Evaluation of electrolytes, blood urea nitrogen (BUN), and creatinine should be performed if a history of renal impairment is present. Serial liver enzyme studies should be available to assess the extent of any hepatic dysfunction from chemotherapy or progression of the leukemia. Chest radiograms and an echocardiogram should be ordered in consultation with the pediatric oncologist and cardiologist if the history or physical examination suggests congestive heart failure or pulmonary findings.

The preoperative visit is an important time for teaching. An explanation of what to expect upon arrival in the operating room, including a review of the monitoring equipment, may help to relieve the anxiety associated with fear of the unknown. She can be assured that there will be no surprises and every effort will be made to ensure her comfort both before and after surgery. If she dreads leaving her parents, she can be reassured that they can be with her until her intravenous catheter is in place or central venous catheter accessed and she is sleepy from titrated intravenous sedation. If establishing venous access is frightening and the facility allows, her parents can stay with her during an inhalation induction. If she dislikes the loss of control she feels after sedation, she can be reassured that sedation will not be used until anesthesia is induced at the start of surgery and that intravenous induction will facilitate a rapid onset of sleep. If she is worried because this procedure is necessary with its implication of mortality, then an oral premedication can be offered. Oral midazolam, 0.5 to 0.7 mg/kg of a 5-mg/mL solution up to 15 mg maximal dose in 10 mL of concentrated grape Kool-Aid, which masks the drug's bitter taste, is quite effective. The onset is 10 minutes, and the peak effect occurs in 30 minutes. If more profound sedation is indicated, pentobarbital, 4 mg/kg up to 200 mg, can be ordered.

ANESTHETIC MANAGEMENT

Unless the patient arrives in the operating room with intravenous access or catheter placement is anticipated to be easy, other techniques for induction of anesthesia should be considered. These include inhalation induction with a volatile anesthetic, usually halothane, or rectal administration of a short-acting barbiturate. Intramuscular administration of drugs such as a short-acting barbiturate or ketamine is performed very infrequently at our institution but may be considered if all other possibilities have been exhausted and thrombocytopenia is not present.

Endotracheal intubation is necessary for adequate airway protection and ventilation in the prone position. Muscle relaxation may facilitate intubation and positioning. Renal impairment may determine the muscle relaxant chosen. Muscle relaxation is not mandatory if the patient's cardiovascular reserve will tolerate potent inhalational agents, but assisted ventilation is advised while the patient is prone. Maintenance of anesthesia is generally accomplished with a balanced technique of volatile agent, oxygen with or without nitrous oxide, and a narcotic. It should be mentioned that prolonged use of nitrous oxide has been associated with bone marrow suppression.[10, 11] This has not been shown with short-term use. Morphine, meperidine, or fentanyl are the most commonly used opiates. Since marrow harvesting takes 1 to 2 hours and postoperative discomfort is mild, narcotics should be titrated carefully. In addition, it has been observed that patients who have had CNS relapse and received high-dose intrathecal chemotherapy tend to have prolonged awakening times. Extubation is generally performed when the patient is awake in the supine or lateral position; however, extubation under deep anesthesia is quite acceptable and may also be accomplished after reversal of neuromuscular blockade.

Although general anesthesia is utilized most often, especially in children, regional techniques, particularly caudal anesthesia, can be used. In contrast to regional anesthesia performed in adults, regional techniques in children are usually combined with a light general anesthetic. After induction, the caudal space can be accessed very easily while the child is in the lateral or prone position with the knees flexed. A total dose of approximately 0.5 to 0.75 mL/kg of 0.25% bupivacaine with 1:200,000 epinephrine may be injected after a negative test dose of 0.1 mL/kg. The block is usually established within 20 minutes; however, if a caudal epidural is combined with a general anesthetic, the anesthesiologist may use a volatile agent initially in order to facilitate surgery starting and titrate to a lower concentration as the block takes effect.

All techniques have advantages and disadvantages. Advantages of a regional technique include good postoperative analgesia, more rapid awakening, and less myocardial depression from lower concentrations of volatile agents. Relative contraindications may include preharvesting anticoagulation with heparin and the presence of a neuropathy.

Because the anatomic landmarks are so easily palpated, the caudal is generally the preferred route to the epidural space in children. That is not to say that an epidural is difficult, caudal anesthesia simply has a lower risk of inadvertent subarachnoid puncture and is more readily and easily performed in the majority of children.

The major challenge during maintenance of anesthesia for autologous bone marrow harvesting is to preserve hemodynamic stability. An estimate of the patient's blood volume and allowable blood loss facilitates the anesthesiologist's strategy in fluid and blood administration. Crystalloid is used initially to replace fluid deficits and blood loss and provide normal fluid maintenance. As the aspiration procedure progresses, careful monitoring of the vital signs and serial intraoperative hematocrits, either by venipuncture or capillary sample, serve as a guide for blood replacement.

The risks of transmitting disease and compromising immune defenses combine to make it desirable to avoid transfusion of homologous blood. The percentage of pediatric patients requiring transfusion for this procedure varies among institutions and ranges from 50% to 95% . Preoperative hypervolemic hemodilution has recently been described to reduce the need for homologous blood.[12] Ultimately, however, these patients will need blood and blood components during the support period following ablative therapy.

POSTOPERATIVE PAIN MANAGEMENT

Pain from donor sites is reported to be mild and can be controlled with acetaminophen, with or without codeine. If a single-dose caudal epidural was accomplished intraoperatively, postoperative analgesia should be present for 6 to 8 hours.[13] If a caudal was not used and if oral medications cannot be used, intravenous morphine as an infusion at 20 µg/kg/hr or patient-controlled analgesia (PCA) would be useful analgesic methods. The control in self-administering her own medication may make PCA especially attractive to this patient.

REFERENCES

1. Henderson ES, Lister TA: *Leukemia,* ed 5. Philadelphia, WB Saunders Co, 1990.
2. Kersey JH, Weisdorf D, Nesbit ME, et al: Comparisons of autologous and allogeneic bone marrow transplantation for treatment of high-risk refractory acute lymphoblastic leukemia. *N Engl J Med* 1987; 317:461.
3. Ramsay N, LeBien T, Nesbit M, et al: Autologous bone marrow transplantation for patients with acute lymphoblastic leukemia. *Blood* 1985; 66:508.
4. Johnson FL, Pochedly C (eds): *Bone Marrow Transplantation in Children,* ed 1. New York, Raven Press, 1990.
5. Selvin B: Cancer chemotherapy: Implications for the anesthesiologist. *Anesth Analg* 1981; 60:425–433.
6. Burrows F, Hickey P, Colan S: Perioperative complications in patients with anthracycline chemotherapeutic agents. *Can Anaesth Soc J* 1985; 32:149–157.
7. Spivey WH: Intraosseous infusions. *J Pediatr* 1987; 111:639–643.
8. Tocantins LM, O'Neil JF: Infusion of blood and other fluids into circulation via the bone marrow. *Proc Soc Exp Biol Med* 1940; 45:782–783.
9. Hickman RO, et al: A modified right atrial catheter for access to the venous system in marrow transplant recipients. *Surg Gynecol Obstet* 1979; 148:871–875.
10. Lassen HCA, et al: Treatment of tetanus. Severe bone-marrow depression after prolonged nitrous-oxide anesthesia. *Lancet* 1956; 1:527.
11. Skacel PO, Hewlett AM, Lewis JD, et al: Studies on the haemopoietic toxicity of nitrous oxide in man. *Br J Haematol* 1983; 53:189.
12. Perez de Sa V, et al: Hemodilution during bone marrow harvesting in children. *Anesth Analg* 1991; 72:645–650.
13. Krane EJ, Jacobson LE, Lynn AM, et al: Caudal morphine for post-operative analgesia in children: A comparison with caudal bupivicaine and intravenous morphine. *Anesth Analg* 1987; 66:647–652.

71

Mental Retardation and Dental Surgery

An obese (70 kg), 12-year-old severely retarded girl is scheduled for dental restoration on an outpatient basis. She is combative, and the nurse was unable to draw a blood sample for preoperative laboratory studies. She has no clearly defined syndrome or inborn error of metabolism.

Recommendations by George M. Hoffman, M.D.

The child with mental retardation (MR) often presents with multiple cognitive, motor, and sensory deficiencies and may have primary or secondary pathology in multiple organ systems. The unpredictable behavior of many children with MR poses the greatest challenge for the anesthesiologist.

MENTAL RETARDATION

MR encompasses disorders of the central nervous system (CNS) that result primarily in decreased cognitive function. Mild MR, defined as an IQ less than 70 or 2 SD below the mean, affects 3% of the general population.[1] These children overconsume medical and surgical services because of associated anomalies and behavioral problems that place them at higher risk for adverse health consequences. With an increasing life expectancy, even severely retarded individuals will present for multiple procedures from infancy to adulthood; thus in a busy pediatric hospital one will frequently encounter the mentally retarded patient in the day surgery area.

Many different etiologic classification systems have been proposed, and all suffer from inaccuracy and arbitrariness (Table 71–1). While environmental or polygenic factors are probably responsible for most mild MR, a specific pathophysiologic diagnosis can be made in approximately 50% of children with severe MR who have IQs less than 60. The most common genetic etiologies for severe

TABLE 71–1.

Classification of Mental Retardation by Etiology*

Etiology	Severity	Familial	Seizures	Behavior Disorder	Systemic Involvement	Examples
Genetic	Variable, severe, IQ < 50	Common	Common	Common	Common, primary and secondary	Trisomy 21; Fragile X syndrome; PKU†
Multifactorial	Moderate	Sometimes	Sometimes	Sometimes	Sometimes, usually secondary	Neural tube defect; Prader-Willi syndrome; microcephaly
Environmental	Variable, mild, IQ > 75	No	Sometimes	No	Less likely	Intrauterine infection; intracranial hemorrhage; cranial trauma

*Adapted from Accardo PJ, Capute AJ: Mental retardation, in Oski FA, DeAngelis CD, Feigin RD, et al (eds): *Principles and Practice of Pediatrics.* Philadelphia, JB Lippincott, 1990.
†PKU = phenylketonuria

MR include Down syndrome, or trisomy 21, and fragile X syndrome, the latter contributing to the 50% greater incidence of severe MR in males.

Mild MR is more likely to reflect mild CNS impairment resulting from intrauterine or perinatal insults or genetic variability. Associated organ involvement is unlikely, and minimal or no preoperative laboratory testing is appropriate.[2] Conversely, severe MR more likely reflects the presence of a biochemical abnormality resulting from a single genetic or chromosomal abnormality in which associated organ system dysfunction and severe behavioral disturbance are more common. With increasing multiorgan pathology, the appropriate medical workup might be more involved.

PREOPERATIVE ASSESSMENT

Preoperative evaluation of the child with MR should be directed toward answering two questions: what is the specific diagnosis, and what is the functional level of the child? Knowledge of the specific diagnosis will clarify the involvement of other organ systems; understanding the functional level will aid in planning an induction that is least likely to be traumatic to the patient or physician.

The anesthesiologist should have an understanding of the patient's behavioral repertoire both at baseline and in response to prior medical interventions. Recent changes in behavior might suggest an intercurrent infection, changes in drug levels, or perhaps a complication of head trauma that may be occult in the patient unable to verbalize specific complaints. The possibility of pregnancy should be seriously considered in the postmenarchal female since the incidence of sexual abuse is probably higher in the mentally incapacitated individual.

Other specific areas of questioning relate to associated disease in the more severely affected individual. The frequency and type of seizures should be noted, with predisposing events sought. Many patients have an increase in seizure frequency with minor upper respiratory infections (URIs). Because of discoordination of upper airway and pharyngeal musculature due to underlying disease or sedative medication, recurrent aspiration of oral secretions is not uncommon and results in chronic reactive airway disease.

THE INSTITUTIONALIZED CHILD

The medical history of an institutionalized child may be both more complicated and less accessible, given the lack of a consistent informant. Obtaining important historical data can require days of planning prior to the actual preoperative assessment. A phone call to the institution prior to the patient's visit to the hospital will facilitate access to these records. At this time, the anesthesiologist should request that the patient's favorite care giver accompany her to the hospital. It is helpful to plan for this individual to be present both during induction and recovery for the most difficult patient.

PREOPERATIVE ORDERS

Generally, medications previously prescribed should be continued preoperatively, including the morning of surgery, with minor alterations in eating and drinking guidelines if necessary. CNS stimulants such as methylphenidate (Ritalin) or amphetamines prescribed to control distractable behavior may dramatically increase anesthetic requirements. Anticonvulsants such as phenytoin and phenobarbital induce hepatic microsomal enzyme systems, thereby increasing the clearance of drugs with low hepatic extraction ratios such as thiopental. They also have pharmacodynamic effects that increase the apparent anesthetic requirement by induction of both acute and chronic tolerance. Other anticonvulsants such as carbamazepine (Tegretol) may cause chronic hepatocellular enzyme elevations that are of unclear significance. The purpose of continuing these medications preoperatively is to maintain therapeutic drug levels into the postoperative period when oral intake of medications might be impaired.

Plans for preoperative fluids should be explicitly communicated. Recent work in healthy children strongly suggests that intake of clear fluids 2 to 4 hours preoperatively does not increase and may decrease the number of patients at risk for acid aspiration syndrome while decreasing the severity and incidence of preoperative irritability.[3] The psychological benefits of allowing fluid intake in the retarded child with disturbed behavior must be seriously considered.

Premedication should be directed toward facilitating a nontraumatic anesthetic induction. Careful review of prior responses to premedication can be helpful in selecting the child in whom disinhibition might be a problem; "paradoxical" reactions to "cough" medicine and antihistamines can be a clue. In such a child, the use of a sedative-hypnotic premedication such as a barbiturate can cause increased behavioral disorder until the patient actually falls asleep. While an anxiolytic drug such as midazolam can be helpful in the frightened patient[4] disinhibition can certainly occur with the benzodiazepines. Accordingly, a higher dose, 0.5 mg/kg to a maximum of 10 mg of midazolam, should be administered orally. The use of ketamine for premedication has a long track record of success,[5] with excellent akinetic properties and a unique ability to maintain functional residual capacity and upper airway tone.[6] Its efficacy when given orally has recently been documented as an adjunct to permit outpatient gynecologic examination[4] and to facilitate induction[7] in the uncooperative adult with MR.

If induction via the intravenous route is eventually anticipated, as I would recommend, application of a local anesthetic cream at the time of premedication will allow sufficient time for the onset of analgesia.[8] Whatever the initial premedication plan, a "backup" plan is necessary. The efficacy of ketamine, 4 mg/kg, with or without midazolam, 0.1 mg/kg, administered intramuscularly is superb when nothing else has worked.

INDUCTION AND MAINTENANCE OF ANESTHESIA

If loss of consciousness has not occurred by preinduction, then the presence in the operating room of the favored care giver is invaluable in facilitating mask or intravenous induction.[9] Monitoring during induction can be minimized to a precordial stethoscope and pulse oximeter if the patient is tenuously cooperative.[10] The individual patient's ability to cooperate with an inhalation induction or even mask application for denitrogenation must be thoughtfully anticipated. The strong, poorly controllable older child or adult will be even less controllable during the excitement phase. For relatively fast, stable induction by mask, the author recommends halothane over isoflurane even in postadolescent patients.[11] While the fast recovery characteristics of propofol are ideal for day surgery cases,[12] one must be prepared to deal with pain on injection without sacrificing the intravenous catheter or the patient's dignity. I prefer the predictability of an intravenous induction with thiopental.

After the patient has lost consciousness, anesthesia can be deepened with a potent vapor to permit tracheal intubation. Only the most brief dental procedures would justify the continued maintenance of an unprotected airway. For postadolescents and patients receiving potential hepatotoxic medications or anticonvulsants, the use of isoflurane should be considered. Muscle relaxation may be used at the anesthesiologist's discretion.

The decision to use an oral or nasal endotracheal tube should be discussed with the surgeon. Nasal tubes are more likely to produce bacteremia but may be more stable. Because of the increased size and friability of lymphatic tissue in children, bleeding from the adenoidal bed can be a significant problem with nasotracheal intubation. The amount of trauma to the posterior portion of the nasopharynx can be reduced by passing the endotracheal tube over a fiber-optic bronchoscope inserted through the nasopharynx under direct vision or over a flexible suction catheter used to gently negotiate the passage beyond the turbinates and around the velopalatine angle. Attempts at "blind" nasal intubation in children more frequently result in bleeding and soft-tissue injury than in expeditious tracheal intubation. The anesthesiologist must carefully secure the endotracheal tube, the 15-mm adapter, and the breathing circuit to prevent disconnection as the table is turned.

A relatively low inspired anesthetic concentration can be maintained if adequate regional anesthesia is employed by the surgeon. However, prolonged postoperative nerve blockade may increase the incidence of self-induced oral and lingual trauma in this patient population and thus may be best avoided. Combinations of nitrous oxide, volatile agents, barbiturate or propofol infusions, and muscle relaxants all have appropriate use if the goal is rapid recovery. Intravenous fluids should be administered with the expectation that no further oral intake will be possible during the day of surgery. To obviate the need for oral postoperative medications such as anticonvulsants, consideration should be given to administering a parenteral dose intraoperatively. If no regional anesthetic is used, analgesia with ketorolac or very low-dose narcotic may be helpful to provide postoperative comfort without respiratory depression or further disinhibition.

Tracheal extubation is usually accomplished after the stomach is suctioned and confirmation that all surgical packs have been removed from the oropharynx. The anesthesiologist should anticipate a potentially stormy emergence due to disinhibition and be prepared to stay with the patient in the early recovery period.

POSTOPERATIVE CARE

Early introduction of a familiar care giver is recommended over pharmacologic measures to control postemergence excitement. If the patient is uncontrollable in the presence of the care giver, the anesthesiologist should consider the administration of additional analgesia.

REFERENCES

1. Accardo PJ, Capute AJ: Mental retardation, in Oski FA, DeAngelis CD, Feigin RD, et al (eds): *Principles and Practice of Pediatrics*. Philadelphia, JB Lippincott, 1990.
2. O'Connor ME, Drasner K: Preoperative laboratory testing of children undergoing elective surgery. *Anesth Analg* 1990; 70:176–180.
3. Schreiner MS, Triebwasser A, Keon TP: Ingestion of liquids compared with preoperative fasting in pediatric outpatients. *Anesthesiology* 1990; 72:593–597.
4. Amaranath L, et al: Outpatient sedation: An essential addition to gynecologic care for persons with mental retardation. *Am J Obstet Gynecol* 1991; 164:825–828.
5. Bach V, et al: Ketamine: An update on the first twenty-five years of clinical experience. *Can J Anaesth* 1989; 36:186–197.
6. Malaquin JM: The effect of ketamine on the functional residual capacity in young children. *Anesthesiology* 1985; 62:551–556.
7. Goldstein IC, Dragon AI: Oral ketamine facilitates induction in a combative mentally retarded patient. *J Clin Anesth* 1990; 2:121–122.
8. Cooper CM, Gerrish SP, Hardwick M, et al: EMLA cream reduces the pain of venepuncture in children. *Eur J Anaesth* 1987; 4:441–448.
9. Hannallah RS, Rosales JK: Experience with parents' presence during anaesthesia induction in children. *Can Anaesth Soc J* 1983; 30:286–289.
10. Coté CJ, Goldstein EA, Coté MA, et al: A single-blind study of pulse oximetry in children. *Anesthesiology* 1988; 68:184–188.
11. Larsson LE, et al: Halothane, enflurane and isoflurane anaesthesia for adenoidectomy in children, using two different premedications. *Acta Anaesthesiol Scand* 1987; 31:233–238.
12. Morton NS, Wee M, Christie G, et al: Propofol for induction of anaesthesia in children. A comparison with thiopentone and halothane inhalational induction. *Anaesthesia* 1988; 43:350–355.

72

Hemophilia and Fracture

A 12-year-old boy sustained a compound fracture of the tibia when he fell from a minibike. Despite a compression dressing, the wound is bleeding briskly. His past history is significant in that he is a known hemophiliac and human immuno-deficiency virus (HIV)-positive. The hematocrit is 32%; no other laboratory data are available. The orthopedist indicates that debridement and closed reduction should be accomplished as soon as possible.

Recommendations by Robert C. Pascucci, M.D.

Patients with *classic hemophilia* (hemophilia A, factor VIII deficiency), *factor IX deficiency* (Christmas disease, hemophilia B), and *von Willebrand disease* (von Willebrand Factor [vWF] deficiency) present similar problems to the clinician during episodes of acute bleeding or surgery. This discussion will be limited to the child with specific factor VIII deficiency, with some reference to the other disease processes when appropriate. The specific diagnosis for an individual patient must, of course, be established by history or laboratory testing to ensure optimal management.

HEMOPHILIA A

Classic hemophilia is inherited as an X-linked recessive disorder.[1] The plasma of these patients may contain normal levels of factor VIII antigen (VIII:Ag), but it is deficient in factor VIII activity (VIII:C). Expressed as a fraction of normal adult activity (100% factor VIII:C = 1 unit/mL plasma), the deficiency of factor VIII:C may be severe (less than 1%), moderate (1% to 5%), or mild (5% to 50%). The majority of affected individuals have severe disease. Spontaneous bleeding is uncommon in the milder forms and in the first year of life, but both spontaneous and trauma-induced bleeding, particularly recurrent hemarthroses, become a fact of life for these children as they grow and become ambulatory. Trauma with hemorrhage and impending surgery demands temporary correction of the coagulopathy, usually by administration of the deficient factor.

PREOPERATIVE MANAGEMENT

In addition to the routine preoperative evaluation, an accurate assessment of the severity of this patient's disease and his usual therapeutic requirements must be made. The child and his family are often involved in a home treatment program and have in-depth knowledge of the disease and its management. They may well be able to provide all needed information regarding the child's usual factor VIII level, the amount of factor VIII typically required for hemostasis, and the best sites for intravenous access.

Laboratory testing will demonstrate a prolonged partial thromboplastin time (PTT), indicating a factor VIII:C level less than 40% of normal. Specific assay of the factor VIII:C level, if available, will provide more precise information. The prothrombin time (PT), platelet count, and fibrinogen should be normal. If they are not, factors other than the hemophilia may be at play. Factor VIII inhibitors, circulating IgG antibodies directed against the factor VIII molecule, are seen in approximately 10% of hemophiliacs at some time. Their presence can be anticipated by a careful review of the patient's history. If time permits, an assay for inhibitor activity can be performed.

The standard treatment of classic hemophilia in the perioperative period has been and still is the administration of adequate quantities of factor VIII to ensure at least 50% activity, 0.5 units/mL, in the plasma at all times.[2] As evidenced by this unfortunate case, however, the necessity for repeated infusions of factor VIII, typically obtained from concentrates prepared from multiple donors, has led to HIV infection in as many as 90% of patients with severe hemophilia.[3, 4] Although progression to frank acquired immunodeficiency syndrome (AIDS) seems to be more delayed in children than adults, there is little doubt that AIDS will eventually develop in the majority of patients who required transfusion therapy in the early 1980s, the peak infectious period.[4-7]

Several modifications in the preparation of factor concentrates have been introduced to significantly increase their safety. Heat treatment of the products together with more rigorous screening of donors has reduced or eliminated the risk of HIV transmission. Pasteurization or solvent-detergent treatment of the concentrates adds additional safety by elimination of hepatitis viruses as well as HIV.[6] An even more purified product containing little else than the factor VIII protein itself may be obtained by treating concentrate with a monoclonal antibody to factor VIII (Monoclate; Hemofil).[8, 9] These latter products are so purified as to be useful only for classic hemophilia because they lack vWF and so are not effective for the treatment of patients with von Willebrand disease. Finally, recombinant factor VIII has been developed and appears to be as effective as conventional plasma-derived factor VIII.[10] This recombinant product, soon to be commercially available, will likely become the new standard of factor replacement therapy for this disease.

Another therapeutic option is available for patients with von Willebrand disease and to those with the mild form of classic hemophilia: pretreatment with desmopressin (DDAVP).[11] Administration of 0.3 to 0.4 μg/kg DDAVP, either intravenously or subcutaneously, has been shown to produce threefold rises in factor VIII:C levels within 60 to 75 minutes in many patients. The response of an individual patient or kindred is usually consistent and reproducible.[12, 13] The drug is sometimes administered in combination with an antifibrinolytic, especially for operations in the oral cavity, because desmopressin is a known activator of plasminogen.[14] If the desired result is obtained, drug administration may be repeated at 24-hour intervals.

The initial dose of factor VIII is calculated to raise the factor VIII:C concentration to 100%. Subsequent doses are given every 8 to 12 hours to prevent the level from falling below 50%; a normal PTT is assurance that this goal has been achieved. A number of formulas are in use to calculate the dose of factor VIII. One easily remembered version is that 1 unit of factor VIII per kilogram will raise the plasma level by 2% (0.02 units/mL). As an example, if this child weighs 40 kg and has a usual factor VIII level of 2%, he would receive an initial dose of 1,960 units and then half that amount every 8 to 12 hours:

$$\text{Wt (kg)} \times \frac{\text{Desired change in level}}{2} = \text{No. units}$$

$$40 \times \frac{98}{2} = 1,960$$

Factor IX replacement for patients with Christmas disease proceeds in a manner analogous to that for classic factor VIII deficiency. Factor IX may be obtained from fresh or frozen plasma or from commercial factor IX concentrates. As with the factor VIII preparations, these concentrates have undergone significant refinements in recent years with the development of techniques for heat treatment, solvent-detergent treatment, or immunopurification that have led to concentrates essentially free from infectious and thrombotic risk.[15, 16] The level of factor IX needed to provide hemostasis is lower than that of factor VIII in hemophilia A, 30% rather than 50%, and the biologic half-life is sufficiently long to allow administration every 24 hours. One unit of factor IX per kilogram will increase the plasma level by 1% to 1.5%.

The factor product chosen should be administered intravenously shortly before induction of anesthesia. In trauma patients such as this boy, complete assessment to ascertain other injuries, particularly intra-abdominal and intracranial hemorrhage, is necessary. Blood samples for type and crossmatch and other laboratory tests are sent, sufficient analgesia to allow patient comfort during the move is provided, and the child is transferred to the operating room for surgery.

INTRAOPERATIVE MANAGEMENT

Adequate restoration of intravascular volume must be ensured prior to induction of anesthesia. Regional, spinal, and epidural anesthesia are not advisable in this patient because of the risk of hematoma formation with potential nerve compression. Assuming normal airway anatomy, a rapid-sequence induction technique using cricoid pressure to avoid regurgitation is appropriate. Care should be taken to minimize trauma to the airway. A cuffed endotracheal tube of proper size should be placed orally; nasal intubation is relatively contraindicated because of the risk of epistaxis. Tracheal bleeding may be a problem despite gentle handling. Should significant bleeding occur, irrigation of the tube with half-strength bicarbonate solution will lyse red cells and help avoid airway obstruction by clotted blood.

No unusual intraoperative monitoring is required. Universal precautions with special care to ensure hand, skin, and eye protection should adequately shield the anesthesiologist from the risk of HIV infection. The choice of anesthetic agents is determined by the anesthesiologist's preference and the hemodynamic state of the patient. Intravenous access must be sufficient to allow large-volume replacement. A tourniquet applied above the operative site will help minimize blood loss. Unusual bleeding despite adequate factor VIII replacement should prompt further investigation of the coagulation system to ascertain other deficits or to determine the presence of factor VIII inhibitors.

Significant postoperative pain may be anticipated, and plans should be made for its relief even as the anesthetic is begun. A narcotic-based technique with postoperative patient-controlled analgesia (PCA), narcotic infusion, intermittent doses of a long-acting agent such as methadone, or other techniques for ensuring adequate analgesia is recommended.

POSTOPERATIVE MANAGEMENT

Before the patient is extubated, airway protective reflexes should be present and significant airway bleeding controlled. Undue coughing and bucking stimulated by the endotracheal tube may induce such bleeding, and can be diminished by judicious use of narcotics and intravenous lidocaine. The pulse in the operated extremity should be palpated distally to ensure adequate flow.

Continued administration of factor VIII during the postoperative period is recommended, with the goal of maintaining a factor VIII:C level of 50% for 7 to 10 days. One half the initial dose every 8 to 12 hours will usually accomplish this goal. Some hematologists feel that a slow, continuous infusion of factor accomplishes this goal more consistently.[17]

REFERENCES

1. Dallman PR: Blood and blood-forming tissues: Disorders of coagulation, in Rudolph AM, Hoffman JIE, Rudolph CD, et al (eds): *Rudolph's Pediatrics,* ed 19. E Norwalk, Conn, Appleton & Lange, 1991, pp 1162–1165.
2. Madhok R, Forbes CD: HIV-1 infection in haemophilia. *Baillieres Clin Haematol* 1990; 3:79.
3. Gjerset GF, et al: Treatment type and amount influenced by human immunodeficiency virus seroprevalence of patients with congenital bleeding disorders. *Blood* 1991; 78:1623.
4. Roberts HR: The treatment of hemophilia: Past tragedy and future promise. *N Engl J Med* 1989; 321:1188.
5. Becherer PR, Smiley ML, Matthews TJ, et al: Human immunodeficiency virus-1 disease progression in hemophiliacs. *Am J Hematol* 1990; 34:204.
6. Stockman JA III: Transfusion medicine: The problem of HIV infection. *Curr Probl Pediatr* 1991; 21:41.
7. Ujhelyi E, et al: Age dependency of the progression of HIV disease in haemophiliacs; predictive value of T cell subset and neopterin measurements. *Immunol Lett* 1990; 26:67.
8. Lusher JM, Salzman PM: Viral safety and inhibitor development associated with factor VIIIC ultra-purified from plasma in hemophiliacs previously unexposed to factor VIIIC concentrates. The Monoclate Study Group. *Semin Hematol* 1990; 27(suppl 2):1.
9. Smith KJ, et al: Initial clinical experience with a new pasteurized monclonal antibody purified factor VIIIC. *Semin Hematol* 1990; 27(suppl 2):25.
10. Schwartz RS, et al: Human recombinant DNA-derived antihemophiliac factor (factor VIII) in the treatment of hemophilia A. Recombinant Factor VIII Study Group. *N Engl J Med* 1990; 323:1800.
11. Mannucci PM: Desmopressin (DDAVP) for treatment of disorders of hemostasis. *Prog Hemost Thromb* 1986; 8:19.
12. Mannucci PM, Vicente V, Alberca I, et al: Intravenous and subcutaneous administration of desmopressin (DDAVP) to hemophiliacs: Pharmacokinetics and factor VIII responses. *Thromb Haemost* 1987; 58:1037.

Hemophilia and Fracture

491

13. Rodeghiero F, Costaman G, DiBone E, et al: Consistency of responses to repeated DDAVP infusions in patients with von Willebrand's disease and hemophilia A. *Blood* 1989; 74:1997.
14. Aledort LM: Treatment of von Willebrand's disease. *Mayo Clin Proc* 1991; 66:841.
15. Michalski C, Bal F, Burnoff T, et al: Large-scale production and properties of a solvent-detergent–treated factor IX concentrate from human plasma. *Vox Sang* 1988; 55:202.
16. Smith KJ: Immunoaffinity purification of factor IX from commercial concentrates and infusion studies in animals. *Blood* 1988; 72:1269.
17. Bona RD, Weinstein RA, Weisman SJ, et al: The use of continuous infusion of factor concentrates in the treatment of hemophilia. *Am J Hematol* 1989; 32:8.

73

Rheumatoid Arthritis and Cervical Laminectomy

A 13-year-old girl with rheumatoid arthritis is scheduled for cervical laminectomy and fusion. Jaw mobility is limited, and when she attempts to extend her neck, she loses sensation in her right arm. She has had no previous surgery. Current medications are prednisone and aspirin. Hemoglobin, 9 g/dL; hematocrit, 27%.

Recommendations by Michael Smith, M.D.

Few patients raise the level of concern among anesthesiologists more than those who have airways potentially difficult to manage and to intubate. When airway problems are combined with a multisystem disease such as juvenile rheumatoid arthritis (JRA) complicated by symptoms of cervical nerve entrapment, the concerns are compounded. An understanding of the other manifestations of JRA, careful preoperative assessment and preparation, and fastidious technique in the operating room are essential in providing a safe and comfortable anesthetic and surgical experience for the patient.

JUVENILE RHEUMATOID ARTHRITIS

Children with JRA have a chronic, relapsing, and extremely variable systemic disease characterized by synovitis as well as associated extra-articular manifestations. The arthropathy is often mild, but in approximately 25% of patients it progresses to destruction of joint cartilage and erosion of contiguous bone, which leads to joint subluxation, ankylosis, and deformity seen in adults.[1] The presentation of JRA in children falls into one of three broad clinical classifications. Fifty percent of patients develop pauciarticular disease affecting fewer than five major joints. However, a serious complication of this form of JRA is chronic uveitis. Only rarely are the temporomandibular joints (TMJ) and cervical spine involved; therefore, there are few specific anesthetic considerations.

The other two types of JRA are polyarticular-onset disease, which accounts for 40% of patients, and systemic-onset disease, seen in 10% to 15%. In these groups, five or more major joints are involved, including the axial skeleton, and there are varying degrees of involvement of other systems. In systemic-onset disease, the extra-articular manifestations can be severe in acute stages of the disease and may even precede the arthropathy by months or years.[1] The joint involvement in this group follows the pattern of polyarticular-onset disease. It is most likely that this patient has presented with one of the latter forms of JRA, and certain features of the disease deserve more attention.

The large joints, namely, the knees, ankles, wrists, elbows, and then fingers are involved first. The joints may be warm, tender, swollen with effusions, and stiff. Cervical spine arthritis develops in 60% to 70% of patients. It is complicated quite early by apophyseal ankylosis and by fusion of vertebrae, usually C2 and C3, but more levels may be involved to create a fusion-en-bloc.[1, 2] Restricted neck movement, flexion deformities, loss of extension, and torticollis are common features. Atlantoaxial subluxation is a frequent radiologic finding, but neurologic symptoms, as in this patient, are extremely rare.[1-3]

TMJ involvement occurs in 65% of patients. It usually presents as an earache and may significantly limit mouth opening.[4] Five percent of patients have severe secondary mandibular hypoplasia and retrognathia. Cricoarytenoiditis is uncommon in children but is manifested by local pain, hoarseness, and stridor and may lead to airway obstruction.[5, 6]

During periods of acute exacerbation, the extra-articular manifestations of systemic-onset disease include a high spiking fever and the classic macular rash of JRA. Generalized lymphadenopathy, impressive hepatosplenomegaly, and abdominal pain may also occur. Cardiac involvement, recognized in 5% to 10% of cases, is usually limited to pericarditis with minor effusions, although acute tamponade and acute aortic insufficiency are described.[1, 7] A transient pneumonitis and minor pleural effusions are not uncommon, but interstitial pulmonary fibrosis is rare in children. Periodic proteinuria is seen, but significant renal dysfunction is a late and unusual complication. Chronic anemia is common in these patients and may become more profound in acute stages of the disease. Children often develop a patchy vasculitis and involvement of the central and peripheral nervous systems to varying degrees.

The course of the disease is one of remissions and exacerbations over several years. Chronic destructive joint complications develop in 25% of patients. The principles of management are to preserve joint function and control symptoms with as conservative a program as possible.

PREOPERATIVE EVALUATION

The complications and treatment of the arthritis in this patient require that she be seen in consultation sufficiently in advance of surgery to allow adequate evaluation, preoperative preparation, and instruction in the planned anesthetic management. It is most likely that fiber-optic nasotracheal intubation will be undertaken.

With respect to her airway, the active mobility of her neck must be assessed. A neutral, symptom-free position should be identified and a rigid, custom-molded neck brace or collar of thermoplastic be made to wear to the operating room (Fig 73–1). The relative size of her mandible, her mouth opening, which will be further restricted by the neck brace, the prominence and condition of her teeth, and the patency of her nasal airway must be evaluated. A history of trauma to her nose and any episodes of epistaxis may be informative. In the presence of a sore throat, hoarseness, or stridor, a preoperative indirect laryngoscopy should be performed to identify active cricoarytenoiditis or glottic narrowing. Flexion and extension cervical x-ray films should be obtained and reviewed to evaluate C1–2 subluxation.

Active pulmonary and cardiac disease should be diagnosed clinically and by review of a chest x-ray, electrocardiogram (ECG), or echocardiogram if a pericardial effusion is suspected. Pulmonary function tests may be indicated. If a murmur is heard, a cardiologist's opinion must be sought. In the presence of hepatomegaly or symptoms of a bleeding diathesis, liver function and coagulation tests should be performed. She is anemic at 9 g/dL, but this is quite consistent with her chronic disease.[1] Although her oxygen-carrying capacity is reduced, no further active preoperative intervention is required in the absence of significant pulmonary or cardiac disease.

Her current medications, aspirin and prednisone, require comment. Aspirin induces a relative coagulopathy by irreversibly causing platelet dysfunction through its interference with the cyclooxygenase enzyme pathway. In higher doses, salicylates also interfere with the vitamin K–dependent function of factor VII.[1, 8, 9] Hence, both bleeding time and the prothrombin time may be prolonged, and surgical blood loss is likely to be higher than usual. For minor procedures, this is not a problem. This patient, however, may require an iliac bone graft for her fusion, and it would be advisable to discontinue the aspirin therapy 10 days to 2 weeks prior to surgery and substitute acetaminophen for pain control.[1] Regardless, adequate blood components must be available for the procedure.

Corticosteroids are the most potent anti-inflammatory agents for treatment of the rheumatic dis-

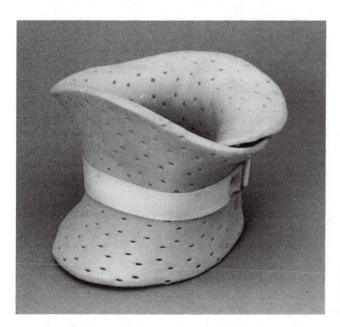

FIG 73–1.
Photograph of rigid, custom-molded thermroplastic collar recommended for this patient.

eases, but they are also associated with many complications. Cushingoid features, growth retardation, protein wasting, osteoporosis, fluid retention, hypertension, gastrointestinal irritation, carbohydrate intolerance, and myopathy are some of the more important. This patient's maintenance prednisone will have suppressed the hypophyseal-pituitary-adrenal axis, and supplemental steroids will be necessary to meet the stress response of the perioperative period.[1, 7] In recent years, lower-dose schedules of steroid replacement have been used to adequately prevent acute adrenal insufficiency and have provided more physiologic serum cortisol levels.[10–13] Current recommendations are that 50 mg/m^2 hydrocortisone hemisuccinate be administered intravenously 1 hour preoperatively and subsequently 25 mg/m^2 intravenously every 6 hours. Depending on the duration and extent of surgery, the supplemental steroids can be tapered to her oral maintenance dose after 48 to 72 hours. During this time, full fluid replacement and electrolyte balance must be maintained.

The patient's mood and level of cooperation should be assessed preoperatively. Most likely, the anesthetic plan will be to gain control of her airway by awake fiber-optic or blind nasal intubation, and she must be assured that she will be sedated and comfortable and instructed that this management is the safest approach. It may be apparent at this time that some preoperative sedation such as oral midazolam, 0.5 mg/kg, would be appropriate.

ANESTHETIC MANAGEMENT

An early morning operating time should be requested. Further preparation for surgery includes placement of an intravenous catheter the evening prior to the procedure to ensure adequate hydration. The patient should fast after midnight and receive oral cimetidine or ranitidine the evening before and on the morning of surgery. The morning dose should be accompanied by intravenous metoclopramide to ensure low gastric volume and acidity.[14] The supplemental steroids should be administered as recommended above and premedication given if necessary. The neck brace must be applied before she leaves the ward.

Several anesthetic strategies have been described for these patients.[15–17] In one series, a technique for posterior cervical fusion under local anesthesia is described. This approach is generally inappropriate in children.[18] Ketamine monoanesthesia and general anesthesia using the laryngeal mask airway have been used in patients with JRA, but there is no guarantee of airway control in the prone position, and these techniques are relatively contraindicated here.[19, 20] Although blind nasotracheal intubation under sedation or general anesthesia and intubation over a wire passed retrograde from the cricothyroid membrane have been traditional approaches, for the experienced anesthesiologist fiber-optic nasotracheal intubation is now the best available management. All efforts should be made to provide a supraglottic airway because tracheostomy is a high-risk procedure in this patient and in the prone position a relatively insecure method of airway control.

Details of technique and schedules for sedation for fiber-optic bronchoscopy and intubation are well reported in the literature,[7, 21–27] but several points are worth stressing. The operating room must be quiet for the patient's arrival and full noninvasive monitoring applied early. An arterial catheter should be necessary only in the presence of significant cardiac or pulmonary disease. Somatosensory evoked potentials (SSEP), despite the frequency of false-positive and -negative readings, may be a very useful monitor of cervical spinal cord function.[28] The neck collar must remain in place for the duration of airway instrumentation and positioning.

Intravenous atropine or glycopyrrolate should be administered early to dry secretions and to protect against vagal reflexes. Sedation is begun with incremental doses of intravenous midazolam, 0.05 mg/kg, and fentanyl, 0.5 µg/kg, or morphine, 0.05 mg/kg.

Effective topical anesthesia is critical to success of the procedure. Topical anesthesia of the nasal airway is accomplished first with 4% cocaine, 2 mg/kg, and anesthesia of the pharynx induced by gargling 4% lidocaine, 2 mg/kg. Sedation may be titrated further to allow introduction of the 3.5-mm endoscope. Airway obstruction, should it occur, may be treated by a nasopharyngeal airway, retraction of the tongue, or reversal of the sedation. The endoscope is introduced first by itself and slowly advanced until the glottis is seen. Additional topical anesthesia to the larynx and trachea is administered via the working channel with 2% lidocaine, up to 5 mg/kg. Once the trachea is entered, a smaller-than-usual, lubricated endotracheal tube is advanced over the endoscope with the bevel turned posteriorly and positioned above the carina. A 6.0-mm cuffed tube would be chosen for this patient.

With the airway secured, additional intravenous or inhalation agents can be administered to deepen the anesthesia sufficiently to prevent coughing but allow the patient to breathe spontaneously until she is positioned for surgery. The patient should be "log-rolled" into the prone position with specific personnel assigned to support the head and neck, still splinted by the collar. When the head is placed in the neutral position on a Mayfield headrest, the collar can be removed and fine adjustments to her position made. Bolsters must be placed under her hips and shoulders to free her abdomen. All pressure points and active joints must be protected and positioned carefully. Because her arms will be placed at her sides, intravenous access must be confirmed to be adequate and secure.

From this point almost any anesthetic technique can be used, but there may be an advantage to retaining spontaneous ventilation as a monitor of spinal cord function. Prompt replacement of significant blood and fluid losses must be undertaken. Patients with pulmonary disease or abdominal visceromegaly may require assisted or controlled ventilation. If the patient has a reduced cardiac reserve, agents impairing myocardial contractility will be tolerated poorly.

After the completion of surgery, spontaneous ventilation should be restored, and cautious intravenous sedation with narcotics or lidocaine can be administered to prevent coughing. Once the neck collar has been reapplied, the patient can be carefully moved to her bed. Her level of anesthesia should now be allowed to lighten in the operating room or the recovery unit, and she must be sufficiently awake to protect her airway prior to extubation.

The requirements for postoperative care and monitoring will be determined by her overall condition and by her tolerance of the surgery and anesthetic. At the very least, vigilant observation of her airway, ventilation, and cardiovascular stability must be continued until she is fully stable.

In summary, this patient with JRA presents several challenging implications for her anesthetic management. In addition to her cervical vertebral symptoms and pathology, the extra-articular manifestations of the disease and medical treatment must be considered. Although other techniques may be quite suitable, management of her airway by fiber-optic nasotracheal intubation with modest sedation and local anesthesia is recommended.

REFERENCES

1. Cassidy JT, Petty RE: *Textbook Pediatric Rheumatology,* ed 2. New York, Churchill Livingstone, Inc, 1990.
2. Espanada G, Babini JC, Maldonado-Cocco JA, et al: Radiologic review: The cervical spine in juvenile rheumatoid arthritis. *Semin Arthritis Rheum* 1988; 17:185.

3. Smith PH, Sharp J, Kellgren JH: Natural history of cervical subluxations. *Ann Rheum Dis* 1972; 31:222.

4. Grosfeld O, Czarnecka B, Drecka-Kuzan K, et al: Clinical investigations of the temporomandibular joint in children and adolescents with rheumatoid arthritis. *Scand J Rheumatol* 1973; 2:145.

5. Jacobs JC, Hui RM: Cricothyroid arthritis and airway obstruction in juvenile rheumatoid arthritis. *Pediatrics* 1977; 59:292.

6. Goldhagen JL: Cricoarytenoiditis as a cause of acute airway obstruction in children. *Ann Emerg Med* 1988; 17:532.

7. Smith MF: Skin diseases and connective tissue disorders, in Katz JK, Steward DJ (eds): *Anesthesia and Uncommon Pediatric Diseases,* ed 2. Philadelphia, WB Saunders Co, 1992.

8. Davies DW, Steward DJ: Unexpected excessive bleeding during operations: Role of acetyl salicylic acid. *Can Anaesth Soc J* 1977; 24:452.

9. Amrein PC, Ellman L, Harris WH: Aspirin-induced prolongation of bleeding time and perioperative blood loss. *JAMA* 1981; 245:1825.

10. Symreng T, Karlberg BE, Kagendal B, et al: Physiological cortisol substitution of long term steroid-treated patients undergoing major surgery. *Br J Anaesth* 1981; 53:949.

11. Korolenko OA, Aliakin LN: Anesthesia tactics in the care of children with rheumatoid arthritis receiving hormonal therapy (Russian). *Anesteziol Reanimatol* 1989; 6:58.

12. Cassidy JT, Petty RE: Preventing acute adrenal insufficiency, in Cassidy JT, Petty RE (eds): *Textbook of Pediatric Rheumatology,* ed 2. New York, Churchill Livingstone Inc, 1990, p 76.

13. Kenny FM, Preeyasombat C, Midgeon CJ: Cortisol production rate. II. Normal infants, children and adults. *Pediatrics* 1966; 37:34.

14. Manchikanti L, Kraus JW, Edds SP: Cimetidine and related drugs in anesthesia. *Anesth Analg* 1982; 61:595.

15. Reginster JY, Damas P, Franchimont P: Anaesthetic risks in osteoarticular disorders. *Clin Rheumatol* 1985; 4:30.

16. Jenkins LC, McGraw RW: Anaesthetic management of the patient with rheumatoid arthritis. *Can Anaesth Soc J* 1969; 16:407.

17. Crosby ET, Lui A: The adult cervical spine: Implications for airway management. Review article. *Can J Anaesth* 1990; 37:77.

18. Zigler J, Rockowitz N, Capen D, et al: Posterior cervical fusion with local anesthesia. The awake patient as the ultimate spinal cord monitor. *Spine* 1987; 12:206.

19. D'Arcy EJ, Fell RH, Ansell BM, et al: Ketamine and juvenile chronic polyarthritis (Still's disease). *Anaesthesia* 1976; 31:624.

20. Smith BL: Brain airway in anaesthesia for patients with juvenile chronic arthritis (letter). *Anaesthesia* 1988; 43:421.

21. Raine J, Warner JO: Fiberoptic bronchoscopy without general anaesthetic. *Arch Dis Child* 1991; 66:481.

22. Shelly MP, Wilson P, Normal J: Sedation for fiberoptic bronchoscopy. *Thorax* 1989; 44:769.

23. Hemmer D, Lee TS, Wright BD: Intubation of a child with a cervical spine injury with aid of a fiberoptic bronchoscope. *Anaesth Intensive Care* 1982; 10:163.

24. Daum RE, Jones DJ: Fiberoptic intubation in Klippel-Feil syndrome. *Anaesthesia* 1988; 43:18.

25. Kleeman PP, Jantzen JP, Bonfils P: The ultra thin bronchoscope in management of the difficult paediatric airway. *Can J Anaesth* 1987; 34:606.

26. Schnapf BM: Oxygen desaturation during fiberoptic bronchoscopy in pediatric patients. *Chest* 1991; 99:591.

27. Suderman VS, Crosby ET: Elective intubation in the unstable cervical spine patient. *Can J Anaesth* 1990; 37(suppl):122.

28. Grundy BL: Intraoperative monitoring of sensory evoked potentials, in Nodar RH, Barber C (eds): *Evoked Potentials II.* Boston, Butterworth Publishers Inc., 1984, p 624.

74

Drug Overdose

A 13-year-old girl who was found in her bedroom "asleep" on the floor is brought to the emergency room by ambulance. She is pale and listless, does not respond to commands, but does withdraw from painful stimuli. Her respirations are shallow at a rate of 14 min. An empty diazepam bottle was found beside her. Her mother states that the prescription for 30, 10-mg tablets was filled the previous day. She further states that her daughter was depressed about breaking up with her boyfriend. The emergency room physician plans to insert a nasogastric tube and lavage the patient's stomach. He requests an evaluation of the need for airway protection.

Recommendations by Desmond J. Bohn, M.B., B.Ch., F.R.C.P.C.

Diazepam was first synthesized in 1959 and since its introduction in 1963 has become one of the most commonly prescribed drugs in the Western world. It has achieved popularity as a psycho-therapeutic agent with relatively few cardiorespiratory side effects. Drowsiness and central nervous depression are less frequent with diazepam than with comparable doses of barbiturates. Because of the wide difference between its therapeutic and toxic levels, it has largely displaced barbiturates as the tranquilizer of choice, and there has been a consequent fall in the number of deaths caused by self-administered overdoses of barbiturates.

Diazepam is formed by manipulation of the benzodiazepine ring. It is relatively lipid soluble and water insoluble. After oral administration, it is rapidly and completely absorbed in the gastro-intestinal tract and reaches peak blood concentrations within 2 hours. After a single dose, the clinical effects seem to wear off rapidly owing to rapid tissue distribution rather than to biotransformation. The major breakdown product of diazepam is nordiazepam (dimethyldiazepam), which is formed by the removal of a methyl group. This compound has appreciable pharmacologic activity and is itself biotransformed, even more slowly than diazepam, to yield oxazepam, which is rapidly glucuronidated and excreted as the major urinary metabolite of diazepam. Estimation of serum levels of diazepam is performed by ultraviolet spectrophotometric analysis, which does not differentiate between diazepam and its breakdown products. Alternatively, gas chromotography, which accurately measures serum concentrations of diazepam, can be employed.

INITIAL ASSESSMENT

This girl conforms to a fairly well-recognized pattern of acute diazepam overdose. It probably represents an overreaction to emotional stress rather than a genuine suicide attempt but nevertheless represents a serious degree of drug poisoning. The benzodiazipines are generally of a lower order of toxicity than other sedative-hypnotics. Oral ingestion of up to 1,500 mg with only minor toxicity has been reported. Although diazepam ingestion alone rarely results in deep coma with cardiorespiratory depression, it is not infrequently combined with other more toxic central nervous system (CNS) depressants or with alcohol. Since the introduction of more conservative measures of treating acute drug poisoning that are based on supportive and symptomatic treatment with less emphasis placed on aggressive methods of eliminating the drug from the body, the morbidity and mortality from secondary complications such as aspiration, electrolyte imbalance and pulmonary edema have declined. Management of this patient, as with any case of acute drug ingestion, should be based, in the first instance, on confirming the diagnosis while excluding other forms of coma, assessing the severity of the poisoning, and identifying the drug involved. Active treatment is based on instituting measures to prevent further intestinal absorption of any ingested drug by the use of activated charcoal and a cathartic while providing supportive therapy for the cardiorespiratory system where necessary.

The history and circumstances in this case all point to an acute overdose of diazepam; however, it is important that other causes of a depressed level of consciousness be excluded before a presumptive diagnosis is made. In this age group, these would include trauma, CNS infections, endocrine disorders (especially diabetes), and disorders of metabolism. With this in mind, a history from the parents would be important, as would a full neurologic examination. Evidence of localizing signs such as unequal pupils, hyperactive reflexes, or extensor plantar responses would indicate other CNS pathology. Any urine passed should be tested for evidence of glycosuria, and laboratory evaluation should include blood sugar, blood urea nitrogen (BUN) and electrolyte determinations. In addition to CNS effects, overdose of diazepam can also cause respiratory depression, which is occasionally severe enough to require assisted ventilation. More rarely, hypotension also occurs.

It seems highly likely, from both the history and the physical findings, that this is a straightforward drug ingestion. Therefore, the next priority is to assess the degree of CNS depression and, specifically, the need for airway protection. A coma scale has been devised by Reed et al.[1] for assessing patients with acute drug overdose:

- 0—Asleep, but can be aroused.
- 1—Comatose, but responsive to painful stimuli. Reflexes intact, no respiratory or circulatory depression.

- 2—Does not withdraw from painful stimuli. No respiratory or circulatory depression. Reflexes intact.
- 3—Most reflexes absent. No respiratory or circulatory depression.
- 4—Most or all reflexes absent. Significant respiratory or circulatory depression, or both.

At the outset, it is important to establish the degree of coma because the level of consciousness will fluctuate, depending on whether or not there is further absorption of the drug from the gastrointestinal tract. This particular girl is in a grade 1 coma—drowsy but responsive to painful stimuli. The clinical picture is certainly compatible with the history of ingestion of 300 mg of diazepam. A greater degree of coma would lead to suspicion that the overdose of diazepam was associated with other CNS depressants or with alcohol.

The emergency room physician intends to perform nasogastric lavage. This maneuver can be performed safely only if the patient has well-preserved gag and cough reflexes that will enable her to protect her own airway. In the absence of these reflexes, the airway should be protected with a cuffed endotracheal tube. In this particular instance, with the patient in a grade 1 coma, it is likely that both pharyngeal and layrngeal reflexes will be preserved. When assessing the need for airway protection in a comatose patient, a basic rule to keep in mind is that if the patient is sufficiently obtunded to tolerate laryngoscopy and endotracheal intubation, airway protection is required. Inserting either a tongue spatula or a suction catheter into the back of pharynx will elicit a cough or gag reflex. In the event that this patient should require an endotracheal tube, a 6.5-mm cuffed tube would be appropriate. If an endotracheal tube is required for airway protection, it is also important to have it in place after lavage as well as prior to the procedure because of the very real danger of vomiting and aspiration. In the event that this patient is "light" enough to have retained her own airway protective reflexes, nasogastric lavage should still be performed with the patient lying on her side in the head-down position. Following lavage, activated charcoal should be left in the stomach.

DRUG IDENTIFICATION

It is important at this time to definitely identify the type of intoxication. Of particular importance is the history, from the parents, that the empty diazepam bottle was found in the patient's vicinity. In many cases of diazepam overdose there is a second drug involved; therefore, relatives should be closely questioned about whether any other drugs were available in the house. An estimate of the actual quantity of drug ingested can also be helpful, but bear in mind that these estimates, either from relatives or the patients themselves, are often unreliable. Analysis of stomach contents obtained from nasogastric lavage will enable the drug or drugs involved to be positively identified. An emergency toxicology screen should be performed to include barbiturates, diazepam, tricyclic antidepressants, phenothiazines, and alcohol. Actual serum levels of diazepam are available either by gas chromatography or by spectrophotometric analysis. In a published series of benzodiazepine overdose, serum diazepam concentrations ranged from 1 to 9 μg/mL.[2] Even with serum concentrations in the upper limit of this range, no patient was in a more severe coma than grade 1. However, the routine measurement of diazepam plasma levels does not provide clinically useful information.

SUPPORTIVE THERAPY

In acute drug ingestion, supportive therapy is based on providing cardiovascular and respiratory stability. Although ingestion of diazepam, even in large doses, is not associated with major cardio-respiratory depression in normal patients, two deaths ascribed purely to diazepam overdose have been reported.[3] Therefore, careful evaluation of any degree of respiratory depression and/or hypotension is mandatory.

The patient's respirations are "shallow," at a rate of 14/min. This might indicate a mild degree of respiratory depression. Evidence of carbon dioxide retention such as sweating and tachycardia should be sought and arterial blood drawn for gas analysis to evaluate alveolar ventilation.

Assessment of the cardiovascular system should include not only pulse and blood pressure but also the adequacy of tissue perfusion as evidenced by peripheral skin temperature. Clinically significant hypotension is uncommon with diazepam ingestion alone and, when present, should alert the clinician to the possibility of ingestion of other drugs. If there is no significant depression of the cardiovascular system, an intravenous infusion of saline or Ringer's lactate should be initiated to provide maintenance fluids. There is no indication to attempt to increase renal excretion of the drug by producing a diuresis because this is totally ineffective, may prove dangerous, and can lead to both fluid overload and electrolyte abnormalities. If cardiovascular depression has occurred, it is likely that one is dealing with something more than a straightforward diazepam overdose. In this situation, severe poisoning may cause cardiovascular depression by either effects on the vasomotor center or loss of peripheral vasomotor tone. The first step in treatment would be expansion of intravascular volume with 10 mL/kg of colloid or crystalloid solution. Monitoring the central venous pressure would enable the clinician to assess the effect of therapy on intravascular volume. Failure to respond to volume loading with 10 mL/kg would indicate the necessity for inotropic support. Dopamine, starting at a dosage of 5 μg/kg/min, would not only increase cardiac output but also cause a selective renal vasodilatation. Disturbances of cardiac rhythm are extremely rare with diazepam intoxication.

FURTHER MANAGEMENT

With adequate supportive therapy, acute diazepam poisoning is not life-threatening. As with many other forms of drug overdose, more harm than good can be done by adopting aggressive measures to encourage drug excretion. Therapy is confined primarily to removing any unabsorbed drug from the gastrointestinal tract by nasogastric lavage and instilling activated charcoal into the stomach in a dosage of 15 to 30 g. This will have the effect of binding any unabsorbed drug onto its surface, thereby decreasing further absorption. The dose can be repeated every 2 to 6 hours, except in the presence of ileus. A saline cathartic (magnesium or sodium sulfate) or sorbitol should be given with the first dose only.

Administration of the newly introduced benzodiazepine antagonist flumazenil may be warranted. The recommended initial dose is 0.2 mg administered over 30 seconds. Additional doses, to a maximum cumulative dose of 5 mg, appear safe. Most patients respond to a cumulative dose of 1 to 3 mg and larger doses do not reliably produce additional effects. Patients who do not respond to a cumulative dose of 5 mg within 5 minutes have likely ingested other depressants. Re-sedation is common when large doses of benzodiazepines have been ingested, necessitating careful observation. If re-sedation occurs, additional flumazenil can be administered. No more than 1 mg should be given at any one time and the dose should be limited to 3 mg/hour.

While evidence of respiratory depression exists, the patient should be admitted to the intensive care unit where she can be closely observed and the level of coma evaluated at regular intervals. Temperature, respiration, blood pressure, pupil size, and the response of the patient to verbal and noxious stimuli should be monitored. In the normal event, diazepam-induced coma does not last more than 12 to 24 hours. After this time, the patient could be transferred to the open ward for psychiatric assessment.

REFERENCES

1. Reed CE, Driggs MF, Foote CC: Acute barbiturate intoxication: A study of 300 cases based on a physiologic system of classification of the severity of the intoxication. *Ann Intern Med* 1952; 37:290–303.
2. Cardoni AA: Benzodiazepine overdose, in Edlich RF, Spyker DA (eds): *Current Emergency Therapy.* Rockville, Md, Aspen, 1985.
3. Litovitz T: Fatal diazepam toxicity? *Am J Emerg Med* 1987; 5:472–473.

75

Cotrel-Dubousset Instrumentation for Scoliosis

A 14-year-old, 51-kg girl with scoliosis but otherwise healthy is scheduled for posterior spinal fusion and Cotrel-Dubousset (C-D) instrumentation. The thoracolumbar curve is 65 degrees. The orthopedist prefers moderate hypotension and an intraoperative wake-up test. Somatosensory evoked potentials will be monitored as well. Hemoglobin, 12.2 g/dL; hematocrit, 37%.

Recommendations by Robert M. Brustowicz, M.D.

The information provided implies that the etiology of the scoliosis is idiopathic, as is 70% of all scoliosis. As such, a careful history would most probably reveal that the patient has no other medical problems except for those related to her scoliosis. The extent of those problems is related to the location and severity of her curve. Thoracic and thoracolumbar curves over 90 degrees can produce significant effects on the cardiopulmonary system.[1]

PREOPERATIVE EVALUATION

The Cobb method is conventionally used for measuring the spinal curve. The degree of curve refers to the angle between the upper surface of the "top-end" vertebra and the lower surface of the "bottom-end" vertebra. The "end" vertebrae are those that are maximally tilted. The curve is described as facing to the right or to the left, depending on the side of convexity. Figure 75–1 demonstrates a left thoracic curve of 30 degrees.

The degree of physical impairment should be assessed by inquiring into the patient's normal level of activity. For patients who have no other medical problems, the preoperative measurement of pulmonary function tests and arterial blood gases is usually not necessary unless the patient has a

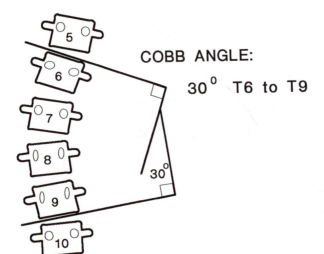

COBB ANGLE:

30° T6 to T9

FIG 75–1.
A schematic presentation of the Cobb method for measuring spinal curves. Illustrated is a 30-degree left thoracic curve. (Courtesy of Dr. John B. Emans, Assistant Clinical Professor of Orthopedics, Harvard Medical School.)

curve over 90 degrees. Other preoperative laboratory tests that should be obtained include a complete blood count, urinalysis, chest x-ray, and coagulation profile.

Even though somatosensory evoked potentials (SSEP) will be monitored intraoperatively, many surgeons still insist upon a "wake-up test" to confirm that there has not been any damage to the motor pathways. Therefore, the mechanics of the wake-up test[2] should be discussed with the patient preoperatively. For most laypeople, the term "wake-up" is associated with "wide awake" and is frightening. Therefore, it is important to stress to the patient that during the test she will still be asleep and that while she may or may not remember anything, she will not feel pain. She should be told that after the surgeon has straightened her back the level of anesthesia will be diminished slightly and she will be asked to move her hands and then her toes. Once this is successfully completed, the anesthesia will be restored to its original level. This procedure should be practiced a few times during the initial preoperative evaluation and again just prior to surgery.

Concern about disease transmission by contaminated blood has led many patients to donate blood prior to surgery. It is important to inquire whether the patient has made any arrangements for predonation and, if so, to be certain that the autologous blood is available for surgery. The possibility of intraoperative normovolemic hemodilution should also be discussed.

THE SURGICAL PROCEDURE

The C-D system that is to be used on this patient was developed in Paris by two orthopedic surgeons, Drs. Cotrel and Dubousset. The system is a double-rod system with cross-links that provide extraordinary strength (Fig 75–2). Although not unique to this system, ambulation on the first postoperative day is possible, and when compared with the traditional Harrington instrumentation, patients spend less time hospitalized. The C-D system not only decreases the amount of curvature of the scoliosis but also permits the surgeon some degree of control of the residual lordosis and kyphosis in the instrumented spine. The "rib hump" that is especially prominent in patients with thoracic

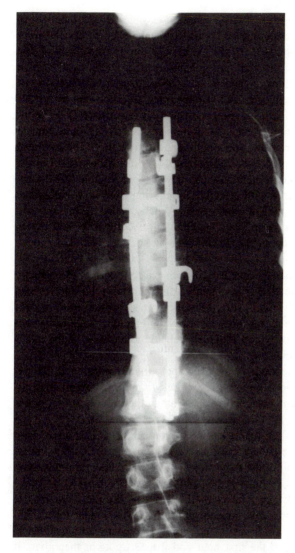

FIG 75–2.
Cotrel-Dubousset Instrumentation in situ. Note the cross-links that contribute to the system's strength. (Courtesy of Dr. John B. Emans, Assistant Clinical Professor of Orthopedics, Harvard Medical School.)

curves is also diminished. The major disadvantage is that inserting the instrumentation is technically difficult and the operative time may be prolonged.

INTRAOPERATIVE MANAGEMENT

There are many ways to successfully manage this patient intraoperatively. The appropriate selection of techniques is based on understanding the needs of the patient, the surgeon, and the neurophysiologist.

Since most healthy patients are admitted the morning of surgery, premedication with intravenous midazolam, 0.05 to 0.10 mg/kg, is very useful. It has a rapid onset and allows the patient to be comfortable while the electrodes for SSEP monitoring are applied. When evoked potentials are to be monitored, there are some very important points that must be kept in mind when planning the anesthetic. It is important to communicate with the neurophysiologist or neurologist to determine exactly what they are measuring and the limitations of their system. SSEP measure the function of neural transmission in the afferent spinal cord pathways. This is most often accomplished by repeatedly stimulating the posterior tibial nerve and measuring the conduction characteristics of the stimulations at some point cephalad to the site of the surgery. Measurements of latency, how long it takes the signals to travel to the point of measurement, and amplitude, the strength of the averaged signals, are used to assess spinal cord function. It has been reported that SSEP measured from the scalp can be completely ablated by as little as 0.02% halothane in 100% oxygen,[3] while SSEP measured at the CZ position (midline) are compatible with effective monitoring even with halothane, 0.75 MAC, or isoflurane, 1.0 MAC, each with 60% nitrous oxide.[4] When inhaled agents are used with nitrous oxide, our experience has been an inconsistent suppression of cortical evoked potentials. However, under the same circumstances, cervical evoked potentials measured at the C7 position are routinely spared.

Regardless, it must be remembered that only the integrity of the sensory pathways is actually measured and it is only *assumed* that motor function is also intact. Unfortunately, there have been cases where this assumption has proved false.[5] This is why the wake-up test is often used in conjunction with SSEP monitoring. Currently, there is a growing body of literature suggesting that monitoring motor evoked potentials intraoperatively can provide a reliable assessment of the integrity of the motor pathways in anesthetized patients.[6]

Once the electroencephalographic (EEG) electrodes have been appropriately positioned, the patient is brought to the operating room. Conventional monitors are applied, and glycopyrrolate is administered to minimize secretions. Use of an antisialagogue in patients in the prone position is important because excessive salivation can loosen the tape securing the endotracheal tube.

If the patient is still anxious, an additional 0.05 mg/kg of midazolam can be administered. Fentanyl, 10 to 15 μg/kg, is then administered. The patient must be carefully monitored with a precordial stethoscope during this time. Oral intubation of the trachea is accomplished after administration of appropriate doses of thiopental and curare. Tincture of benzoin is applied to the face to make certain that the tape securing the endotracheal tube adheres well. Curare is my preferred muscle relaxant because it also helps to lower blood pressure. Anesthesia should be maintained with fentanyl and nitrous oxide–oxygen prior to the wake-up test. The fentanyl is usually administered in increments up to a maximum dose of 15μg/kg in the first hour and 2 to 3 μg/kg/hr thereafter. If necessary, blood pressure is controlled with 5-mg doses of labetalol after the patient is placed in the prone position. Inhalation agents are rarely used. A narcotic-based anesthetic not only avoids much of the controversy surrounding the effects of inhalation anesthetics on cortical evoked potentials but also makes the wake-up test easier.

The eyes should be protected with a nonirritating petroleum ointment and taped closed with paper tape. A second large-gauge intravenous catheter, arterial catheter, and central venous catheter are inserted, as are a nasogastric tube, esophageal stethoscope, and Foley catheter. Since urine output is an unreliable sign of hydration in patients in the prone position, a central venous pressure (CVP) catheter is particularly useful for evaluating the patient's state of hydration. The value obtained as soon as the patient is placed prone is used as the baseline. The CVP is also useful during the wake-up test, when the patient may breathe spontaneously and generate significant negative intrathoracic pressures. A low or negative CVP might place the patient at risk of venous air embolism, and the surgeon would be asked to flood the field and the exposed epidural veins. Complications from CVP insertion can be minimized by inserting the catheter through an antecubital vein.

An arterial catheter is essential for monitoring blood pressure and for drawing samples for arterial blood gas analysis and serial hematocrit determinations. Experience has shown that healthy patients do not need fluid boluses prior to positioning on a Relton-Hall frame to prevent hypotension. Avoiding large fluid infusions at the start of the procedure also makes blood pressure control easier. To help maintain the patient's temperature, all intravenous fluids should be warmed prior to infusion.

The actual move to the frame must be a carefully planned and coordinated venture if the patient is not to be traumatized, extubated, or have one of the catheters pulled out. Because the electrocardiogram is also disconnected, the anesthesiologist must listen to the heart sounds through the esophageal stethoscope or be certain that the arterial blood pressure is being continuously transduced. The patient should be preoxygenated prior to the move. It is important to keep her head stable and move it *with* the rest of the body. To achieve this goal, the following procedure is useful. With the patient located to the right of the frame, the anesthesiologist's pronated left hand is positioned with the forearm along the left side of the head and the palm on the sternum. The right hand then presses the patient's head from the right side against the anesthesiologist's left forearm. With the head thus secured, the patient can be turned with the head firmly supported. Once the patient is prone, the endotracheal tube should be reconnected and its position confirmed. Special care should be taken to ensure that there is no pressure on the eyes and that the electrocardiogram leads are not being pressed into the patient. An oral or nasal temperature probe is inserted at this time.

Proper positioning on the frame is critical. The thoracic cage should not be impinged upon in any way, and the abdomen should hang freely. To achieve this, the rostral supports are located at the lateral aspects of the upper thoracic cage below the clavicles but as far cephalad as possible. The caudal supports should be located at the anterolateral aspect of the pelvic girdle between the iliac crests and the greater femoral trochanters[7] (Fig 75–3). Proper positioning also helps minimize blood loss. With the abdomen hanging free, intra-abdominal pressure is decreased, as is the pressure on the inferior vena cava. This encourages venous return through the vena cava and not the vertebral venous plexus. Passing a nasogastric tube to decrease intra-abdominal pressure and avoiding high inflating pressures and positive end-expiratory pressure (PEEP) during ventilation will also decrease bleeding. Hyperventilation, however, should be avoided since this decreases blood flow to the spinal cord.

With the patient properly positioned, the stretcher is placed just outside the operating room with a board on top of the mattress. This precaution is taken in the unlikely event that a firm surface is needed for cardiopulmonary resuscitation (CPR). Effective CPR is virtually impossible in the prone position.

The first of the hourly arterial blood gases should now be measured. Ionized calcium and serum electrolyte levels are also monitored since they tend to fluctuate with large intraoperative fluid shifts. Moderate hypotension to a blood pressure of approximately 100 systolic or 70 mean may be induced to reduce blood loss. If hemodilution is also planned, the degree of both must be very closely monitored and neither allowed to go to extremes.

While surgeons often provide a 20-minute warning before requesting the wake-up test, many

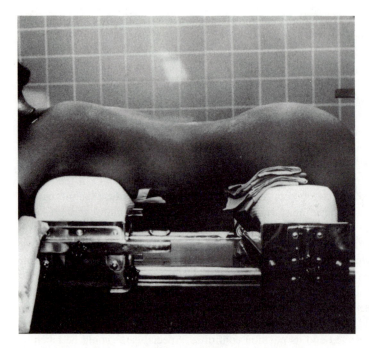

FIG 75–3.
A patient properly positioned on the operative frame. The rostral supports are positioned to allow for good chest excursion, and the caudal supports allow the abdomen to hang freely.

times they forget. Fortunately, C-D instrumentation requires the insertion of two rods. Usually the time from the insertion of the first rod to insertion of the second is about 20 to 40 minutes. By observing the surgery, the anesthesiologist can project when the wake-up will be requested. If the neuromuscular blocking agent is titrated so that the patient has 2/4 on the train-of-four just prior to the wake-up test, it can usually be accomplished without reversing the neuromuscular blockade. The CVP should be checked prior to the wake-up test. Low or negative values dictate that the surgical field be flooded with saline to minimize the potential for air embolism. Nitrous oxide administration should be discontinued and mechanical ventilation discontinued after the end-tidal nitrous oxide concentration has diminished significantly. The anesthesiologist should wait for the patient to breathe spontaneously or with minimal assistance. This usually takes anywhere from 30 seconds to 10 minutes. The patient is asked to move her hands first. This confirms that the level of anesthesia and neuromuscular blockade are such that they will not inhibit her response. Next the integrity of the spinal cord is tested, and she is asked to wiggle her toes. Someone other than the orthopedic surgeon is under the drapes watching the patient. Once the patient demonstrates good bilateral movement, the nitrous oxide is reinstituted, and midazolam, 0.05 mg/kg, and methadone, 0.08 mg/kg, are administered. Methadone is an excellent postoperative analgesic when properly titrated in the post anesthesia care unit.

If the patient demonstrates substantial neuromuscular blockade, one fourth of the usual dose of neostigmine and glycopyrrolate should be administered. This dose can be repeated, if necessary. If the patient demonstrates good neuromuscular function but appears narcotized, naloxone in 0.02-mg increments can be judiciously administered. Patients who have been "reversed" are much more likely to "buck" on the endotracheal tube during the wake-up test; therefore it is advisable to have a syringe of thiopental readily available. The orthopedic surgeons should be standing close by ready to stabilize the patient. If the patient does not move her toes despite these maneuvers, the degree of distraction of the spine must be diminished and the test repeated.

BLOOD TRANSFUSION

Although the operative blood loss often exceeds 1 unit, there are several techniques available to avoid the use of homologous blood. Three techniques that may be appropriate are preoperative blood donation, acute normovolemic hemodilution, and intraoperative blood salvage.

Predonation not only provides exactly matched blood for the procedure but also provides a patient actively engaged in erythropoiesis. Although the anesthesiologist's role is limited to transfusion of blood donated preoperatively, there are facets of the program with which he should be familiar. Children as young as 7 years and weighing as little as 23 kg have been able to donate blood, although 48 to 50 kg is the more commonly accepted lower weight limit. Optimally, donations begin 4 to 6 weeks prior to surgery and can continue weekly until 72 hours before surgery. A healthy patient can donate as often as every 3 days.[8] Although oral iron is currently prescribed, the use of recombinant human erythropoietin may increase the number of autologous units that can be donated.[9]

Contraindications to autologous donations generally include a hematocrit less than 33%, bacteremia, seizures, or a positive test for human immunodeficiency virus (HIV) or hepatitis B surface antigen. Relative contraindications include sickle cell trait, cardiac disease, and chronic respiratory disease. Overnight express delivery services make it possible for the blood to be collected at a site convenient for the patient and then be shipped to the hospital where surgery is performed. If the scheduled surgery is delayed, the expiration dates of the autologous blood should be checked. Units of whole blood or packed cells that would expire by the new surgical date should be converted to frozen red blood cells.

The fact that autologous blood is being administered should not dampen our vigilance. Adverse reactions are still possible. Over 60% of fatal transfusion reactions are the result of clerical errors.[10]

Another strategy that can be employed to minimize homologous transfusion requirements is acute normovolemic hemodilution (ANH). There are two advantages to ANH. The red blood cell loss is decreased when the hematocrit is lower and fresh autologous blood is available for transfusion. The amount of blood to be withdrawn (V) is calculated on the basis of the patient's estimated blood volume (EBV), initial hematocrit (H_0) and the desired hematocrit (H_f) and the average of H_0 and H_f (H_{AV}):

$$V = EBV \times \left(\frac{H_0 - H_f}{H_{AV}} \right)$$

The recommended limits of hemodilution,[11] precautions, and a protocol for the technique[12] can be found elsewhere. While a safe and effective procedure, it should only be performed by anesthesiologists familiar with the technique and in appropriately selected and monitored patients.

The third autologous transfusion technique is intraoperative blood salvage and reinfusion.[13] Postoperative blood salvage is also possible, and several devices exist for collecting postoperative drainage for reinfusion.[8, 13]

POSTOPERATIVE MANAGEMENT

At the conclusion of surgery, as the patient is returned to the supine position on the bed, the head should be supported in a manner similar to that previously outlined. Once transferred, the patient's neuromuscular blockade is reversed, and she is extubated.

Once she is in the postanesthesia care unit, additional methadone is administered if her respiratory status is adequate. The drug is administered in 0.02-mg/kg increments.[14] Methadone has a prolonged half-life, often providing adequate analgesia for hours.

These patients need to be closely observed until their fluid status stabilizes. Ventilatory support is usually not required during this time, although a face mask or nasal prongs are used to provide humidified oxygen. As soon as possible, in the recovery area, a chest x-ray should be taken to rule out a hemothorax/pneumothorax and confirm the position of the CVP catheter.

REFERENCES

1. Kafer ER: Respiratory and cardiovascular functions in scoliosis and the principles of anesthetic management. *Anesthesiology* 1980; 52:339–351.
2. Hall JE, Levine CR, Sudhir KG: Intraoperative awakening to monitor spinal cord function during Harrington instrumentation and spinal fusion. *J Bone Joint Surg [Am]* 1978; 60:533–536.
3. York DH, Chabot RJ, Gaines RW: Response variability of somatosensory evoked potentials during scoliosis surgery. *Spine* 1987; 12:864–876.
4. Pathak KS, Ammadio M, Kalamchi A, et al: Effects of halothane, enflurane, and isoflurane on somatosensory evoked potentials during nitrous oxide anesthesia. *Anesthesiology* 1987; 66:753–757.
5. Gugino V, Chabot RJ: Somatosensory evoked potentials. *Int Anesthesiol Clin* 1990; 28:154–164.
6. Edmonds HL, Paloheimo MPJ, Backman MH, et al: Transcranial magnetic motor evoked potentials (tc-MMEP) for functional monitoring of motor pathways during scoliosis surgery. *Spine* 1989; 14:683–685.
7. Relton JES, Hall JE: An operation frame for spinal fusion: A new apparatus designed to reduce haemorrhage during operation. *J Bone Joint Surg [Br]* 1967; 49:327.
8. Stehling L: Autologous transfusion. *Int Anesthesiol Clin* 1990; 28:190–196.
9. The National Blood Resource Education Program Expert Panel: The use of autologous blood. *JAMA* 1990; 263:414–417.
10. Miller AC, Scherba-Krugliak L, Toy PT, et al: Hypotension during transfusion of autologous blood. *Anesthesiology* 1991; 74:624–628.
11. Robertie PG, Gravlee GP: Safe limits of isovolemic hemodilution and recommendations for erythrocyte transfusion. *Int Anesthesiol Clin* 1990; 28:197–204.
12. Stehling L, Zauder HL: Acute normovolemic hemodilution. *Transfusion* 1991; 31:857–868.
13. Williamson KR, Taswell HF: Intraoperative blood salvage: A review. *Transfusion* 1991; 31:662–675.
14. Berde CB, Holzman RS, Sethna NF, et al: A comparison of methadone and morphine for postoperative analgesia in children and adolescents. *Anesthesiology* 1988; 69:A768.

Index

A